GLAISTER'S

MEDICAL JURISPRUDENCE
AND TOXICOLOGY

EDGAR RENTOUL

M.B.E., J.P., M.A., LL.B., M.B., Ch.B., M.R.C.Path.

Late Lecturer in Forensic Medicine, University of Glasgow

HAMILTON SMITH

B.Sc., Ph.D., A.R.I.C., M.R.C.Path.

Lecturer in Toxicology, University of Glasgow

GLAISTER'S
MEDICAL JURISPRUDENCE
AND TOXICOLOGY

EDITED BY THE LATE

EDGAR RENTOUL

AND

HAMILTON SMITH

Foreword by GILBERT FORBES

Thirteenth Edition

CHURCHILL LIVINGSTONE
EDINBURGH AND LONDON 1973

ISBN 0 443 00894 9

First Edition	-	-	*1902*
Reprinted		-	*1909*
Second Edition	-	-	*1910*
Third Edition	-	-	*1915*
Fourth Edition	-	-	*1921*
Fifth Edition	-	-	*1931*
Sixth Edition	-	-	*1938*
Seventh Edition	-	-	*1942*
Eighth Edition	-	-	*1945*
Revised Reprint	-	-	*1947*
Ninth Edition	-	-	*1950*
Revised Reprint	-	-	*1953*
Tenth Edition	-	-	*1957*
Eleventh Edition	-	-	*1962*
Twelfth Edition	-	-	*1966*
Thirteenth Edition	-	-	*1973*

Printed in Great Britain by
Butler & Tanner Ltd, Frome and London

FOREWORD

THIS famous textbook was first published in 1902 under the pen of John Glaister, Sr, who occupied the Regius Chair of Forensic Medicine in the University of Glasgow, with distinction, from 1898 until 1931. When his son, John Glaister, Jr, succeeded him in the Chair he took over the textbook, improved it greatly, and saw it through successive editions up to the 11th Edition, which appeared in 1962. Dr Edgar Rentoul, a faithful member of the staff, became involved in the revision necessary for the preparation of the later editions and, most appropriately, he appeared as co-author of the 12th Edition, as by this time the senior author had retired, and Dr Rentoul was responsible for virtually the whole of the work.

Tragically, when the preparation of the 13th Edition was nearing completion and after the 12th Edition had gone out of print, Dr Rentoul died, and within a matter of months Professor Glaister did also. Fortunately, when this most unusual situation was arrived at, where both of the authors of a book have died when it was on the point of being published, help was forthcoming from Dr Jocelyn Rentoul and Dr Richard Young, who had been assisting Dr Rentoul in the rewriting, and who were familiar with his manuscript and notes. They, with some editorial help, supervision and advice from Dr W. D. S. McLay, Chief Medical Officer of the City of Glasgow Police, were able to put the final touches to the outstanding chapters and to submit the manuscript for publication.

I know that this edition will maintain the high standard which has been set by previous editions, and that its appearance will receive a welcome from the whole of the English-speaking medical world, where this book has always been accepted as a standard authority. While the usual care has been taken to bring this edition up to date on matters medical and legal, the section on Toxicology has been entirely rewritten by Dr Hamilton Smith, a Lecturer on Toxicology in this Department. He has received assistance from Dr John S. Oliver, also a Toxicologist here.

Because of the almost unique circumstances surrounding the production of the 13th Edition, and because this book has always been associated with the Department of Forensic Medicine in Glasgow

University, it was felt by the publishers that the present head of the Department should offer a word of explanation to the readers. It would have been tragic if, when so nearly completed, the 13th Edition had had to be abandoned because of the death of the authors, and I have much pleasure in acknowledging the handsome way in which Dr Jocelyn Rentoul, Dr Richard Young, Dr W. D. S. McLay, Dr Hamilton Smith and Dr John S. Oliver have rallied round and put the finishing touches to a work which is perhaps some sort of memorial to the late Dr Edgar Rentoul, who laboured so mightily to produce a book which would be a credit to Glasgow University.

1973   GILBERT FORBES
M.B., B.Sc., F.R.C.S. (Glas.), F.R.C.S.(Ed.), F.R.C.Path.
Regius Professor of Forensic Medicine
University of Glasgow.

PREFACE

THE preparation of this new edition was a suitable opportunity for the major revision of the medical jurisprudence and the complete rewriting of the toxicology. Much of the older material has been replaced and new techniques and concepts included.

The major changes made include the following. The law has been brought up to date. New material on identification, e.g. by teeth marks, is included. The chapter on the medico-legal aspects of death has been reconstructed and the chapter on wounds has been split into three new chapters. Blood and blood-stain examination has been re-written. The section on toxicology has been rewritten and restyled to present the toxic materials alphabetically. The appendix has been changed to present a selection of common techniques, explained in relatively simple terms, so that some idea may be obtained of the processes being described in court. The list of simple tests is omitted as this is properly the field of the skilled chemist, but a selected collection of data is included which may be of use to the analytical toxicologist for comparison purposes.

I would like to acknowledge the considerable assistance given by Dr W. D. S. McLay. He has been particularly helpful in providing information and photographs of the many interesting cases in which he has been involved. I also wish to thank the City of Glasgow Police for the use of photographs taken at the scenes of various crimes.

Lastly I should like to acknowledge the many others who have contributed advice, materials and help during the preparation of this edition.

HAMILTON SMITH

Department of Forensic Medicine
The University of Glasgow
1973

CONTENTS

Chapter 1

GENERAL MEDICAL COUNCIL, MALPRAXIS, LEGAL PROCEDURE, AND NATIONAL INSURANCE (INDUSTRIAL INJURIES) ACTS

Chapter 2

MEDICAL EVIDENCE

Chapter 3

IDENTIFICATION

Chapter 4

THE MEDICO-LEGAL ASPECTS OF DEATH

Chapter 5

DEATH CERTIFICATION AND CREMATION

Chapter 6

ASPHYXIA

Chapter 7

DEATH FROM LIGHTNING, ELECTRICITY AND BURNING

Chapter 13

MEDICO-LEGAL ASPECTS OF SEXUAL FUNCTIONS AND CRIMINAL ABORTION

Chapter 14

INFANTICIDE OR CHILD MURDER

Chapter 15

RAPE AND OTHER SEXUAL CRIMES

Chapter 16

MENTAL DISORDER IN ITS MEDICO-LEGAL ASPECTS

Chapter 17

LAW RELATING TO POISONS

Chapter 18

GENERAL ACTIONS OF POISONS, EVIDENCE AND TREATMENT OF POISONING

Chapter 19

TOXIC MATERIALS

Chapter 20

FOOD POISONING

Chapter 21

PLANT IRRITANTS, ARROW POISONS, STINGS AND BITES 718

Appendix 1

ANALYTICAL TOXICOLOGY

Appendix II

USEFUL WEIGHTS AND MEASURES

Appendix III

NORMAL LEVELS OF TRACE ELEMENTS

Appendix IV

PHARMACEUTICAL AND TRADE NAMES

Appendix V

PROSECUTION AND PUNISHMENT OF OFFENCES INVOLVING ALCOHOL UNDER THE ROAD TRAFFIC ACT, 1972

INDEX

Chapter 1

GENERAL MEDICAL COUNCIL, MALPRAXIS, LEGAL PROCEDURE, AND NATIONAL INSURANCE (INDUSTRIAL INJURIES) ACTS

MEDICAL Jurisprudence, Legal Medicine, or Forensic Medicine, is the subject concerned with the application of medical knowledge to certain branches of the law, both civil and criminal. Since members of the medical profession are liable to be called upon to render professional assistance, of the most varied character, in medico-legal cases which may later compel their attendance at court, it is highly important that they should appreciate and understand both the medical and legal aspects of the subject. This involves on the part of the practitioner a knowledge of the medical aspects of the various criminal acts which may come under his consideration, of the medical bearing of various Acts of Parliament, and of the law of evidence. He must also be familiar with the Acts which are concerned with the control of doctors and their relations with the public.

THE MEDICAL ACTS 1956 TO 1969

The Medical Act 1956 consolidated enactments relating to medical practitioners taken from twenty statutes of which the earliest was the Physicians Act, 1540, and the latest was the Medical Act, 1950. The Medical Act, 1956 (Amendment) Act, 1958, made minor alterations as to the experience required for full registration. The Medical Act, 1969, has made major alterations in the law relating to medical practitioners.

The objects of these Acts are:

1. The establishment of the General Medical Council.
2. The maintenance of an official Register of medical practitioners.
3. The supervision of standards of proficiency required for qualification for registration.
4. The exercise of discipline over the Medical Profession.
5. Publication of the British Pharmacopoeia (but see p. 9).

The General Medical Council

The Council consists of forty-seven representatives, of whom eighteen are appointed by the Universities in the United Kingdom having medical faculties, ten by the Medical Corporations, eight by Her Majesty in Council, three of whom must not be registered medical practitioners or holders of qualifying diplomas, and eleven by election by the medical profession. The Council is divided into branch councils for England, Scotland, and Ireland.

The Register of Medical Practitioners

This is kept by the Registrar and it is his duty to record the names, qualifications, addresses and dates of registration of the persons registered.

The Register consists of the Principal List and the Overseas List which contains the names of those who are entitled to be registered but who are resident overseas.

There is a separate register for those who hold Commonwealth or foreign qualifications and are practising medicine in hospitals or other institutions approved by the Council.

The names of those provisionally registered for the purpose of obtaining the required experience are specially marked in the Register. The General Council is given power to make regulations regarding the payment of fees for the entry of a name in the Register and for the retention of a name on the Register in years following the initial entry. The Council also is given the right to make regulations authorising the Registrar to erase from the Register the names of persons who fail to pay the prescribed fee after due warning. The fees payable by registered practitioners are detailed in THE GENERAL MEDICAL COUNCIL (Registration (Fees) (Amendment) Regulations) ORDER OF COUNCIL, 1970. The fees at present payable are:

(a) on provisional registration under section 17 or section 23 of the Act of 1956 . . . . £10
(b) on full registration under section 7 of the Act of 1956
  (i) in the case of a person who is or has at any time been provisionally registered under section 17 of the Act of 1956 or by virtue of any provision of the law of the Republic of Ireland made for the purposes similar to the said section 17 . . . . £15
  (ii) in the case of any other person £25
(c) on full registration under section 18 of the Act of 1956
  (i) in the case of a person who is or has at any time been provisionally registered under section 23 of the Act of 1956 . . . . £20
  (ii) in the case of any other person £35

The annual retention fee is £5. The Registrar must arrange for the publication annually of the Medical Register containing the names of all those on the Principal List on 1st January in that year.   This enables the public to identify the qualified practitioner, but does not prevent them from seeking medical assistance from unregistered persons.

The most important limitations which the Acts impose upon the unregistered practitioner are that he is forbidden to use any title which he does not possess, or to pretend that he is a qualified doctor.   He cannot recover fees in a court of law, poisons may not be supplied by him, or dispensed by a pharmacist on his prescription, and he cannot sign valid certificates.   He is also precluded from holding medical appointments in the public service, and from practising under the National Health Service Acts, or from holding Crown appointments. He may not, apart from urgent necessity, attend maternity cases unless under the direction and personal supervision of a duly qualified medical practitioner, and he cannot, by virtue of the Venereal Disease Act, 1917, treat venereal diseases.   Further, only duly qualified and registered medical practitioners, if they so desire, are exempted from serving on juries.

Cases where the pretence of qualification is made are relatively rare. During 1960, however, a man who had previously been employed as a miner, shop assistant, seaman, and farm labourer pleaded guilty to charges arising out of his posing as a qualified medical practitioner. During a period of approximately twenty days he made out eight hundred prescriptions, including six for dangerous drugs and two hundred and three for scheduled poisons.[1]

It is the act of registration which renders the practitioner legally qualified to practise, and not his medical qualifications.   Therefore, it is most important that all who become medically qualified should be registered.   The qualifications for registration are detailed in the Medical Acts, 1956 and 1969.   Registration can only be obtained by application after passing a qualifying examination and producing a certificate of subsequent experience in medicine and surgery.   The subsequent experience required is employment in a resident capacity in an approved hospital or institution.   The time is prescribed by the Council after approval by the Privy Council.   The certificate is granted by the body who granted the qualifying diploma.   In order that people who have obtained qualifying diplomas may be employed in the capacities necessary to obtain the prescribed experience, provisional registration was introduced.   Persons provisionally registered have their names appropriately marked in the Register and the provisions which make it an offence for anyone falsely to pretend to be registered are extended to apply to provisional registration.

The supervision of standards of proficiency required for qualification for registration

The standards required and the duties and powers of the Council in this connection are contained in sections 10 and 11 of the Medical Act, 1956, with minor modifications contained in the Medical Act, 1969.

The Council can require any body granting a qualification for registration to supply the Council with information concerning the courses of study and examinations, the age at which such courses and examinations must be taken and the requisites for obtaining qualification. They can appoint inspectors to attend qualifying examinations and visitors to study the sufficiency of the courses of instruction. If the Council consider that the standards are insufficient they can report this to the Privy Council and if after considering the report of the General Medical Council and any objections made to it by the appropriate Medical School, the Privy Council can make an order declaring that the qualification of the Medical School concerned shall no longer be registrable.

The disciplinary function

The Council, by enactment strengthened by decision of the courts of law in their interpretation of the Medical Acts, has attained the position of a court of justice. It performs this function by means of the Medical Disciplinary Committee. This committee consists of the President and eighteen other members of the Council, of whom at least six must be elected members of the Council and at least two must be persons who are neither registered medical practitioners nor the holders of qualifying diplomas. The members of the Committee are appointed by the Council. A Penal Cases Committee decides in advance which cases shall come before the Medical Disciplinary Committee for inquiry. When acting as a court of medical discipline and conduct, the Disciplinary Committee conforms in procedure to that of a court of law, and has the power to compel attendance of witnesses, to administer the oath, and to compel production of documents. An Assessor is appointed by the Disciplinary Committee for the purpose of advising them on questions of law arising in proceedings before them. The functions of the Assessor are defined in rules drawn up by the Lord Chancellor. The verdicts are either guilty or not guilty 'of serious professional misconduct'.

The powers of the Disciplinary Committee are based on Section 33 of the Medical Act, 1956, and Section 13 of the Medical Act, 1969.

Section 13 states:

(1) For subsection (1) of section 33 of the Act of 1956 (erasure from register for conviction of crime or for infamous conduct in any professional respect) there shall be substituted the following subsections—

'(1) Where a fully registered person—

    (a) is found by the Disciplinary Committee to have been convicted (whether while so registered or not) in the United Kingdom or the Republic of Ireland or any of the Channel Islands or the Isle of Man of a criminal offence: or

    (b) is judged by the Disciplinary Committee to have been (whether while so registered or not) guilty of serious professional misconduct.

the Committee may, if they think fit, direct that his name shall be erased from the register or that his registration therein shall be suspended (that is to say, shall not have effect) during such period not exceeding twelve months as may be specified in the direction.

(1A) Where a direction for the suspension of a person's registration in the register has been given under this section the Disciplinary Committee may—

    (a) from time to time direct that the period of suspension specified in the original direction shall be extended or further extended for such further period from the time when it would otherwise expire as may be specified in the direction: or

    (b) at any time while the suspension continues to have effect direct that the person's name shall be erased from the register:

but the Committee shall not extend any period of suspension under this section for more than twelve months at a time.

(1B) Where a direction under this section for the suspension or suspension for an extended period of a person's registration in the register takes effect, the Registrar shall make a note of the fact in the register; and while a person's registration in the register is suspended by virtue of this section he shall be treated as not being registered therein notwithstanding that his name still appears therein.'

The expression 'infamous conduct in any professional respect' is no longer to be used in the Medical Acts and enactments and the words 'serious professional misconduct' replace this expression wherever it has been used.

In any inquiry concerning serious professional misconduct, findings of fact made in any matrimonial proceedings in the High Court or Court of Session must be accepted as conclusive evidence by the Disciplinary Committee.

Where a University or other Qualifying body has struck off the name of a qualified person it can notify this to the General Council along with the findings on which its decision was based and the Disciplinary Committee can accept the findings as conclusive of the facts found.

Cases in which a practitioner has been convicted in the Courts. Convictions of registered medical practitioners are habitually reported to the Council by the police authorities. In considering a conviction, the Disciplinary Committee has to determine whether the gravity of the offence which the practitioner committed, or the cumulative gravity of offences committed by him on more than one occasion, makes it necessary in the public interest to erase his name from the Register.

The Committee are legally bound to accept a conviction as conclusive. It is therefore not open to a practitioner to contend before the Committee that he was in fact innocent of an offence of which he has been convicted, and that he was convicted only because he pleaded guilty in order to avoid publicity or for any other reason.

Erasure from the Register has been directed in consequence of convictions for the following offences, among others:

(*a*) Procuring or attempting to procure abortion or miscarriage;

(*b*) Driving or being in charge of a motor vehicle when under the influence of drink or drugs, or being found drunk, or being drunk and disorderly or incapable;

(*c*) Contravention of the Dangerous Drugs Acts and Regulations;

(*d*) Forgery, fraud, larceny, embezzlement, and cognate offences; and

(*e*) Offences involving indecency.

The verdict, 'guilty of infamous conduct in a professional respect', was defined in the Court of Appeal in the following terms: 'If it is shown that a medical man, in the pursuit of his profession has done something with regard to it which would be reasonably regarded as disgraceful or dishonourable by his professional brethren of good repute and competency, then it is open to the Council to say that he has been guilty of "infamous conduct in a professional respect".' When the Committee has determined that a person's name is to be erased from the Register, it is the duty of the Registrar to serve notice of the determination of the Committee. Any registered practitioner on whom such notice has been served has the right to appeal to Her Majesty in Council within twenty-eight days of the service of the notification.

A medical practitioner's name cannot be removed from the Register merely at his own request, without compliance with certain provisions.[2]

From time to time the Council have enlarged the scope of matters embraced within the meaning of the words, 'infamous conduct in a professional respect'. The following summary of the resolutions and decisions of the Council upon forms of professional misconduct, brought before the Council in the exercise of its disciplinary jurisdiction over the members of the medical profession, has been published by the Disciplinary Committee of the General Medical Council for the guidance of medical practitioners.

The summary of instances of professional misconduct does not constitute a complete list of the offences which may be punished by erasure from the Register, and the Medical Disciplinary Committee is in no way precluded from considering and dealing with any form of professional misconduct which may be brought before them, although it may not appear to come within the scope or precise wording of any of the categories set out below.

Cases raising questions of infamous conduct in a professional respect: Adultery, or improper conduct or association, with a patient. Any medical practitioner who abuses his professional position by committing adultery or improper conduct with a patient, or by maintaining an improper association with a patient, is liable to erasure. In this connection the Act specifically provides that in any inquiry held by the Committee any finding of fact which has been made in matrimonial proceedings in the High Court or the Court of Session, or on appeal from a decision in such proceedings, in the United Kingdom or the Republic of Ireland, shall be conclusive evidence of the fact found.

Advertising and canvassing. In the opinion of the Committee, the practices by a medical practitioner

(1) of advertising, whether directly or indirectly, for the purpose of obtaining patients or promoting his own professional advantage; or, for any such purpose, of procuring, or sanctioning, or acquiescing in the publication of notices commending or directing attention to the practitioner's professional skill, knowledge, services or qualifications, or depreciating those of others; or of being associated with, or employed by, those who procure or sanction such advertising or publication: and

(2) of canvassing, or employing any agent or canvasser, for the purpose of obtaining patients; or of sanctioning, or of being associated with or employed by those who sanction, such employment,

are discreditable to the medical profession and are contrary to the public interest. Any practitioner resorting to any such practice is liable to erasure.

The question of advertising is a difficult one. It has been the practice in the Glasgow Medical School to advise students when they qualify and are on the Register that they should not allow their names to be used on television or radio programmes. This principle was carefully observed by the older practitioners in all branches of medicine and it still appears to us to be wise. There have been however in recent years many instances of prominent members of the profession allowing their names to be used in programmes which would certainly and indirectly promote their own professional advantage without any action having been taken by the Disciplinary Committee.

There is therefore at the present time a tendency to relax the restrictions on what would formerly have been considered as advertising. It is not possible to say how far this trend will go and while we deplore it there is no doubt that it has the approval of the public to whose entertainment it contributes, and even possibly of a majority of the profession.

Professional certificates, reports and other documents. Medical practitioners are in certain cases bound by law or may be from time to time called upon to give professional certificates, reports, and other documents of kindred character: for example, under the National Health Service and National Insurance Acts, in relation to birth, illness, death, or cremation, for the purpose of excusing attendance in the Courts or in public or private employment, and for many other purposes.

Any practitioner who signs or issues in his professional capacity any certificate, report, or other document of a kindred character containing statements which he knows, or ought to know, to be untrue, misleading or otherwise improper, is liable to erasure.

Association with unqualified or unregistered persons practising medicine (covering); Relations with persons performing functions relevant to Medicine, Surgery, and Midwifery.

(1) Any medical practitioner who by his presence, advice, or co-operation (whether by the administration of anaesthetics or the issue of certificates or otherwise) knowingly enables or assists a person not registered as a medical practitioner to practise medicine, or to attend or perform any operation on a patient in respect of any matter requiring medical or surgical discretion or skill, is liable to erasure.

(2) Any medical practitioner who
  (i) Knowingly enables any person other than a certified midwife to attend a woman in childbirth, otherwise than in a case of sudden or urgent necessity or under the direction and personal supervision of a registered medical practitioner (such attendance being contrary to the Midwives Act, 1951), or
  (ii) Employs and leaves in charge of any 'open shop', or other place where scheduled poisons may be sold to the public, any assistant not legally qualified to sell such poisons,
  is liable to erasure.

(3) Nothing in the foregoing paragraphs is to be regarded as affecting or restricting in any way (i) the proper training of medical and other

bona fide students, or (ii) the legitimate employment of nurses, mid-wives, physiotherapists, dispensers, and other persons trained to perform specialised functions relevant to Medicine, Surgery, and Midwifery, provided that the medical practitioner concerned exercises effective supervision over any person so employed and retains personal responsibility for the treatment of the patient.

Other matters. Medical practitioners have been judged to have been guilty of infamous conduct in a professional respect on the following grounds, among others:

(1) Treating or attending patients while under the influence of drink;
(2) Abuse of dangerous drugs, or of the privileges conferred on medical practitioners by the Dangerous Drugs Acts and Regulations;
(3) Commercialisation of a secret remedy;
(4) Gross and/or prolonged neglect of duties, and disregard of personal responsibilities to patients; and
(5) Improperly obtaining or attempting to obtain payments from the National Health Service or otherwise to which they were not entitled.

The Council does not of itself initiate proceedings against members of the medical profession. It takes action only in cases of criminal conviction, or of judicial censure, officially brought to its notice, or in cases of formal complaints, supported by evidence, brought before it by responsible persons or bodies. When a member of the medical profession is convicted in a court of law, the fact is reported to the Council. After consideration of the facts by the Penal Cases Committee, the delinquent may be summoned to appear before the Medical Disciplinary Committee, or alternatively, he may be sent a warning that the matter has been noted and that there should not be a repetition of the offence.

These are all examples of Infamous Conduct. The extent to which the new offence of Serious Professional Misconduct will alter the policy of the General Medical Council cannot be determined.

Production of the British Pharmacopoeia

The duty of publishing the Pharmacopoeia was imposed on the Council by section 47 of the Medical Act, 1956. Section 98 of the Medicines Act, 1968, however makes provision for the assignment to Her Majesty of the Council's copyright in the British Pharmacopoeia.

General Dental Council

The Dentists Act, 1957, provides for the establishment of a General Dental Council and the dissolution of the former Dental Board of the United Kingdom.

The principal duties of this Council comprise:

1. The setting up of an Education Committee, which assumes the previous functions of the General Medical Council relating to courses of study and examinations.
2. Disciplinary duties, carried out by a Disciplinary Committee, assisted by a legal assessor.
3. Duties connected with the Dental Register.
4. The regulation of proceedings before the Council and Disciplinary Committee.

The Act applies to the United Kingdom and may be cited as the Dentists Act, 1957.

NATIONAL HEALTH SERVICE ACTS, 1946 AND 1949
NATIONAL HEALTH SERVICE (SCOTLAND) ACT, 1947

These Acts contain provisions for the preparation and publication, by Executive Councils, of lists of medical practitioners, dentists and pharmacists who undertake to provide their respective services under the Acts.   Provision is also made for the constitution of Tribunals with the power to order the removal of the names of practitioners, dentists or pharmacists from these lists.   The Tribunals consist of a chairman and two other members.   In England, the chairman is appointed by the Lord Chancellor and must be a barrister or solicitor.   In Scotland, he is appointed by the Lord President of the Court of Session, and must be a practising advocate or solicitor.   One of the other members is a person appointed, in England, by the Minister of Health, and, in Scotland, by the Secretary of State, after consultation with representatives of the Executive Councils.   The other member, referred to as the practitioner member, is a member of the profession concerned, for example, medical, dental, or pharmaceutical, and is appointed, in England, by the Minister of Health, and, in Scotland, by the Secretary of State, after consultation with the appointed representatives of that profession.

The purpose of these Tribunals is to inquire into cases where representations are made in the prescribed manner to the Tribunal by an Executive Council, or by any other person, that the continued inclusion of any person in any list prepared under these Acts would be prejudicial to the efficiency of the services in question.   The Tribunal, on receiving representations from an Executive Council shall, and in any other case may, inquire into the case and, if they are of the opinion that the continued inclusion of the said person in any list to which the representations relate would be prejudicial to the efficiency of the said services, shall direct that his name be removed from that list, and may also, if they think fit, direct that his name be removed from, or not be included in, any corresponding list kept by any other Executive Council under these parts of these Acts.

An appeal lies, in England, to the Minister of Health and, in Scotland, to the Secretary of State, from any direction of the Tribunal.

An instance of a name being removed from the Medical List occurred in 1953.   This action by the Tribunal was occasioned by the finding of irregularities in prescribing and dispensing for patients.[3]

VENEREAL DISEASE ACT, 1917

This Act was passed to prevent the treatment of venereal disease otherwise than by duly qualified medical practitioners, and to control the supply of remedies for the purpose of treatment.

CANCER ACT, 1939

Under this Act, it is illegal to take any part in the publication of an advertisement offering to treat any person for cancer, or to prescribe any remedy for it, or to give any advice for its treatment, or to refer to any article in terms calculated to lead to its use in the treatment of cancer. The Act is not intended to apply to those who publish as a reasonable necessity to bring the advertisement to the notice of certain specified persons such as a local authority, those controlling hospitals, medical practitioners, nurses, chemists, students of these professions, or sellers of surgical appliances.

MALPRAXIS

Malpraxis means failure in the exercise of a reasonable degree of skill and care on the part of a medical practitioner in his treatment of a patient.   The public who entrust themselves to the care of registered practitioners are entitled to demand and to expect from them the exercise of reasonable skill and care.

The most authoritative statement of the law of medical negligence was given by Lord Clyde and has been followed in the case of McHardy v. Dundee General Hospitals Board of Management.[4]

Lord Clyde stated: 'In the realm of diagnosis and treatment, there is ample scope for genuine difference of opinion, and one man clearly is not negligent merely because his conclusion differs from that of other professional men, nor because he has displayed less skill or knowledge than others would have shown. . . . To establish liability by a doctor where deviation from normal practice is alleged, three factors require to be established. First of all it must be proved that there is a usual and normal practice; secondly, it must be proved that the defender has not adopted that practice; and thirdly (and this is of crucial importance) it must be established that the course the doctor adopted is one which no professional man of ordinary skill would have taken if he had been acting with ordinary care.'[5]

The result of medical negligence is a claim by the injured party against the doctor for compensation for his injuries. The following are examples of cases in which claims have been made against doctors:

> Amputation of the wrong finger.
> Use of the wrong chemical.
> Too tight plaster.
> Failure to release a tourniquet.
> Failure to make X-ray examination in suspected fracture.
> Failure to anticipate the risk of tetanus.
> Inhalation of a tooth or tooth fragments.
> Failure to remove instruments or swabs at operation.

The case of Whiteford v. Hunter and Gleed[6] is of interest. Put briefly, the facts of this case are that a seventy-year-old plaintiff sued a surgeon and a general practitioner for damages on the ground of their negligence in wrongly diagnosing his condition. They had told him that he was suffering from cancer and had only nine months to live. He thereupon gave up his business and went to America to die. An American surgeon had then operated upon him for a bladder complaint which he declared was the sole and obvious cause of the condition. The plaintiff claimed that he had suffered pecuniary loss and mental agony as a result of defendant's mistake. Mr Justice Birkett held that no negligence could be attributed to the general practitioner. With regard to the surgeon it was now admitted that the diagnosis was wrong. The surgeon had done nothing afterwards to confirm or verify it. His Lordship said he was clearly of opinion that the surgeon was negligent in not making a microscopic examination; he was lacking in his duty in taking no step to check or verify his diagnosis, and also in not making a cystoscopic examination. Judgment was entered against the surgeon for £6,300. A stay of execution was granted with a view to appeal, which was upheld. Mr Justice Asquith, in giving judgment, said that a doctor was not liable in negligence by reason only that he had made a mistake in diagnosis. An appeal was made to the House of Lords, who unanimously dismissed Mr Whiteford's appeal and finally cleared Mr Hunter, the surgeon, of negligence.[6]

Under circumstances when the negligence shown is so gross in character as to amount to recklessness, criminal prosecution may result. In these cases the nature and degree of the negligence must be such as to convince the jury that it should be punished. It is clear, therefore, that what might amount to negligence in a civil action would not necessarily warrant a conviction on a criminal charge.

In the case of R. v. Bateman,[7] the Lord Chief Justice said that in a civil action for negligence, the extent of a man's liability depends on how much damage he causes; in a criminal trial it depends on how negligent he was.

The case of R. v. Wight provides a good example of a criminal prosecution. The accused, a medical practitioner, was charged with having caused the death of a woman while delivering her with forceps, he being at the time under the influence of alcohol. It was shown in evidence, however, that the cause of his condition was not alcohol but chloral hydrate. He was convicted and sentenced to three months' imprisonment. The comments of the judge indicated that no medical man was entitled to practise his profession while under the influence of any drug or other narcotic substance, and that had alcohol been proved the cause of the prisoner's condition, a much more severe sentence would have been passed.

At the Central Criminal Court a doctor admitted responsibility for the death of a child to whom he had administered an anaesthetic. He was sentenced to twelve months' imprisonment. The circumstances were that during the operation the doctor was seen to remove the connecting tube between the anaesthetic apparatus and the child and to put the tube into his own mouth. The doctor did not switch from an empty to a full cylinder of oxygen and for three or four minutes the child's brain was deprived of oxygen. This was the direct cause of the child's death a month later.[8]

Lord Ellenborough has held that if a person acting in a medical capacity be guilty of misconduct arising either from gross ignorance or criminal inattention by which the patient dies, he is guilty of manslaughter.

The rarity of criminal prosecutions may be taken as an indication of how serious a degree of recklessness has to be committed before members of the profession are brought within reach of the law, and how rarely criminal negligence is found in medical practice.

LIABILITY OF HOSPITALS AND NURSING HOMES

It has long been established as a rule of law that a master is liable for the wrongful or negligent acts of his servants.

Hospitals and nursing homes are therefore clearly liable for the negligent acts and omissions of their non-medical staffs.

The medical staffs were, however, held to be in a different position because between them and the managers of hospitals there was no true relationship of master and servant. The reason for this lay in the fact that the managers of hospitals had no right of interference or direction as to the way the work was to be done. The contract was not one of service but an agreement to render services, and the obligations of the hospital authorities were fulfilled when they appointed personnel who were fully qualified and competent.

With the passing of the Health Service Acts and the disappearance of the voluntary hospital, conditions have changed and the courts have held that it is the duty of the hospitals to provide treatment for their patients and are thus responsible for negligent acts of those whom they have appointed to carry out that treatment.

Legal opinions on this matter were given in the following cases: Cassidy v. Ministry of Health,[9] Jones v. Manchester Corporation,[10] and Hayward v. Board of Management of Royal Infirmary of Edinburgh.[11]

LEGAL CRIMINAL PROCEDURE

ENGLISH PROCEDURE

In England there is a Director of Public Prosecutions. The duties of this official, under the direction of the Attorney-General, are, among others, to institute, undertake, or carry on criminal proceedings at any stage and in any court, and to give advice and assistance to persons, whether officials or not, concerned in a criminal proceeding. He undertakes all cases of murder, and cases of importance or difficulty, or in which, owing to special circumstances or the refusal or failure to proceed with a prosecution, intervention on the public behalf is necessary for the prosecution of the offender.

The Beeching Commission reported in 1969 (Cmnd. 4153) on the structure and administration of the English courts. They recommended the abolition of fixed Assizes and the substitution of a centrally administered Court system capable of adapting to changes in the patterns of population, crime, and litigation.

The essence of the Courts Act, 1971, which sets up the new structure, is flexibility in the administration of justice, the whole being under the central control of the Lord Chancellor.

English Criminal Courts

Magistrates' Court of Petty Sessions. This is a Court of Summary Jurisdiction, or a Court of First Instance.

Two or more Justices of the Peace or one professional magistrate, either sitting alone or with other Justices, preside in the court, which tries petty offences and passes sentence. In all serious charges, before a prisoner can be committed for trial the witnesses in the case give their evidence on oath before a body of Justices, who elect their chairman, and in the presence of the accused, and in open court. The accused is entitled to give evidence on oath and to call witnesses. When making preliminary inquiry as to whether an accused person shall, or shall not, be committed for trial by a jury, the Justices are termed 'examining magistrates' or 'examining Justices'. The evidence is recorded in writing, and after being read over to the respective witnesses is signed by them and by the presiding Justice. The evidence of each witness so recorded is termed a deposition and these depositions form the basis of the evidence led at any subsequent trial of the accused person, the various witnesses being expected to adhere to their respective depositions. From the evidence given, it remains for the Justices to decide whether or not the accused shall be committed for trial. If there is not a prima facie case established against the accused he is discharged, but this is not synonymous with acquittal since he may be arraigned again on the same charge.

In any case where a medical witness has given evidence in a court in which an accused person is committed for trial, he, in common with other witnesses, is bound over to give evidence at the trial.

Crown Court. This court, a part of the Supreme Court, replaces Quarter Sessions and Assize Courts. It exercises jurisdiction over all cases heard 'on indictment'—i.e. before a judge and jury. When hearing appeals from magistrates' court findings or where a convicted person has been committed by the magistrates for sentence, the Crown Court judge sits with not less than two and not more than four Justices of the Peace.

The procedure at a trial in the Crown Court may be summed up shortly. The prisoner having tendered a plea of 'not guilty', and the jury having been sworn, the prosecuting counsel opens the case against the prisoner by outlining briefly the facts to which the witnesses he is about to call will testify. He next calls and examines his witnesses in turn. This part of the examination of a witness is called the examination-in-chief. Each witness, at the conclusion of this examination, may be cross-examined by counsel for the accused, or by the accused himself if not represented by counsel, after which prosecuting counsel may re-examine each witness on points brought out in cross-examination, but he may not examine the witness on any fresh subject of evidence. If the witness is to be asked further questions, these must be put by the judge. After the witnesses have been called, the case for the Crown is closed. If counsel for the defence calls witnesses, he will conduct their examination-in-chief, and counsel for the prosecution will cross-examine them. Thus the position of counsel with reference to the defence witnesses is reversed.   At the conclusion of the evidence, prosecuting counsel addresses the jury, thereafter defending counsel addresses the jury, and finally, the judge sums up.   The jury then retire to consider their verdict.

Queen's Bench Division of the High Court.   An appeal from the inferior criminal courts lies to this court, by a stated case on a point of law.

Court of Criminal Appeal.   In certain circumstances, a convicted person may appeal to the Court of Criminal Appeal, presided over by the Lord Chief Justice of England, and not less than, but usually, three judges of the Queen's Bench Division of the High Court.   It may decide by a majority.   The court has a wide range of jurisdiction and can quash a sentence and substitute the one it thinks ought to have been passed, and it can substitute a verdict for that, in fact, returned where it is justified by the evidence.   Thus it can increase sentences or penalties.

House of Lords.   An appeal lies to the House of Lords from the judgment of the Court of Criminal Appeal, but only where the Director of Public Prosecutions, or the prosecutor, or defendant obtains a certificate of the Attorney-General that the decision involves a point of law of exceptional public importance, or that it is desirable in the public interest that a further appeal should be brought.   Such appeals are few. On appeals, only lords who hold, or have held, high judicial office act as judges.

The Coroner and the Coroner's Court

The office of the Coroner is of great antiquity and there is now no record of its origin.   The Brodrick Committee has recently made a searching inquiry into the office and function of the Coroner (Cmnd. 4810).

By the Coroners (Amendment) Act, 1926, s. 1, no person is qualified to be appointed a County Coroner or a Borough Coroner unless, with certain exceptions, he is a barrister, solicitor, or legally qualified medical practitioner, of not less than five years' standing in his profession.

Every Coroner must appoint a deputy Coroner who possesses the necessary qualifications of a Coroner.

The jurisdiction of a Coroner is restricted to the district to which he has been appointed.

His main duty is to inquire into the circumstances of certain deaths occurring within his jurisdiction.

There is an obligation upon him to make an inquiry when he is informed that a dead body is lying within his jurisdiction, and there is reasonable cause to suspect that such a person has died either a violent or unnatural death, or has died a sudden death of which the cause is unknown, or that such person has died in prison, or in such place or under such circumstances as to require an inquest. (Coroners Act, 1887, s. 3.)

It should be clearly understood that it is contrary to the common law of England for anyone to bury the body of a person dying from a violent death, or to dispose of a body so as to prevent the holding of an inquest, or to obstruct the Coroner and his jury before the Coroner has had an opportunity of holding an inquest upon such body.

He obtains information by means of his officer.   The Coroner's officer is not a statutory official, but his duties are onerous since he is primarily responsible for collecting relevant information on the Coroner's behalf. He is closely connected with the detailed arrangements for inquiries and inquests.   Frequently a police officer is permanently detailed for this purpose.

The Coroner's inquiry may take the form of a private inquiry or of an inquest in the Coroner's Court with or without a jury.

Whichever method of inquiry is adopted medical evidence forms an important part of the proceedings, and as a verdict arrived at without medical evidence has little value it is now the practice to call medical evidence at every inquest.

The relationship of medical witnesses to the Coroner is governed by the Coroners Act, 1887, and the Coroners (Amendment) Act, 1926.

Under the Coroners Act, 1887, s. 21, the Coroner in the course of his inquiry may summon as a witness any legally qualified medical practitioner who attended the deceased at his death or during his last illness. If a doctor has not attended the deceased, the Coroner may summon any legally qualified practitioner, who is at the time in actual practice in or near the place where the death occurred, and may obtain evidence from him as to the cause of death.

If a Coroner considers that information to be obtained by a post-mortem examination will make an inquest unnecessary he may instruct a registered medical practitioner to make a post-mortem examination and to report the result to him in writing.

Under the Coroners (Amendment) Act, 1926, s. 22, the Coroner at any time after he has decided to hold an inquest, can request any suitably qualified practitioner to make a post-mortem examination of the body, or to make such special examination of the body or parts of the body as he may think necessary to provide evidence concerning the cause of death.

The Coroners Rules, 1953, provide more specific instructions with regard to post-mortem examinations.   The principal provisions are:

1. The post-mortem examination should be made, whenever practicable, by a pathologist having suitable qualifications and experience. He should have access to suitable laboratory facilities.
2. The person making a post-mortem examination shall report to the Coroner in the form set out in the First Schedule of these rules or in similar form.
3. Unless authorised by the Coroner, the person making a post-mortem examination shall not supply a copy of his report to any person other than the Coroner.
4. Every post-mortem examination shall be made in premises which are adequately equipped for the purposes of the examination (dwelling houses and licensed premises are excluded).   Such premises to be recognised as adequately equipped must be supplied with proper heating, running water, and lighting facilities, and containers for the storage and preservation of material.

When there is sworn testimony that, in the belief of a witness, the death of a deceased person was caused partly, or entirely, by the improper or negligent treatment of a medical practitioner, or other person, that medical practitioner or other person shall not be allowed to perform or assist at any post-mortem or special examination made for the purposes of an inquest on the deceased.   The medical practitioner or other person concerned has, however, the right, if he so desires, to be represented at the post-mortem examination.

The foregoing is of great practical importance to practising members of the medical profession, and has made the evidence of pathologists increasingly important at Coroners' inquests.

When the Coroner has reasonable cause to suspect that the deceased has died a violent or unnatural death, or has died in prison or in such place or in such circumstances as to necessitate the holding of an inquest in accordance with the requirements of any Act, other than the Coroners Act, then he must hold an inquest.

The Coroner must summon a jury, which consists of seven and not more than eleven members, in cases where there is reason to suspect that:

(a) the death was caused by murder, manslaughter, or infanticide;
(b) the death occurred in prison or in such circumstances as to require an inquest under any Act other than the Coroners Act, 1887;
(c) the death was caused by an accident, poisoning, or disease, notice of which is required to be given to a government department, or to any inspector or other officer of a government department under any Act;

(*d*) the death was caused by an accident arising from the use of a vehicle in a street or public highway;

(*e*) the death occurred in circumstances the continuance or possible recurrence of which is prejudicial to the health or safety of the public or any section of the public.

The Coroner, before holding an inquest, must view the body. The jury do not need to view the body unless the Coroner so directs or a majority of the jury so desires.

Witnesses can be compelled to attend an inquest and give evidence but the summons of a Coroner is limited to his sphere of jurisdiction. If it is necessary to compel the attendance of a witness who is outwith the Coroner's jurisdiction this can be done by obtaining a Crown Office subpoena. Evidence is given on oath and counsel and solicitors who attend inquests in a representative capacity may question witnesses.

In cases of murder, manslaughter, and infanticide, the evidence must be recorded in writing and signed both by witnesses and Coroner. These statements of evidence are termed depositions, and can be used in subsequent legal proceedings (see pp. 15 and 21). It is, however, essential that they should be taken in the presence of the accused person if they are to be used at a criminal trial.

When the evidence is completed it is customary for the Coroner to sum up for the jury, who then give their verdict. The Coroner can accept a majority verdict provided that the minority is not larger than two. The verdict is in simple form and embodies such facts as the identity of the deceased, the cause, time, and place of death, and classifies the death as 'natural' or 'violent'. It further classifies the death as 'not criminal' or 'criminal'. If some part of the inquest is unanswered, an open verdict is returned.

When, as a result of the verdict, some person is charged with murder, manslaughter, or infanticide, or of being an accessory before the fact to a murder, the Coroner must issue a warrant to arrest such person, if a warrant has not already been issued. He must also bind the witnesses by recognisance. The warrant of commitment should include a direction as to the court in which the accused is to appear. The Coroner is bound to attend a court where a case is being tried on an inquisition taken before him.

The Coroner while acting in his court is in the position of a judge and is therefore immune from actions at the instance of any individual, e.g., no action can be taken by an individual for slander in the Coroner's summing up. This immunity is effective only while the Coroner is acting within his jurisdiction.

It is the duty of every Coroner to make an annual return to the Secretary of State of all cases on which he has held an inquest.[12]

Relation of medical men to Coroner and Inquest

There are certain questions which affect the medical profession with respect to their relation to the Coroner. Probably the most important is whether or not it is the duty of a medical practitioner in attendance upon a person who has died from a violent or any unnatural cause to report the fact to the Coroner. Although there does not appear to be any statutory obligation, a medical practitioner would appear to owe a duty as an ordinary citizen to report violent, or unnatural death, a sudden death, the cause of which is unknown, or the kind of death into which the Coroner is obliged by statute to inquire. This would include deaths which result from the administration of an anaesthetic. It is commonly, but erroneously, thought that the Births and Deaths Registration Act, 1953 (see p. 141), restricts the practitioner's duty to report suspicious deaths to the authorities and that he has discharged his duty merely by completing the death certificate and delivering it to the Registrar. This Act has not relieved the practitioner from the duty which he already owed before this Act was passed. In all cases of doubt an informal conversation with the Coroner will provide a clear indication of what he considers is the proper line of conduct having regard to the circumstances of the specific instance under review.

In 1914, Mr Justice Avory, in delivering judgment in the case of a woman who died from the effects of an illegal operation, and who had been seen by a number of doctors prior to her death, said, 'It may be the moral duty of the medical man, even in cases when the patient is not dying, or not unlikely to recover, to communicate with the authorities when he sees good reason to believe that a criminal offence has been committed. However that may be, I cannot doubt that in such a case as the present, where the woman was, in the opinion of the medical men, likely to die, and, therefore, her evidence was likely to be lost, it was his duty, and that some one of these gentlemen ought to have done it in this case'.

Medical practitioners when summoned to appear as witnesses must obey the summons or become liable to penalty.

SCOTTISH PROCEDURE

The prominent characteristic of criminal procedure in Scotland is the existence of the office of Public Prosecutor.

The Lord Advocate, the Solicitor-General, and four Advocates-Depute are the public prosecutors, on behalf of the Crown, before the High Court of Justiciary. In each county there is a Procurator-Fiscal for whose appointment the Lord Advocate is responsible. He initiates the prosecution of crimes and offences in the Sheriff Court, and conducts such prosecution either personally or by depute. The Lord Advocate and the Advocates-Depute, who are responsible for the direction of criminal proceedings, preside at the Crown Office, Edinburgh. When a Procurator-Fiscal has collected all the evidence in any case, it is sent to the Crown Office. There, the evidence is fully reviewed and decision is taken with regard to the nature of further proceedings and as to the court in which the case will be tried. It may be that no further proceedings will be authorised through insufficiency of evidence or other good reason. The most serious cases are tried before the High Court of Justiciary, but in less serious cases they will probably be disposed of by the Sheriff.

In Scotland, the legal advisers at the Crown Office assess the adequacy of evidence in any given case and instruct proceedings. In this way the evidence to be led at a trial is not available to the public and to potential members of a jury who may be called upon subsequently to pass a verdict.

In contrast, the usual English procedure necessitates the disclosure of the evidence at the Magistrates' Court prior to the actual trial, and thus the evidence becomes known to the public.

The duty of bringing all accused persons to a bar of justice falls primarily upon the Procurator-Fiscal as local Public Prosecutor. In addition, he is charged with the duty of inquiring into the cause of sudden or suspicious deaths, which inquiry takes the form of precognition of witnesses, both lay and medical. This is ordinarily a private inquiry. After he has performed this duty, it is his further responsibility to report and certify the cause of death to the Registrar of the district in which the death took place.

Some explanation of the term 'precognition' is necessary. A precognition is a statement from a person who will probably be called by the Crown as a witness in a case. This statement embodies the facts to which the potential witness will testify at a trial, and is recorded by a Procurator-Fiscal or one of his deputes. The statement, which is not given on oath or signed by the witness, is usually made at the office of the Procurator-Fiscal and, as will be noted, is obtained with much less formality than the English deposition, already described. A witness is not bound by the terms of his precognition, the object of which is to form a basis for the preparation of the prosecution, and to facilitate the leading of evidence at the trial. A precognition taken in this way cannot be used to contradict what he says when giving evidence. Solicitors acting for an accused person may also take precognitions and thus prepare the case for the defence. It should be clearly understood that in criminal prosecutions every person competent and compellable as a witness for the prosecution may be compelled in the preliminary investigations to disclose what he knows concerning the crime under investigation. This does not apply to the opinion of experts. If a person is unwilling to submit to precognition by the Procurator-Fiscal in the ordinary way, he may be compelled to attend before a magistrate, and may be imprisoned if he refuses to answer pertinent inquiries.

By the Summary Jurisdiction (Scotland) Act, 1954, any witness who, after being duly cited fails, without reasonable excuse after receiving at least twenty-four hours' notice, to attend for precognition by a Procurator-Fiscal or Burgh Prosecutor at the time and place mentioned in the citation served on him, or refuses when so cited to give information within his knowledge in regard to any matter relative to the commission of the offence in regard to which such precognition is taken, shall be deemed guilty of contempt of court and be liable to be summarily punished forthwith for the same by fine or imprisonment.

In civil actions, the court will not order persons against their will to submit to precognition.   There is no duty or obligation on any person to give information before the trial regarding any matter which may form the subject of litigation or to allow himself to be precognosced with a view to his being called as a witness.   The statements which a witness voluntarily makes on precognition are in the same position with regard to privilege as statements made on oath in the witness-box (see p. 55).

If a medical witness assumes the attitude that his function is to aid the ends of justice, his duty becomes clear.   Should, therefore, the prosecution or the defence desire to precognosce a medical witness who has been called by the defence or the prosecution, he should not have the slightest hesitation in submitting both his findings in, and views on, the case at issue, just as he has done for the side who first requested his professional services.   The same facilities should be at the command of either the prosecution or the defence.

Duties of the Procurator-Fiscal

The Procurator-Fiscal is charged statutorily with the duty of making public inquiry into the causes of fatal accidents, and, in special circumstances, of sudden deaths.   The former is held under the Fatal Accidents Inquiry (Scotland) Act, 1895, as amended by the Fatal Accidents and Sudden Deaths Inquiry (Scotland) Act, 1906, and the Criminal Procedure (Scotland) Act, 1938, and the latter under the Fatal Accidents and Sudden Deaths Inquiry (Scotland) Act, 1906.   The Procurator-Fiscal presents a petition to the Sheriff craving him to hold a public inquiry in regard to the cause of the death and the circumstances of the accident, and the Sheriff in granting the petition pronounces an order, directing that a public inquiry be held, and grants warrant to cite witnesses at the instance of the Procurator-Fiscal.   In the last mentioned Act it is enacted that, in any case of sudden or suspicious death in Scotland, the Lord Advocate may, whenever it appears to him to be expedient in the public interest, direct that a public inquiry into such death and the circumstances thereof shall be held.

The Inquiry is held by a Sheriff and jury, the jury consisting of seven jurors, of which neither an employer of the person regarding whose death the Inquiry is held, nor any person engaged under the same employer as the deceased, can be a member.   After hearing the evidence, of which part is frequently medical, and following the summing up by the Sheriff, the jury returns a verdict which sets forth when and where the accident and the death took place, together with the cause or causes of the accident and death, and additional facts as to fault or negligence of anyone, or defects in mode of working in the case of accidents.   The verdict is usually unanimous, but it may be returned by a majority.   It is the duty of the Fiscal at the close of the inquiry to transmit all the documents, including reports and productions, with a copy of the verdict, together with the usual schedule for the Registrar of deaths of the district, to the Crown Agent.

The duties of the Procurator-Fiscal, therefore, include the sphere of action of the Coroner in England.   In carrying out his duties in connection with the investigation of crime, when serious cases are reported to him, he, or one of his deputes, will proceed to the scene and there make an examination.   In such cases as rape, child-murder, or concealment of pregnancy, where invaluable evidence of the commission of the crime may be lost by delay, he arranges for early medical examination of the assaulted person or of the accused.   When death results from violence, he ensures that a post-mortem dissection of the body is made by experienced medical men who, as soon as possible, furnish him with a report of the autopsy together with their opinion as to the cause of death.   In the event of a serious assault to the danger of life, and where death after an interval takes place, he will obtain evidence respecting the treatment of the injured person during that interval.   In cases of assaults likely to prove mortal, he must proceed with a Sheriff so that the deposition of the dying person may be taken (see p. 48).   The inquiry into the cause of sudden deaths by the Procurator-Fiscal is to eliminate possible crime.   In deaths from accident, and in all cases of sudden deaths reported to him, he precognosces witnesses, among whom is a medical witness who reports on the cause of death, without a post-mortem examination when the cause of death can be so ascertained, otherwise after a post-mortem dissection.

As a medical witness may require to appear in any of the law courts, the following indicates the names of these courts, and the class of cases therein:

Police Court: for certain common law and statutory offences of a minor kind, or as the court of first instance in remits to a higher court.

Sheriff Court: in which the Sheriff may act alone, or with a jury. The jurisdiction of this Court is of a very extensive character since it is concerned with both civil and criminal cases. Certain common law and statutory offences of less serious character are tried before a jury, and the conduct of the prosecution is in the hands of the local Procurator-Fiscal. All except very few crimes may be tried, and as much as two years' imprisonment may be given when the trial is on indictment, namely, when the trial is heard before a jury.

The High Court of Justiciary: which ordinarily sits in Edinburgh also sits quarterly or oftener in certain large towns, when it is popularly called the High Court, or the High Court on Circuit. This Court deals with major crimes. The judges of the court are the Lord Justice-General, the Lord Justice-Clerk, and fourteen other judges. A single judge, sitting with a jury composed of fifteen members, presides. Appeals from this court lie to the Criminal Appeal Court.

Court of Session: is the Supreme Civil Court in Scotland and, in certain cases of importance, an appeal to the House of Lords from this Court may be made. The Court of Session has an establishment of eighteen judges but at present only seventeen have been appointed. These are the same as those composing the High Court of Justiciary, but as civil judges they are termed Lords of Session. The Lord Justice-General has the title of Lord President of the Court of Session. The Court has a wide and exclusive jurisdiction and is primarily concerned with actions connected with considerable sums of money, divorce and nullity, and civil trials by jury. The Inner House, when sitting as an appellate court, hears appeals from the Outer House of the Court, together with certain appeals from the Sheriff Court. The Lord President presides over the First Division, and the Lord Justice-Clerk over the Second Division of the Inner House.

Criminal Appeal Court: this Court was instituted by the Criminal Appeal (Scotland) Act, 1926, and to it an appeal from the High Court of Justiciary is permitted on special grounds. The right of appeal is given only to the accused, and is usually based on questions of law.

House of Lords: is the ultimate Court of Appeal in civil causes.

Procedure in investigation of a serious crime. The police lay information of the crime, for example, murder, before the Procurator-Fiscal, and provide him with a list of the witnesses in the case. The prisoner on apprehension is brought before a Police Magistrate on the given charge, by whom he is remitted to the Sheriff. By this time, the report on the post-mortem examination of the body of the victim, together with all other relevant reports in the case, are in the hands of the Procurator-Fiscal, who has previously made the requisite arrangements for these necessary investigations. The Fiscal then proceeds to precognosce the witnesses. The Sheriff gives the prisoner an opportunity, in the presence of his law agent, if he is legally represented, of emitting a declaration concerning the charge preferred against him, the prisoner having been duly warned that he need not say anything, but that if he chooses to do so his statement will be written down, and used at his trial. When the accused is brought before the Sheriff for examination on any charge, and he or his agent intimates that he does not desire to emit a declaration in regard to such a charge, no declaration is taken.

When the Fiscal has concluded his investigations, the precognitions of witnesses, together with the medical reports, are now forwarded to the Crown Office, where they are placed before one of the Advocates-Depute. After reviewing all the documents, the Lord Advocate or one of his Deputes makes an order on the following lines: that no further inquiry is necessary; to continue the inquiry; to prosecute in the manner suitable to the circumstances of the crime. Depending upon the nature and gravity of the crime, the order may be 'Sheriff summarily', or 'Sheriff and jury', or 'Indict', which necessitates trial before the High Court of Justiciary, or the High Court on Circuit.

Indictment. When the Lord Advocate orders trial, either before a Sheriff and jury or in the High Court, an indictment or charge is carefully drawn up, setting out the nature of the crime, the place and time of its perpetration, and the productions or exhibits in the case. Productions may comprise garments, weapons, or documents, etc., which are to be produced at the trial as evidence against the accused. An indictment may be either written or printed, or partly written and partly printed, and consists of the following sections:

1. (a) Name and designation of accused; (b) name of Lord Advocate; (c) the charge, which condescends upon (1) time, (2) place, (3) and manner; (d) aggravations.
2. Numbered list of productions.
3. Numbered list of witnesses.

The indictment is signed by the Lord Advocate or by one of his Deputes or, when the trial takes place before a Sheriff, by the Procurator-Fiscal, who prefixes to his signature the words 'By authority of Her Majesty's Advocate'.

At the trial the productions bear a number and have individual labels attached to them. On these labels will be found the signatures of the principal witnesses who will speak to their identity. These have been signed by the witnesses on a previous occasion following identification. Therefore, all that any of these witnesses has to do, in order again to identify an article when giving evidence, is to examine the label for the presence of his or her signature.

The indictment is served upon the accused prior to trial, together with a notice calling upon him to appear and answer the charge.

The precognitions and reports in the case form the brief of the prosecutor at the trial of the accused, and from them he leads the evidence of the witnesses.

Another step in the procedure prior to trial is what is termed the pleading diet. This consists of the accused or his solicitor intimating a plea of 'guilty', 'not guilty', or 'not guilty' with the intimation of a special defence, in relation to the charge preferred, in the presence of the Sheriff in court.

Procedure at trial in Scotland. In Scotland, the procedure at the trial of an accused person is very similar to that in England. There are, however, a few differences.

In Scotland, when the court has assembled, the diet is called against the prisoner, who is asked by the judge to plead to the indictment against him. Should he plead guilty the judge passes sentence. If he plead not guilty, then a jury of fifteen is impanelled and put on oath by the clerk of court. By custom, the first person selected by ballot usually becomes the foreman. The prosecutor then calls the first witness who, after being put on oath by the judge, is examined by the prosecutor. At the conclusion of this examination-in-chief the witness is next cross-examined by counsel for the prisoner at the bar, or the 'panel', as the prisoner is commonly called. The witness may then be re-examined by the prosecutor on points brought out in cross-examination. Thereafter, the judge may, as at any time during the course of the preceding examinations, ask questions of the witness. Any juror, through the medium of the judge, may also ask questions. In this manner witnesses for the Crown give their evidence, and, when the last has been heard, the case for the prosecution is closed. Next, witnesses for the defence, including the prisoner himself, may be called. If they are called, the position of respective counsel is reversed with respect to the leading of evidence. At the conclusion of all the evidence, the prosecutor addresses the jury, then counsel for the prisoner addresses them, the evidence is summed up by the judge, and the jury finally delivers the verdict. Counsel for the prisoner is entitled to have the last word with the jury before the summing-up of the judge. Notes of the evidence must be taken by the judge during the trial and a complete record is made by official shorthand writers, previously sworn. The jury may return a verdict without retiring from the box, or after retiral, and the verdict which is announced by the foreman, may either be unanimous or by a majority.

When the case is heard by a Sheriff and jury, the local Procurator-

Fiscal prosecutes, and the accused may be defended either by counsel or by a solicitor.

Differences in English and Scottish court procedure

It will be apparent that procedure in Scotland differs from that in England. An English jury is composed of twelve persons, a Scottish jury of fifteen. The former may fail to return a verdict, or, if a verdict is returned, it must be one of two only, namely, 'guilty' or 'not guilty'. The latter must return one of three verdicts, 'guilty', 'not guilty', or 'not proven'. The Scottish jury can return a simple majority verdict. The English law used to require a unanimous verdict and if this could not be obtained the jury were discharged. The position was altered by section 13 of the Criminal Justice Act, 1967. The jury must now attempt to reach a unanimous verdict; if they have not done so after a period of two hours' deliberation, the jury can accept a majority verdict provided that if there are twelve jurors, ten of them agree: if the jury has been reduced to ten jurors nine of them must agree. If the jury has been reduced to nine the verdict must be unanimous.

The National Insurance (Industrial Injuries) Acts, 1946–65

These Acts substitute for the Workmen's Compensation Acts, 1925 to 1945, a system of insurance against personal injury caused by accident arising out of, and in the course of, a person's employment and against prescribed diseases and injuries due to the nature of a person's employment. These are detailed in the First Schedule, Part I to the 1946 Act.

Industrial injuries contributions are collected from employers and workers. These contributions, together with sums provided by taxation, form the Industrial Injuries Fund.

Three types of benefit are provided by this fund.

(i) 'Death benefit' where an injured person dies as a result of an industrial accident or prescribed disease and the benefit is paid to his dependants in the form of a pension or gratuity.

(ii) Injury benefit where, during the period an insured person is incapacitated for work as a result of an accident or prescribed disease, benefit is paid at a flat rate with allowances for dependants, up to a maximum period of 26 weeks from the date of the accident or development of the disease.

(iii) Disablement benefit, awarded if the injured person still suffers from a substantial or lasting 'loss of faculty' after cessation of injury benefit.

'Loss of faculty' means the partial or total loss of the normal use of organs or parts of the body, or the destruction or impairment of bodily or mental functions. It includes disfigurement.

The degree of disablement is assessed as a percentage.   Where disablement is 20 per cent or more, benefit takes the form of a pension. Where the assessment is under 20 per cent, benefit is provided as a lump sum.

Claims are made to the Ministry and routine questions are decided by an insurance officer.   Where, however, there are special difficulties, the insurance officer may refer the case to a local appeal tribunal which consists of a chairman, a lawyer appointed by the Minister, and two members representing employers and workers.   In all cases there is an appeal from decisions of an insurance officer to the local appeal tribunal.

The Crown appoints a barrister with high legal qualifications as Industrial Injuries Commissioner.   Appeals can be made to him from decisions of the local appeal tribunal.

Questions of disablement are decided by medical boards.   These boards normally consist of two doctors.   An appeal lies to a medical appeal tribunal which consists of a legal chairman and two doctors, usually specialists in the type of disablement involved.

Questions as to whether employment is insurable employment or not are decided by the Minister.   An appeal on points of law lies to the superior courts.

Law Reform (Personal Injuries) Act, 1947

This Act repeals the Employers Liability Act, 1880, and abolishes the defence of common employment.   It also amends the law relating to the liability in damages for breach of statutory duty and to the measure of damages for personal injury or death.   By section 3 of the new Act, the measure of damages for personal injuries is related to such awards as may have been made under the National Insurance (Industrial Injuries) Act, 1946.

References

1. *British Medical Journal*, **1,** 357, 1960.
2. R. v. G.M.C., *ex parte* Kynaston [1930], 1 K.B., 562.
3. *Lancet*, **2,** 681, 1953.
4. S.L.T. (Notes), 1960, 19.
5. Hunter v. Hanley, 1955, S.C., 200.
6. Whiteford v. Hunter and Gleed, 1948, *Lancet*, **2,** 232; [1950] W.N. 553; 94, S.J. 758.
7. R. v. Bateman [1925] All E.R. Rep. 45.
8. *Lancet*, **1,** 464, 1959.
9. Cassidy v. Ministry of Health [1951], 2 K.B., 343.
10. Jones v. Manchester Corporation [1952], 2 Q.B., 852.
11. Hayward v. Board of Management of Royal Infirmary of Edinburgh, 1954, S.L.T., 148.
12. PURCHASE, W.B. & WOLLASTON, H.W.   *Jervis on the Office and Duties of Coroners*, 9th ed.   London: Sweet & Maxwell, 1957.

Chapter 2

MEDICAL EVIDENCE

MEDICAL evidence resolves itself into two forms, namely:

Documentary, and
Oral.

As documentary evidence, however, must eventually be spoken to on oath in the witness-box, the above distinction is more theoretical than practical.

DOCUMENTARY EVIDENCE

This may take the following forms:

The medical certificate.
The medical report.
Notes or memoranda.
Dying declarations and depositions.

The medical certificate

This is the simplest form of documentary evidence, and may, for example, consist in the certification, by a duly qualified and registered practitioner, of the inability of attendance in court of a witness or juror, by reason of illness.   In England no particular form of words is required. A simple statement of facts, embodying the name, address, designation, and nature of the illness, of the witness or juror, signed by a practitioner, is all that is necessary.   In Scotland something more is required to render the certificate legal.   The statement of facts must be attested 'on soul and conscience'.   Without this attestation no certificate or report in a Scottish court is admissible.   Certificates of death, however, do not require such form of attestation, as they are in the form scheduled in the Registration Acts.

The medical report

This form of evidence is given at the instance of the Procurator-Fiscal by a medical witness in circumstances such as the following:

In a case where injuries have been inflicted upon an assaulted person. As the result of a post-mortem examination of the body of a person who has died suddenly, or under suspicious circumstances, or from culpable violence, or from any other form of violent death.

For purposes of the Fatal Accidents Inquiry (Scotland) Act.

For purposes of an inquiry regarding the death of a person while in prison, under the Prisons (Scotland) Act.

As the result of the examination of a body after exhumation.

Following an examination of stains on clothing.

Following toxicological examination in cases of poisoning.

In Scotland such reports must be signed 'on soul and conscience'.

Reports upon the examination of assaulted persons should include an accurate description of the character, number, situation, measurements, and direction of the injuries found, together with an opinion of the class of weapon which has been used in their production.

When a post-mortem examination of a body is required, procedure differs in England and Scotland. In England, the request of the Coroner to undertake the examination is the authority for performing it (see p. 17). In Scotland, the procedure is so different that some detailed consideration is necessary.

The Procurator-Fiscal presents a petition to the Sheriff in the following terms:

'GLASGOW,   , 19   .
'Unto the Honourable the
SHERIFF OF THE COUNTY OF LANARK.
'The Petition of   Procurator-
Fiscal of Court for the Public Interest,
'*Humbly Sheweth,*
'That from information received by the Petitioner it appears that   died at or in   on the   day of
'That the circumstances call for investigation and a dissection of the body is necessary.

'May it therefore please your Lordship to grant warrant to cite witnesses for precognition in the premises, and to grant warrant to   , to dissect said body and to report.
'According to Justice, etc.
'(Signed)
'Procurator-Fiscal'.

'
19   .   Grants warrant as craved.
'(Signed)
'Sheriff'.

The above warrant is transmitted to the doctor or doctors named in it, together with the information as to where the body is lying. At the mortuary, witnesses who have been summoned for the identification of the body will be in attendance along with a representative of the police. The warrant entitles those named in it to have possession of the body until the examination has been completed. When death is due to culpable violence by an assailant, two medical men are named in the warrant, and both are responsible for the performance of the examination. If they are agreed upon the findings both will sign the report, but if they should fail to agree, which is unusual, each will write a report.

Identification of body

Before commencing the examination of the body, it is the duty of the medical examiners to establish its identity. For this purpose, identification may be either personal or legal.

Personal identification is made by two persons who are usually near relatives or close friends of the deceased. Their names, designations, and addresses must be recorded by the examiners for inclusion in their report. Thus the body is identified as a given person who was well known to the witnesses during life.

Under certain circumstances, however, it is not possible to secure personal identification, and in this event the body has to be identified in the legal sense, namely, that the body in question is the body which was found or seen by those called upon to identify it, and not as the body of a given person known to them during life.

Full particulars of these witnesses must be embodied in the medical report, and special care must be taken to record in the report any possible identifying features present on the body, in order to facilitate subsequent identification of the body as that of a particular person.

No one, except the practitioners instructed to conduct the examination and their assistants, is allowed to be present at a post-mortem examination except with consent of the Crown. The presence of a doctor who has attended the case or who represents the interests of an accused person may be sanctioned by the Crown authorities, but only on condition that he is present as an onlooker, and will not interfere in any way with the examination. No formal intimation is given that the autopsy is to be held, but in all cases where any person is in custody on suspicion of causing death, this examination is made as a matter of course, so that an accused person or his advisers cannot be in doubt as to the necessity of making immediate application for permission to send a medical representative to witness the examination if they so desire. Such application should be made to the Procurator-Fiscal. He will communicate with the Crown Agent for the instructions of Crown counsel. If an independent post-mortem examination is desired, for the purposes of the defence, it can be made after the Crown examination.

It is expedient for one examiner to perform the manual work and the other to observe the findings and take notes of the facts observed during the examination.

External examination.   A careful external examination of the body must be made.   The appearances indicative of the time of death and the position in which the body has lain after death should be noted, together with any marks of violence, or other marks, which might point directly or indirectly to the cause of death.

If identity of the body has not been established as that of a known individual, all identifying features, such as height, approximate age, sex, colour of the eyes and hair, condition and number of teeth, bodily deformities or abnormalities, scars and tattoo marks, together with other characteristic features, should be carefully noted, so that subsequent identification may be established.   In the ordinary course of events, the examiners need not extend their observations to the clothing, but it would fall within their duty to note carefully, for example, the wrappings in which the body of a newly born child was found, or the clothing or wrappings of a body which has been discovered in an advanced state of decomposition.   Clothing should be examined separately for stains, cuts, or perforations, in cases of injury.   It is advisable that this examination should be made in the laboratory, where suitable facilities are available, and should form the subject of a separate report.   When garments are considered to have an important bearing on the investigation of a case, by instructions of the Procurator-Fiscal, they are brought by the police to the laboratory where detailed examination can be made.

The points to be ascertained with regard to the time of death include the rectal temperature, the presence and extent, or absence, of rigor mortis, the incidence, extent, colour, and degree of fixation of post-mortem lividity, and the presence, character, and extent of putrefaction. The points relating to the likely cause of death must include any lesion which is indicative of violence.   All wounds must be measured accurately, their characters described in detail, and their position fully recorded.   Such data will prove invaluable in the determination of the class of weapon which has been responsible for the wounding, and may throw light on the important question as to whether the wounds are due to accident, suicide, or homicide.   When injuries are situated in the line of the usual incisions necessary for post-mortem examination, such incisions must be modified to enable the lesions to be examined in their entirety.   When bruises or similar marks are present, all of them, after measurement, should be incised, to verify the presence of extravasated blood, since questions may arise in court regarding their possible confusion with post-mortem lividity (see p. 115).   Full notes should be made of ligature marks, and evidence of bruising and abrasions on the neck. The hands should be inspected for defensive wounds, blood-staining, weapons, or other objects. Common sites, and other parts of the body surface, should be carefully examined for puncture marks which might have been caused by a hypodermic needle, and the possibility of the presence of wounds which have been produced in the process of embalming should not be overlooked. When evidence of burning or corrosion is present, full particulars of the incidence, character, extent, and degree should be recorded. The condition of the natural orifices of the body should be ascertained. The possibility of fractures being present should be verified or eliminated.

The foregoing is merely illustrative of some of the points which must receive attention, but the circumstances of each case should suggest the important lines of investigation, and these will receive detailed description, at a later stage, in the consideration of the various medico-legal forms of death.

Internal examination. When the external examination has been completed, the examiners proceed to the internal examination which must include an examination of all the organs and parts of the body, despite the fact that the apparent cause of death has been previously found in one of them, since evidence contributory to the cause of death may be found in one or more of the others. The importance of this cannot be too strongly insisted upon, as inadvertent omission of a complete examination may readily invalidate a report.

A doctor was asked to examine the body of a man for whose death two men were in custody on a charge of murder. He stated that he found certain marks about the head and upper part of the body, but he attributed death to 'failure of the heart's action, due to shock'. Owing to the unsatisfactory character of the evidence, a re-examination of the body was made, and the doctor had to admit that in the first examination he had overlooked a dislocation of the first and second cervical vertebrae with fracture of the odontoid process and rupture of the lateral ligaments. This case indicates very emphatically that every post-mortem examination for medico-legal purposes must be completely and carefully performed.

Notes on post-mortem technique

Having extended the head, a median incision, reaching from a point about one inch below the symphysis menti to the symphysis pubis and avoiding the umbilicus, is made. The abdominal portion of the wound should first be opened and clearance of the tissue from the ribs effected from below upwards. The lower ends of the recti muscles should be severed to allow greater retraction of the abdominal flaps. To open the thorax, the costal cartilages are severed obliquely and the sterno-clavicular joints disarticulated or sawn through. The sternum is removed by separating the underlying tissue from below upwards. The skin and under-tissue on each side of the neck are reflected outwards. A block is placed under the neck, and the knife is passed round the inner margin of the lower jaw. The attachments of the tongue are separated, and the tongue pulled down through the opening. Using gentle downward traction of the tongue and by dissection, the pharynx, epiglottis, larynx, trachea, and upper part of the oesophagus are freed. The great vessels of the neck are next severed at the root of the neck. The trachea and oesophagus are now pulled downwards and the mass of thoracic viscera is raised out of the chest cavity. The aorta is severed together with the oesophagus before these structures pass through the diaphragm. The oesophagus should be severed between a double ligature to prevent escape of stomach contents. The pericardium is next severed at its diaphragmatic attachment and the inferior vena cava divided. The mass of thoracic viscera may now be removed entire for detailed examination. As an alternative method the heart and lungs may be removed separately.

With regard to the abdominal cavity, this should be inspected carefully before the contents are disturbed. When this is completed, the small intestine should be removed from its mesentery from the caecum upwards to the duodenum, where a double ligature should be applied before severance of the intestine. The large bowel is next removed, and a double ligature applied before it is divided at the junction of the sigmoid and rectum. The abdominal organs are then removed individually.

In abortion cases, particularly, the removal of the female pelvic viscera is of importance, and the following method is recommended. Retract the bladder from the pubic arch, and separate the peritoneum and areolar tissue. Carry an incision round the level of the pelvic brim and continue downwards to the pelvic outlet. The legs of the subject are then abducted widely and an incision is commenced under the symphysis pubis and continued downwards and backwards on each side of the labia minora to the posterior border of the vagina. The dissection commenced within the pelvis is continued until a communication with the external incisions is established. The entire genital tract, together with the bladder and rectum, is then removed.

To remove the brain, the first step is to sever the scalp transversely, from ear to ear, and reflect the anterior part of the scalp forwards to the superciliary ridges, and the posterior part backwards to a point just below the occiput. A coronet is then applied, to steady and control the head, and the skullcap is removed by a circular line of severance, using a saw. The line of severance follows a point just above the superciliary ridges in front and through the occiput behind. The skullcap should be completely severed prior to removal and leverage should not be used since such force may fracture the skull or extend an existing fracture. The skullcap removed, the dura mater is cut along the line of skull severance and also along the falx cerebri. When the surface of the brain has been exposed, the fingers of the left hand are inserted between the dura and the frontal poles of the cerebrum and the latter are gently raised. Vessels, nerves, tentorium cerebelli, and spinal cord are severed. The brain, which has been pulled backwards gradually, is now resting on the left hand, and with the use of both hands is transferred to a platter for examination and dissection.

In conducting a post-mortem examination it is advisable to have a basin containing warm water at hand in order to keep gloves and instruments clean.

The foregoing simple points may prove to be of some help, but, for those who are inexperienced in practice, further theoretical guidance from works dealing with post-mortem technique should be obtained.[1] Those who undertake post-mortem examinations should familiarise themselves with the appearances of healthy and diseased organs.

The average weight of adult organs and those of the newborn child, together with some useful post-mortem room data, in connection with weight, measurement, and temperature conversions will be found on pp. 754 and 755.

Examination of stomach. In all cases, attention should be directed to the stomach contents. The odour, especially if alcoholic, should be noted. In accident cases, in death from culpable violence, and in any other case in which an assessment of the degree of possible intoxication may have a bearing, a generous sample of blood should be obtained for the purpose of determining the alcoholic content by analysis (see p. 609). A sample of urine should also be taken for the same purpose. The analyst prefers, when possible, to get at least 60 ml of blood or urine. The stomach contents will give indication of the extent of digestion which has taken place and, in an approximate manner, the interval of time since the ingestion of the last meal prior to death. An ordinary meal leaves the stomach in about four hours. Maile and Scott,[2] following radiological surveys, have shown that a large meal may be retained for five hours and that a meal, not necessarily large, but containing a considerable quantity of butter or cream, is retained in the stomach for a longer period. Concentrated carbohydrates, such as sugar, leave the stomach much more quickly than natural carbohydrates, such as banana or potato. Fat in abnormal proportions causes the stomach emptying time to be prolonged in marked degree.

Some important points. The membranes should always be stripped from the base of the skull, and the bone carefully examined for evidence of fracture.

GMJ—D

The vertebral column should be examined for fracture or dislocation.

Incisions should be made between the ribs when examination for fracture is undertaken, since this procedure enables the examiner to test the mobility of each rib in turn.

Parts of the body, necessary for further detailed dissection, should be removed and placed in containers to which a 5 to 10 per cent solution of formalin in saline has been added.

In every case of fatal wounding the dimensions of the wound or wounds should be recorded, together with the depth and direction of the track.   These particulars may have a bearing, not only in relation to the weapon which caused the wound, but to the relative positions of the assailant and assaulted person when the injury was inflicted.

When blood or other fluid is found within a cavity, the quantity should be measured and recorded.

The eyes should be examined for evidence indicative of impaired vision, for example, an artificial eye or corneal opacity.   This is of great importance sometimes, especially in cases of vehicular accident.

The finger-nails should be inspected for evidence of blood-staining and for small portions of epidermis, indicative of struggle.

In cases of suspected strangulation, manual or otherwise, the structures of the mouth and neck should be removed for detailed dissection and histological examination.

The coronary arteries should always be examined carefully.

The entire length of the aorta should be opened and examined for evidence of degenerative changes.

In cases of head injury following vehicular accident, specimens of hair, close to the edges of the wounds, should be removed.   Comparative examination of hairs found on the suspect vehicle may be necessary at a later stage in the investigation (see pp. 100 and 104).   In such cases, the wounds and scalp generally should be examined for glass or paint fragments.   When found, these should be retained.

In cases of suspected carbon monoxide poisoning and in burning cases, separate specimens of blood should be taken from the left and right sides of the heart for laboratory examination.

In cases of culpable violence, a specimen of blood should be retained for blood-grouping purposes (see p. 353).

When there is any doubt as to whether an injury was inflicted before or after death, tissue should be removed for histological examination. This is of special importance in connection with bruises (see pp. 246 and 257 and Fig. 112).

In fatal cases associated with rape, a specimen of pubic hair and vaginal swabs should be taken (see pp. 438 and 436).

In cases of burning, a specimen of mucus from the air passages should be examined microscopically for the presence of carbon particles.

In cases of drowning, when the stomach contents indicate the swallowing of unusual fluids, a specimen should be retained for examination.

In cases of firearm wounding a surface scraping should be removed from any area of blackening surrounding the wound of entry, together with a specimen of hair, adjacent to the wound, on any hair-bearing surface. Microscopical examination of the particles and of the hairs may prove important with regard to the assessment of the range of fire. Bullets retained in the body must be located (see pp. 210 and 293).

The notes made during the currency of a post-mortem examination should be scrutinised carefully before the body is closed.

Effects of keeping bodies in refrigerating chamber

Under these circumstances, if the body has been exposed to a low temperature soon after death, the onset of rigor mortis will be retarded. If exposed at a later stage, when rigor is passing off, putrefaction will be retarded. Bodies which have been kept in a cold chamber most frequently show reddish, patchy colorations on the body surface, especially in the hypostatic regions and sometimes in the organs, the blood is of a brighter reddish colour, and surface injuries, such as bruises and abrasions, have an intensified appearance. We have frequently noted these manifestations, and consider that a necessary allowance should be made in their interpretation. Prior to autopsy, bodies which have been chilled should be removed from the cold chamber and placed on the table for about two hours. This will allow the tissues to become softer and easier to manipulate.

Effects of embalming

Embalming of a body is effected by the injection of a preserving fluid, containing formaldehyde and methyl alcohol, into one of the large arteries either by gravity or by positive pressure. It is necessary to drain a considerable quantity of the blood from a vein so that there will be a replacement by the embalming fluid. Openings into both the chest and abdominal cavities are also made and a quantity of the solution is injected into them. The object of embalming is to preserve the body by the destruction of micro-organisms. It is important to note that both post-mortem dissections and the removal of specimens from bodies for investigation should be completed prior to embalming, since the tissues of the body will be hardened and the detection of certain poisons made difficult, if not impossible, by the process.

Procedure in suspected poisoning

In cases where poisoning is the suspected cause of death, special precautions are adopted. Careful attention should be paid to the condition of the mouth, the oesophagus, and the gastro-intestinal tract. The lower end of the oesophagus, about three inches above the cardiac orifice of the stomach, should be tied with a double ligature, and severed between the ligatures.   A double ligature should be placed round the upper part of the duodenum, and the stomach, with contents, removed. Next, the whole of the large and the small intestines are removed by division between double ligatures.   The various parts should be placed in separate glass jars, labelled, signed, and sealed.   In further jars are placed the liver, kidneys, spleen, and specimens of blood and urine, in addition to other organs and tissues as the circumstances of the specific case dictate (see p. 541).   When these containers are formally handed over to the analyst, a receipt should be obtained.   Should the stomach and intestines be opened and examined in the post-mortem room, care must be taken to keep the various parts separate and free from contamination not only from each other but from the other organs.   It is only by such procedure that an opinion, as to the possible interval of time which has elapsed between the ingestion of the poison and death, can be expressed after the results of chemical analysis have been considered.   This is of particular importance in cases of metallic irritant poisoning, such as arsenical poisoning.   The necessity for taking all the important parts of a body in a case of poisoning will be obvious when it is explained that after analysis by the Crown experts, the remainder may be requested by the accused for examination by experts nominated by him for his defence.   In cases of suspected arsenical poisoning, specimens of hair, skin, bone, and nails should also be removed for analysis (see p. 542).

Exhumations

It is sometimes necessary in cases of suspected crime, in cases of civil actions for damages, in certain instances of life insurance, where the cause of death is disputed, and in other contingencies, to disinter bodies for the purpose of determining the actual cause of death.   In any case of comparatively recent interment it is an unsavoury operation, and one not unattended by danger.

In England, at common law, a Coroner may order a body to be disinterred for the purposes of inquisition.   If exhumation is required for other purposes, the licence of the Home Secretary must be obtained under section 25, Burial Act, 1857.

In Scotland, a Sheriff, after petition, may grant a warrant.   In a civil case, a petition is presented to the Sheriff, or to the Court of Session, usually to the former, by the party desiring the exhumation.   Thereafter, the relatives are informed that such a petition has been made, and a date is arranged for hearing any objections.   After the hearing, the petition may or may not be granted, but it it is granted, the name of the practitioner, or practitioners, is put on the warrant for exhumation, and authority given to the graveyard authorities to have the body exhumed.

The necessary preparations having been made with the authorities of the graveyard, the body is disinterred, and the examination made. The coffin should be identified by the undertaker, and the grave-digger should identify the grave.

Certain precautions should be adopted in exhumations. For example, the examination should be made during the lightest period of the day and, when possible, the dissection conducted in the open. It may be necessary to have a temporary screen erected. When the examination is made inside a building, the accommodation used should permit of free ventilation. When the coffin has been raised to the surface, adequate time should be given for the drainage of fluid from the interior of the coffin, and after the body has been removed from the coffin, it should be exposed to the air for a short period to permit the dissipation of foul gases. Care should be taken to ensure that the gloves worn are in perfect condition.

The dissection is made in the same manner as that of the routine post-mortem examination.

In cases of suspected arsenical poisoning it is important to preserve a portion of the earth from above the coffin, against a possible defence that the poison, which may be found in the body, was imparted to it by the soil. A piece of the shroud enveloping the body, together with a portion of the wood from the coffin, should also be retained in such cases for the purpose of eliminating the presence of arsenic (see p. 543).

Important and decisive information respecting the cause of death, may be obtained from an examination of a body following exhumation.

Report on a post-mortem examination

From the result of a post-mortem examination the report of the examiners is framed.

The opinion expressed by the examiners in their report must be founded solely on the facts comprehended within the report, and not upon facts which are not specified in detail in the description of the organs as found.

The examiners should send to the Procurator-Fiscal, within two days after the examination, their report of the examination, embodying their opinion of the cause of death, and the reasons for that opinion, which should be stated clearly. Along with the report the warrant, still in their possession, should be returned to the Procurator-Fiscal. If further investigation is necessary, the report, by arrangement, may be delayed until the investigation is completed.

The examiners should frame the terms of the report in simple but clear terms, remembering that it may in all probability be read in court for the information of the court, counsel, and jury.   The report should be as brief as possible, compatible with clearness.   It is not necessary to describe each organ in detail, and it is sufficient to say, where the organs of a cavity have been found healthy, that 'all the organs of this cavity were examined, and found healthy'.   Should one or more organs only be found diseased or injured, after description of the facts found with respect to these, it is more advisable to say that 'the other organs of this cavity were examined and found healthy', than to describe their normal appearances.   While in certain circumstances it may be impossible to avoid the use of technical terms, the examiners should try to give them popular interpretation, within brackets.   Conciseness, brevity, and clear language are of high value in the expression of the opinion, since without these attributes the issues may readily become confused, and the report occasion dubiety, and unnecessarily prolonged cross-examination.

Examiners should avoid the use of such terms as 'about', or 'nearly', when measurement is in question, or of comparative or superlative adjectives with respect, for example, to amounts of fluid or blood, when such can be determined.   The report should be exact in its terms.   The original notes made at the examination should be retained, together with a copy of the report sent to the Procurator-Fiscal, for future reference in the preparation of evidence.

Framing a report is often a matter of some difficulty for the less experienced, and for this reason the following skeleton basis for a report is given:

FORM OF MEDICAL REPORT

Preamble

Date and place from which report is written.

Warrant for the examination, by whom granted, together with place of examination.

Names, ages, designations, and addresses of witnesses who have, in the presence of the examiners, identified the body.

External examination

External appearances of body indicative of time of death.

Presence or absence of external marks of violence.   Their site, character, dimensions, and relation to each other, and of any other markings bearing upon the cause of death.

Internal examination

Description of—

Brain, its membranes, condition of calvarium, and of base of skull.

Spinal column, and, if necessary, condition of spinal cord and membranes.

Description of organs and contents of thoracic cavity—
General disposition of organs.
Presence of fluid in pleural cavities.
Condition of pericardium, heart, and large blood-vessels.
Condition of larynx, trachea, oesophagus, lungs, ribs, etc.

Description of organs and contents of abdominal cavity—
General disposition of organs.
Presence of abnormal fluid in abdominal cavity.
Condition of stomach, intestines, liver, spleen, kidneys, urinary bladder, pancreas, aorta, etc.

Description of organs and contents of female pelvis—
Vaginal tract.
Uterus and appendages.

The reasoned opinion of the cause of death based upon the facts found.
In Scotland, attestation of the report 'on soul and conscience'.
Signatures and medical qualifications of examiners.

NOTE. In reports, all numbers, except the date of report, should be expressed in words, and not in figures.
All interpolated words, or deleted words, should be initialled by the signatories. At the foot of each page, the number of words deleted should be indicated and initialled by the signatories.
When the report occupies more than one page, the signatures of the examiners should be appended to each page.

The following report embodies greater detail and applies many of the points suggested:

Place.
Date.

By virtue of a warrant of the Sheriff of   , and at the instance of   , Esquire, Procurator-Fiscal of the said County, we, the undersigned, on this date and within the mortuary of (*here name institution or police station*) made a post-mortem examination of the body of (*insert full name, if known*), which was identified in our presence by the following persons:

1. A. B., 22 years, son of the deceased, residing at 24 Blank Street, Glasgow, and
2. B. C., 58 years, confectioner, cousin of the deceased, residing at 261 Blank Street, Glasgow.

External examination

The body was that of a well-nourished and well-developed person. Death-stiffening, or rigor mortis, was present generally. The only mark of violence visible on the body surface was an incised, or clean-cut, wound situated one and a half inches below the level of the left collar-bone, and two and a quarter inches from the middle line of the breast-bone. There was faint bruising at the edges of the wound. It measured three-quarters of an inch in length and a quarter of an inch in breadth. It was oval in shape.

Internal examination

Head. The brain and its coverings were found normal. The skull was intact.

Chest. On opening the chest cavity, a considerable quantity of clotted blood was found lying in the tissues below the breast-bone, and extending into the left side of the chest. Within the pericardium, or heart-bag, fluid and clotted blood, amounting to 300 ml, was found. There were, in addition, 200 ml of blood in the left side of the chest. Before the organs of the chest were removed, careful inspection of the direction of the wound on the front of the chest was made. This inspection showed that the wound had a direction downwards, from left to right, and that it had penetrated the chest wall, between the first and second ribs. Dissection showed that the wound continued through the heart-bag, and into the main artery of the body, the aorta, which leads from the left chamber of the heart. The wound penetrated this vessel at a point one and a quarter inches above the point where the vessel leaves the heart. The wound in the wall of the heart-bag measured three-eighths of an inch in length, and in the blood-vessel, a quarter of an inch. These two wounds lay, with relation to one another, in a slightly oblique line, the latter just below the level of the former. The structure of the heart was normal. The lungs were healthy.

Abdominal cavity. The organs of this cavity were examined individually, and, with the exception of the liver, which was somewhat fatty, were found healthy.

Opinion. From the foregoing examination we are of opinion: (1) that the cause of death was wounding of the aorta, or principal artery of the body; (2) that the wound, which penetrated the chest and injured the pericardium and aorta, was produced by a sharp-pointed, sharp-edged instrument of at least some inches in length; and (3) that the injury must have been inflicted with some measure of force.

These are attested on soul and conscience.

(Signed)

(Qualifications)

Human Tissue Act, 1961

This Act makes provision for the use of parts of bodies of deceased persons for therapeutic purposes and purposes of medical education and research.   Section 1 permits the person lawfully in possession of the body to authorise removal of any part of the body for therapeutic, educational, or research purposes if the deceased during his last illness has made such a request either orally or in writing in the presence of two or more witnesses.

This section also permits the person lawfully in possession of the body to authorise removal of parts of the body for these purposes if after making reasonable inquiry he has no reason to believe that the deceased had expressed an objection to his body being used in this way or that the surviving spouse or surviving relative objects.

Progress in the field of transplantation surgery has been baulked by the provisions of this Act, but social and ethical repugnance at the thought of interchanging body parts must be remembered.   Bills have been introduced into Parliament to promote, for example, kidney transplantation but have yet to become law.   A clear account of the position is to be found in the Report of Law Reform Committee on the Law relating to Organ Transplantation (London, General Council of the Bar, 1971), which is discussed by the legal correspondent of the *British Medical Journal* (*British Medical Journal*, **3**, 716, 1971).

Procedure for bequeathing a body for anatomical examination

A person wishing to leave his body to a medical school, writes either to H.M. Inspector of Anatomy, Ministry of Health, Whitehall, S.W.1, or to the Licensed Teacher of Anatomy at the medical school which he wishes to benefit, stating his desire; upon which the necessary forms will be sent to him.

He should then leave clear instructions in writing and inform his executors of his wishes.   If no particular institution is named, the Inspector of Anatomy will send the body to the next Metropolitan School due to receive one.

When death occurs, the executor completes the form already received and posts it along with the medical certificate of the cause of death to the Inspector, who will then issue a warrant to an undertaker to remove the body and place it in the charge of some particular Licensed Teacher of Anatomy.

During the examination of the body care is taken that every particle removed from it is placed in the coffin in which it will ultimately be buried.

The burial is conducted by a clergyman of the faith which the deceased professed during life. The undertaker must present the burial certificate to the Inspector of Anatomy.

It must be understood that no individual has a right of property in his body after his death and if any near relative objects to the body being used for anatomical dissection, H.M. Inspector of Anatomy will refuse to issue a warrant for its removal to a medical school.

Reports on nature of stains

Reports regarding the nature of stains upon clothing and upon many other articles may be required. No warrant is necessary for this examination. In Scotland, the examination is made at the request of the Procurator-Fiscal, who sends a police officer, with the articles to be examined, to the laboratory of the examiner. This officer receives from the examiner a receipt for the articles, and, in turn, a receipt is required from him when the productions are returned on completion of the examination. This is for the purpose of maintaining their identity and the sequence of events so that the chain of evidence given subsequently in court may be complete.

Work of this character should be undertaken only by experts. The report on the examination embodies such particulars as the nature of the instructions received and from whom, the date the articles were received and from whom, together with a detailed description of the articles examined and the wording on the labels attached. Further details in relation to the presence or absence of stains, their number and situation, relative to their position on the article and to one another, their shape, colour, and other physical characteristics must be included. With regard to the technique employed in the examination of the stained material, it is not necessary to enter into detail in the report. It is sufficient to state that after an examination by chemical analysis or microscopic or spectroscopic examination, certain substances were or were not found. Then follow the opinions, the attestation 'on soul and conscience', if in Scotland, and signature. The evidence of what has been found should be preserved by the examiner for subsequent production in court, should this be requested.

The following is a more or less general example of such a report:

Place.
Date.

Acting upon instructions received from A. B., Esquire, Procurator-Fiscal, County Buildings, Glasgow, I, the undersigned, on 24th June 1961, received from C. D., Detective-Inspector, Southern Division, City of Glasgow Police, the undernoted article for examination and report thereon: A blue cloth jacket, labelled 'Found in the possession of E. F., 216 Blank Street, Gl anasgow,d referred to in the case against E. F.'

Examination. The following reddish-coloured stains were present upon the garment:

1. On left lapel of jacket (outer surface)—
   (a) A circular, red-coloured stain, close to the junction of the neck seam and lapel, which measured a quarter of an inch in diameter.
   (b) A similar stain, one and a half inches below (a), which measured half an inch in diameter.
   (c) A triangular-shaped, smeared stain, situated close to (b), which measured one inch and a half by half an inch; and
   (d) Adjacent to (c), a group of seven small and indefinite stains.
2. On left side of jacket (inner surface)—
   (e) A stain, half an inch in length, shaped like an 'exclamation mark', situated three inches above the level of the top button-hole, and at the same distance from the free edge of jacket.
   (f) A stain, which measured a quarter of an inch in length, of similar shape to (e), situated one inch above the level of the top button-hole, and two and a quarter inches from the free edge of jacket.
   (g) A circular stain, situated one inch from (f), which measured half an inch in diameter; and
   (h) An irregularly-shaped stain, situated five inches below (f) and in direct line, which measured one inch at its point of greatest breadth.

Portions from the stains lettered (a), (c), (f), and (h) were excised, and after suitable preparation, were examined chemically, microscopically, and microspectroscopically. They were also examined serologically.

Opinion. As the result of the foregoing examination I am of the opinion that—

1. Stains lettered (a), (c), (f), and (h) are composed of human blood;
2. The 'exclamation mark' stains resulted from forcible projection of the blood against the garment.

These are attested on soul and conscience.

(Signed)
(Qualifications)

Photographs are automatic records of appearance and may be used in evidence to assist oral description of the objects photographed. Medical reports used for legal purposes in Scotland must be certified 'on soul and conscience' and must be sworn to in court as true reports by the author of them. They must exclude facts elicited by the writer on hearsay.

Notes or memoranda

Notes or memoranda may be used in a court of law by a medical witness but, if used, they may be scrutinised by cross-examining counsel for the purpose of cross-examination, since they are then treated as productions, or exhibits, in the case. It is necessary, therefore, to know under what circumstances reference to them is permissible. Such notes may be used by a witness for the purpose of refreshing his memory if:

The notes were made at the time of, or shortly after, the occurrence of the event to which they refer, and were made by the witness, or by another and reviewed at the time by the witness.

On the other hand, they may not be used if:

They were made only after a lapse of time following the event to which they refer, they were made by another and not supervised by the witness at the time, or they are used for the purpose of bringing forward facts which the witness has forgotten.

It must be clearly understood that the use of notes or memoranda is restricted solely to the purpose of refreshing the memory of a witness with regard to some point which may arise in the course of his evidence. Having refreshed his memory on the point in question by reference to the notes, he must then be able to testify from his own recollection.

Casualty surgeons should if possible take accurate notes of the condition of a patient on first being seen by him. This will make the subsequent giving of evidence very much easier for him. Subsequent treatment may considerably alter the picture and it may be impossible to recall the condition of the patient if notes have not been made. Unfortunately this is also the most difficult time to take accurate records as they are nearly always being made under pressure.

Dying declarations and dying depositions

Since it may become the duty of a medical practitioner to record statements made by dying persons, which may be of great importance in the attainment of justice, it is necessary for him to know his duty in this connection. It is important to realise that a dying declaration is inadmissible if on its face it is incomplete.[3]

England. The principle on which evidence of this description is admitted is 'that such declarations are made in extremity when the party is at the point of death, and when every hope of this world is gone; when every motive of falsehood is silenced, and the mind is induced by the most powerful considerations to speak the truth; a situation so solemn and so awful is considered by the law as creating an obligation equal to that which is imposed by a positive oath administered in a court of justice'.[4]

In the ordinary course of events these statements are taken in the form of a dying deposition. The procedure is conducted by a Justice of the Peace and the deposition is taken on oath in answer to his questions. The statement is reduced to writing, read over to the deponent, and signed by him, if he is able, and by the examiner. If the deponent cannot write, that fact and its cause should be recorded. The writing itself must be produced at the trial, and be sworn to by two witnesses, of whom one should be the examiner, as correct and as made voluntarily when the deponent was in his sound mind.

If a witness is dying and there is no time to arrange for administration of the oath and a formal deposition being taken, his evidence may be written down as a declaration by any credible person.

The conditions necessary for the acceptance of dying declarations and dying depositions as valid evidence are:

1. The case must be a criminal one.
2. The case must be one of homicide.
3. The death of the deceased must be the subject of the charge, and the circumstances of the death the subject of the declaration or deposition.
4. The words used must be those of the deceased and if questions have been put these must be given together with the answers.
5. The person making the statement must be actually dying, must believe that he is dying, and must express no hope of recovery. It is not necessary that he should have stated his expectation of immediate death, if this can be inferred from other circumstances.
6. The person who made the statement must be dead.

The use of depositions as evidence is also controlled by statute. The Criminal Law Amendment Act, 1867, makes provision, in the case of indictable offences, for the taking of depositions out of court where information is likely to be lost owing to the probable death or continuing illness of a witness. If the deponent dies, or is unlikely ever to be able to give evidence in court, then the deposition is acceptable as evidence.

Scotland. The law of Scotland gives a wider validity to dying declarations and depositions than the law of England.

It holds that a dying deposition or a dying declaration of a person who subsequently dies is admissible as evidence whether that person were the party injured or not, if in life he would have been a competent witness.

The circumstances necessary for this type of evidence to be valid in Scotland therefore are:

1. The declarant or deponent must be a competent witness in a criminal trial.
2. He must be a material witness.
3. His life must be in danger.
4. His mind must be sufficiently clear to give reliable evidence.

It should be noted that there does not appear to be any legal obligation on a medical attendant to record the declaration of a dying man, but as he is often the only person present who is capable of undertaking the duty, he should in the interests of justice do so in an emergency. Where there is time, it is his duty to ensure that notice is given to the legal authorities so that in Scotland a Sheriff, or in England, a Justice of the Peace, may attend and take the statement in the form of a dying deposition.

ORAL EVIDENCE

Oath and affirmation

Whatever form medical evidence may assume, it must ultimately take the form of oral evidence, which can only be valid in court when given upon oath or affirmation.   In Scotland, the oath is administered to the witness by the judge, who, standing in his place and speaking the words of the oath, requests the witness to repeat the words after him.   This is done clause by clause.   The words of the oath in Scotland are as follows: 'I swear by Almighty God, as I shall answer to God at the great Day of Judgment, that I will tell the truth, the whole truth, and nothing but the truth.'

In Scotland the Criminal Procedure (Scotland) Act, 1965, made provision for the taking of minutes of admission when facts are agreed by both parties to a case.   The agreed evidence is read in court and this removes the necessity for the witness to appear in court and give oral evidence.   This is a valuable piece of legislation and its more frequent use would save the time of the courts and also that of medical practitioners.

In England section 9 of the Criminal Justice Act, 1967, enabled a similar procedure to be used.   The English courts make frequent use of this provision.

Certain judges omit the words 'as I shall answer to God at the great Day of Judgment'. The words are repeated by the witness while holding up his right hand.

In England, the witness is sworn by an officer of the court, by repeating the following words: 'I swear by Almighty God that the evidence I shall give to the court touching the matters in question shall be the truth, the whole truth, and nothing but the truth.'

In the Coroner's Court the oath taken is: 'I swear by Almighty God, that the evidence I shall give to this inquest on behalf of our Sovereign Lady the Queen, touching the death of . . . shall be the truth, the whole truth, and nothing but the truth.'

In regard to affirmation, by virtue of the Oaths Act, 1888, every person upon objecting to being sworn, and stating as the reason either that he has no religious belief, or that the taking of an oath is contrary to his religious belief, shall be permitted to make his solemn affirmation instead of taking an oath in all places, and for all purposes where an oath is or shall be required by law. This affirmation has the same legal force and effect as the oath. The form of an affirmation is as follows: 'I, A. B., do solemnly, sincerely, and truly declare and affirm', and then follow the words of the oath prescribed by law, omitting any word of imprecation.

Medical evidence

In giving evidence there are certain principles which should never be forgotten by the medical witness. The language used in the witness-box should be clear, concise, and as untechnical as possible. Such terms as 'syncope', 'comatose', 'highly vascular', 'oedematous', and others should not be used. It is unreasonable to expect a jury to know what is meant by the terms 'pericardium', 'meninges', and 'calvarium', but the substitution of 'heart-bag', 'brain-coverings', and 'skullcap', or 'vault of skull', will make matters clear.

The language should be concise. Adjectives of degree, especially superlatives, should be used sparingly, and only when absolutely necessary, since their use may be regarded as biased opinion, and this discounts the value of the evidence. The voluble witness is often a godsend to opposing counsel with a weak case, since the witness saying more than is required is apt to say more than he means, and in doing so increases his vulnerability while under cross-examination. Categorical answers, when possible, are the best, and when not possible, answers should be concise and clear.

The replies of a witness should invariably be courteous. This is not difficult during examination-in-chief, since both witnesses and examiner are in accord, but it frequently becomes less easy during cross-examination, when the object of the cross-examiner is to weaken or, if possible, negative the evidence given in the previous examination. However trying the situation may be, the witness should keep the fact clearly before him that he is giving expression to honest opinion, and that he has but consistently to hold by what he has formerly said, and to give fully the reasons for his belief, to convince the court of his sincerity. It is usually with reference to opinions or inferences that differences between counsel and witness arise.

It may be of assistance to the witness under cross-examination to bear in mind that it is the business of the cross-examiner to make the best case he can for his client. Calm but persistent restatement of former evidence will sooner or later break down even the most pressing cross-examiner, and a witness may rely upon the judge interfering when he considers that counsel is overstepping the bounds of legitimate cross-examination. In short, if the witness can preserve himself free of the assumption that cross-examining counsel is his natural enemy, and if he does not, therefore, assume the mental attitude appropriate to that view, he will leave the witness-box, if otherwise he has been well pre-pared, with credit. There are occasions, however, upon which it is absolutely necessary for a medical witness to maintain a very firm attitude, and to decline strongly to have words attributed to him which have not been stated. Occasionally cross-examining counsel may ask a question, which is based upon a statement which he desires the witness to understand he has already made in reply to a previous question, the answer to which tends to put an entirely different complexion upon the tenor of his evidence. If the witness is collected he will detect the misstatement and at once challenge it. Should counsel persist in stating that the witness made the statement, the witness should appeal to the judge who, by having reference made to the notes of the shorthand writer, in court, will quickly settle the issue.

Evidence should always be given distinctly, deliberately, and audibly. It has often been said by judges that no witnesses are so difficult to be heard and to be understood as medical witnesses; difficult to be heard from want of clearness in articulation, and difficult to be understood by reason of the nature of the evidence.

The general rule is that ordinary lay witnesses must speak only to matters of fact and not of opinion. A medical witness, however, usually speaks both to matters of fact and of opinion, and therefore is regarded by the court as an expert witness. Under certain circum-stances he may only be called upon to give evidence on matters of opinion and not of fact. A skilled witness should not be asked to give an expression of opinion which is a direct answer to the issue under trial since this is a matter to be decided by the judge or jury as the case may be. As a general rule, subject to certain exceptions, hearsay evidence is not valid evidence, and a witness, therefore, must speak only to facts which come within his own personal knowledge. Any opinion which he expresses from a given series of facts must be his own opinion. The published opinions of writers on the subject may be adopted by skilled witnesses and made a part of their evidence. A skilled witness may be taken as concurring in his evidence with the opinion expressed in full by a preceding skilled witness. An expert may speak to the recognised authority of a particular writer, and may adopt as his own opinions, specified parts of a published work. The passage is then regarded as being supported by the weight of the author as well as of the witness. The published work need not be produced in court, and it does not matter whether the author is living or dead. This is not an unimportant point since, quite frequently, cross-examining counsel will quote certain passages from standard books, with the intention of rebutting evidence given by a witness in his examination-in-chief, and ask the witness whether he agrees or disagrees with opinions of the author. In such a case a witness is well advised never to offer any reply until he has been permitted to read for himself the quotation as given in the book together with the context.

Any statement which a witness has made on precognition, but which he has modified in the witness-box, cannot be challenged on the ground that he made a different statement on a former occasion, although this does not apply to a deposition in England (see pp. 15, 19 and 21).

Members of the medical profession should understand clearly that evidence given by them is absolutely privileged and that no witness can be compelled to answer any question which might have the effect of incriminating him, or which would tend to degrade his character socially or professionally. To this general rule there is an exception. By the Criminal Evidence Act, 1898, a person charged, and tendering evidence on his own behalf, may be asked any question in cross-examination notwithstanding that the answer might incriminate him in relation to the offence charged.

In a trial for rape a medical witness was asked, in cross-examination, if he had been in the way of having connection with the woman said to have been ravished. He hesitated for some time whether to answer or not, when it occurred to him to ask if he must answer the question, and on being assured that he need not do so unless he chose, he said, 'Then I refuse to answer.'

Certain principles should always be remembered by medical witnesses. These are:

Study the case, and be conversant with the facts, and the literature on the subject.
Always have adequate reasons for opinions.
Be fair and unbiased, concede points which should be conceded.
Answer 'I do not know' when you do not know.

Never express an opinion on the merits of the case.   That is the function of the judge or jury as the case may be.

Do not 'sit on the fence'.   A doctor who will not commit himself to his opinion is not worth calling as a witness.

If a medical witness has made a thorough examination, is conversant with his subject, has made an accurate report on his findings, is truthful, unbiased, remains composed, and is fair in all his opinions, his integrity and professional reputation will remain untarnished, even under the most exacting cross-examination.

PROFESSIONAL SECRECY AND PRIVILEGE

From the days of Hippocrates until the present, members of the medical profession have bound themselves not to divulge professional secrets.

The declaration taken by medical graduates of the University of Glasgow is: 'I do solemnly and sincerely declare that, as a Graduate in Medicine of the University of Glasgow, I will exercise the several parts of my profession, to the best of my knowledge and abilities, for the good, safety, and welfare of all persons committing themselves, or committed to my care and directions; and that I will not knowingly or intentionally do anything or administer anything to them to their hurt or prejudice for any consideration or from any motive whatever.   And I further declare that I will keep silence as to anything I have seen or heard while visiting the sick which it would be improper to divulge. And I make this solemn declaration in virtue of the Provisions of the Promissory Oaths Act, 1868, substituting a Declaration for Oaths in certain cases.'

Lord Riddell[5] sums up the legal position of doctors, in relation to professional secrecy.

'A doctor being in a fiduciary capacity must preserve his patient's confidences unless relieved from the obligation by some lawful excuse, for example, legal compulsion, the patient's consent, the performance of a moral or social duty, or protection of the doctor's interests.   A doctor shares with other citizens the duty to assist in the detection and arrest of a person who has committed a serious crime.   Everyone recognises the necessity and importance of medical confidences.   Everyone recognises that they are sacred and precious.   But we must recognise also that the rules regarding them exist for the welfare of the community, and not for the aggrandisement or convenience of a particular class. We must recognise also that they must be modified to meet the inevitable changes that occur in the necessities of various generations.'

Legal decisions have shown that secrecy is an essential condition of the contract between a medical man and his employers, and breach of secrecy affords a relevant ground for an action of damages. This, therefore, may be taken as a general expression of the law.

There are certain circumstances in which the doctor is protected from any legal action which might be taken against him for disclosure of information.

1. In a Court of Law

It seems clear that a medical witness, in court, cannot claim any privilege and that he must disclose, when a judge so rules, any secret information which he may have obtained in the course of his professional relationship to a party involved in any case. Medical practitioners must therefore reckon upon their liability to be called upon to make such disclosures when necessary. At the same time, a medical witness should always be reluctant, in a court of law, to disclose such secrets, and he should ask for a ruling of the court before he makes such a disclosure. Under certain circumstances, permission may be given the witness to write his answers to certain questions, thus obviating divulgence in public. Such action will, at least, convince the public that the medical profession guards that which has been committed to its members as confidential, and that it is most reluctant to divulge unless compelled by law to do so.

The general question of professional secrecy in relation to medical witnesses was fully commented on by the judge in the case of Kitson v. Playfair. He stated that the medical profession had no right to legislate on the matter. They might make their own rules, for their guidance as professional men, but they could not impose upon the public their self-made laws. Although the judge was the person who had to rule whether or not a witness was to answer a question, he would exercise discretion in ordering a witness to answer or not. There might be some matters which the judge thought most unreasonable to be divulged by a professional man, and he might refuse to permit it, and allow the witness to say, 'I refuse to answer.' Each case had been considered by its own particular circumstances and by the ruling of the judge who happened to preside on the occasion. The judge would decide according to law. There was always a rule to set a judge right if he went wrong.

The observations of Mr Justice Horridge, in the Divorce Court in 1921, regarding the reluctance of a medical witness to give evidence with regard to venereal disease on the ground that he, with other medical men, had undertaken these duties at a clinic on the distinct understanding that professional secrecy would be observed, reaffirmed the claim of courts of law to compel the disclosure of professional confidences. In the same year, also in the Divorce Court, a similar point was raised before Lord Mersey, who said that there was no statement in the Acts relating to venereal diseases to the effect that the information was confidential, and that he did not consider the production of a card would be against public policy.

2. Where the interests of the community conflict with those of the patient

In criminal offences disclosure is justified in cases of murder and serious crimes, especially where there is an element of prevention as well as detection.

The opinion expressed by Lord Justice-Clerk Inglis, regarding the conduct of Dr Paterson, one of the medical witnesses in the Pritchard poisoning case, is important to practitioners. Dr Paterson, a witness for the Crown, stated in the witness-box that when called to see Mrs Pritchard for the first time, he had formed the opinion that she was under the influence of antimony. His lordship said that Dr Paterson was under the decided impression, when he saw Mrs Pritchard on these occasions, that somebody was practising upon her with poison. He thought it consistent with his professional duty, and his duty as a citizen of this country, to keep that opinion to himself. His lordship could not say that Dr Paterson had done right, and he would be sorry to lead the jury to think so. He cared not for professional etiquette or professional rule. There was a rule of life and a consideration that was far higher than these, the duty of every citizen of this country which was owed by every right-minded man to his neighbour, to prevent the destruction of human life in this world. In that duty he could only say that Dr Paterson had failed.

The judge in Kitson v. Playfair also stated that there was a general rule existing in the medical profession, that when they saw, in the course of their medical attendance, that a crime had been committed, or was about to be committed, they were in all cases to go off to the Public Prosecutor, he was bound to say that it was not a rule which met with his approbation, and he hoped it would not meet with the approbation of anybody else (see p. 388). There might be cases when it was the obvious duty of a medical man to speak out, for instance, in cases of murder. A man might come with a wound which it might be supposed had been inflicted in the course of a deadly scuffle. It would be a monstrous thing if the medical man screened him, and tried to hide the wound which might be the means of connecting the man with a serious crime. That was a different thing altogether. Communications between a doctor and his wife, or children, were said to be privileged when it was necessary to reveal them in order that the wife or children might be protected. He thought that that required a great deal of limitation, because cases might be imagined where the wife might be living under circumstances in which she did not want any such protection at all, and giving to her a secret belonging to a patient would be only a wanton violation of the rule.   This was a very delicate question.

It is generally agreed that a doctor may divulge professional secrets for the purpose of protecting himself or his family.

Privileged statements

Since this subject is important to members of the medical profession, and is intimately associated with that of professional secrecy, it should next receive consideration.   A privileged communication can be defined, in a general manner, as a communication made bona fide upon any subject-matter in which the party communicating has an interest, or in reference to which he has a duty, if made to a person having a corresponding interest or duty, although it contain incriminatory matter which, without the privilege, would be slanderous or actionable.

When privilege is claimed, the facts alone must determine the issue.

It would appear that a doctor must not disclose to an insurance company information as to the cause of death of a deceased person without the consent of the nearest surviving relative.   A request for such information may be made by a company which has accepted an insurance without examination.   It is open to the company to refer the matter to the Industrial Insurance Commissioner, and then the family practitioner will be requested to make an affidavit for the consideration of the court over which the Commissioner presides.   This avoids attendance at this court and the statement, so made, is protected by privilege since the proceedings are quasi-judicial.

Another important case, involving the subject of privilege, was that against the late Sir Patrick Heron Watson for damages for alleged slander.

The question at issue was: Does the privilege which protects a witness from an action of slander in respect of his pertinent evidence in the witness-box also protect him against the consequences of statements made to a solicitor and counsel in preparing the proof for trial?

This case decided that the preliminary examination of a witness by a solicitor was within the same privilege as that which he would have if he had said the same thing in his sworn testimony in court.

From what has been said with regard to professional secrecy and privileged statements, the importance of medical practitioners being members of a Medical Defence Society, which will represent them when legal difficulties arise in the course of their professional relationships, becomes clearly established.

Presence of medical witnesses in court

In England.   It is usual for medical witnesses to be present in court, and they may hear the evidence of one another.

In Scotland. Except by arrangement, medical witnesses are not allowed to be present in court when medical evidence is being given by others, unless the witnesses have already given their evidence when, thereafter, they may remain in court. Expert witnesses who are to speak to matters of opinion may by agreement of counsel remain in court while witnesses are deponing to matters of fact, but they are not permitted to remain while expert witnesses are giving evidence on matters of opinion.

Unless special permission is granted, medical witnesses for the defence are not allowed to remain in court when medical witnesses for the Crown are giving evidence.

Attitude of medical examiner towards examination of assaulted, accused, and other persons. Permission for the examination must be obtained from the person who is to be examined. With regard to persons under the age of sixteen, permission must be obtained from a parent or guardian, since those under that age are not sufficiently adult to give permission. In exceptional instances, however, for example, a young person under sixteen who has no parent, relative, or guardian, the permission of such young person would be regarded as acceptable. In all cases the permission for examination must be freely given, since there is no power which can compel a person to submit his or her body for examination against consent. An assaulted person, by laying a charge, is presumed to be willing to afford all evidence, even to examination of the body; nevertheless, consent must be obtained. It is advisable, when the examination is to be uncorroborated, to have a suitable person in attendance when consent to the examination is given, and while the examination is proceeding. The object of the examination should first be explained, and the examinee informed that the findings will be embodied in a medical report.

When accused persons have to be examined, the question of obtaining necessary consent is a matter of extreme importance, since the possible consequences might be the discovery of facts which would be used against the accused person at the trial. It is not sufficient that the person to be examined offers no resistance or objection, for that may result solely from ignorance of his or her rights. The proper procedure is to inform the accused, in the presence of a third party, that the examiner has been asked by the authorities to make an examination, but that he can only do so after obtaining consent, which can be withheld, and that he will report the results of the examination whatever they may be. Should consent be refused, the duty of the examiner is to report this fact.

Should consent be given, the examination of either an assaulted or accused person will be directed along the lines of the specific investigation necessary in the circumstances of the individual case.   Few, if any, questions should be asked, and thoughts should not be expressed aloud. All relevant findings should be carefully noted and subsequently embodied in the report.   Judgment should not be biased by any state-ments made, and opinions should be based solely upon the results of the examination.   Statements made by an accused person should not be embodied in the report.

There has been a change in recent years in the attitude of the legal authorities to the examination of suspected persons.   It may be that such an examination can now be made even without their consent.   In the case of H.M. Advocate v. Hay[6] evidence concerning marks on the victim's breast which were considered to be bite marks was an important part of the evidence.   Dental impressions were taken from twenty-nine persons including Hay, by consent, on two occasions.   Hay then became a definite suspect.   The Crown authorities desired to take more careful impressions and measurements in order to strengthen their case.   They were afraid that Hay might refuse or take action to alter his dental picture.   The Procurator-Fiscal applied to the Sheriff for a warrant to take the third impression.   This was granted by the Sheriff and the impressions were taken.   The competency of this evidence was chal-lenged at the trial.   This separate point was considered by three judges and they decided that the procedure had been fair and regular.   The Court of Criminal Appeal later upheld this judgment and stated that even if the evidence had been obtained unlawfully it should have been admitted.

It would appear, therefore, that there is a tendency at the present time to reduce the emphasis on the rights of the individual and emphasise rather the interests of the State in securing a conviction.   How far this tendency will go it is at present impossible to say.   It is interesting to speculate on what would have happened if Hay had been more mature and had refused to provide the third dental impression.

The legal consequences of want of knowledge of, or inattention to, the necessity of obtaining consent may be serious.   In a case tried at Manchester, where a woman was accused of abandoning her infant a few hours after its birth, the judge said in his summing-up of the case 'that no medical man may suppose himself armed with authority to proceed contrary to the express will of the person he is instructed to examine'.   In another case, a doctor, acting on the verbal request of the Coroner and an inspector of police, proceeded to examine a female to ascertain whether or not she had recently been delivered of a child. The woman refused to be examined and offered to send for a medical man whom she knew to make the examination, but the doctor proceeded to examine her.   The jury returned a verdict for the plaintiff, and assessed damages at £200.

Admission to hospital does not necessarily imply consent on the part of a patient to any form of subsequent examination or procedure. It is expedient, therefore, for hospitals to use printed forms of consent for presentation to, and signature by, patients.

References

1. FARBER, S. *The Post-Mortem Examination.* Baltimore: Thomas, 1937. BOX. *Post-Mortem Manual.* London: Churchill, 1919, and other works.
2. MAILE, W.C.D. & SCOTT, K.J.L *Lancet,* **1,** 21, 1935.
3. Waugh v. R., [1950], A.C. 203.
4. R. v. Woodcock, 1789, 1 Leach, 504.
5. LORD RIDDELL. *Medico-Legal Problems.* London: Lewis, 1929.
6. Hay v. H.M. Advocate, 1968, J. C. 40.
Also referred to LEWIS, W.J. *Law of Evidence in Scotland.* Edinburgh: Hodge, 1925.

Chapter 3

IDENTIFICATION

THE question of personal identity frequently arises in the law courts not only in the identification of criminals but also in the identification of other persons and dead bodies.

The detection of criminals by identification falls essentially within the province of the police, but in matters pertaining to identification of the dead, and in problems touching upon identification generally, the services of the medico-legist are likely to prove important.

Identification of criminals

The establishment of the identity of criminals will first be considered.

Anthropometry or Bertillon's system

In addition to descriptive data of prisoners, the Bertillon system depends on exact measurements of the body. These measurements are recorded on cards which are retained in specially arranged cabinets in the Bureau of Identification.

Ancillary to his main system, Bertillon developed a method for the scientific indexing and filing of the descriptions of certain facial characteristics of criminals. This was called 'portrait parle' and laid the foundation for the modern descriptive indices of convicted criminals in use throughout the world today.

For methods employed in the classification of the measurements the reader may consult the work referred to.[1] The chief disadvantage of the system lies in possible inaccuracy when taking the measurements.

Dactylography or finger-print identification

The method of identifying criminals by means of their digital or palmar prints is used universally and can be divided into two main branches:

1. The filing of criminals' finger-prints for criminal records;
2. The searching and identification of chance impressions from scenes of crime.

The papillary ridges which cover the inner surfaces of the hands sometimes run in 'parallel' curves, and in certain areas, such as the bulbs of the fingers and parts of the palms, they form various patterns. It is because of the occurrence of these patterns that the essential features of the system are impressions which are taken from the bulbs of the fingers and thumbs. It is a simple matter to record the impressions on paper by means of printer's ink, thus permitting of easy examination by means of a hand lens, in order that the pattern may be classified for search and filing purposes.

On the official finger-print form, the imprints of the fingers and

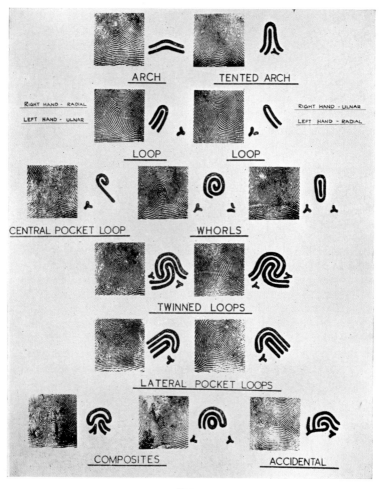

FIG. 1

Principal patterns, formed by papillary ridges, used in finger-print classification.   Cores and deltas are shown in diagrammatic form

(By courtesy of the City of Glasgow Police)

thumbs are taken in two different ways, and from the method used are called 'rolled' and 'plain' impressions.   First, the rolled impressions are taken by rolling each digit from one side to the other.   The resulting print ensures, as far as possible, the recording of all the detail necessary in classification.   Plain impressions are taken of all ten fingers for the purpose of checking that the rolled impressions have been taken in the proper order.   These plain impressions are taken by simply placing the inked fingers and thumbs directly on to the form, without any rolling movement.

Galton was the first to devise a system of classification of the finger-print patterns, and along with Henry[2] classified all these patterns into four main types, Arches, Loops, Whorls, and Composites (Fig. 1).

Various systems for the classification and filing of finger-prints exist,

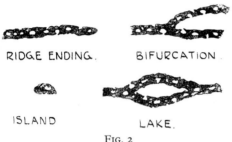

RIDGE ENDING.   BIFURCATION.

ISLAND   LAKE.

FIG. 2

Ridge characteristics (Galton details)

many of these systems being based on the Henry method.   It is felt, however, that the classification of finger-prints is a matter for finger-print experts, and details in this connection are omitted.   It is interesting to note, however, that even in large collections, like that at New Scotland Yard, where over a million sets are filed, the system is so perfect that when the finger-prints of a person have been recorded and classified, their location is readily obtained for comparison with the same individual's finger-prints, should these be taken by the police on some future occasion, irrespective of what name the person may take.

Prints from the soles of the feet are as reliably identifiable as finger or palm prints, and many Eastern countries utilise this method of identification in relation to chance foot-prints found at the scene of crime.   Toe-prints have been accepted as evidence of identification in British courts.

The final identification of any finger or palm print is not made by comparison of patterns, but by comparison of the numerous details or characteristics which occur throughout the ridge areas, and of the sequence in which these characteristics occur.   The characteristics of a print, known originally as the 'Galton details', may take the form of ridge endings, bifurcations, lake formations, or island formations (Fig. 2).

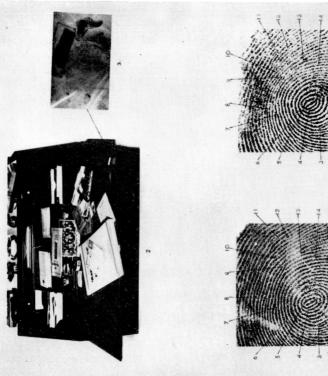
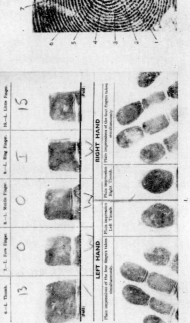

Fig. 3

The accuracy of the finger-print and palm-print system of identification is based on the facts—

1. that the patterns and characteristics are present and constant from before birth until decomposition after death, remaining the same except for accidental damage as long as the body survives;
2. that no two separate finger or palm prints have exactly the same arrangement and formation of papillary ridges;
3. that in practical experience throughout the world, no two finger or palm prints have been found which were identical in the sequence of their ridge details; and
4. that mathematical calculations indicate the extreme improbability of chance duplication.

For legal purposes, it is generally accepted that the chances of two finger-prints disclosing sixteen ridge characteristics which are identical and occur in the same sequence are less than one in ten thousand million million. To prove the identity of a single finger-print in court it is necessary to have sixteen ridge characteristics identical and occurring in the same sequence as sixteen ridge characteristics in the comparison print.

In England prior to the Criminal Justice Act, 1948, the procedure with regard to apprehended persons was that, if the person did not object to his finger-prints being taken, they could be taken by the officer arresting or by any other police officer after the person had been charged. When the person refused to have his finger-prints taken, he was remanded in custody and sent to prison where, under the Penal Servitude Act, 1891, his finger-prints could be taken on a warrant granted by a magistrate. The Criminal Justice Act, 1967, section 33 and the Magistrates Courts Act, 1952, section 40 (1) enact that where any person not less than fourteen years of age has been taken into custody and charged with an offence before a Magistrates' Court, the court may, on the application of an officer of police not below the rank of inspector, order that the finger-prints of that person shall be taken

---

On 2nd June 1947, a dwelling house in the city was entered by means of forcing the vestibule door with bodily pressure and a quantity of linen and jewellery was stolen. Search was made for finger-prints, and an impression of a right thumb of the whorl type was found inside the lid of a writing bureau in the sitting-room (2). This was photographed (3) and compared with the finger-prints of all persons having legitimate access to the bureau, with a negative result. The impression was then classified and searched in the Single Finger Print Collection. It was identified as the right thumb-print of ——, G.C.R.O. 116/42. This man was arrested, charged with the housebreaking, and finger-printed (1). He intimated a plea of 'Not Guilty', and productions were prepared for court. Enlarged photographs of the digital mark on the writing bureau and the right thumb-print on the finger-print form were prepared. On each of these sixteen identical ridge characteristics occurring in the same sequence were marked (4).

Accused was convicted and sentenced to two months' imprisonment.

by a constable. Finger-prints taken in pursuance of such an order are taken either at the court or, if the person is remanded in custody, at any place to which he is committed. A constable may use such reasonable force as may be necessary for that purpose. Where finger-prints of any person have been so taken, if the person is acquitted or discharged, or if the information against him is dismissed, the finger-prints and all copies and records of them must be destroyed.

In Scotland, at common law, the police may competently take finger-prints of arrested persons who are in police custody without the consent

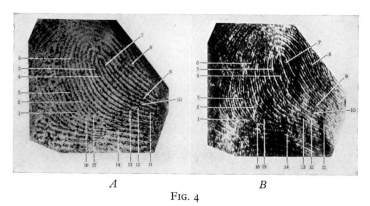

A B

FIG. 4

Comparison of finger-print on bottle in cellar, No. 2 Dalton Square (A), with photograph of dermis of right thumb of Body No. 1 (B). Sixteen points of agreement are marked (see Ruxton Case, p. 96)

of such persons and without a warrant. Without consent, finger-prints of a person who has not been arrested may not be taken by the police, and they may not be taken without consent in the case of a person who is not in police custody, for example, a person who has been arrested but has subsequently been released on bail.

Since the doctor and the police investigator have to work frequently in close co-operation in the elucidation of certain cases, it is highly important that the former should realise the necessity for the adoption of strict precautions to prevent any unwitting interference with finger-prints left by a criminal at the scene of crime. He should therefore refrain from handling or touching any object until the finger-print expert has completed his examination. The prints left at the scene of crime may be visible or almost invisible. The latter may be developed artificially by dusting the area, by means of a camel's-hair brush, with light or dark coloured powders, depending on whether the surface on which the latent print is situated is dark or light, the object being to provide a contrast. Following development the prints may be photographed. Latent prints may also be examined by oblique lighting.

Of importance to those who are attempting the identification of a dead body is the fact that even after the epidermal covering layer of the finger-tips has been shed, as the result of putrefaction, the characteristics of the exposed surfaces of the dermis are identical with those of the voided epidermis, since the ridges of the papillary layer of the dermis or true skin are the primary cause of the ridge pattern of the epidermis. Dermal impressions may lack clear definition, and it may be necessary to employ enlargements of direct photographs of the dermis. Many difficulties may arise when an attempt is made to obtain direct impressions. When the print-bearing surfaces are either sodden or hardened, modification of the ordinary ink method of recording prints must be used to meet individual circumstances. Hardened skin may be rendered pliant by the use of oil or Vaseline which should be massaged into the tissues. Excess must be removed. Injection of the print-bearing portions of the fingers with special paraffin-wax may be resorted to in an attempt to restore contour. In one case of drowning, the terminal phalanx of a thumb was removed and boiled in water, with marked success, in that the process, although reducing the size of the specimen, rendered the skin almost normal in character. When the shed epidermis is available, it should be preserved carefully between two sheets of glass for subsequent examination by a finger-print expert. Successful photographs of the print may be obtained by photographing from the back of the glass by means of transmitted light. The identification of dead bodies by means of finger-prints is, of course, only possible when there are prints available for comparison purposes.[3]

Identification by teeth marks

This form of identification has proved of value. Two men were tried at Cumberland Assizes on a charge of theft. On examination of the premises, a piece of cheese, with teeth marks upon it, was discovered. A cast of the teeth of one of the suspects was made and found to fit exactly the impressions on the cheese. Expert evidence was given by a dentist, who stated that no two sets of teeth are exactly alike. The prisoner requested that his mouth should be examined again to ascertain if his teeth would fit the impression on the cheese. On complying with the request, it was found that, since the original impression had been taken, he had removed a stump.[4]

Assailants can sometimes be identified from the teeth marks they have inflicted on their victims. These are usually seen on the breasts of girls when they are referred to in the circles where they most commonly occur as love bites. The characteristic mark consists of a central area of bruising with a surrounding area which may show discrete bruises and abrasions. They occur frequently on those who enjoy the more aggressive forms of love making.

Occasionally, however, these marks are found on the bodies of girls who have been murdered during a sexual assault. They are then of great importance as they may provide the main evidence of identification of the assailant.

It is important that those who perform autopsies in these cases should recognise the characteristic lesions. This may be difficult as the marks caused by the mouth may be scarcely recognisable amongst lesions caused by other forms of violence. When an examiner considers that there are bite marks on the body of a victim he should immediately call for the help of a dentist with forensic experience. Photographs and impressions must be taken of the bites and it may be necessary to do this over a period of time and during this time the less disturbance of the body the better.

Bite marks on the breast of the victim provided the principal evidence incriminating the accused in the case of H.M. Advocate v. Hay heard in the High Court of Justiciary, 1968. This case is described in detail in the *Journal of the Forensic Science Society*, 1968, Vol. 8, No. 4, and this should be read by anyone who is likely to be involved in cases of this type.

It is worth considering the accuracy of identification by mouth marks on a body. This requires the co-operation of a forensic medicine expert, an experienced dentist, and expert photographer and an expert on surface markings. It seems to us that the main function of the forensic medicine expert is to make the decision that the marks in question are made by a human mouth either sucking or biting. We think that this should probably be the limit of his evidence. The dentist must provide the evidence in detail about the shapes of the marks found and the shapes of the teeth which made them and he must be able to give an estimate of the probability of these particular shapes occurring in individuals. He must base his opinion on the marks which he has seen and on the work of the expert photographer. We consider that in cases where only bruising is present a definite opinion should not be given. The mechanism of production of a bruise makes this too dangerous. Where, however, abrasions are present the position is different. If it can be stated that these are due to a human bite and they show shapes which an experienced dentist can identify as having been caused by an unusual mouth pattern and there is a suspect who has that pattern then there is a probability that the bites have been caused by the suspect. The degree of probability will depend on the features of the mouth pattern and on how many of these have been transferred to the body. It is here that the evidence of the dentist becomes vital and it is also the position where the forensic medicine expert cannot give a valuable opinion. There does, however, appear to be some conflict of dental opinion on this matter. Perhaps somebody will eventually work out the mathematics of the probability involved.

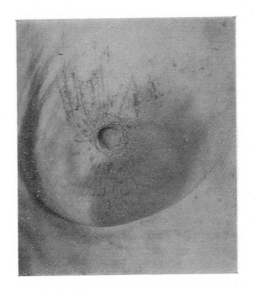

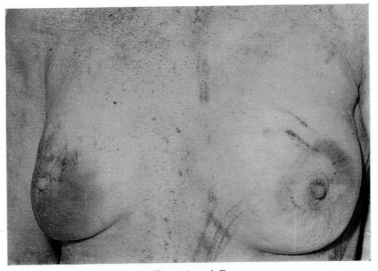

FIG. 5A and B
Typical bites on breast

Anyone who is interested should certainly read the prosecution and defence evidence given in the Hay case and the subsequent controversy in the *Journal of the Forensic Science Society*, 1969, Vol. 9, Nos. 3 and 4.

Dr S. S. Kind has discussed 'The Nature of the Process of Identification' in the *Journal of the Forensic Science Society*, 1964, Vol. 4, No. 3, and concludes: 'Forensic scientists are routinely faced with immediate practical problems in identification and have little time to consider the logical processes behind their methods. Nevertheless, I believe it is necessary to render our methods more efficient by taking greater cognizance of the logical steps in our schemes of identification and not to become lost in the beauty of our instrumentation.'

This warning note should be remembered by all who provide the courts with scientific evidence and also by the courts who have to weigh this evidence and who may at the present time have passed from a period when they were too reluctant to accept scientific evidence to one where they are reluctant or unable to subject it to proper scrutiny.

ERRATUM:

The caption to Figures 6A and 6B opposite should read: 'Detail of bite marks from Figures 5A and 5B'.

Identification by wounds on the body

On rare occasions the presence of wounds on the body may assist in associating a suspected criminal with a given crime.

In Glasgow, a thief broke the plate-glass window of a jeweller's shop, stole some jewellery and escaped. On examination of the window, a small, almost circular, piece of skin was found adhering to the edge of the broken piece of window. The police rounded up all the thieves whose speciality was shopbreaking, and their hands were examined. On the finger-tip of one of the men an unhealed wound was found. It was almost circular in shape, and when the piece of preserved skin was applied it was found to fit almost exactly.

A young girl of thirteen was brought to the police by her mother who alleged that the girl had been criminally assaulted. Examination of her genitals showed both swelling and bruising. The hymen was ruptured, and the underclothing soaked with blood. Examination of the scene of the crime showed a considerable amount of blood on the floor of the stair landing. A man was apprehended, and the girl identified him as her assailant. On examination of the prisoner, a recent rupture of the fraenum of the penis was found. Although his trousers had been recently washed, the inner surface showed the presence of blood in the seams, and the soles and nails of his boots also gave

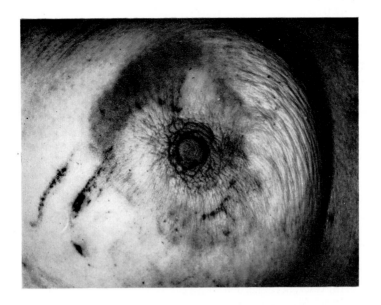

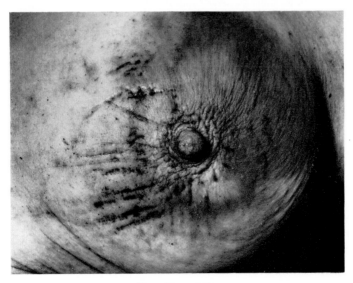

FIG. 6A and B
Bites with models of teeth for comparison

unmistakable evidence of blood.   The accused strenuously denied the accusation, but at his trial he pleaded guilty.

Dust and debris

Dust and debris removed from the surfaces of clothing, pockets, and the turn-ups of trouser legs may, when submitted to careful microscopical examination, give some indication of the occupation of a person. Deposits from the ears, nostrils, and from under the nails should also be examined, since particulate matter found in the atmosphere of certain factories and workshops may be found in these regions.   Debris from pockets may disclose certain habits.   The turn-ups of trouser legs may contain some forms of vegetation which may provide important information in some cases, so may debris associated with bodies retrieved from water, or with footwear or motor cars.   Not infrequently the services of a botanist, zoologist, entomologist, or chemist may prove essential in the investigation.   Spectrographic analysis of traces, often insufficient in quantity for the application of ordinary chemical tests, may yield highly important results.

Among many of our cases in this connection, two may be cited.   In one of the cases, in connection with a contravention of the Criminal Law Amendment Act, a young girl was the subject of a sexual offence which took place in an outdoor lavatory in a quiet country district.   Certain stains upon the overcoat of the accused were found on analysis to be of the same chemical composition as the material covering the walls in the lavatory.   The second case was one of murder.   A young woman was strangled.   Her coat and one stocking were stained with a yellowish-green pigment which in all respects was the same as the pigment found upon the sleeve of the accused, and on the door of an outside lavatory in which the body had been placed (see Fig. 65).   Reconstruction experiments demonstrated the fact that there was only one position in which her body could have been carried into the lavatory to deposit it in the position found, and that in doing so the position of the pigment staining on the garments belonging to the two participants in the experiments was closely similar to that on the garments submitted for examination in the case.   With regard to photomicrography of particulate matter, photographs should be taken both by transmitted and reflected light. For detail, infra-red photography by reflected light is recommended.

Two newer techniques have become available for the identification of fragments of material.   These are activation analysis and infra-red spectrography.

Activation analysis.   This technique allows the determination of elements in quantities far below the limits of conventional analytical methods.   These depend on the behaviour of electrons on the outer part of the atom. The nucleus cannot be affected by conventional physical or chemical methods. It can, however, be studied by induced radio-activity. This is usually done by exposure in a nuclear reactor and the activity is measured in a Geiger counter or a scintillation counter. This technique should prove extremely valuable in identifying traces of paint, particles of glass, and possibly gun-shot residues.

Infra-red spectrometry. In this technique a beam is directed through the sample and a graph obtained. The graph shows the absorption which is dependent on the bonding between the atoms. The graph gives a finger-print style of identification and has to be compared with a large number of known graphs.

An example is shown where a very small piece of tissue was found at the back of a couch in a room where a baby was thought to have had his genitalia mutilated by a knife and no other traces could be found. The fragment provided the infra-red spectrograph shown as Figure 7A. This was somewhat puzzling as a spectrograph of a skin control gave the picture shown in Figure 7B. A dusting of talcum was then applied to the control skin and this gave the spectrograph shown in Figure 7C, which compares with a high degree of accuracy with the fragment of tissue in question.

Tattoo marks

The practice of tattooing is common among certain classes of persons, and is very prevalent among sailors and soldiers. The process consists of the injection of bright pigments into the true skin to form various patterns or designs. The extent of such marks varies among individuals. It may extend over the major portion of the body or be confined to small areas. The devices assume the most varied character.

In many cases the presence of such marks on the body may lead to the identification of an individual not only during life but after death. The nature of the devices may prove of assistance in establishing identity since, in a number of cases, in addition to the initial letters of the name of the person tattooed, further identifying details may be available from the nature of the emblems.

Tattoo marks produced by unstable pigments tend to fade and disappear after variably long intervals, but stable pigments produce permanent marks. Carbon, indian ink, vermilion, and prussian blue are the most permanent pigments. Cinnabar, cochineal, aniline dyes, and ordinary ink, are much less permanent. Tattoo marks made professionally are composed of stable pigments which are injected by several methods and are permanent. Various means have been devised for the elimination of these marks, but the only perfect method is

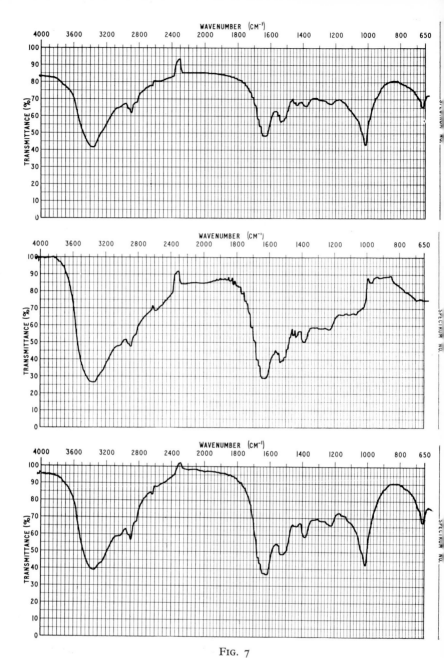

FIG. 7

A. Spectograph of tissue sample found at back of couch.
B. Spectograph of skin control.
C. Spectograph of skin control dusted with talcum.

surgical removal, when the resultant scar is minimal. A tattoo design may be altered, or a second may be superimposed.

Tattoo marks on unidentified putrefied bodies may be photographed with sharp definition if the loose epidermis is first removed and the design on the dermis is recorded. This method is of special value in the case of bodies recovered from water (Figs. 8 and 9). The use of the ultra-violet lamp or of infra-red photography may prove helpful in revealing latent tattoo marks.

Teeth

An examination of the teeth may prove of high value in regard to identification, more particularly if dental work has been carried out. The state of the teeth, if the professional records of a dentist are available, is of the greatest importance, and the following, among other, particulars should be noted:

The number and position of teeth present in, and missing from, each jaw.
Whether extraction of the teeth has been recent or remote.
The presence and position of cavities, fillings and crowns.
Whether a denture has been worn, and a denture known to have been made for the particular person fits the mouth.
The quality of any dental work found present.
The existence of any recognisable peculiarity of the jaws or teeth.

The following case[5] has been reported. A woman was found unconscious in the black-out, having been hit on the head by a passing motor van. She was wearing dentures. The upper one remained in her mouth, but the lower one was missing. The police traced the van. The driver denied hitting anyone, although marks were present on the van. In the back of the vehicle was the missing denture. The police took the dentures to a dentist who was asked if he could identify them as made for a patient some years previously. The upper denture was immediately recognised and the lower, which was broken, was found when held together to fit into normal occlusion. The finding of the lower denture in the van, and proving that it belonged to the upper one, provided evidence that the woman had been knocked down by the van.

Identification of living and dead persons

Since many of the features used in the identification of dead bodies are equally applicable to the establishment of identity of living persons, to obviate repetition, these aspects of the subject will be discussed together.

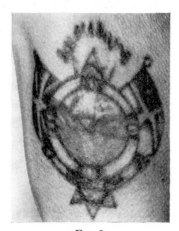

FIG. 8   FIG. 9

Appearance of tattoo marks following shedding of epidermis
after thirty-seven days' immersion in water.   The arms showed
green putrefactive change.   Although the skull was completely
denuded of tissue, these marks established identity

(By courtesy of the late Dr Robert Richards,
Aberdeen University)

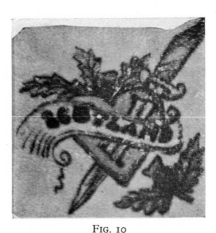

FIG. 10
Tattoo mark

The solution of identity, reviewed broadly, depends upon a consideration of the following features:

Age.
Sex.

Stature.

Deformities, peculiarities, and individual characteristics.

Age

Evidence of age for medico-legal purposes may be required in several types of cases, for example:

1. As an aid to identification.
2. In rape and sexual offences.
3. Capacity for procreation.
4. Maturity of a fetus.
5. Age of marriage.

In the instance of young children, a fairly accurate opinion as to age may be arrived at from the state of eruption of the teeth, the general development, height, and weight of the body, and the condition of ossification of the bones. The assessment of age based solely on the state of eruption of the teeth may occasionally prove misleading, but further allusion will be made to this point when consideration is given to the ages at which the first and second dentitions appear. One may also be led astray by the condition of development, height, and weight, more especially in the case of children born and reared in cities, by reason of malnutrition or illness, which disturb these factors prejudicially, and it will be found that the difficulty does not become lessened as age increases. The time of onset of puberty in girls and of virility in boys is very variable, and although from a large mass of cases we may be able to formulate some average age at which it appears, the calculation does not apply to the individual. It is also necessary to remember the possibility of precocious sexual development which is a condition of childhood characterised by genital development which approximates adult proportions during the first decade, whereas precocious puberty is sexual precocity with further maturation of the child as manifested by spermatogenesis and menses.[6] We are aware of a case of a male child who, from a clearly visible moustache, well-developed sexual organs, growth of suprapubic hair, and other signs, might readily have been mistaken for a young man. The epiphyses of the long bones on X-ray examination were found to be united to the diaphyses by osseous union. His age, as attested by the mother, the medical man who attended the birth, and the certificate of birth, was only ten years and seven months. He was charged with indecent conduct towards a girl.

Kerr[7] records a case of pubertas praecox in a girl aged six years and ten months, who at the age of three and a half years began to menstruate. The menstrual periods occurred four times annually and each lasted from one to two days. Her appearance was that of a well-developed girl of twelve to fourteen years. The breasts were enlarged, and there was prominence of the mons veneris on which there was some dark, fine hair.   The uterus on bimanual examination was of almost adult size.   She probably suffered from pineal syndrome due to neoplasm or hyperplasia of the pineal gland.   Such precocious development is usually attributable to suprarenal disease, commonly tumour.

Approaching middle life, the greatest difficulty in the assessment of age from external appearances is experienced, the result of the cumulative effect of inherited conditions and the vicissitudes of life upon the individual.   Prematurely old men and comparatively active old men are quite frequently seen.   It is clear, therefore, that in the assessment of age, little reliance can be placed on external manifestations, and that dependence must rest upon general developmental and growth changes in the skeleton.

The importance of developmental changes is clearly illustrated in the assessment of fetal age.   This is sometimes important in connection with charges of criminal abortion, infanticide and concealment of pregnancy or concealment of birth, since it is important for the authorities to know whether certain structures found are the product of conception and, if so, what stage in development has been reached.   As will be appreciated later, when the subject of infanticide is reviewed, the estimation of fetal age in medico-legal work is of frequent importance (p. 412).   It is necessary, therefore, to recognise the stage of development of the products of conception.   The following data will prove of assistance in arriving at an opinion.

Development of fetus

End of fourth month.   Length = 12½ to 17½ centimetres (5 to 7 inches), weight is from 85 to 255 grams (3 to 9 ounces), and the skin is fairly dense.   The pupillary membrane is distinct.   The nails on fingers and toes begin to appear.   The genital organs are sufficiently developed to enable sex to be recognised.   Downy hair appears on the body and scalp.   A small quantity of meconium may be found in the intestine.

End of fifth month.   Length = 15 to 25 centimetres (6 to 10 inches), and weight about 170 to 340 grams (6 to 12 ounces).   The nails are now distinct.   Growth of hair commences, and skin may show sebaceous secretion.   Dental germs appear in the maxillae.   Ossification centre is found in the calcaneus.

End of sixth month.   Length = 22 to 30 centimetres (9 to 12 inches), and weight about 690 grams (1½ lb).   Skin, now divisible into cutis vera and epidermis, is wrinkled.   Eyelids still closed by pupillary membrane. Umbilical cord is situated a little above pubis.   Hair 'of eyebrows and eyelashes begins to form. Testes are found lying close to kidneys.

End of seventh month. Length = 32 to 37 centimetres (13 to 15 inches), and weight 1·3 to 1·8 kilograms (3 to 4 lb). Nails do not yet reach extremities of fingers. Pupillary membrane difficult to detect. Testes found in process of descent towards scrotum, and in the vaginal process of peritoneum. Fetus capable of life if born (viable). Centre of ossification is present in the talus.

End of eighth month. Length = 35 to 42 centimetres (14 to 17 inches), and weight about 1·8 to 2·2 kilograms (4 to 5 lb). Sebaceous secretion begins to be formed on skin. The nails now practically reach the extremities of the fingers. Pupillary membrane has now entirely disappeared. One testis, usually the left, may be found in scrotum, and the other well advanced in downward descent. Centre of ossification appears at lower end of femur.

End of ninth month. Length = 45 to 60 centimetres (18 to 42 inches), and weight from 2·8 kilograms (6½ lb) upwards, the average weight being about 3·1 kilograms (7 lb). Umbilical cord inserted about three-quarters of an inch below centre of body. Hair is found on scalp and on portions of body. Sebaceous secretion is likely to be found in flexures of joints, and more or less over the whole body. Both testes are in scrotum. The finger-nails are fully formed and developed. The child is mature. The centre of ossification at lower end of femur is about the size of a pea. Small centre in cuboid bone, and possibly an ossification centre in upper epiphysis of tibia.

The fact that the length of the fetus in centimetres is equal to the square of the number of months of gestation, provides a method for arriving at the approximate age of a fetus. After the fifth month of gestation has been reached, the length of the fetus in centimetres, divided by 5, gives the age of the fetus in months. From the fourth month onwards, the length of the fetus in inches is approximately equal to the number of months multiplied by 2.

Teeth. An examination of the state of eruption of the temporary or deciduous teeth in infants will offer a reliable indication of age in most cases, since the respective periods of eruption of the different teeth are fairly constant. It must be remembered, however, that these teeth may appear either abnormally early, indeed, in rare cases some of them may be present at birth, or their appearance may be abnormally delayed. We have examined a boy of eleven who did not then possess, and never had possessed, any teeth. Precocious dentition has been frequently recorded.   The teeth which usually signalise this precocious dentition are the central incisors.

The following dental charts indicate approximately the period at which the different temporary and permanent teeth appear:

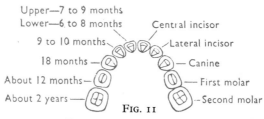

Upper—7 to 9 months
Lower—6 to 8 months   Central incisor
    9 to 10 months   Lateral incisor
    18 months   — Canine
About 12 months —   — First molar
About 2 years —   --Second molar

FIG. 11

Temporary or deciduous teeth

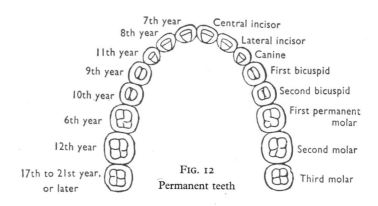

        7th year   Central incisor
    8th year   Lateral incisor
    11th year   Canine
    9th year   First bicuspid
    10th year   Second bicuspid
    6th year   First permanent molar
    12th year   Second molar
17th to 21st year,   Third molar
    or later

FIG. 12
Permanent teeth

The temporary teeth are twenty in number, and the permanent teeth thirty-two.   The former begin to be shed from the fifth to the seventh year.

It will be evident that the first permanent molars appear about the sixth year, the second molars about the twelfth year, and the third molars about the eighteenth year, earlier or later.   There is greater uncertainty respecting the time of eruption of the third molars than of the other teeth.   In odd cases they do not appear till adult age is well advanced.

In the younger subject, age from permanent teeth can be assessed relatively, but not with absolute accuracy, as the formation and eruption of teeth vary in individual subjects.

Times of appearance of centres of ossification in the epiphyses and their fusion with diaphyses

An approximately accurate estimate of age is given by the centres of ossification, and the progress of that ossification in the unification of the bones.

Flecker has carried out considerable research on the subject. He holds the view that a perusal of the various anatomical authorities shows a considerable discrepancy regarding the ages at which the various

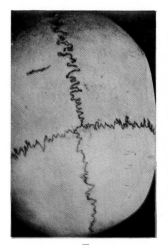

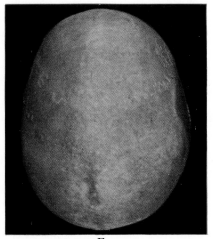

Fig. 13	Fig. 14
Absence of closure of sutures of skull	Closure of sutures of skull

centres of ossification in the epiphyses appear, and at which the epiphyses fuse with their respective diaphyses. For detailed information the reader is referred to Flecker's work[8] and to standard works on anatomy.

According to Brash,[9] growth changes in the skeleton, although providing a very reliable basis for the estimation of age, do not permit of an exact determination, but only within a range, since there is variation in relation to growth and age. In referring to this point he states that, 'before puberty, when the skeleton begins to consolidate, so many active growth changes are going on—including the development of the growing (epiphyseal) ends of the limb bones, and the progressive calcification and the eruption of the teeth—that it is relatively easy to determine probable age within a year or so. From puberty until the consolidation of the skeleton (at twenty-two or twenty-three, or at the most twenty-five years), a fairly close estimate—within a range of two to three years

—may still be made, mainly on the progress of the union of the epiphyses. Thereafter the range must lengthen; and after thirty years, when the mature skeleton already begins to show signs of "ageing"— including the beginning of the progressive closure of the cranial sutures —it will be hardly safe to estimate more closely than in decades.'

The development and consolidation of the bones of the skeleton which ossify in cartilage occur, as a rule, about two years earlier in the female than in the male, but the obliteration of the sutures of the vault of the skull sets in a little later and proceeds more slowly in the female than in the male.

When all the epiphyses of the limb bones are completely united it indicates a minimum age of twenty-two to twenty-five years, but after apparent adult age has been attained, and particularly toward later adult life, some indication of age may still be ascertained. For example:

The absence of any sign of closure of any of the sutures of the skull points to a strong probability that the age does not exceed thirty years. The following are recognised average times for the closure of skull sutures:

Sagittal ⎫
Coronal ⎬ Commence about thirty.
Lambdoid ⎭

Parieto-mastoid ⎫ Commence between thirty-five and forty.
Squamous ⎬ Increase slowly till fifty.

Spheno-parietal ⎫ Commences about thirty.
⎬ Completed at seventy.

Evidence of commencing union of the sutures is first seen on the inner surface of the bone. Franchini[10] after a very comprehensive investigation stated that the obliteration of sutures may be of subsidiary help in association with other appearances but the variations are such that it is impossible to rely on it alone for determining the age of the subject.

Beyond middle age, ossification of the laryngeal cartilages and in the hyoid bone may usually be found, although commencing ossification of the larynx may be present at an earlier age.

Ossification of the costal cartilages is usually associated with advancing years, but may be present in younger subjects.

The xiphoid process usually fuses with the body of the sternum about the age of forty, and in advanced life the manubrium is occasionally joined to the body by bone, although only the superficial parts of the intervening cartilage is converted into bone.

After middle age the angle of the lower jaw tends to become more obtuse, its alveolar margin shows some evidence of absorption of bone, and the teeth still present may be found in a loosened condition.

With respect to the age of a body of which only mutilated remains are available for examination, a fairly accurate estimate of age can frequently be arrived at. The ability to do this will depend very largely upon the parts available for examination, with respect to their amount, nature, and variety. The Ruxton case, which will be considered later, illustrates several of the points already touched upon in addition to further aspects which find a place in the subject of identification of the dead. This case involved a very wide and varied field of investigation, and the results are regarded as highly instructive in the practical application of available methods for the identification of mutilated and dismembered remains.

Sex

Difficulty about this question may arise in the examination of bodies when decomposition is so far advanced that the external and internal sexual organs have disappeared, either from exposure to air or water, after burial in the ground, as the result of mutilation and dismemberment, or when only portions of a body are available for examination.

Brash states that, in the examination of bones, occasionally the skull and limb bones present general features which are in some respects equivocal for the diagnosis of sex. This necessitates a careful assessment of the balance of the anatomical features before anatomical proof becomes available for the correct opinion as to sex.

The more outstanding general characters, apart from the genital organs and breasts, which differentiate the sexes may be summed up as follows: The male is generally of larger build and greater muscular development than the female, although the effeminate male and the masculine female must be remembered. The adult male is broader at the shoulders than at the hips, the adult female broader at the hips than at the shoulders. The waist is marked in woman and ill-defined in man, and the gluteal regions in the former are full and rounded whereas in the latter they are flatter and contractile. The legs of the female are more rounded and the wrists, ankles, and nails more delicate. Hair only covers the mons veneris in the female, but in the male it covers the pubis and may extend upwards on to the abdomen, and more or less over the anterior surface of the chest. The hair of the male head is shorter, thicker, and coarser than that of the female. The larynx of the male is more prominently developed than that of the female.

In the case of mutilated remains, identity is simplified when those parts of the body bearing sexual characters are available. In this connection it is well to remember that the unimpregnated uterus is one of the organs of the body to resist rapid putrefaction, and consequently when abdominal remains are available, this organ and its appendages should be looked for carefully.   When the uterus and its appendages are absent, it becomes necessary to rely upon the general appearances of the parts, the disposition of the hair, the presence or absence of the mammae, the presence or absence of linae albicantes, as indicative of previous pregnancy, and any parts of the external genitals which may remain.   The prostate gland is resistant to putrefaction, and it should always be looked for since its presence indicates male sex.

When sexual characteristics of the soft parts are unavailable, it becomes necessary to base the diagnosis of sex on the secondary sex characters displayed by bones.

By consideration of the character of the long bones with reference to muscle-attachments, and especially of the character of the pelvis, skull, and sternum taken as a whole, an opinion may usually be arrived at with considerable accuracy.   Generally the bones of the female skeleton are lighter, are not so large, and muscle-attachment marks are not so pronounced as in the male.   Apart from certain measurements of the long bones, the pelvis, skull, sternum, and sacrum must be reckoned as the chief means of differentiating sex in a skeleton.   The principal points of differentiation are shown on facing page.

The sexual characters of the pelvis are of the highest importance in the sexing of skeletal remains.   Since the female pelvis is constructed for the function of child-bearing, most usually it presents very distinctive features which contrast with the pelvis of the male.   Despite this fact, there are frequent instances in which a pelvis shows variable secondary characters, mixed male and female characters, and in such cases an opinion regarding sex must be limited to one of greater or lesser probability.

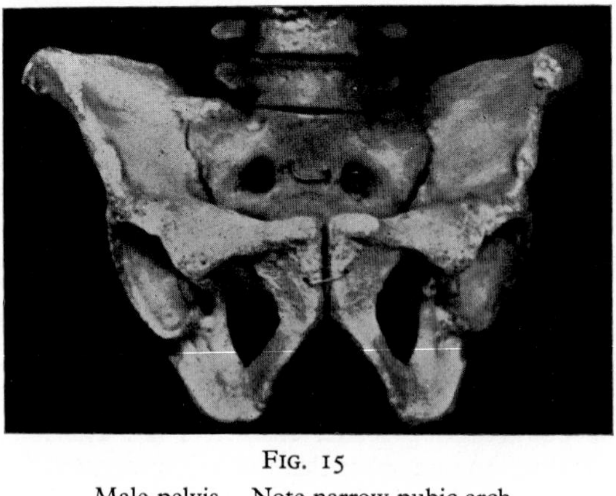

FIG. 15
Male pelvis.   Note narrow pubic arch

The Pelvis

Male	*Female*
Bony framework massive	Bony framework less massive
Deep	Shallow and more capacious
Walls not splayed	Walls splayed
Pubic arch narrow, not more than about 70 degrees	Pubic arch wide, practically right-angled
Great sciatic notch narrow	Great sciatic notch almost a right angle or even greater
Obturator foramen ovoid	Obturator foramen more triangular
Preauricular sulcus not marked.	Preauricular sulcus pronounced.
Iliopectineal line well marked and rough	Iliopectineal line rounded and smooth
Body of pubis approximately triangular	Body of pubis approximately square
Ramus of pubis is like a continuation of body of pubis	Ramus of pubis has a pinched or narrowed appearance and is squat in character
Acetabulum is large, averaging 52 mm in diameter, and faces laterally	Acetabulum is small, averaging 46 mm in diameter, and faces forward as well as laterally
Sacrum is relatively narrow and long, and its curve is more or less equal over the entire length	Sacrum is relatively wide and short, and its curve is practically confined to a point commencing below centre of third vertebra
Promontory fairly prominent	Promontory less prominent.
... ...	Transverse, oblique, and antero-posterior diameters greater than in male
... ...	Pelvic outlet is roomy and admits the passage of the clenched fist

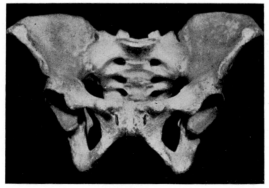

FIG. 16

Female pelvis. Note wide pubic arch

Sacrum

Fawcett[11] advocates a method for sexing the sacrum.　It consists of comparing the transverse diameter of the first sacral vertebra with the transverse diameter of the base of the sacrum.　The formula used is:

$$\frac{CW \times 100}{BW} = \text{Index of body}$$

CW = corpus width,
BW = basal width.

Readers are referred to the original article.[11]

	White races (adults)	
	Male	Female
Number . . .	134	79
Age range . . .	25–49	22–54
	Corporo-basal index	
Mean	45·041	40·486

The Skull

Male	Female
... ...	Usually smaller
Mastoid processes massive	Less pronounced
Superciliary ridges marked	Less marked
Fronto-nasal junction prominent	Less prominent
Sites of muscular insertions at base well marked	Less pronounced

The sex of a subject can frequently be determined from the general characters of the skull, but here again a variability in the sexual characters may be encountered.

In arriving at a conclusion regarding the sex of a pelvis or of a skull, it is necessary that the balance of all the characters should be considered with care.

Sternum

The proportion between the manubrium and the body of the sternum, according to several authorities, is definitely influenced by sex.　Ashley has formulated the '149 Rule'.　By this rule,[12] if the combined midline length of manubrium and mesosternum in Europeans equals, or exceeds, 149 millimetres, the sternum is probably masculine, if less than 149

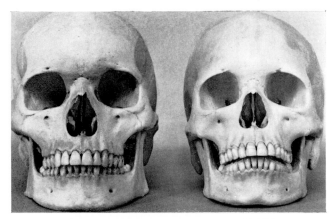

MALE   FEMALE

FIG. 17

Skulls—Anterior view

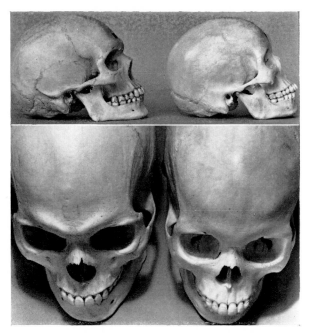

MALE   FEMALE

FIG. 18

Skulls—Lateral and supraorbital views

millimetres, probably feminine. It has been estimated that, by this rule, accuracy is obtainable in 80 per cent of cases.

Sexing of the limb bones

According to Brash, the measurements of the limb bones are reliable and conclusive if within a certain range, and the two most important bones for this purpose are the humerus and femur. There is, however, a considerable variation in the lengths of the bones in each sex which occasions a considerable overlap in the range of the length of each bone in the two sexes. He is of the opinion, however, that an indication of probability of sex, more or less great, may be obtained from such measurements. The table below shows the mean measurements of the maximum lengths of the humerus and femur from a particular series.[13]

Maximum length (mean)				Humerus	Femur
Male .	.	.	.	326·18 mm	459·3 mm
Female	.	.	.	298·66 ,,	426·27 ,,

Other figures for the femur are:[14]

Male, 447·24 mm   Female, 409·19 mm

The sizes of the heads of the humerus and of the femur offer even more significant sex characters than the lengths of these bones, The average measurements of the humeral head (with cartilage in position), according to Dwight,[15] are:

	Head of humerus	
	Vertical	Transverse
Male (average) . .	48·7 mm	44·6 mm
Female (average) . .	42·6 ,,	38·9 ,,

According to his measurements, the boundary between male and female lies between 45 and 46 millimetres for the vertical diameter and between 41 and 42 millimetres for the transverse diameter.

Parsons' measurements of the vertical diameter of the head of the femur (including cartilage) have shown that when the measurement exceeds 48 millimetres it indicates a male bone and when less than 44 millimetres, a female bone.

Karl Pearson has formulated a method for 'sexing' femora on a basis of values which may be assigned as shown in the table opposite.

The probability of a correct result is greatly increased by the summation of these marks. The measurements are in millimetres, and it should be noted that Parsons' figures and those of Pearson for the

Rules for 'Mathematical' Sexing of Femur (Pearson)

Measurement	Female	Female?	?	Male?	Male
Vertical diameter of head . .	41·5	41·5–43·5	43·5–44·5	44·5–45·5	> 45·5
Popliteal length .	<106	106–114·5	114·5–132	132–145	>145
Bicondylar width .	< 72	72–74	74–76	76–78	> 78
Trochanteric oblique length . .	<390	390–405	405–430	430–450	>450
Mark assigned to each . . .	+2	+1	o	−1	−2

vertical diameter of the head correspond closely when 3 millimetres (representing cartilage) are deducted from the former, since the latter measurements are of dried bone devoid of cartilage.

Of the above measurements, the maximum bicondylar width is considered highly important especially for sex differentiation. The popliteal length, that is, the measurement from the apex of the popliteal surface to the centre of the intercondylar line, is much less reliable since this measurement cannot always be appreciated with accuracy. The maximum bicondylar width is taken parallel to the infra-condylar plane, that is, with the bar of the calipers touching the lowest points of both condyles in the infra-condylar plane, and the arms of the calipers touching, respectively, the external condyle, externally, and the internal condyle, internally, at the maximum distance. The trochanteric oblique length is the vertical distance from the top of the great trochanter to the infra-condylar plane.

Stature

The calculation of stature comes to be a matter of necessity when an examiner is called upon to deal with a part or parts of a body or skeleton.

When certain of the long bones are available, more particularly the humerus or femur, reliable estimations of stature may be made by the employment of certain formulae. In the case of a dismembered body, estimation of stature becomes possible by direct measurement, provided the parts of the body, including at least one of the lower limbs, are available and an accurate reconstruction of the body is possible. It will be obvious that this is a preferable method of estimation to the use of formulae when the circumstances of the case permit. In assembling parts of a body with a view to direct measurement, it is necessary to arrange the parts in their correct and natural positions as securely as possible so that the measurement of the reconstructed body may be determined accurately. After measurement, a small deduction of 1·25 centimetres from the male and 2 centimetres from the female length, the amount by which, on the average, the body lengthens after death, should be made in order to arrive at the probable living stature. It must also be remembered that information regarding the height of missing persons supplied to the police by relatives and friends, especially in the case of women, may prove to be rather misleading, since the estimate given may in the first place be inaccurate, either because the actual measurement has not been taken during life or on account of added height by reason of the hair and footwear.

If bones only are available for examination, the formulae now employed, because of their comprehensiveness and accuracy, are those of Karl Pearson,[16] Dupertuis and Hadden,[17] and Trotter and Gleser.[18] These are based on a mathematical study of measurements of limb bones and statures. The formulae employed for the reconstruction of female stature differ from those of male stature. The bones frequently used for measurement are the femur, humerus, tibia, and radius. Should it be necessary to refer to such formulae, recourse should be had to the original works.

Body deformities and peculiarities

The presence of congenital deformities, such as hare-lip, cleft palate, polydactylism, syndactylism, defective development of the ribs and acquired deformities, including mallet-fingers and hammer-toes, together with evidence of joint diseases and fractures, are important aids in establishing the identity of persons. Moles, naevi, scars, and tattoo marks, when present, should be noted carefully since their presence may be of considerable value in this respect. Amputations, also, have frequently played a part in identification. Little requires to be said about these conditions with the exception perhaps of scars.

Scars. A surface scar always follows an injury of the true skin or dermis, and scar tissue is usually devoid of hair and sweat glands. Scar tissue is formed in about four weeks following moderate injury, and in the course of time the newly formed connective tissue undergoes cicatricial contraction by the diminution in size of the blood-vessels and cells, together with the consolidation of the young avascular fibrous tissue. When sepsis has supervened or when there has been considerable loss of tissue due to trauma, the resultant scar-tissue formation may be considerable in amount. The healing of an uncomplicated incised wound occasions relatively little scar formation, except in instances where the wound, although gaping, has not been stitched. Scars increase in size if the part on which they are situated increases as the result of growth. A well-developed scar never disappears spontaneously, but scars resulting from wounds in which there has been no appreciable loss of tissue may become very difficult to detect. Scars can be removed artificially, but a new scar is created as the result.

The age of a scar can only be arrived at in a very approximate manner, due to the variable periods which different wounds take to heal. A recent scar is of reddish colour, and with increasing age becomes progressively whiter and glistening. The duration of each stage, however, is liable to wide variation. The other factors attendant upon scar formation include the original extent of the wounding, the amount of tissue destruction, the manner of healing, and the health of the subject. The furthest a medical witness should be prepared to go in appraising the age of a scar must depend upon the circumstances of the individual case before him, and he should give a wide margin in his computation of age. Scars may result from various causes and these include, for example, lineae albicantes of an old pregnancy, healed ulcers, varicose and others, also vaccination. Extensive and disfiguring scar formation frequently results from burning. The well-known keloid condition needs no description. In the case of a living person, when it is important to discover a suspected scar or scars, not readily visible, certain methods may have to be employed. On account of the relative or complete avascularity of scar tissue, depending upon its degree of maturity, any influence which will produce marked increase in the activity of the cutaneous circulation in the surrounding skin will prove of assistance. The application of heat, or the use of surface friction, will produce the desired result. The employment of filtered ultraviolet light may in some cases be beneficial in revealing the presence of faint scarring (p. 73). A magnifying glass may prove serviceable.

Mutilation and dismemberment

In approaching the medico-legal aspects of the investigation of cases in which there has been mutilation and dismemberment of a body or bodies, a number of salient questions must receive special consideration. These are:

Are the remains of human or animal origin?
If human, do they represent one or more bodies?
What is the sex?
What is the age?
What is the stature?
Do the mutilation and dismemberment indicate, by their character, the use of anatomical and medical knowledge? For example, disarticulation at the joints as opposed to the use of a saw.
Has there been purposive removal of identifying features?

Do any features still remain which are likely to facilitate identification?

What is the state of the parts in relation to the process of putrefaction?

Are all the parts in a similar state so far as preservation or putrefaction is concerned?

Are there any marks indicative of the application of ante-mortem violence?

Do the remains show evidence suggestive of an attempt to destroy them?

Are there any articles associated with the remains which might lead to identification?

What was the cause of death?

In certain cases other subsidiary questions will probably arise, but the answers to the foregoing questions usually assume a high degree of importance.   Much could be written under each of these headings, but the subject-matter will be dealt with in more practical form by giving an illustration, in some detail, of the application of the medico-legal methods employed in the Ruxton case.

The legal importance of the establishment of the identity of remains, however, should first be mentioned.   In law, it is not necessary that there should be a dead body in order that a charge of murder may be presented against some person or persons; but where no body or part of a body, which is proved to be that of the person alleged to have been killed, has been found, the accused person should not be convicted either of murder or manslaughter, unless there is evidence either of the killing or of the death of the person alleged to have been killed.   In the absence of such evidence there is no onus upon the prisoner to account for the disappearance or non-production of the person alleged to be killed.   (Halsbury's *Laws of England.*)

THE RUXTON CASE

The case[19] is notable primarily on account of the extent and character of the mutilation of the two victims.   This provided a problem of reconstruction demanding for its solution anatomical work in detail not previously required in such cases.   On account of the purposive removal of identifying features a novel comparison of skull and portraits was used which, with other circumstantial evidence, helped to place identification beyond doubt (Fig. 23).

Facts of the case

On September 29, 1935, human remains were discovered in the bed of Gardenholme Linn, below the bridge on the Moffat–Edinburgh road.

Some of the remains were tied up in bundles around which were pieces of cotton sheeting, and associated with some of the parts were a blouse, a pair of child's rompers, pieces of newspaper, straw, and pieces of cotton-wool. Over a succession of days, further portions of human remains were recovered in and around the linn. On October 28, a left foot was found on the roadside some nine miles south of Moffat, and

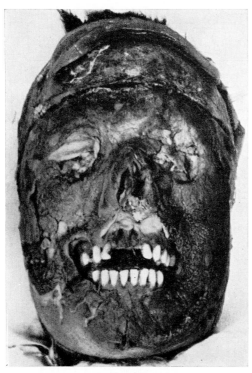

Fig. 19

Ruxton case. Head of Body No. 1 showing mutilations

on November 4, a right forearm with hand was also discovered by the roadside about half a mile south of the linn. Seventy portions of human remains had been recovered by this time. All the remains were decomposing and maggot-infested.

Subsequent to the discovery of the remains, it was ascertained that Mrs Ruxton and her nursemaid, Mary Rogerson, had disappeared from the house of Dr Ruxton in Lancaster on September 15, 1935. They were never seen alive again.

The dismembered remains

Among the remains were the following parts:

Two heads, each with a portion of neck (including cervical vertebrae) attached;

Two portions of trunk (thorax and pelvis), which fitted together to form a trunk; and

Four upper arms (separated at shoulder and elbow), two right and two left, which could be matched in pairs;

Three forearms and hands, one right and two left, including a pair;

Four thighs (separated at hip and knee), two right and two left, which could be matched in pairs; and

Four legs, two with feet, a pair, and two without feet, also a pair.

Attached to each of the thighs forming one of the pairs was a patella, and two other patellae, forming a pair, were found with the detached

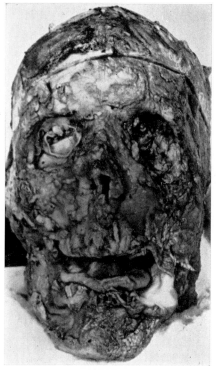

FIG. 20

Ruxton case.   Head of Body No. 2 showing
mutilations

soft parts.   The left foot and the right forearm with hand, subsequently found, completed two sets of limbs with the exception of one foot.   In addition to the limb segments, the soft parts included three female breasts which had been mutilated, a uterus with appendages, and two irregular skin-covered pieces of tissue which were portions of female external genitals.

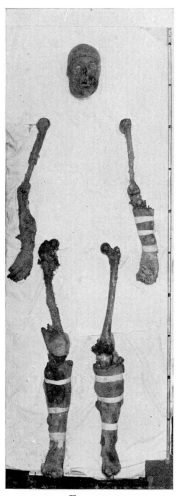 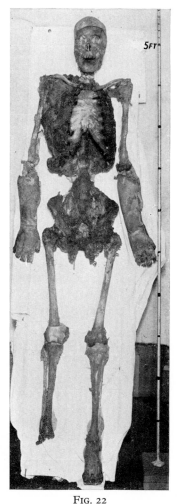

Fig. 21

Body No. 1 reassembled

Fig. 22

Body No. 2 reassembled

Note the scale, the lower end of which was adjusted to the level of the left heel, is marked at 6-inch intervals and in inches at the top.

Nature of the mutilations and dismemberment

Both heads had been mutilated by the removal of the ears, eyes, nose, lips, and skin of the face; and teeth had been extracted, probably after death. The terminal joints of the fingers had been removed from two of the hands. A large amount of tissue had been removed from the

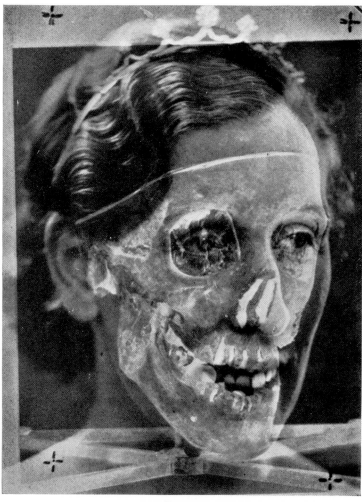

FIG. 23

Positive portrait of Mrs Ruxton and negative of Skull No. 2 photographically superimposed by Professor J. C. Brash. Note the coincidence of the registration marks by means of which the superimposition was effected

surfaces of the bodies, and many of the missing portions might have led to the identification of the bodies, and have borne marks of violence or signs suggestive of the cause of death. The reader is referred to Figures 21 and 22, which will give some conception both of the extent and character of the mutilations. The bodies had been neatly dismembered into portions convenient for transport, and the dismemberment had been effected by disarticulation with a knife. An obvious attempt had been made to efface any evidence which would lead to ready identification of the bodies, and it seemed evident that the person responsible had some medical as well as anatomical knowledge. This view was strengthened by the facts that there was very little damage to the joints, that the teeth had been extracted after death with some degree of skill, and that the uterus with its appendages had been removed from one of the bodies.

The available parts were then assembled to show the remains of two bodies as shown in Figures 21 and 22.

A comparison of the size and shapes of the skulls was made by superimposing photographs of the skulls and portraits of Mrs Ruxton and Mary Rogerson.

The remains of the two bodies were then compared with all the known facts about Mrs Ruxton and Mary Rogerson. The results are detailed in the tables on pages 96 and 97.

Dr Ruxton was arrested and charged with murder. In his house, human blood-stains were found in the bathroom, on the stair rails and banister, on stair carpets and pads, and on a suit of clothes belonging to him. Particles of human tissue were found in the drains. He was found guilty of murder and hanged.

Additional murder cases involving problems of identification of human remains

In 1949, John George Haigh was found guilty of the murder of Olive Durand-Deacon. He placed the body in a drum which he filled with sulphuric acid, later pouring out some of the acid and pumping fresh acid into the drum in order to fill it up again. At a later date he poured the whole of the contents of the drum away over some earth in a yard. Later on, when the ground over which Haigh had poured the acid from the drum was examined, there were found, not only human remains, but also an artificial denture belonging to the victim, together with other indications that the body which Haigh had tried to dissolve in the acid was in fact the body of Mrs Durand-Deacon. A dental surgeon identified the dentures as those supplied by him to Mrs Durand-Deacon. They had certain peculiarities which made it quite clear to him that the dentures were supplied to Mrs Durand-Deacon.[20]

In 1953, John Christie was convicted of the murder of his wife.

	Mary Jane Rogerson	Body No. 1—female
Age	20 years (October 8, 1935)	Certainly between 18 and 25. Probably between 20 and 21
Stature	About 5 ft	4 ft 10 in. to 4 ft 11½ in. (without shoes)
Hair	Light brown	Hair from scalp and body light brown
Eyes	Blue. 'Glide' in one	Removed
Complexion	Light. Freckles on nose and cheeks	Ears, nose, lips, and most of skin of face removed; complexion of remainder of skin consistent
Teeth	Old extraction of six teeth, four of them named	Old extraction or loss of eight teeth, including the four named
Neck	Short neck	Very small larynx very highly situated
Tonsils	Subject to tonsillitis	Microscopic evidence consistent with recurrent tonsillitis
Vaccination marks	Four on left upper arm	Four on left upper arm
Finger-nails	Maidservant	Trimmed but not regularly manicured; scratches indicating some form of manual work
Scars	1. Abdominal scar—appendix operation 2. Operation for septic thumb which had left a mark	1. Trunk missing 2. Terminal segment right thumb denuded of tissue; no scar on left thumb
Identifying peculiarity	Birth-marks (red patches) on right forearm near elbow	Skin and soft tissues removed from upper third of forearm, and lower two-thirds of front only
Size and shape of feet	Left shoe as evidence	Cast of left foot fitted shoe
Form of head and face	Two photographs in different positions	Outlines of photographs of skull in same positions fitted
Finger-prints	Numerous imprints from house at 2 Dalton Square	Positively identified as the finger-prints of both hands and palmar impressions of left hand
Breasts	Age 20, unmarried	Single breast, appearance and structure consistent

	Isabella Ruxton	Body No. 2—female
Age	34 years 7 months (October 3, 1935)	Certainly between 30 and 55. Probably between 35 and 45
Stature	5 ft 5 in. to 5 ft 6 in.	5 ft 3½ in. (without shoes)
Hair	Soft texture, mid-brown with patch of grey slightly to right of top of head	Scalp completely removed; a few adherent hairs light to medium brown. Eyelashes dark brown. Available body hair mid-brown
Eyes	Deep-set; grey-blue	Removed
Complexion	Fair	Ears, nose, lips, and skin of face removed
Teeth	Denture replacing three named teeth in gap which would show during life; old extraction of one other named tooth	Old extraction or loss of fifteen teeth, including the four named
Fingers and nails	Long fingers. Recognisable nails—bevelled, brittle, growing tight at corners, rounded at ends, regularly manicured	Terminal segments of all fingers removed
Legs and ankles	Thick ankles. Legs of same thickness from knees to ankles	Soft tissues removed from legs
Left foot	Inflamed bunion of left big toe	Hallux valgus of left foot; tissues removed over metatarso-phalangeal joint down to bone and joint opened. X-rays showed exostosis of head of metatarsal
Size and shape of feet	Left shoe as evidence	Cast of left foot fitted shoe
Nose	Bridge uneven	Removed, but bone and cartilage arched
Form of head and face	High forehead, high cheek-bones, rather long jaw. Two photographs in different positions	Corresponding features. Outlines of photographs of skull in same positions fitted
Breasts	Pendulous breasts : three children	Appearance and structure of pair of breasts consistent
Uterus	Three children	Separate uterus. Could not be assigned but structure consistent

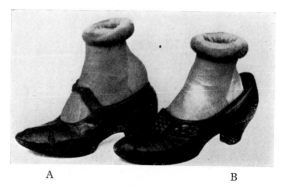

FIG. 24

The Feet and the Shoes. A, Flexible cast of Foot No. 2 in
Mary Rogerson's shoe. B, Flexible cast of Foot No. 1 in
Mrs Ruxton's shoe. It is obvious that neither foot fits the
shoe in which it has been placed

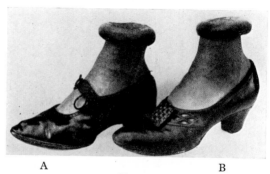

FIG. 25

The Feet and the Shoes. A, Foot No. 1 in Mary Rogerson's
shoe. B, Foot No. 2 in Mrs Ruxton's shoe. The fit of
each foot to the shoe in which it has been placed appears
to be perfect

The preliminary investigations before the trial were not limited to the
death of Mrs Christie, but included the deaths of three other women
found murdered in the same house and the identification of two female
skeletons recovered from the garden. As the case is a long and complicated one which introduces many lines of investigation connected
with the identification of human bodies, the reader is referred to the
publication by Camps.[21]

A very instructive case was that against Harry Dobkin in 1942; the
following were the facts. A demolition worker clearing debris, following bombing damage, found in a cellar of a chapel in Kennington Lane,
London, the remains of a woman partly covered by a paving stone.

Medical evidence was to the effect that the body, which had been cut up by someone without anatomical knowledge, had been dead for about twelve to fifteen months, that death had been due to strangulation, and that twenty-four points in the proof of identity had been discovered. Following dismemberment of the body the parts had been buried in lime, and these included the skull.   Apart from the assessment of sex, age, and stature, a dentist identified his fillings in the teeth of the upper jaw, the uterus showed a large fibroid, and inquiry at two London hospitals showed that Mrs Dobkin had been examined at their out-patient departments, had been diagnosed as suffering from a fibroid tumour of the uterus, and had refused operation.   Mrs Dobkin's dentist was satisfied that following extraction some buried roots of teeth were still present, and radiological examination of the jaw of the victim showed the roots in the expected position.   A photograph of the dead woman was superimposed on a photograph of the skull found in the cellar of the chapel and the superimpositions fitted.

Harry Dobkin was found guilty of the murder of his wife.

It is commonly and erroneously believed that quicklime accelerates the destruction of human remains.   Experiments have shown the contrary, namely, that lime, whether quick or slaked, has a definite preservative effect.

Occasionally portions of human remains are submitted to a medico-legal expert by the police for the purpose of determining whether or not a crime has been committed.   Frequently these are easily recognised as anatomical specimens and an opinion can be given immediately.   Some-times a very careful examination must be made and there may even be difficulty in deciding that the remains are human.

When in the course of demolition operations bones are found, these are usually submitted to the police who consult forensic pathologists. They expect the pathologist to be able to give an opinion as to the probable time of death.   This is one of the most difficult problems with which a forensic pathologist can be faced.   We have, from time to time, examined bones from graveyards when the time of interment was known and as a rule we have ventured to give opinions to the police based on this experience.   This is, however, at best an unsatisfactory procedure.   Bernard Knight[22] has made a valuable study of this problem.   He used five principal methods in arriving at an estimation:

the nitrogen content,
the amino acid content,
the benzidine reaction,
ultra-violet fluorescence,
the anti-human serum reaction.

Knight found that almost all samples of bone less than fifty years old showed a nitrogen content of more than 3·5 grams per cent.

If by the use of thin layer chromatography less than seven amino acids can be demonstrated, the bones are probably more than one hundred years old.

The precipitant test appears to be positive for about ten years. This however depends greatly on the technique and sera which are used.

Positive benzidine tests can persist up to about one hundred and fifty years.

Ultra-violet fluorescence of freshly cut limb bones persists throughout the bone up to a period of approximately one hundred years. From then on there is progressive loss from the periphery.

These methods of investigations are available to nearly all forensic pathologists and should be very helpful to them in solving this very difficult problem.

Hairs and fibres

Hairs. It may be necessary to examine specimens of hair removed from:

the head of victims of murder and assault,
the surfaces of vehicles involved in hit-and-run accidents,
the surfaces of weapons suspected of having been used for murder or assault,
the clothing and bodies of persons involved in sexual offences especially rape and bestiality,
the containers and vehicles involved in fur thefts.

A rather exceptional case was where a comparison was made, in a murder case, between short beard hairs found upon the cutting edges of a safety-razor blade, discovered among bracken, and three-day-old hairs shaved from the face and chin of the accused man while in custody. Gross and detailed structure of these specimens were so similar that they were consistent with a common source of origin.

As a result of macroscopic and microscopic examination it is possible to distinguish human hair from animal hairs and from fibres. Detailed examination of human hairs may indicate very strong probability that they have come from the same source. It is not, however, possible to identify an individual definitely by examination of hairs.

The examination of hairs should include the following particulars:

1. colour to naked eye and on microscopic examination.
2. length, ascertained by actual measurement.
3. texture.
4. approximate breadth by micrometer.
5. hair-tip or hair-end characters whether intact, cut or torn.
6. condition of bulb if present, whether forcibly pulled out, degenerated, or cut across by a sharp instrument or crushed by a blunt one.

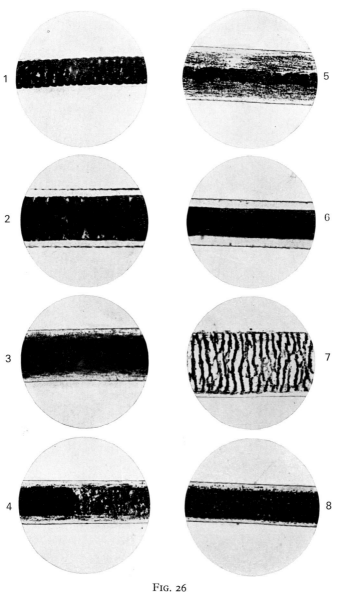

FIG. 26
Various hairs

1. Sheep	3. Goat	5. Horse	7. Rat
2. Cat	4. Dog	6. Cow	8. Rabbit

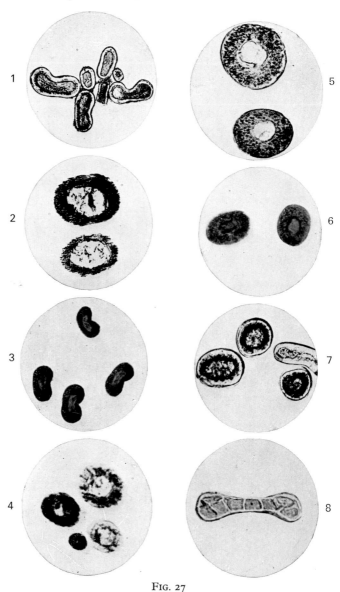

FIG. 27

Cross-sections of hairs

| 1. Squirrel | 3. Goat | 5. Horse | 7. Rat |
| 2. Cat | 4. Dog | 6. Cow | 8. Rabbit |

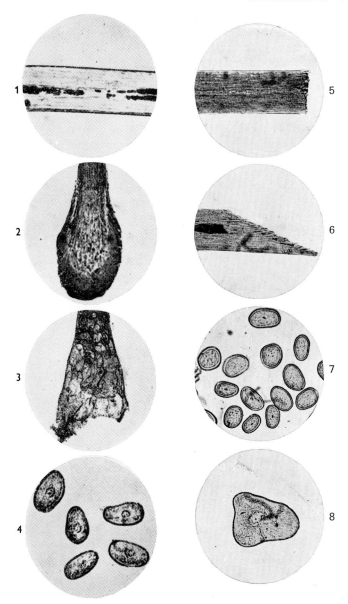

FIG. 28

Certain hair features

1. Grey hair
2. Healthy bulb
3. Degenerate bulb
4. Sections of pubic hair
5. Hair cut by sharp blade
6. Severed by blunt blade
7. Sections of head hair
8. Section of moustache hair

7. character of cuticle, extent and character of cortex, presence or absence of medulla and, if present, the character and breadth.
8. whether hairs are dyed or undyed.
9. contour of transverse sections in respect of points set down in (7).

Hairs from different parts of the human body sometimes present differentiating characteristics, as, for example, the hairs of moustache, eyebrow, eyelash, and pubic hair.

It should be possible to differentiate human from animal hairs. Examination of the structure of animal hairs shows that the pigment in

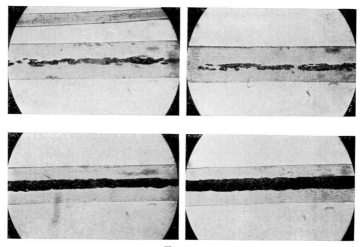

FIG. 29

Comparison of hairs adherent to a motor car (left), with those removed from the head of a person fatally injured (right)

the cortical layer is coarser, and the medulla broader and less regular. It is advisable to build up a collection of animal hairs, especially those of domestic animals, so that comparison with given specimens may be readily available.

The dyeing of hair is a common practice. Hair may be made darker or lighter. The number of different hair dyes and tinting materials available is innumerable, and a large variety of shades can be produced by their use. Alteration in the colour of hair may be effected in a variety of ways by the use of decolorants, vegetable dyes, dyes with a metallic base, or by synthetic organic dyes. Hydrogen peroxide is the most commonly employed decolorant, henna the most frequently used vegetable dye; and of the dyes with a metallic base, lead and bismuth form the bases in many instances. Of the synthetic organic dyes, phenylenediamine is the principal example, and serious cases of dermatitis together with toxic manifestations have been produced by its use (p. 532). The detection of hair dyes is important in some cases, and its presence is indicated usually by a lack of uniformity in the colour of the hair, which is often lacking in lustre and brittle in character. The natural colour of the more recently grown hair at the roots strikes a contrast with the shade of the remainder of the hair on the scalp, and

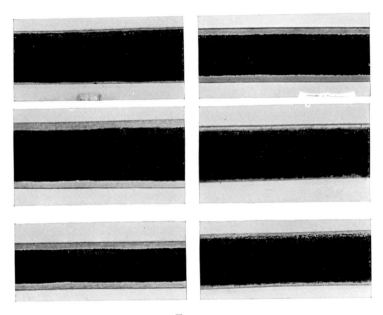

FIG. 30

Comparison of silver fox hairs. Top—Hairs from silver fox furs alleged to have been stolen. Middle and Bottom—Hairs found in cartons and sack thought to have contained the stolen furs (see Fig. 32)

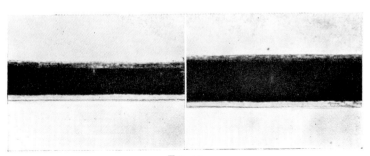

FIG. 31

Hair comparison in bestiality case. Left—Hair from clothing of accused man. Right—Hair from hind quarters of a mare

this is well demonstrated by the use of filtered ultra-violet light, when dyed hair appears lustreless and like tow.   The use of infra-red photo-micrography, especially when the hair has been dyed or bleached, is an

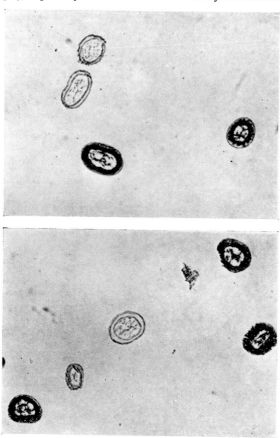

FIG. 32

Comparison of transverse sections of silver fox hairs.   Top—Hairs from furs alleged to have been stolen.   Bottom—Hairs from cartons thought to have contained the stolen furs (see Fig. 30)

important adjunct in the examination of hair.   Comparison of the colour of the hair on the head with that of the hair on other parts of the body will frequently indicate the presence or absence of dye in the former.   The scalp may occasionally show staining due to the dye which has been employed.   On applying appropriate chemical tests, the nature of many of the dyes commonly used can be detected.   A portion of the hair may be steeped in diluted nitric acid, and this will give a solution which can be tested by qualitative chemical methods.

On examining dyed hairs microscopically, the intimate structure appears hazy and shows a uniformity in general shade which is not seen in hairs of natural colour.   This haziness is more marked when the darker dyes have been employed, but when bleaching substances have been used, such as hydrogen peroxide, the substance of the hair shows a typical bleached appearance which differs from the character of natural white hairs.

Technique for the Preparation of Hairs for Microscopic Examination[23]

Preparation of specimens for examination in longitudinal plane

Prior to mounting the specimens, it is necessary to use some cleansing reagent to remove adherent debris which may mask structural detail. One of the most efficient consists of equal parts of ether and absolute alcohol.   The specimens should be placed in a small test tube with this solution and gently shaken.   The hairs are then removed from the tube and dried between sheets of filter-paper.   Before mounting, they should be steeped in a good quality benzol or oil of turpentine, which acts as a clearing agent.   After drying, the specimens are mounted preferably in Gurr's De Pex mounting medium, or Euparal, long cover-slips applied, and the slides allowed to stand for twenty-four to forty-eight hours, if time will permit, for clearing purposes.   By so treating the hairs, they become permanent specimens.   In some cases, debris adherent to human hairs may prove valuable by giving a hint as to the site of the body from which the hairs have come.   For example, the presence of sweat, vaginal or menstrual secretion, seminal fluid, faecal or food material, nasal secretion or cerumen, are important indications. It is therefore expedient to make a routine preliminary microscopical examination of the hairs before washing and finally mounting them.

Preparation of cross-sections of hairs

The following are the stages recommended:

1. Cleanse hairs in equal parts of ether and absolute alcohol.
2. Place in a solution of 2 per cent alcohol to which has been added an equal quantity of 5 per cent liquor ammonii fortis or ammonium hydrate.   Steep for five minutes.
3. Soak in 10 per cent potassium hydrate for one or two minutes. Maintain temperature at 50°C.
4. Wash specimens in a solution composed of equal parts of 5 per cent sulphuric acid and absolute alcohol for some minutes.
5. Wash in xylol or benzol for a few minutes.
6. Dry hairs between sheets of filter-paper.

7. Steep hairs in liquid paraffin-wax for fifteen minutes.
8. Block specimens in paraffin.
9. Cut sections about 8 to 10 μ in thickness.
10. Float sections on water at temperature of 40°C.
11. Place on albuminised slides and put in incubator at temperature of 37°C for twenty-four hours.
12. Dissolve paraffin-wax with xylol, dry slides, and add Gurr's De Pex mounting medium, or Euparal.

The objects of stages 1 to 5 are to cleanse, soften, and dehydrate the hairs; step 7, to ensure adherence of paraffin during blocking stage; step 10, to uncurl the sections; and step 11, to ensure adherence of the sections to the slides.

A variety of paraffin-waxes of different melting-points should be available in the ovens, since success lies in the selection of a wax of suitable melting-point, having regard to the thickness and consistency of the hairs to be sectioned. For general purposes a wax of melting-point at 52°C should prove satisfactory. During the various stages, the hairs are immersed in the form of a bundle. The bundle is made by binding the strands together at intervals with fine silk thread. When only a single hair is available, the various stages may be carried out in a watch-glass, and the specimen embedded by means of fine forceps.

Examination of fibres

Cotton. This is the seed hair of the genus *Gossypium*. When undyed, it has a whitish colour.

Flax. This is the bark of *Linum usitatissimum* and has either a grey or cream colour. When the fibres are damped, they curl or turn in a clockwise direction.

Hemp. This is the bark of *Cannabis sativa* and is creamy-white or grey. When the fibres are damped, they curl or turn in an anti-clockwise direction.

Jute. This is the bark of *Corchorus capsularis* or *Corchorus olitorius*. It is yellowish-brown or yellowish-white.

Manila hemp. This is made from the leaf of *Musa textilis* and is of light brown colour.

Sisal hemp. This is made from the leaf of the genus *Agave* and is of light yellow colour.

We have been requested to examine fibres in a large variety of cases,

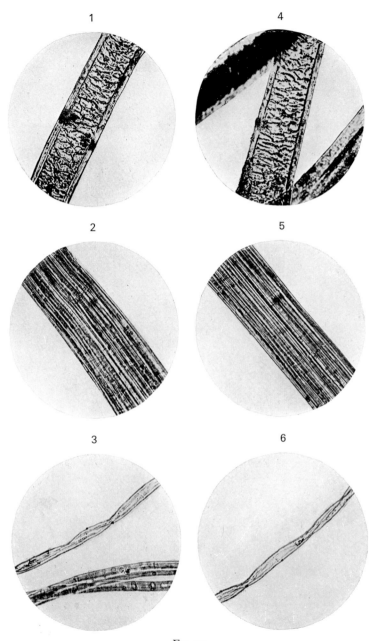

FIG. 33

Comparison of fibres

1. Fibre from large foot mat
2. Fibre from large rug
3. Fibres from large rug
4. Fibres on trousers worn by accused
5. Fibre on black sock worn by accused
6. Fibre from under surface of heel of right boot worn by accused

Characters and Identification of Fibres

Cotton	Flax	Hemp	Manila hemp	Jute	Wool	Silk	Linen
Flattened, twisted fibres with thickened edges. Irregularly granulated cuticle. Blunt apex. No transverse markings. Fibres show a spiral twist. Fibres swell in a solution composed of copper sulphate and sodium carbonate dissolved in ammonia. Insoluble in strong sodium hydroxide, but soluble in strong sulphuric acid and partially soluble in hot, strong hydrochloric acid.	Apex tapers to fine point. Transverse sections are polygonal, and show a small cavity. The fibres consist of cellulose and give blue or bluish-red colour when treated with a weak solution of potassium iodide saturated in iodine and sulphuric acid. The fibres, which show transverse lines and are usually seen in grouped formation, dissolve in a solution composed of copper sulphate and sodium carbonate in ammonia.	Fibres show transverse lines and consist of cellulose. Large oval cavities seen in transverse sections. Ends usually blunt, and there is often a tuft of hair at the knots. Stain bluish-red with phloroglucine and yellow with both aniline sulphate and a weak solution of potassium iodide saturated with iodine and sulphuric acid.	Fibres are smooth without transverse or longitudinal marking. The cavities are large and uniform. The walls are lignified. The tips are fine-pointed.	Fibres are quite smooth without either longitudinal or transverse marking. The fibre has a typical, large cavity, which is not uniform in size, but varies with the degree of contraction of the walls of the fibres which are lignified. The ends are blunt. The fibres are stained red with phloroglucine and yellow with aniline sulphate, also with iodine and sulphuric acid.	These fibres can easily be distinguished from vegetable fibres, since the former show an outer layer of flattened cells and imbricated margins. The interiors are composed of fibrous tissue, but sometimes the medulla is present. They do not dissolve in a solution composed of copper sulphate, sodium carbonate and ammonia. Stain yellow with iodine and sulphuric acid, also with picric acid. Do not dissolve in sulphuric acid. Smell of singeing on burning.	Manufactured silk is almost structureless, microscopically. Fibres stain brown with iodine and sulphuric acid, yellow with picric acid. They dissolve in sulphuric acid, but dissolve slowly in a mixture of copper sulphate, sodium carbonate and ammonia.	Fibres are straight and taper to a point. Cortical area shows transverse lines which frequently intersect, simulating a jointed appearance. The medullary region shows a thin, dense line. They do not dissolve in concentrated sulphuric acid. If placed in 1 per cent alcoholic solution of fuchsin and then in a solution of ammonium hydroxide, they assume a bright red colour.

for example, in cases of burglary, when fibres from the garments of accused persons have been found adherent to the surfaces of broken windows, or when incriminating fibres have been discovered upon, or close to, safes which have been blown, and also in cases of fatal motor car accidents, in connection with cars thought to have been involved. In one case a bundle of fibres, similar to those composing a carpet at the scene of a burglary, was found embedded in debris attached to the heel of footwear worn by a man accused of the burglary (see Fig. 33).

When making an examination of fibres, it is advisable to examine them after bleaching, in addition to examining them in their natural state, since detail, masked by colour, may then be seen clearly. For the purpose of bleaching, only a portion of the fibres should be utilised, and hydrogen peroxide or, preferably, a solution composed of equal parts of bleaching powder and sodium carbonate dissolved in water should be used.

The table on p. 110 may be found useful in the identification of various fibres.[24]

References

1. *Signaletic Instructions*, American ed., 1896, trans. McClaughry.
2. HENRY. *Classfication and Uses of Finger-prints.* 1928.
3. GLAISTER, J. & BRASH, J.C. *Medico-legal Aspects of the Ruxton Case.* Edinburgh: Livingstone, 1937.
4. *British Medical Journal*, **1**, 343, 1906.
5. *Medico-legal Review*, **13**, pt II, 99, 1945. Also *British Dental Journal*, **78**, 76, 1945.
6. BERGMAN, B. *J. Pediat.*, **31**, 142, 1947.
7. KERR, W.L. *Br. med. J.*, **2**, 620, 1937.
8. FLECKER, H. *J. Anat.*, **67**, 118, 1932.
9. See Reference No. 3.
10. FRANCHINI. *Boll. Soc. ital. Biol. sper.*, **22**, 151, 1946.
11. FAWCETT, E. *J. Anat.*, **72**, 633, 1938.
12. ASHLEY, G.T. *J. forens. Med.*, **3**, 27, 1956.
13. *Philosophical Transactions of the Royal Society*, **189**, 1935, 1897.
14. PEARSON & BELL. *A Study of the Long Bones of the English Skeleton,* Part I, *The Femur.* Drapers' Company Research Memoirs. Cambridge University Press, 1919.
15. DWIGHT, T. *Am. J. Anat.*, **4**, 19, 1905.
16. PEARSON, K. *Phil. Trans. R. Soc., A.*, **192**, 169, 1899.
17. DUPERTUIS, C.W. & HADDEN, J.A. *Am. J. phys. Anthrop.*, N.S. **9**, 15, 1951.
18. TROTTER, M. & GLESER, G. *Am. J. phys. Anthrop.*, N.S. **10**, 463, 1952.
19. See Reference No. 3.
20. *Trial of J. G. Haigh. Notable British Trials.* Edinburgh: Hodge, 1953.
21. CAMPS, F.E. *Medical and Scientific Investigations in the Christie Case.* London: Medical Publications Ltd, 1953.
22. KNIGHT, B. *Medicine Sci. Law*, **9**, No. 4, 1969.
23. SMITH, S. & GLAISTER, J. *Recent Advances in Forensic Medicine.* London: Churchill, 1938.

24. Additional information can be obtained from: LUCAS, A.: *Forensic Chemistry*. London: Arnold, 1946. WILDMAN: *Animal Fibres of Industrial Importance: Their Origin and Identification*. Wool Industries Research Association, 1939. VON BERGEN & KRAUSS: *Textile Fibre Atlas*. New York: American Wool Handbook Company, 1942.

Chapter 4

THE MEDICO-LEGAL ASPECTS OF DEATH

DEATH may be defined as complete and persistent cessation of respiration and circulation. This simple statement would have been considered to be an adequate definition throughout the period when the previous twelve editions of this book have been in existence. Recently, however, developments in medicine have complicated the picture. The two main factors are:

1. The widespread use of strong hypnotic and tranquillising drugs. They can produce states where although the definition is still relevant it becomes extremely difficult to tell whether respiration and circulation have ceased. There have been a number of cases in recent years when bodies of people who have been examined by qualified medical practitioners, sometimes in hospitals, have been transported to mortuaries where they have been found to be alive by the mortuary attendants. This gives the profession a bad image and should be avoidable. We have personal knowledge of a case where the mortuary attendant thought that a woman, who had been sent to the mortuary after having been examined by a doctor in a large teaching hospital and declared dead, was still alive; he instituted resuscitative measures, the woman was returned to hospital and survived. There is rarely much difficulty in diagnosing death in the terminal stages of an illness in which the doctor has been in attendance. The difficulty arises when a doctor is confronted for the first time with an apparently completely non-reacting body whose condition may be due to illness or the deep coma produced by drug overdosage or death. In these cases a rapid decision should not be made and certainly the examination should not be done in an ambulance or under any conditions where there is inadequate light and space.

SIGNS OF DEATH

A doctor would be justified in stating that death has occurred if the following signs of death were present:

   (i) Cessation of heart beat (auscultation over five-minute period).
   (ii) Cessation of respiration (observation over ten-minute period).
   (iii) Skin pallor on parts of the body, other than dependant parts, due to cessation of circulation. In cases of death due to drowning and exposure, exposed parts of the body may remain pink long after the cessation of circulation.

   (iv) Loss of corneal reflex (also lost in deep coma).

   (v) Clouding of cornea, when eyes assume a glazed appearance.

   (vi) Pupil light reflex abolished (pupil reacts to atropine (dilatation) and physostigmine (contraction) for one hour after death).

   (vii) Tone of the eyeball reduced.

   (viii) Fragmentation and stasis of blood in the retinal vessels ('cattle trucking'). Seen on ophthalmoscopy. May occur in leukaemia during life.

2. The second modern factor which has made the old definition inadequate is the development of advanced resuscitative techniques by which the circulation and respiration are maintained by machines. The need for a more specific definition of death has been made all the more necessary by the requirements of the transplant surgeons.

Shapiro[1] has defined death as the irreversible loss of the properties of living matter and he made a definite distinction between the properties of the whole person and those of his component parts. He holds that when the properties of the whole patient are irreversibly lost the patient is legally dead and there can be no objection to the preservation and removal of the properties of living matter in the component parts. If the transplantation of organs is to continue the medical profession will require to operate under a definition of this kind. We are still left with the decision as to when the properties of the whole patient are irreversibly lost and it is about this that there may be differences of opinion.

Anyone who considers that it is always easy to arrive at a decision as to when irreversible changes have taken place should read the account of the revival of a boy who had been under water for twenty minutes and suffered apparently irreversible changes and yet survived with complete recovery.[2]

CHANGES AFTER DEATH

1. Cooling of the Body

After death heat production ceases and the loss of heat is continuous until the body reaches the environmental temperature. The actual temperature of the body at any time after death and the rate of cooling depend on a variety of factors which may or may not be determinable and will be discussed in detail in the section concerned with timing of death.

2. Hypostasis or Post-mortem Lividity

This condition may be observed on all bodies irrespective of cause of death. It is seen, although with difficulty, even in deaths from haemorrhage.

Hypostasis is due to the engorgement of the capillaries by gravitation of the blood. It occurs in the dependent parts of the body other than those exposed to pressure caused by collars, constriction by waistbands garters, or corsets, or contact with the surface on which the body lies. The absence of hypostasis in these areas is due to occlusion of the capillaries.

Hypostasis affects also the internal organs, and it is seen in the case of a body left on its back, on the posterior parts of the lungs, the posterior wall of the stomach, the lowermost parts of the intestinal tract, and the kidneys. This can be confused with pathological conditions.

In medico-legal work, especially in cases where there are marks of violence, the incidence of hypostasis must be carefully noted. It can indicate the position in which a body has lain, and sometimes movement of the body. It must be differentiated from bruising. This is done by incising the tissues in the area of discolouring. Bruises will then show blood extravasated in the cutaneous and subcutaneous tissues, whereas hypostasis will be seen as discrete points of blood oozing from capillaries. In all cases where violence is suspected, tissue sections should be examined microscopically (p. 32).

3. General Muscular Flaccidity of the Body

In this condition there is complete relaxation of the muscles for two to three hours after death. Contact flattening of the muscles occurs. The soft, convex portions of the body, for example, the buttocks and calves, which lie on contact with the hard surface, become flattened with pressure and lose their convexity. Alterations in the position of a body after death may be indicated by the presence of areas of contact flattening on parts of the body which no longer lie in contact with a solid surface (Fig. 34).

4. Rigor Mortis

The condition of general muscular flaccidity of the body is replaced by a progressive rigidity which affects the muscular system and includes both the voluntary and involuntary muscles of bodies of all ages.

Szent-Györgyi[3] has investigated the chemistry of muscular contraction. He is of the opinion that one of the principal factors concerned in the maintenance of suppleness and plasticity of muscle is the degree of hydration of the protein. This in turn is dependent on the amount of adenosine triphosphate which is adsorbed in the myosin of the muscle. After death, the adenosine triphosphate is gradually decomposed, dehydration takes place and this results in the condition known

as rigor mortis.   The subsequent relaxation is due to the final dis-
organisation of muscle.

The earliest manifestations of rigor mortis will be found in the muscles
of the eyelids and those of the lower jaw.   Rigidity of the eyelids usually
precedes that of the jaw muscles, which are affected in about three to
four hours after death.   The rigidity next appears progressively in the
muscles of the neck, the face, the thorax, the upper extremities, the
trunk of the body, and the muscles of the lower extremities.   Rigor

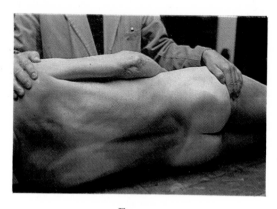

FIG. 34

Hypostasis, or post-mortem staining, and areas of contact flattening

mortis brings about slight shortening of the muscle fibres.   The
muscles in which rigor mortis first appears are those from which it
usually first disappears.   Rigor also affects the involuntary muscles, and
might be mistaken for hypertrophy, for example, in the instance of the
heart.   It is probable that the chemical changes described by Szent-
Györgyi as responsible for the rigidity are progressing simultaneously
throughout the various parts of the body although the manifestations
tend to occur in the sequence described, the sequence being determined
by the muscle bulk involved.

The period of invasion can be stated only in broad terms, since there
are so many modifying factors.   As a rule, general stiffening will be
established after ten to twelve hours, although in some cases the period
may be shorter.

When rigor is established, the jaw, neck, and extremities become
fixed in position, and movements at the joints are possible only within
a very limited degree unless the rigidity of muscle is overcome by effort.
When force has been used in this way, the rigidity of muscle does not
subsequently recur.   In the majority of cases, rigor will have commenced to pass off in about thirty-six hours, but, in cold weather and
for other reasons, a much longer interval may elapse.

Under certain circumstances, however, rigor mortis may appear unusually early, or its appearance may be considerably retarded. The stronger muscularly the person is at the time of death, the later is the time of onset, and the longer the duration. The more feeble or exhausted the muscular condition, the more rapid is the time of onset, and the shorter the duration. In long-continued, febrile and chronic diseases, and in some convulsive disorders, for example, status epilepticus and strychnine poisoning, this may be the case. It is accelerated by gross violence or exertion shortly before death.

If a body, already the subject of newly established rigidity, is exposed to a temperature of 75°C., the rigidity becomes more pronounced, since the albuminates in the muscles become coagulated. If, on the other hand, a body is exposed immediately after death to a temperature at, or below, freezing-point, the onset of rigor mortis is retarded so long as this temperature continues. When the temperature is gradually elevated to 10°C., or 50°F., rigor comes on rapidly, but disappears more quickly than had the body not been subjected to such a condition.

Conditions simulating rigor mortis. Heat stiffening occurs in bodies exposed to intense heat by burning, or immersion in hot liquids, and is due to coagulation of the albuminates in the muscles. Rigor mortis does not supervene in such cases, and the primary rigidity persists until the onset of putrefaction. When heat stiffening affects a body, the position of the limbs simulates the general attitude of a boxer, and to this condition the term 'pugilistic attitude' has been aptly applied (p. 215).

Stiffening of the body as the result of exposure to cold may simulate rigor mortis. When the general stiffness of the body is due to freezing, passive flexion of the joints may be accompanied by faint crepitant sounds due to the fragmentation of the frozen synovial fluids. When the body thaws, this stiffening passes off, and true rigor may become established unless it has previously supervened (p. 230).

Instantaneous rigor or cadaveric spasm

This condition is of considerable medico-legal importance, and is unconnected with rigor mortis. It occurs at the moment of death, and the muscles of the hand are most usually affected. We have seen it several times in cases of suicidal cut-throat, and suicidal shooting, when the weapon was so firmly grasped in the hand that considerable force was required to disengage it. In cases of drowning, the finding of articles grasped firmly in the hands of the victims is not unusual. This condition is due initially to a voluntary vital act, probably accompanied by a high degree of emotion, immediately preceding death.

A full explanation of this condition has yet to be ascertained. That it is not simply an unusually early local onset of ordinary rigor mortis seems clear, since the muscles involved do not share in the general primary flaccidity of the muscular system, else the weapon would fall out of the hand, or the postural attitude of the body would be lost.   The condition of the nervous system at the time of death would appear to play an important part.   Cadaveric spasm may affect only certain groups of muscles, or all the muscles, of a limb or limbs.

When a weapon, or other article, is found firmly clutched in the hand of a dead person, it is proof that it was in the hand of the person during life, and that the grasp occurred at, or about, the moment of death (see Fig. 35).   Nothing can simulate instantaneous rigor, or cadaveric spasm, and it cannot be produced by any method after death.   Personal experiments have been unsuccessful.

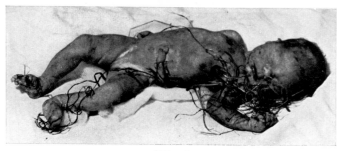

FIG. 35

An unusual case of instantaneous rigor, or cadaveric spasm, in a newly born child who died from the effects of incomplete respiration.   Note the grass tightly grasped in the left hand.   Birth occurred in the open

5. CONDITION OF CADAVERIC BLOOD

Considerable attention has been given to this subject by Yudin.[4]   In a review of 500 cases he found that when a person died from a severe disease, for example, cancer, tuberculosis, or sepsis or trauma with prolonged shock, the blood formed coagulum that could not be dissolved, remaining firm until putrefaction.   On the other hand, when death had been sudden, whether due to severe acute trauma, such as concussion, suffocation, or electrocution, or following a short attack of angina pectoris, or apoplexy, then the blood quickly coagulated into ordinary clot, but, within a quarter to one and a half hours, dissolution of the clot took place with liquefaction.   This has been confirmed by our own experience.

6. PUTREFACTION

This follows rigor mortis and is manifested by gradual loss of rigidity in the muscles: this is frequently termed secondary flaccidity.

Putrefaction is the last stage in the resolution of the body from the organic to the inorganic state.

The factors responsible for the process of putrefaction are micro-organisms, the action of warmth, the presence of air, and the presence of moisture.

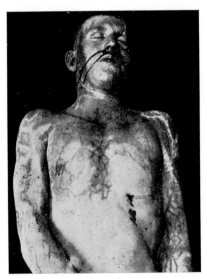

FIG. 36

Discoloration of superficial veins due to
putrefactive changes

The organisms chiefly responsible are *B. coli*, Staphylococcus, non-haemolytic Streptococcus, *Streptococcus viridans*, *Cl. welchii*, diphtheroid and proteus types. The most commonly found are the commensals of the respiratory and alimentary tract.

External signs of putrefaction

The following summary indicates the usual progress of putrefaction.

Greenish coloration over the right iliac fossa.

Extension of greenish colour over the whole of the abdomen, and other parts of the body.

Discoloration and swelling of the face.

G M J—I*

Swelling and discoloration of the scrotum, or of the vulva.

Distension of the abdomen with gases.

Brownish coloration of the surface veins giving an arborescent pattern on the skin.

Development of bullae, of varying size, on the surfaces.

Bursting of bullae, and denudation of large irregular surfaces due to the shedding of epidermis.

Escape of blood-stained fluid from the mouth and nostrils.

Liquefaction of the eyeballs.

Increasing discoloration of the body generally, and greater and progressive abdominal distension.

Presence of maggots.

Shedding of the nails, and loosening of the hair.

Facial features unrecognisable.

Conversion of tissues into a semi-fluid mass.

Bursting open of the abdominal and thoracic cavities.

Progressive dissolution of the body.

The evolution of gases of putrefaction, for example, sulphuretted hydrogen, phosphoretted hydrogen, and ammonia, together with the liquefaction of the tissues, are the responsible factors in the rupture of the natural cavities of the body.

The colour changes seen on the body surfaces result from blood changes due to bacterial action.

Putrefaction of internal organs

With regard to putrefaction of the organs, these may be divided into two classes:

(A) Those which putrefy early.
(B) Those which putrefy late.

(A) Brain.
    Lining of trachea and larynx.
    Stomach and intestines.
    Spleen.
    Liver.
    Uterus (pregnant or in puerperal state).

(B) Oesophagus.
    Diaphragm.
    Heart.
    Lungs.
    Kidneys.
    Urinary bladder.
    Uterus.
    Prostate gland.

The organs composed of muscular tissue resist putrefaction longer than the parenchymatous organs, with the exception of the stomach and intestines, which, by reason of their contents at the time of death, may decompose quickly. The rate of the process also depends, in some measure, upon the amount of fibrous tissue which an organ contains.

Wide variations in the order of putrefaction are frequently met, and the specific factors present in each case must be the subject of special consideration.

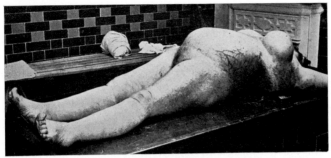

FIG. 37

Distension of abdominal cavity and breasts due to the formation of putrefactive gases

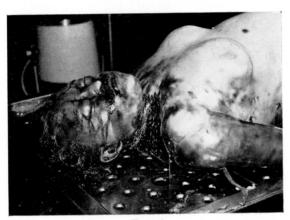

FIG. 38

Putrefactive changes affecting the face

Factors which modify rate of putrefaction

These may be divided into:

External factors.
Internal factors.

External.   The principal external factors are:

Presence or absence of micro-organisms;
Presence or absence of air;
Temperature of the environment;

Presence or absence of moisture;
Character of medium in which the body lies.

Presence or absence of micro-organisms and air.   The presence of air promotes, and its absence retards, decomposition.   Under uniform circumstances, a nude body will decompose more rapidly than one which is clothed.   Porous, light soils accelerate decomposition, while clayey, dense, or water-logged soils retard it.

Occasionally bodies show unusually rapid external manifestations of decomposition characterised by a bloated and swollen state of the skin and underlying tissues of an emphysematous nature.   We have quite frequently isolated *Cl. welchii* in such cases.

Temperature of environment.   Putrefaction begins at about 50°F., and is most favoured by temperatures ranging from 70° to 100°F. The process is retarded by temperatures between 100° and 212°F. since the fluids are dried up, and there is a probability of mummification of the body tissues.   Bacterial development is retarded at extremes of temperature (p. 129).

Presence or absence of moisture.   Moisture is essential for decomposition of an animal substance, and normally the body contains sufficient for the process.   Additional moisture, however, may aid the rapidity of the action.   This is one of the reasons why bodies decompose more quickly in water than in the earth.   If warmth is added, the rate of decomposition is much accelerated.

Type of medium in which the body lies.   These media are three in number: air, earth, and water.   It may be accepted as a general principle that a body decomposes in air twice as quickly as in water, and eight times as rapidly as in earth.   Putrefaction develops rapidly in bodies lying in sewage-polluted water.

Bodies retrieved from water after lengthy immersion very frequently show advanced putrefactive changes involving the face, neck, and chest. This is probably due to exposure of these parts to the air after flotation (Fig 37).

Internal.   The following are the principal factors:

Age;
Sex;
Condition of body at death;
Nature of death.

Age.   Usually the bodies of very old persons do not putrefy rapidly on account of the relative absence of fat.

Sex.   This has but little influence, except in the case of bodies of women dying after child-birth, more especially when death has been caused by septicaemia.   In such cases putrefaction is rapid.

Condition of body at death.   The physical state of a body influences the rapidity of putrefaction to some extent.   Fat, flabby subjects putrefy more quickly than lean bodies, doubtless due to the larger amount of fluid in the tissues and the presence of an excess of fat.

Nature of death.   Bodies of persons dying suddenly in apparent health decompose less quickly than those of persons dying from acute or chronic diseases, especially infective diseases.   Mutilation of tissue favours decomposition on account of the larger area exposed to bacteria. In death resulting from chronic poisoning, and in those who have died from poisoning by such substances as carbolic acid, arsenic, antimony, and chloride of zinc, putrefaction is resisted longer, owing to the preservative action of such substances on the tissues, or to their destructive, or inhibitive, action on the organisms which induce decomposition.

MAGGOTS

Identification[5]

In certain cases, with a view to checking the accuracy of the estimate of time between death and the examination of the remains, identification of maggots found on a putrefied body may prove of value, since having identified them it becomes possible to determine the age reached in the cycle of their development.   By this means, an estimate of the time which has elapsed since the eggs of the flies were deposited on the remains becomes possible within fairly accurate limits.   It is, however, necessary for the examiner to have knowledge of the life histories of the various maggots, and for this reason the examination should be left to an entomologist.   It would be out of place to deal with this subject in great detail in a book of this description, but it is felt that the life histories of certain of the muscid larvae may usefully be included.

Life histories of three types

The common blue-bottle (*Calliphora erythrocephala*).   The eggs are laid readily on meat when it is fresh—less commonly when it is decayed.   The maximum number of eggs laid by a single adult fly is generally 2,000.   They are deposited in groups of about 150, and hatch in from eight to fourteen hours, depending upon the temperature of the environment.   Bodies which have lain exposed after immersion in organically polluted waters may retain surface residues which encourage female Calliphorines to deposit eggs (Fig. 39).   Cold weather delays hatching.   The first larval instar (stage in the life history between two successive castings of the cuticle or outer skin) persists for eight to fourteen hours.   The skin is then shed and the second larval instar, similar to the first although larger, appears.   It persists for two to three days. The third instar is the fully grown maggot, which feeds voraciously for six days.   The larva, now creamy white, migrates during the night to some distance from its food and burrows into the soil,

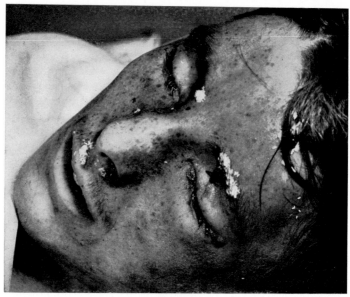

FIG. 39

Body recovered from the sea probably seven to ten days after death.   Calliphorine eggs were deposited, as shown, after body had been in mortuary for twenty-four hours.   Note presence of fly on left eyebrow

(By courtesy of the late Dr Robert Richards, Aberdeen University)

where it pupates.   Owing to the possession by the larvae of a liquefactive ferment, meat parasitised by them rapidly becomes putrid and for this reason, should the infestation be heavy, a body is more advanced in putrefaction than it would normally be.   The pupal stage lasts approximately twelve days.   Calliphorine flies are found from early spring until late autumn.

The green-bottle (*Lucilia caesar*) **and the sheep maggot fly** (*L. sericata*).   These flies, which have a bright metallic lustre, show a life history similar in all respects to that of *Calliphora*.   Their larvae may also invade wounds (myiasis).

The common house-fly (*Musca domestica*).   The female lays about 150 eggs at a time, mainly in manurial matter.   Oviposition on dead bodies is rare.   The eggs hatch in eight to twelve hours, and the first larval stage lasts thirty-six hours.   The second instar persists for one to two days, and the final for three to four days, depending on food, moisture, and temperature.   The pupal stage usually lasts seven days, or less during warm weather.   The full-grown third larva migrates, usually at night, and burrows into the soil to pupate.

Differentiation between the three types

The larva of *Musca* is distinguished from those of *Calliphora* and *Lucilia* by mounting on a slide the thinnest possible section, removed

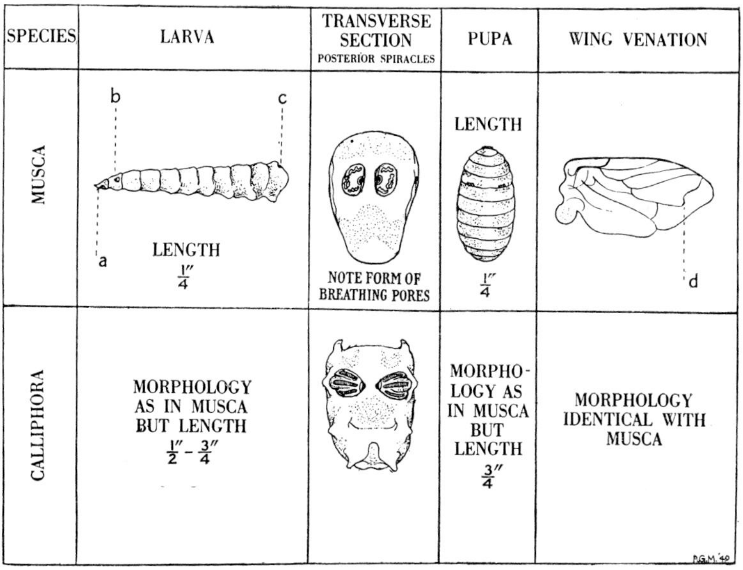

SPECIES	LARVA	TRANSVERSE SECTION POSTERIOR SPIRACLES	PUPA	WING VENATION
MUSCA	b c a LENGTH $\frac{1''}{4}$	NOTE FORM OF BREATHING PORES	LENGTH $\frac{1''}{4}$	d
CALLIPHORA	MORPHOLOGY AS IN MUSCA BUT LENGTH $\frac{1''}{2} - \frac{3''}{4}$		MORPHO-LOGY AS IN MUSCA BUT LENGTH $\frac{3''}{4}$	MORPHOLOGY IDENTICAL WITH MUSCA

FIG. 40

Musca and *Calliphora*.   Differential taxonomic characters

(*a*) Jaw hook.
(*b*) Position of anterior spiracle.
(*c*) Position of posterior spiracle.
(*d*) Characteristic angling of median vein.

from the posterior end of an alcohol-hardened specimen by means of a safety-razor blade, and examining the stigmata or breathing pores with the $\frac{2}{3}$-inch lens.   The contained spiracles are convoluted in *Musca* but straight in *Calliphora* (Fig. 40).

In order to differentiate between the maggots of *Calliphora* and *Lucilia*, it is necessary to examine the anterior end of the specially prepared larva microscopically.   The mandibular sclerite or jaw-hook

(Fig. 40) of *Calliphora* has an internal horizontal process not present in *Lucilia*.

In the Ruxton case, the maggots which infested the remains were identified as those of *Calliphora*, and the estimation of the time since deposit of Calliphorine eggs was as follows:

Stage				Time (outside limit)
Egg .	.	.	.	8 to 14 hours
1st larva	.	.	.	8 ,, 14 ,,
2nd ,,	.	.	.	2 ,, 3 days
3rd ,,	.	.	.	7 ,, 8 ,,
Total	.	.	.	10 ,, 12 ,, (approx.)

The total life of the largest larvae could not have exceeded twelve days, but was probably less. It was unlikely that the eggs had been laid more than a day or two after the deposit of the remains in the linn. The possibility of a laying of eggs by the progeny of the first generation of blue-bottles could be disregarded. That would have required a month, which was quite irreconcilable with the stage of putrefaction of the remains.

The stage of development of the larvae was compatible with the remains having been deposited in the linn about twelve to fourteen days before their examination on October 1. The result of this line of investigation not only corroborated the opinion expressed on other grounds but fitted the hypothesis of the prosecution that the parts of the bodies had probably been placed in the ravine during the early hours of the morning of September 16, 1935 (p. 90). Confirmation of the time of death has similarly been obtained in more recent cases.

Specimens of larvae intended for laboratory examination should be dropped alive into boiling absolute alcohol which kills them instantaneously in the extended state. Several should then be transmitted to the laboratory in a spirit-proof container charged with 50 per cent alcohol.

SAPONIFICATION AND MUMMIFICATION

Putrefaction of the body may be modified in its progress, and in the character of the products formed.

The two principal modifications are:

Saponification.
Mummification.

Saponification

A body upon which moisture has been constantly acting, whether it is immersed in water or in damp soil, may undergo this change.

The cause of saponification is the change of the fatty constituents of the body into new chemical compounds, more or less stable in composition, and the process is brought about by the gradual hydrogenation of pre-existing fats in the body to form higher fatty acids. Adipocere, the term applied to the material resulting from the process of saponification, is a fatty-looking substance which varies in colour from white to yellowish-white, imparts an unctuous feeling to the fingers, melts on heating, burns with a feebly luminant flame, and has a faint mouldy, cheesy odour.

Adipocere in mature form is largely composed of palmitic, stearic, oleic, and hydroxystearic acids. Calcium soaps, proteins, and some other constituents are variable incidental components.

It is not usual for the entire body to be converted into adipocere, although instances have been quite frequently seen (Fig. 41). More generally, the limbs, chest wall, buttocks, or other parts of the body

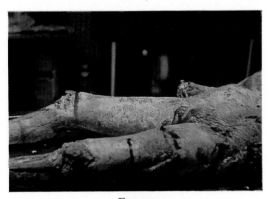

FIG. 41
Adipocere formation

may become saponified. When the face is the seat of this process, the features are well preserved, and when the entire body is involved, the form and contours are well retained.

The change of tissues into adipocere takes a considerable time in temperate climates, but its development in warm climates is much more rapid. It takes several months to effect the change even in limited parts of the body. The process, however, is more rapid in the bodies of infants and young children than in those of adults. Occasional cases of early production of adipocere have been recorded.[6] It is not possible to prescribe any specified time in which adipocere will be produced, on account of variable operative factors.

The necessary conditions for the production of adipocere are a super-

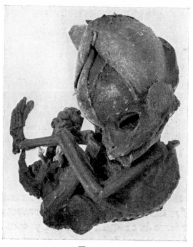

FIG. 42

Mummified fetus found behind a
kitchen fireplace

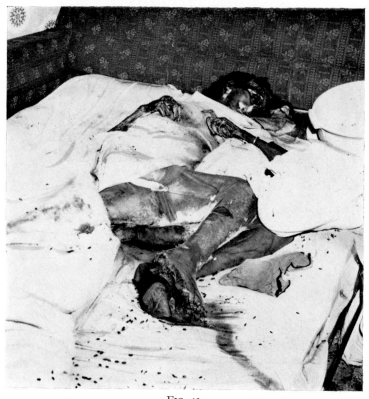

FIG. 43

Mummification—appearance of woman found in bed.
She had been dead for a year.

abundance of moisture and a relative diminution of air and micro-organisms. A warm temperature is a further facilitating factor.

Mummification

This is a common result following embalming in which artificial measures are employed (see p. 37), but in temperate climates it occurs naturally only under certain circumstances.

The factors necessary for the production of mummification are the absence of dampness and the continuous action of a current of dry or warmed air. Dehydration commences before putrefactive changes.

The appearance of a mummified body is quite typical. The whole structure is desiccated, shrivelled, brownish-black in colour, and the anatomical features are well preserved. It is first seen in the fingers, toes, lips, and point of the nose. The skin, which clings closely to the shrunken framework of the body, the hair on the scalp and the

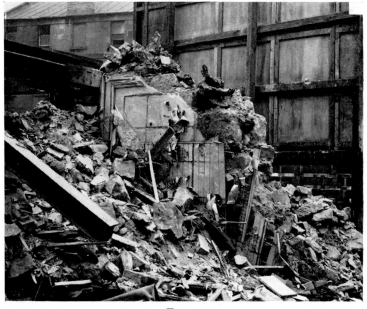

FIG. 44
Dead man's hand protruding from rubble.

FIGS. 44 and 45
The body of a man was found in the chimney of a house undergoing demolition. It was estimated that he had been dead for 50 years. This was based on the finding of a cigarette packet in his pocket, a brand of cigarette which had not been manufactured for 50 years.

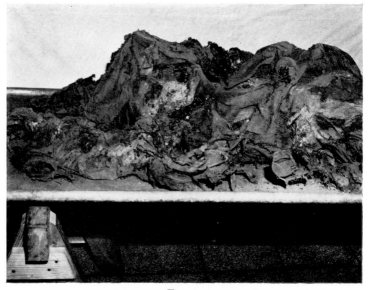

FIG. 45

Mummified body removed from building. His face can be seen in centre of the photograph.

skeletonised features of the face are well preserved.   With its contraction down on to the bony prominences of the face, there is a resultant
Mongolian appearance.   The skin is like leather and a stout knife is
required to deal with it.   A body in this condition is practically
odourless.

Cases are more numerous in the tropics and sub-tropics.   The
mummified bodies of infants are occasionally found in unusual places
of concealment which favour the production of this process, for example,
in drystone walls, suitcases, trunks, and at the back of fireplaces.

Forbes[7] has reported a case of mummified twins found in a 'false
roof' under the slates of a house.   The bodies had probably been
concealed there for a period of from fourteen to seventeen years.   The
skin had entirely disappeared, and the soft tissues were riddled with
roughly circular holes which led into burrows filled with moth eggs and
excreta of moths.   The type of moth responsible for the larvae was the
brown house or false clothes moth—*Borkhausenia pseudospretella*.   The
larvae of this moth eat furs, skins, and dried specimens of animals and
birds.   He states that given time, the soft tissues of the bodies would
probably have completely disappeared.   Larvae were present in the

abdominal, thoracic, and cranial cavities.   No traces of fly infestation were found in the bodies.

TIMING OF DEATH

This is an important function of the medico-legal examiner.   In the course of a murder investigation, evidence of the time of death usually becomes available which is more factually based and usually more accurate than the estimation of the medico-legal examiner.   Nevertheless the police are always anxious as soon as possible after the finding of a body to have an estimate of how long it has been dead and they expect the forensic pathologist to be able to supply them with this information.

The first thing to recognise is that an estimate based merely on the changes in the body after death is liable to serious error.   This does not mean that on occasions forensic pathologists cannot in fact produce a very accurate answer, but when they do, there is an element of inspired guesswork.   After all Jung wrote of Columbus that 'using subjective assumptions, a false hypothesis and a route abandoned by modern navigation, nevertheless [he] discovered America'.

Frequently general practitioners are first on the scene of crime and have the best opportunity of making an estimate of the time of death and it is important that they should be familiar with the factors to be considered.   These are:

> Cooling.
> Hypostasis.
> Rigor mortis.
> Putrefaction.

Cooling

After death heat production ceases and heat loss is continuous, the rapidity of the loss being dependent upon many circumstances, one of the most important being the difference between body and environmental temperatures.   During a period of a few hours following death, but not necessarily during the immediate post-mortem period, the temperature falls comparatively quickly, but later more slowly, the nearer it approaches the environmental temperature.

The principal factors affecting the rate of body cooling are:

1. The temperature of the body at death.
2. The clothing or coverings of the body.
3. The environmental temperature.
4. The medium in which the body is found which may or may not have been constant.

5. Rapidity of movement of air.
6. The condition of the body, e.g., fat content.

The temperature at death for purposes of calculation is usually taken as 99°F (37·2°C). In diseases of bacterial origin the temperature of the body may be considerably higher than this and may even rise above this after death. Severe exertion close to death can also raise the temperature and this situation may well be present in cases of murder. Pontine haemorrhage is the classical example of hyperpyrexia at death. The temperature may be subnormal at death, and is seen in cases of exposure intoxication with barbiturates, salicylates, and alcohol.

The coverings of the body, including clothing, have a marked effect on heat loss.

In water, bodies cool more rapidly than in air.

The rapidity of air movement is always a major factor in the cooling of the living and the dead. Unfortunately it may be one of the most difficult for the forensic pathologist to estimate. The movements of the investigators will cause frequent changes in air movement and prior to their arrival, windows and doors may have been opened or shut by members of the public.

Bodies of the obese retain heat longer then those of thin subjects and bodies of robust persons longer than those of debilitated persons.

Different parts of the body cool at different rates, for example, the trunk surface cools less rapidly than the extremities. Generally, the body surface will feel cold in from eight to twelve hours, but the above factors must be carefully considered.

Several investigators have attempted to devise techniques to take account of their various influences on the rate of cooling. Marshall[8] has constructed the latest and by far the most comprehensive formulae for estimating rates of body cooling. The calculation of cooling curves in the way he indicates will certainly take account of all the factors which are capable of measurement. Unfortunately they involve the use of mathematics which is beyond the capabilities of most of those who are likely to be making these estimations. The procedure which we use in estimating the time of death at a possible murder is:

We feel the jaw. If it is freely mobile, we put a hand in the axilla. If this is warm death has probably occurred within the previous four hours. We confirm this and try to improve on this figure by looking at the level of lividity.

If the jaw is fixed, we test the other limbs. If all are fixed, we put a hand in the axilla. If a little heat can be detected, death has occurred in the mid-period when a body tends to lose 1·5 degrees Fahrenheit per hour. We then take the rectal temperature, using the Fahrenheit scale and apply the formula,

$$\frac{99 - \text{Rectal temperature}}{1 \cdot 5} = \text{hours since death}$$

This will give a fairly accurate answer.

If the body is rigid and we can detect no heat on palpation we again take the rectal temperature and apply the same formula, but we know that we are dealing with a period when the body is approaching the temperature of its surroundings and we explain to the police that any estimate which we can now give is liable to serious error.

Once secondary flaccidity and putrefaction have occurred we prefer not to give an estimate. We have seen a body reach a state of putrefaction within forty-eight hours which we would have estimated as requiring ten to fourteen days to reach that state.

During the course of the post-mortem dissection information can sometimes be obtained about the time of death from a study of the stomach contents and blood alcohol levels.

PROXIMATE CAUSES OF DEATH

All deaths may be attributed to one of three proximate causes, or modes of dying, namely, coma, syncope, or asphyxia. Since life is maintained by the interdependent action of the brain, the heart, and the lungs, the arrest of the function of one of them is quickly succeeded by the arrest of the function of the others, and life ceases. These alone are unacceptable as causes of death on a certificate of death.

Coma

The principal causes of coma are compression of the brain, due to depressed fracture of the skull, cerebral haemorrhage, and tumours of the brain. The effects of poisons introduced into the body, for example, hypnotics and narcotics, and the effects of toxic metabolites produced in disease, such as renal disease and diabetes mellitus, may also produce coma.

A hyperaemic condition of the brain and its covering membranes is commonly found at post-mortem dissection.

Syncope

This term is applied to a sudden cessation of the action of the heart, which may prove fatal. Syncope may be brought about by a large variety of causes, of which the following are examples:

emotion,
rapid evacuation of fluids from body cavities,

injection of fluid into the uterus,
cardiac disease,
blows on the epigastrium and neck,
sudden constriction of the neck over the carotid sinus,
sudden submersion of the body in cold water.

The operative mechanism in some of these cases is obscure, but many are associated with some degree of primary shock.   This causes reflex vasodilatation and a resultant serious fall in the blood-pressure due to the actual diminution of the volume of the blood passing through the heart to the arteries.   The capillaries of the skeletal muscles are chiefly affected, and in these the blood collects instead of returning to the heart, causing a temporary deprivation of the blood from the circulation and cerebral anaemia.

Secondary shock results when there is diminution in the blood volume due to trauma.

The post-mortem appearances are neither prominent nor characteristic.   The cavities of the heart contain comparatively little blood, the organs are pale, and the capillary vessels are congested.

Asphyxia

Asphyxia has been defined as primarily a state, or series of states, induced by an oxygen supply short of tissue needs.[9]

Gordon[10] submits that the cessation of vital functions depends upon tissue anoxia, which may be one of four types, namely:

> anoxic,
> anaemic,
> histotoxic,
> stagnant.

He states that these four types of anoxia initiate the same vicious cycle, and cause cardiac failure leading to death.   He directs attention to the term 'asphyxia' and points out that asphyxia does not constitute a pathological entity, and cannot clearly be recognised on the basis of morbid anatomical observations alone.

This idea provides a useful concept for pathologists in their study of the various mechanisms of death.   We propose to retain the term 'asphyxia' to describe the results of obstructional anoxia.

Asphyxia may be produced in many ways, including the following:

Occlusion of the air-passages by foreign bodies, the effects of scalding or corrosives, angioneurotic oedema, acute inflammation, membranous exudations, acute oedema of the glottis, laryngeal spasm, tumours, and abscesses.

Impediment to respiratory function by pressure on the chest wall, for example, by falls of debris, and in lift and pit-cage accidents.
Strangulation, suffocation, hanging, throttling, drowning.

Generalised anoxia of the tissues may be caused by:

Inhalation of irrespirable gases.
Paralysis of the respiratory nerves or muscles, or of the respiratory centre from injury or disease, or from the action of certain poisons, for example, morphine and barbiturates.
From causes operating from the lungs, or pulmonary circulatory system, for example, lung diseases, pleural effusions, pneumo-thorax, and pulmonary embolism.

When the process of asphyxia is initiated by respiration being suddenly obstructed, either by occlusion of the air-passages or by pressure exerted upon them, the individual gasps for breath, respirations are rapid and deep, the colour of the face darkens and as cerebral anoxia increases convulsions occur. These continue with deepening cyanosis, the face sometimes becoming almost black, until the respiratory centre is poisoned. All movements then cease and death is imminent.

Post-mortem appearances in obstructional asphyxia

External. Lividity of the lips and ears and livid colour of hypostasis. In infants and young children particularly there is usually lividity of the finger- and toe-nails. These colorations vary in intensity from a duskiness to a dark-blue tint. The face is congested and livid in colour, although in some cases it may be pale or slightly dusky. Lividity does not necessarily indicate that death has been caused by respiratory failure, and an asphyxial death need not always show lividity. The tongue may lie in normal position, the tip may be pressed against the back of the teeth, or be protruded either between the margins of the teeth, or beyond them. A frothy and frequently blood-stained fluid may be seen at the corners of the mouth, or at the nostrils, or in both positions. The conjunctivae are commonly congested, and may show a varying number of small punctate haemorrhages (Fig. 56).

Internal. The larynx and trachea may contain a varying amount of slightly frothy mucus. The lungs are engorged and oedematous. On section, a copious, frothy, dark-coloured, blood-stained exudate will be seen. Petechial haemorrhages, due to capillary injury, are commonly present on the parietal, pulmonary, and pericardial pleurae, pericardium, heart muscle, endocardium, and substance of the brain. Some of the marginal portions of the lungs may perhaps show emphysematous changes. The mucous membrane of the trachea is congested.

Microscopically, the lung tissue shows marked dilatation of both capillaries and veins. In infants, interlobar emphysema may be found either in patches, or more or less general in its distribution. The cavities of the right side of the heart are engorged with dark-coloured, imperfectly clotted blood, and the venae cavae are also engorged. The cavities on the left side of the heart are often comparatively empty, but this may be due to contraction of the left ventricle during rigor mortis, the blood readily escaping since the arterial system is relatively empty.

The abdominal viscera show marked venous congestion. The brain is often congested, and an excess of serous fluid is found in the lateral ventricles. The cranial sinuses are usually filled with dark-coloured blood. The blood, generally, is dark in colour and is mostly fluid in the large veins.

There are variations, however, in the intensity of the asphyxial signs which may be present, and these are dependent upon the specific circumstances which may attend a given case. When the asphyxial process is slight and prolonged, the congestive element will be diminished; when intense and short, lividity and congestion are marked; and when, during the process of asphyxia, heart-failure precedes respiratory arrest, the asphyxial signs may be less marked, depending at which stage in the asphyxial process cardiac arrest occurred.

The significance of petechial haemorrhages has been the subject of considerable discussion. It should be appreciated that although petechial haemorrhages are frequently seen in asphyxial deaths, they are by no means restricted to this form of death and are frequently present in deaths due to a variety of other causes. When, however, multiple and fairly large petechial haemorrhages are found on the face, conjunctivae, epiglottis, heart, and lung surfaces, a strong presumption arises that the death is asphyxial.

SUDDEN DEATH

Sudden death has been aptly defined as the termination of life which comes quickly under circumstances when its immediate arrival is unexpected.

In a case of sudden death a medical practitioner should hesitate, unless upon the strongest evidence, to certify the cause of death without a post-mortem examination of the body.

The following is a list of the commoner causes of sudden death in various age groups.

An instance of sudden death is worthy of comment. A boy, aged twelve years, an excellent swimmer, died suddenly at a private swimming club. Having swam several times across the pool, he left the water and, while standing close to the edge, collapsed and died im-

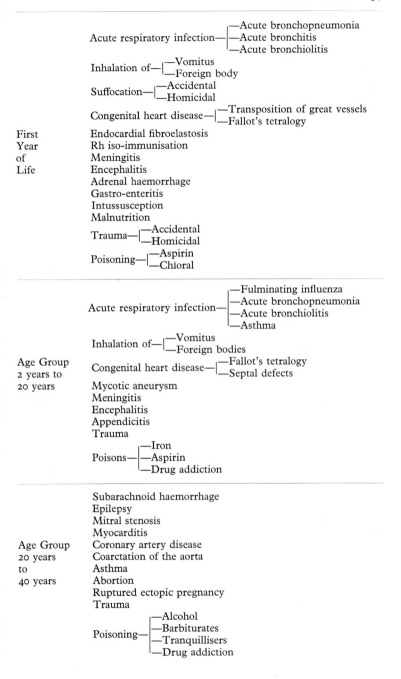

Acute respiratory infection—
—Acute bronchopneumonia
—Acute bronchitis
—Acute bronchiolitis

Inhalation of—
—Vomitus
—Foreign body

Suffocation—
—Accidental
—Homicidal

Congenital heart disease—
—Transposition of great vessels
—Fallot's tetralogy

First
Year
of
Life

Endocardial fibroelastosis
Rh iso-immunisation
Meningitis
Encephalitis
Adrenal haemorrhage
Gastro-enteritis
Intussusception
Malnutrition

Trauma—
—Accidental
—Homicidal

Poisoning—
—Aspirin
—Chloral

Acute respiratory infection—
—Fulminating influenza
—Acute bronchopneumonia
—Acute bronchiolitis
—Asthma

Inhalation of—
—Vomitus
—Foreign bodies

Age Group
2 years to
20 years

Congenital heart disease—
—Fallot's tetralogy
—Septal defects

Mycotic aneurysm
Meningitis
Encephalitis
Appendicitis
Trauma

Poisons—
—Iron
—Aspirin
—Drug addiction

Age Group
20 years
to
40 years

Subarachnoid haemorrhage
Epilepsy
Mitral stenosis
Myocarditis
Coronary artery disease
Coarctation of the aorta
Asthma
Abortion
Ruptured ectopic pregnancy
Trauma

Poisoning—
—Alcohol
—Barbiturates
—Tranquillisers
—Drug addiction

	Coronary artery disease
	Mitral stenosis
	Intra-cerebral haemorrhage
	Dissecting aneurysm
Age Group	Pulmonary embolus
40 years	Acute pancreatitis
to	Perforated peptic ulcer
60 years	Upper alimentary tract haemorrhage
	Rupture of oesophageal varices

Poisoning— ⎰—Barbiturates
⎱—Tranquillisers
—Alcohol

Viral hepatitis

	Bronchopneumonia
	Influenza

Intra-cerebral haemorrhage— ⎰—Hypertensive
⎱—Neoplastic

	Coronary artery disease—rupture of heart
Age Group	Rupture of aorta or other great vessel
over	Subarachnoid haemorrhage
60 years	Hypertensive cardiac failure
	Pulmonary embolus
	Peritonitis
	Hypothermia

Poisoning— ⎰—Barbiturates
⎱—Carbon monoxide

mediately. Post-mortem examination did not disclose any morbid condition. The lower part of the oesophagus contained two large undigested portions of potato, the larger measuring $1\frac{1}{2}$ by $\frac{1}{2}$ inches. The stomach contained a considerable quantity of undigested food, including a piece of potato $1\frac{1}{2}$ by $1\frac{1}{4}$ inches in size. The cause of death was cardiac failure, due to inhibition induced by swimming while the process of digestion was in active operation.

References

1. SHAPIRO, H.A. *J. forens. Med.*, **16**, No. 1, 1969.
2. KVITTINGEN, T.D. & NAESS, A. *Br. med. J.*, **1**, 1315, 1963.
3. SZENT-GYÖRGYI, A. Studies on muscle. *Acta physiol. scand.*, **9**, Suppl. 25, 1945. *Chemistry of Muscular Contraction*, New York: Academic Press, 1947.
4. YUDIN, S.S. *Lancet*, **2**, 361, 1937.
5. The author is indebted to the late DR ALEXANDER G. MEARNS, Department of Hygiene, University of Glasgow, for the notes and drawings in connection with the identification of maggots. See also GLAISTER, J. & BRASH, J.C.: *Medico-legal Aspects of the Ruxton Case*. Edinburgh: Livingstone, 1937. SMITH, S. & GLAISTER, J.: *Recent Advances in Forensic Medicine*. London: Churchill, 1938.

6. POWELL, A.   *Br. med. J.*, **1,** 842, 1917.
7. FORBES, G.   *Police J.*, **15,** 141, 1942.
8. MARSHALL, T.K.   *Medicine Sci. Law*, **9,** 178, 1969.
9. HENDERSON, Y.   *J. Am. med. Ass.*, **101,** 261, 1933.
10. GORDON, I.   *Br. med. J.*, **2,** 337, 1944.

Chapter 5

DEATH CERTIFICATION AND CREMATION

CERTIFICATION of death is a statutory duty imposed upon members of the medical profession which must be performed without fee. Failure to certify is followed by penalty. It is necessary, therefore, that practitioners should fully understand their responsibilities with regard to certification.

The young practitioner will find it profitable to study the printed matter found in each book of blank forms of certificates issued by local registrars.

A dead body should not be disposed of without a registrar's certificate or a Coroner's or Procurator-Fiscal's order. When however burial has occurred without the issue of a certificate of registration of death, the Registration of Births, Deaths and Marriages (Scotland) Act, 1965, section 27 (3) states that the person having charge of the place of interment shall within three days from the date of burial give notice thereof to the Registrar of the registration district in which the death occurred.

England

The principal provisions of the Births and Deaths Registration Act, 1953, are:

Every certificate of the cause of death required to be given shall be in the prescribed form (pp. 142 and 143).

The certificate shall be delivered forthwith, by the registered medical practitioner by whom it is signed, to the Registrar. The Registrar will register the death and issue a disposal certificate.

The practitioner, on signing a certificate, shall give in the prescribed form, to some person required by the Registration Acts to give information concerning the death, notice in writing of the signing of the certificate, and that person shall, except where an inquest is held on the body of the deceased person, deliver this notice to the Registrar (p. 142).

In the case of every still-birth, it is the duty of the person, who would have been required to give information to the Registrar had the child been born alive, to give information to the Registrar of the particulars required to be registered concerning the still-birth, unless there has been an inquest.

Every such person upon giving information shall either deliver to the

Registrar a written certificate, that the child was not born alive, signed by a registered medical practitioner or certified midwife who was in attendance at the birth or who has examined the body of such child, or make a declaration in the prescribed form to the effect that no medical practitioner or certified midwife was present at the birth or had examined the body or that his or her certificate cannot be obtained and that the child was not born alive (p. 144).

It should be noted that the terms 'still-born' and 'still-birth' are defined as applying to any child which has issued forth from its mother after the twenty-eighth week of pregnancy and which did not at any time after being completely expelled from its mother, breathe or show any other signs of life.

It is unlawful to have a still-born child buried without the written sanction of a Coroner or Registrar (p. 140).

A medical practitioner cannot withhold a death certificate, but must certify the cause of death when known, irrespective of the cause. Failure to certify renders the practitioner liable to a penalty of £2.0, and issuing a false certificate makes him liable, on summary conviction, to a fine of £10.0 or on conviction on indictment, to seven years' imprisonment.

When the practitioner is unable to decide between symptoms of natural disease and those due to unnatural causes, it is advisable for him, before granting the certificate in such circumstances, to interview the Coroner, in England, or the Procurator-Fiscal, in Scotland, who will advise the best course to be followed.

The following deaths are reported by the Registrar to the Coroner.

Deaths certified as directly or indirectly due to violence:
Deaths attended by suspicious circumstances:
Sudden deaths:
Deaths whose cause has been stated as unknown.

When a doctor has appended his initials to Statement 'A' on the back of the death Certificate Form, it is the duty of the Registrar of Deaths receiving the certificate to refrain from registering the death until he has been informed by the Coroner what action the Coroner has taken in regard to the death.

In the case of a death which, on information given by a practitioner or others, has been the subject of an inquest, it becomes the duty of the Coroner to send to the Registrar a certificate of the finding of the jury as to the cause of death within the time required by the Registration Acts.

The following are important points in connection with certification of death in England:

A medical practitioner may not issue a certificate unless he has been in attendance upon the deceased during his or her last illness.

DEATH CERTIFICATE FORM USED IN ENGLAND. (Front)

BIRTHS AND DEATHS REGISTRATION ACTS, 1953

Registrar to enter No. of Death Entry.

MEDICAL CERTIFICATE OF CAUSE OF DEATH

For use only by a Registered Medical Practitioner **WHO HAS BEEN IN ATTENDANCE** during the deceased's last illness, and to be delivered by him forthwith to the Registrar of Births and Deaths.

Name of Deceased...

Date of Death as stated to me.........day of..........19.... Age as stated to me.......

Place of Death...day of...........19.... after death by me.

Last seen alive } by me .... Seen* Not seen* } after death by me.

The certified cause of death has* has not* been confirmed by Post-mortem.

These particulars not to be entered in death register.

CAUSE OF DEATH

| I | Approximate interval between onset and death. |

I — Disease or condition directly leading to death†

    a .... *due to (or as a consequence of)*

Antecedent causes. Morbid conditions, if any, giving rise to the above cause stating the underlying condition last.

    b .... *due to (or as a consequence of)*

    c ....

II — Other significant conditions, contributing to the death, but not related to the disease or condition causing it.

I hereby certify that I was in medical attendance during the above named Deceased's last illness, and that the particulars and cause of death above written are true to the best of my knowledge and belief.

Signature...

Qualifications as registered by Medical Council } ....

Residence.. Date....................

* Strike out whichever is inapplicable.
† This does not mean the mode of dying, such as *e.g.*, heart failure, asphyxia, asthenia, etc., it means the disease, injury, or complication which caused death.

COUNTERFOIL

For use of Medical Attendant, who should in all cases fill it up.

Name of Deceased } ....

Date of Death } .... Age..........

Place of Death } ....

Last seen alive } } after death.
Seen* Not seen*

Cause of death confirmed* not confirmed* } by P.M.

Cause of Death :—

I *a*.......................
    due to

   b.......................
    due to

   c.......................

II ....

Signature.........................

Date.........................

* Strike out whichever is inapplicable.

NOTICE TO INFORMANT

I hereby give notice that I have, this day, signed a Medical Certificate of the Cause of Death

of ....

Signature ....

Date ....

This Notice must be given by the Certifying Medical Practitioner to the person who is qualified and liable to act as Informant for the purpose of the registration of the death. As to the person liable to act as Informant, see back.

DUTIES OF INFORMANT

This notice is to be delivered by the informant to the registrar of births and deaths for the sub-district in which the death occurred. **The death cannot be registered until the medical certificate has reached the registrar. Failure to deliver this notice to the registrar renders the informant liable to prosecution.**

The informant must be prepared to state accurately to the registrar the following particulars :

(1) The date and place of death, and the place of deceased's usual residence (2) the full names and surname (3) the correct age (4) the occupation (5) whether deceased was in receipt of a pension, or allowance from public funds and (6), if deceased was a woman who had been married, the date and duration of marriage.

DECEASED'S MEDICAL CARD MUST BE DELIVERED TO THE REGISTRAR.

PERSONS QUALIFIED AND LIABLE TO ACT AS INFORMANTS

The following table shows in full the persons, in the order of their successive liability, who are designated by the Births and Deaths Registration Acts as Informants :—

DEATHS IN HOUSES:
(1) A *relative* of the deceased, *present at the death*.
(2) A *relative* of the deceased, *in attendance* during the last illness.
(3) A *relative* of the deceased, dwelling or being at the time of registration in the sub-district wherein the death occurred.
(4) A person *present at the death*.
(5) The *occupier* } of the house in which the death occurred.
(6) An *inmate* }
(7) The person *causing the disposal of the body*.

DEATHS NOT IN HOUSES, OR DEAD BODIES FOUND EXPOSED :
(1) Any *relative* of the deceased having knowledge of the required particulars.
(2) Any person *present at the death*.
(3) Any person *who found the body*.
(4) Any person *in charge of the body*.
(5) The person *causing the disposal of the body*.

DEATHS IN INSTITUTIONS :
(1) Any *relative* of the deceased who may be available.
(2) The *Chief* (or *Acting Chief*) *Resident Officer*.
(3) A person *present at the death*.
(4) The person *causing the disposal of the body*.

....

DEATH CERTIFICATE FORM USED IN ENGLAND. (Back)

A. Reported to Coroner ?
....

B, Further information offered ?
....

N.B.—If either Statement A or Statement B has been filled up, the fact should be noted in the appropriate place above.

Fill up where applicable.

A.
I have reported this case to the Coroner.
....

Initials of
Certifying Medical } ....
Practitioner

Fill up where applicable.

B.
I may be in a position later to give, on application by the Registrar-General, additional information as to the cause of death for the purpose of more precise statistical classification.

Initials of
Certifying Medical } ....
Practitioner

NOTE.—The Practitioner, on signing the certificate, should fill up, sign and date the Notice to the Informant, which should be detached and handed to the Informant. The Practitioner should then, without delay, deliver the certificate itself to the Registrar of Births and Deaths for the sub-district in which the death occurred. It may be delivered by post ; and the Practitioner is supplied by the Registrar, gratis, with postage-paid envelopes for this purpose.

FORM OF CERTIFICATE OF STILL-BIRTH USED IN ENGLAND

(Births and Deaths Registration Act, 1953, Section 11 (1) (a), as amended by the Population (Statistics) Act, 1960, Section 2 (1))

* I was present at the still-birth of a $\frac{* \text{male}}{* \text{female}}$ child born

* I have examined the body of a $\frac{* \text{male}}{* \text{female}}$ child which I am informed and believe was

born on the............day of.................................19.........to..

(NAME OF MOTHER)

at ....

(PLACE OF BIRTH)

I hereby certify that

    (i) the child was not born alive, and

    (ii) to the best of my knowledge and belief the cause of death and the estimated duration of pregnancy of the mother were as stated below.

CAUSE OF DEATH		
I **I**		
DIRECT CAUSE State fœtal or maternal condition directly causing death	(a)...............................	Estimated duration of pregnancy
ANTECEDENT CAUSES State fœtal and/or maternal conditions, if any, giving rise to the above cause (a) stating the underlying cause last	due to (b)................... due to (c)...................	
II **II**		....
OTHER SIGNIFICANT CONDITIONS of fœtus or mother which may have contributed to but, in so far as is known, were not related to direct cause of death	....	Weeks

        ⎧ 1. The certified cause of death has been confirmed by post-mortem.

†⎨ 2. Post-mortem information may be available later.

        ⎩ 3. Post-mortem not being held.

Signature.. Date..

Qualification as registered by General Medical Council, or ⎫
Registered No. as Certified Midwife ⎭ ....

Residence..

    * Strike out the words which do not apply.

    † Ring appropriate digit.

No other practitioner may sign the certificate on his behalf unless he has also been in attendance upon the deceased during his or her last illness.

With regard to the cause of death, it is desirable that the terms embodied in the Nomenclature of the Royal College of Physicians of London, or in the Registrar-General's Manual of the International List of Causes of Death should be employed.   Vague and ill-defined terms should be avoided.

In all cases of sudden deaths or deaths under any circumstances of suspicion, it is the duty of those who are about the deceased to give immediate notice to the Coroner or his officer or to the nearest officer of police, who then communicates with the Coroner.

In certain cases, a practitioner when signing the certificate may have knowledge that a post-mortem or laboratory examination is to be made, and provision to intimate this information is available on the back of the certificate.

If the certifying doctor has not seen the deceased during the fourteen days before death, and has not seen the body after death, the Registrar must notify the Coroner to this effect.

In all cases the practitioner should verify the occurrence of death before granting the certificate.

When the body of a deceased person has to be removed from England or Wales, notice must first be given to the Coroner in whose jurisdiction the body is lying, and prior to its removal the Coroner's permission must be obtained following inquiry.

Scotland

The relevant current Scottish Act is the Registration of Births, Deaths and Marriages (Scotland) Act, 1965.   This Act also deals with still-births and repeals the Registration of Still-Births (Scotland) Act, 1938.

The relevant sections concerned with the registration of death are contained in Part III of the Act.

Section 23 deals with the duty of relatives, persons present at the death, executors, and any other person who has knowledge of the death to attend at the Registrar's office within eight days and provide him with information concerning the death.   The fulfilment of this duty by any of these persons discharges the duty imposed on the others.

In order that the informant operating under the foregoing section can provide the Registrar with the relevant information it is necessary for doctors to provide death certificates.   The regulations for the granting of these are given in section 24 of the Act.

Subsection (1) states that where a registered medical practitioner has been in attendance on the deceased during his last illness, he must

DEATH CERTIFICATE FORM USED IN SCOTLAND

FORM 11

This certificate is intended for the use of the Registrar of Births, Deaths and Marriages, and all persons are warned against accepting or using this certificate for any other purpose

MEDICAL CERTIFICATE OF CAUSE OF DEATH

To the Registrar of the District of .... died on ....19......

I hereby certify that ....

at ....

and that, to the best of my knowledge and belief, the cause of death and duration of disease were as stated below

Registrar to enter

Dist. No. ....

Entry No. ....

Year ....

CAUSE OF DEATH (Please print clearly)

Not to be entered in death register
Approximate interval between onset and death

Years	months	days

Disease or condition directly leading to death *

I

    (a)

       due to (or as a consequence of)

Antecedent causes

Morbid conditions, if any, giving rise to the above cause, the underlying condition to be stated last

    (b)

       due to (or as a consequence of)

    (c)

II

Other significant conditions

contributing to the death, but not related to the disease or condition causing it

II

* This does not mean the mode of dying such as heart failure, asthenia, etc.; it means the disease, injury or complication which caused death.

Please ring appropriate letter and appropriate figure:—

Certified cause takes account of post-mortem information ... **A**

Information from post-mortem may be available later ... **B**

Post-mortem not proposed ... ... **C**

If deceased was a married woman, and death occurred during pregnancy, or within six weeks thereafter, write "yes", ...

Seen after death by me **1**

Seen after death by another medical practitioner but not by me ... **2**

Signature ....

Date ....

Registered Medical Practitioner

REGISTRATION OF STILL-BIRTHS (SCOTLAND) ACT, 1938
as amended by POPULATION (STATISTICS) ACT, 1960

SECTION 1—(2) Every person upon giving information regarding a still-birth shall—

  (a) deliver to the registrar a certificate in the prescribed form stating that the child was not born alive, and, where possible, the cause or probable cause of death, which certificate shall, if a registered medical practitioner was present at the birth or has examined the body of the child, be signed by him, and otherwise shall be signed by a certified midwife who was present or examined the body ; or

  (b) make a declaration in the prescribed form to the effect that no registered medical practitioner or certified midwife was present at the birth or has examined the body, or that his or her certificate cannot be obtained and that the child was not born alive.

(2a) Every registered medical practitioner or certified midwife who was present at a still-birth or examined the body of a still-born child shall, at the request of any person who by virtue of the Registration Acts is required to give information touching that birth, give to that person a certificate for the purposes of paragraph (a) of the last foregoing sub-section; and the certificate shall, where possible, state (in addition to the other matters referred to in that paragraph) to the best of the knowledge and belief of the person signing it the estimated duration of the pregnancy of the mother of the child.

Persons required to give information for the registration of a still-born child are:—

  (1) the father (of a legitimate child only);

  (2) the mother;

  (3) the occupier of the house in which the birth occurred (in the case of a birth in a hospital, a representative of the hospital);

  (4) the nurse present at the birth.

This Certificate must be delivered to the Registrar of Births, Deaths and Marriages when the Still-birth is registered. It is not an authority for burial or cremation. A list of the persons required to give information for the registration of a still-birth is given on the back of this form.

CERTIFICATE OF STILL-BIRTH

TO BE GIVEN IN RESPECT OF ANY CHILD WHICH HAS ISSUED FORTH FROM ITS MOTHER AFTER THE TWENTY-EIGHTH WEEK OF PREGNANCY AND WHICH DID NOT AT ANY TIME AFTER BEING COMPLETELY EXPELLED FROM ITS MOTHER BREATHE OR SHOW ANY OTHER SIGNS OF LIFE

To the Registrar of the District of ....

* I was present at the still-birth of a *male/female child born

* I have examined the body of a *male/female child which I am informed and believe was born

.... (name of mother)

on ...., 19......, to ....

at .... (place of birth)

I hereby certify that the child was NOT BORN ALIVE and that, to the best of my knowledge and belief, the cause or probable cause of death of the child, and the estimated duration of pregnancy of the mother were as stated below

CAUSE OF DEATH (Please print clearly)

I

Foetal or maternal condition directly causing death .... (a) .... due to

Antecedent causes
Foetal or maternal conditions, if any, (b) .... due to giving rise to the above cause, the underlying condition to be stated last. (c) ....

II

Other significant conditions of foetus or mother contributing to the death, but not related to the disease or condition causing it. ....

Please ring appropriate letter:—

  A Certified cause takes account of post-mortem information

  B Information from post-mortem may be available later

  C Post-mortem not proposed

* Strike out whichever does not apply.

Signature ....

Registered Medical Qualifications (or Regd. No. if a certified midwife) ....

Address ....

	Registrar to enter
	Dist. No. ....
	Vol. No. ....
	Entry No. ....
	Year ....

Not to be entered in register
Estimated duration of pregnancy .... weeks
Weight of foetus (if known) .... lbs .... ozs

Date ....

COUNTERFOIL

Surname of father (or mother) ....

Date of Still-birth ....

Place of Still-birth ....

....

Cause of death

I. (a) ....

   (b) ....

   (c) ....

II. ....

Estimated duration of pregnancy ....

Weight of foetus (if known) ....

P.-M. (ring letter)   A   B   C

Date of certification ....

transmit a certificate in the prescribed form, signed by him, either to the Registrar or the qualified informant as detailed above.

Subsection (2) states that where there is no registered medical practitioner available who was in attendance during the last illness any medical practitioner who can give the cause of death, may sign the certificate.

The doctor must transmit the certificate to the Registrar or the qualified informant within seven days and it is customary for the doctor who has signed the death certificate to hand it to the nearest relative of the deceased and he takes it to the Registrar.

The Registrar will then register the death and issue a certificate of registration.

In cases which have been inquired into by the Procurator-Fiscal, this official must inform the Registrar of the result of the inquiry, but there is no defined time within which the information must be returned to the Registrar.

Contrasted with England, the relation of the practitioner to the duty of certification of deaths is legally different. In England he is bound forthwith to deliver the death certificate to the Registrar. In Scotland, on the other hand, the practitioner is bound to send it to the Registrar within seven days after death.

In the certification of death, general terms, for example, 'Disease of the Heart', must not be employed, and the nature of the disease must be specifically stated.

The suggestions regarding certification, in each book of forms, should be studied carefully. Books of Certificate Forms (Form 11) may be obtained by registered medical practitioners from the Registrar of Births, Deaths, and Marriages of the registration district in which they reside.

For the purposes of the Registration Acts, every birth which occurs will fall into one or other of three classes:

A child who, whatever the duration of pregnancy, breathes or shows any other signs of life after complete expulsion from the mother, is a live-born child and the birth must be recorded in the Register of Births. If the child dies, even within a brief period after birth, both the birth and the death fall to be registered.

The birth of a child before the end of the twenty-eighth week of pregnancy, which did not breathe or show signs of life after complete expulsion from the mother, is not required to be registered.

The birth of a child after the twenty-eighth week of pregnancy which, after complete expulsion from the mother, did not show any signs of life, is a still-birth, and must be registered in the Register of Still-births (p. 147).

Section 21 of the Registration of Births, Deaths and Marriages

(Scotland) Act, 1965, deals with the registration of still-births and states that it is the duty of informants who are qualified to register live births to register still-births in the same way. They must also transmit to the Registrar a certificate stating that the child was not born alive and if possible giving the probable cause of death signed by a registered medical practitioner, or a certified midwife, present at the birth, or who has examined the body. If this certificate cannot be obtained or if a doctor or midwife was not present at the birth the informant must make a declaration to this effect on the prescribed form.

Under the Children and Young Persons (Scotland) Act, 1937, where a person undertakes for reward the nursing or maintenance of a child under nine years and such child dies, it is the duty of such persons to give notice in writing to the Procurator-Fiscal within twenty-four hours of the death. The Procurator-Fiscal will then hold an inquiry into the cause of death unless a certificate by a duly qualified medical practitioner is produced to him certifying that he has personally attended the child during his last illness and specifying the cause of death (p. 221).

Since questions may arise as to the disposal of the remains of a child, born dead before the end of the twenty-eighth week of pregnancy, it may be stated that, apart from the general Public Health Acts, there is apparently no law on the subject.

Important points in death certification

It is particularly important that the practitioner should verify the fact of the occurrence of death before he grants the certificate (p. 145).

It is also important that a practitioner should not grant a certificate of death of a person whom he has not seen for a length of time until he has inquired into the circumstances and examined the body, even although the person is known to him as suffering from a disease which might prove fatal.

Under no circumstances should a practitioner be tempted to sign blank certificates, or to sign a certificate of death of a person while that person, although critically ill, is still alive. This may not only expose him to a charge of false certification, but his action may be deemed 'serious professional misconduct' by the General Medical Council, and may result in the removal of his name from the Medical Register.

CREMATION

The Cremation Acts, 1902 and 1952, and Regulations made thereunder applicable to England and Scotland, deal with the legal aspects of the disposal of dead bodies by incineration. In view of the fact that cremation of a body destroys all evidence of crime, so far as the body is concerned, the procedure, prior to cremation, is more elaborate than that required for ordinary burial. The important regulations are those of 1930 and 1965 for England and those of 1935 and 1965 for Scotland. The procedure and necessary forms are as follows:

1. An application on Form A must be made by the nearest relative or executor. On this he must give the name, age, and date and time of death of the deceased and the place of death. He must also state the name of the practitioner who attended the deceased in his last illness and he must state whether or not death was due to violence, poison, privation, or neglect, and whether death occurred while under an anaesthetic. The Form must be signed and dated by the applicant and then countersigned by a householder who knows the applicant. If the application is not made by the nearest relative or executor the reason for this must be given by the applicant.

2. The applicant must obtain from the doctor who attended the deceased during the last illness and who has seen the body after death Form B duly completed. Form B contains the name, address, and occupation of the deceased and gives the date, time, and place of death. The doctor must answer twenty questions; the most important of these are:

> The time when he last saw the patient alive.
> The interval after death when he saw the body.
> The name of the person who nursed the deceased during the last illness.
> Whether the doctor has any doubt as to the cause of death.
> Has the doctor any reason to suspect that death was due directly to
> > (a) violence,
> > (b) poison,
> > (c) privation or neglect.
> Has the doctor any reason to suspect that a further examination is required.

Finally the doctor must certify on soul and conscience that all the information he has given is true and accurate.

3. Form C is the confirmatory medical certificate. It must be signed on soul and conscience by a practitioner of five years' standing who has studied the information supplied by the doctor who has signed Form B, has consulted him about it, and also has made further inquiry into the death. This further inquiry may take the form of a post-mortem dissection, consultation with some other doctor with knowledge of the case, or consultation with nurses or relatives who looked after the deceased during the last illness. It is

essential that further inquiry is made in one of these ways. The practitioner signing Form C must see the body.

Forms A, B, and C must be transmitted along with the Registrar's certificate of registration of death to the medical referee, who, if he is satisfied after scrutinising the certificates, authorises the cremation on Form F.

When a person dies abroad and the body is transferred to this country for cremation, the medical referee is empowered to accept medical certificates from doctors who possess qualifications substantially equivalent to those prescribed for each certificate by the Regulations.

When a person has died at sea or under circumstances where it is not possible to obtain the required certificates, permission for cremation may be obtained by the medical referee, by application, explaining the circumstances, to the office of the Secretary of State.

When the death has taken place in England and cremation is required in Scotland a certificate must be obtained from the Coroner stating that he has received notice of the intention to remove the body from England and that he does not intend to hold an inquest.

If the Coroner or Procurator-Fiscal has investigated a case and the cause of death ascertained, the medical certificates B and C are unnecessary. They are replaced by Form E which is granted by the Coroner or Procurator-Fiscal, stating that cremation can take place.

Medical referees are appointed by cremation authorities and the appointment must be notified to the Secretary of State.

It is the duty of the medical referee to scrutinise the relevant documents and he must authorise cremation only when he is satisfied that the cause of death has been ascertained, that there is no reason for further inquiry and that all the regulations have been carried out.

He is empowered to make such inquiries as he thinks necessary and he has the power to sign Form C. He also has the power to make a post-mortem dissection or instruct a pathologist to do so. When this is done the appropriate certificate is Form D.

The referee can withhold his authority to cremate without stating reasons.

The medical referee may authorise the cremation of the remains of a still-born child if it has been certified to have been still-born either by the registered medical practitioner who attended at the confinement of the mother or by a registered medical practitioner after a post-mortem examination of the body, and if the medical referee, after such inquiries as he may think necessary, is satisfied that it was still-born and there is no reason for further examination (see p. 147). Where there are any suspicious circumstances in connection with the birth of a still-born child, the medical referee must immediately report the matter to the Procurator-Fiscal of the district in which the birth is alleged to have occurred, and shall not authorise cremation of the remains except with the written permission of the Procurator-Fiscal.

There is provision for the cremation of bodies which have been the subject of anatomical dissection. Usually the application on Form A is made by the nearest relative or executor. It can, however, be made by the head of the school of anatomy. The only other formality required is the completion of Form H.

In July 1944, a doctor was fined £50 at Aberdeen Sheriff Court, when he pleaded guilty to nine contraventions of the False Oaths Act, in connection with the signing of death certificates for cremation. The charge alleged that the doctor had wilfully made the false statements in schedules which had to be completed to satisfy cremation regulations, by stating that he had questioned the doctors who had signed the death certificates, when in fact he had not done so. The Procurator-Fiscal said that when a cremation was to take place, a form certifying the cause of death was signed by the deceased's own doctor and, as a further safeguard, a second doctor had to confirm the cause of death, and thus this second doctor was asked to state in the official form that he had questioned the doctor who had attended the deceased. In none of the cases mentioned had the accused done so. It was a serious matter because the safeguard of the second doctor had not been taken. This case was one of a contravention of the False Oaths (Scotland) Act, 1933, section 2. The president of the General Medical Council announced that the conviction had been proved and the certificates in question came within the warning notice against untrue, misleading, and improper certificates. The Council did not regard the doctor's explanation as affording any excuse for his laxity, and took a grave view of carelessness in the issue of public certificates. As, however, they were prepared to believe that he had signed these certificates, not from any perversity or desire to falsify, but from a mistaken view of his duty and an error of judgment and that the warning he had received would be sufficient, they did not direct the erasure of his name.

The Cremation Act, 1902, applicable to both England and Scotland, contains a penalty section by means of which the Regulations can be enforced. Section 8 enacts that

1. Every person who shall contravene any such regulation, or shall knowingly carry out or procure or take part in the burning of any human remains, except in accordance with such regulations and the provisions of this Act, shall (in addition to any liability or penalty which he may otherwise incur) be liable, on summary conviction, to a penalty not exceeding £50. Provided that any person aggrieved by any conviction may appeal therefrom.

2. Every person who shall wilfully make any false declaration or representation, or sign or utter any false certificate, with a view to

procuring the burning of any human remains shall (in addition to any penalty or liability which he may otherwise incur) be liable to imprisonment not exceeding two years.

3. Every person who, with intent to conceal the commission or impede the prosecution of any offence, attempts to procure the cremation of any body, or, with such intent, makes any declaration or gives any certificate under this Act, shall be liable to conviction on indictment to imprisonment for a term not exceeding five years.

In 1957, at Sussex Assizes, a doctor was fined a total sum of £1,500 on three charges relating to cremation certificates in which he made a false representation that so far as he knew he had no pecuniary interest in the deaths of three persons who were to be cremated.

PRESUMPTION OF SURVIVORSHIP

When more persons than one die at or about the same time from more or less similar accidental causes, it occasionally becomes necessary to solve the difficult problem of survivorship for the purpose of succession to property.

In England, the Law of Property Act, 1925, has done much to overcome the frequent difficulties encountered in such cases.   This Act, stated broadly, lays down that where two or more persons die as the result of circumstances which make it uncertain as to which survived the other or others, then, subject to any order of the court, such deaths shall, for the purposes affecting the title to property, be presumed to have occurred in the order of seniority unless evidence to the contrary is forthcoming.   In the case of intestate spouses modifications have been made to this principle by the Intestate Estates Act, 1952.

The Grosvenor case[1] is worthy of mention since in this connection the words 'subject to any order of the court' were construed to mean that the court could receive evidence, and act upon it in displacement of the statutory presumption.   In another case, two brothers were killed with other people when a bomb fell on a house.   Mr Justice Cohen held that, in the absence of proof, the statutory presumption must apply. The Court of Appeal, however, held that the air-raid deaths were to be taken as simultaneous, but the House of Lords reversed this decision.[2]

In Scotland, this is dealt with under the Succession (Scotland) Act 1964, part VI, S. 31.

(1) When two persons have died in circumstances indicating that they died simultaneously, or making it uncertain which if either, of them survived the other, then, for all purposes affecting title or succession to property, or claims to legal rights, or the prior rights of a surviving spouse.

(a) when the persons were husband and wife, it shall be presumed that neither survived the other; and

(b) in any other case it shall be presumed that the younger person survived the elder unless the next following subsection applies.

(2) If in a case to which paragraph (b) of the foregoing subsection would (apart from this subsection) apply, the elder person has left a testamentary disposition containing a provision, however expressed in favour of the younger, if he survives the elder and, failing the younger, in favour of a third person, and the younger person has died intestate, then it shall be presumed for the purposes of that provision that the elder person survived the younger.

References

1. Grosvenor Case, 1944, *Lancet*, **1**, 129; also *re* Grosvenor, [1944], 1 All E.R. 81.
2. Hickman v. Peacey, [1945], 2 All E.R., 215.

Chapter 6

ASPHYXIA

DROWNING, SUFFOCATION, TRAUMATIC ASPHYXIA, HANGING, STRANGULATION, AND THROTTLING

DROWNING

DROWNING is a comparatively common form of death and is responsible for about 1,500 deaths annually. It is therefore important that what is meant by death by drowning should be clearly defined. A person may be said to have died from drowning into whose air-passages and lungs air has been prevented from entering by any watery, viscid, or pultaceous fluid into which the head has fallen and remained.

There are two types of death from drowning.[1]

1. When the first sudden intake of water occurs the larynx goes into spasm and a minimal amount of fluid enters the lungs. The result of this is progressive tissue anoxia and the death is really one of obstructional asphyxia. When this occurs it is frequently described as dry drowning. It has been estimated that this is the mechanism in about 20 per cent of cases of drowning deaths.

2. In the majority of cases of drowning the person submerges, sucks in water, rises to the surface, expires and submerges again drawing in more water. This process continues until the lungs become steadily heavier and finally water-logged and then the body sinks to the bottom. Some fluid is simultaneously swallowed. It is these actions which produce the classical external and internal signs of drowning.

The process of drowning varies from about two to five minutes. Factors influencing this are the ability to swim, degree of panic, determination to survive, and sheer physical stamina. All of these are affected by the presence of alcohol and other drugs.

The classical signs of drowning

External. The face is usually pale but may sometimes appear pink and life-like due to oxygenation of the blood in the surface capillaries. The most important external sign is the presence of fine foam and froth at the mouth and nostrils. The froth is composed of fine bubbles and results from the churning together of air, mucus, and water. This is very nearly a precise diagnostic sign of drowning. The only conditions which produce a similar froth are, very rarely carbon monoxide poisoning, and organo-phosphorus poisoning. The latter is caused by the

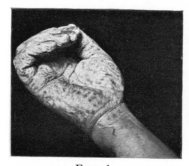

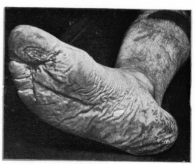

FIG. 46

Sodden condition of skin on palmar aspect of fingers and palm of hand in a case of drowning

FIG. 47

Similar condition to Fig. 46, involving skin on plantar aspect of toes and sole of foot

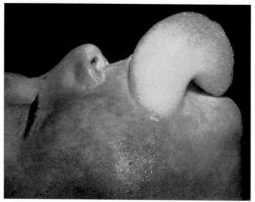

FIG. 48

Foam issuing from mouth in a case of drowning. (By courtesy of Professor C. J. Polson, Leeds University)

great accumulation of fluid in the upper respiratory tract due to the over-stimulation of the parasympathetic nervous system (p. 624)

Cutis anserina occurs when immersion took place prior to molecular death and is caused by the contraction of involuntary muscular fibres. Another skin condition found is bleached puckering. When this occurs on the hands it is known as 'washerwoman's hand'. This is indicative of only fairly prolonged immersion and is caused by the action of the water on thickened epidermis.

Internal. On opening the thoracic cavity the lungs bulge outwards as if formerly they had been retained under pressure. The term 'ballooning' has been applied to this condition. It is the result of increased volume, due to the presence of fluid and air in the bronchi, the latter playing a part since the foam, formed in the process of drowning, acts as a valve which during respiratory effort permits air entry to the lungs but obstructs air exit from them. Usually the lungs appear to be only moderately congested, and sometimes are very pale, due to air and water which has been trapped in the alveoli, forcing the blood from the

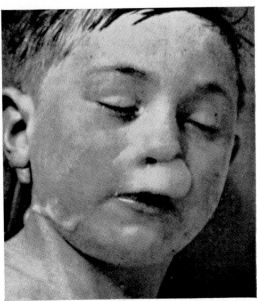

FIG. 49

Froth issuing from nostrils in a case of drowning. (By courtesy of the late Dr Robert Richards, Aberdeen University)

lungs, and compressing the vessels in the interalveolar septa. As the result of the increased volume, the lungs often show impressions of the ribs upon their surfaces. On pressure, they feel rather doughy and readily pit. When the lungs are voluminous, red and grey patches may be seen on the surfaces, due to effused blood which had tracked along the interlobular septa to the surface from ruptured alveoli, and to patchy interstitial emphysema, respectively.

In cases of pulmonary fibrosis and when extensive pleural adhesions are present, the degree of ballooning is reduced.

Petechial haemorrhages are rarely seen on the surfaces of the lungs due to compression of the blood-vessels in the interalveolar septa by the fluid content of the lungs. On section, an oedematous condition, due to the presence of a copious, watery, frothy, blood-stained exudate will

be observed.   This fluid is readily expressed on pressure of the cut surfaces or may exude spontaneously from these surfaces.   The exudation
is usually copious due to the presence of a considerable quantity of water
within the vesicles and bronchioles.   On examination of the trachea,
bronchi and bronchioles, a fine foam or froth will be found on the lining
membrane, occasionally blood-tinged.   Frequently the bronchi are
filled with this fluid, but more usually they are less completely full than
the bronchioles, which contain a considerable quantity.   The presence
of this fine, clear, or occasionally, blood-tinged foamy or frothy fluid
unmistakably points to death by drowning.   It is accounted for by water
entering the air passages and there becoming intimately mixed with air
and mucus.   This is essentially due to a vital act, which is proof of
interference with the function of respiration, by a liquid, during life.

Particulate matter from the drowning medium may be found in the
mouth, pharynx, larynx, trachea, bronchi, or stomach, and may permit
of comparison.

The chambers of the right side of the heart are usually dilated and
contain a considerable quantity of fluid blood, and the associated vessels
show congestion.   In some cases, the heart is globular in shape,
indicative of dilatation of all the chambers.   The abdominal organs and
venous system are congested.

Modifying factors

When putrefaction has occurred the facial appearance is radically
altered.   It rapidly becomes bloated and darkened.   Instead of the
lungs being ballooned and heavy they are found to be small and
collapsed in the posterior parts of the thoracic cavity and surrounded by
blood-stained fluid.

When death has occurred prior to immersion the signs will be related
to the cause of death and none of the signs of drowning will be present.
Occasionally, when there are no signs of drowning and no specific cause
of death is apparent, death is attributed to cardiac inhibition.   It may be
that many of such cases are in fact instances of dry drowning.

The diagnosis of drowning

This may be at one time the simplest and at another time the most
difficult diagnosis with which a forensic pathologist may be faced.

When a body is taken from the water shortly after drowning, the
classical signs are usually present and the cause of death is clear.   When,
however, a body is recovered from the water three weeks or a month
after immersion, then even using all the techniques available there may
still be uncertainty about the cause of death.

A valuable sign, when present, is the presence, in the firmly clenched hand, of objects such as weeds, sand, stones, and other debris which may be related to the water from which the body has been taken. This indicates that the person was alive when in the water, since it is an instance of cadaveric spasm and constitutes a vital act.

Experiments have shown that fluid cannot enter the stomach after death until putrefaction has advanced considerably. The presence of liquid manure, muddy water, and fuel oil are therefore important findings in the diagnosis of drowning.

It was considered that the finding of diatoms in the tissues of the body, particularly in the liver, kidney, and bone marrow, were absolutely diagnostic of drowning.[2, 3] Recently experimental work has cast doubt on this, as some workers have found diatoms after prolonged immersion in bodies which have not been drowned.[4] We have not had sufficient experience of examination for diatoms to give an authoritative opinion, but we tend to think that unfortunately in the cases where we have the most doubt as a result of a detailed post-mortem dissection there is still doubt after an examination for diatoms.

When large quantities of fresh water enter the lungs it rapidly passes into the circulation and causes massive haemolysis. The blood sodium, chloride, calcium, and plasma proteins are diluted and death is supposed to result from ventricular fibrillation. When sea water enters the lungs water diffuses from the blood-stream into the lungs and causes pulmonary oedema. The plasma sodium concentration rises, the blood-pressure falls, and death occurs in asystole.

Although these are probably the biochemical processes which can take place in drowning, biochemical investigations have not proved to be a valuable aid in the diagnosis of difficult drowning cases. It has been suggested that the principal factor in producing electrolyte changes and their effects, is the volume of fluid aspirated per pound body weight. The critical level in causing serious electrolytic change appears to be somewhat above 10 ml of fluid per pound body weight. As approximately 85 per cent of cases of drowning aspirate 10 ml or less of fluid per pound body weight it is unlikely that further investigation of electrolytic changes will prove helpful.[5]

Sometimes in cases where there is almost complete absence of signs of drowning an estimation of the blood and urine alcohol level provides the solution. Where the blood alcohol level is high the resistance to drowning seems to be minimal and death appears to occur in these cases almost immediately on entering the water.

Was drowning due to accident, suicide, or homicide?

In many cases an examination of the body will not throw much light upon the answer to this question. There are, however, certain general indications, attention to which may assist in arriving at an opinion.

Among the causes of accidental drowning may be cited the following:

Children falling into water.
Persons drowned by the upsetting of a boat.
Persons wandering in a fog and falling into a river, or canal.
Persons drowned while bathing.
Intoxicated persons or epileptics falling into water.
Elderly people drowning in baths.
Snorkel swimmers.

The following case of accidental drowning of a woman in a rain-barrel is exceptional. She was preparing for a washing, had evidently been dipping a bucket into the water of the barrel, when she lost her balance and fell in.

Another most unusual case reported to the writer was that of a schoolboy who entered the swimming pond of a bathing establishment, during a competition, for the purpose of retrieving diving plates. These were about 6 inches in diameter with a round hole in the centre. He swam along the bottom of the pond picking up as many plates as possible. One of these plates lay on the top of a grating covering a water outlet at the deep end of the pond. In attempting to retrieve the plate he put his finger not only through the centre hole of the plate but accidentally between two bars of the grating. He was unable to extract his finger, and although other swimmers went down to him they were unable to extricate his finger or to raise the grating. At the same time an attempt was made to empty the pond but the boy was dead before this was accomplished.

Several cases of death have resulted from embedding of the head in mud through diving into water.

There are two separate types of accident which occur in shallow-water diving. Death may result from drowning but in some cases the mechanism is entirely different. The causal factor is the altered gas pressure within the lungs.

Snorkel swimmers who attempt to stay under water as long as possible hyperventilate. In this way they increase the time they can hold their breath. Their residual oxygen may, however, be reduced to such an extent that they lose consciousness after surfacing and drown. The oxygen lack itself may cause lung changes which are similar to those in drowning.[6]

Scuba diving, i.e., diving with self-contained underwater breathing apparatus, is becoming an increasingly popular sport. In the United States there are reputed to be eight million participants. If, however, the necessary precautions are not observed serious accidents can occur, due to the development of excess pressure in the alveoli of the lungs.

One way in which this can occur is during the manoeuvre called 'ditching'; the diver swims to the bottom, discards his equipment, rises to the surface, and then swims down again and replaces his equipment. Pressure at a depth of 9 feet is 1·3 times that at the surface and this results in an expansion of lung volume from 5·5 litres at the bottom of the bath to 7 litres at the surface. No damage results if expiration is carried out while the diver is ascending, but if the breath is held, the pressure in the alveoli may exceed that in the pulmonary vessels by 200 mm Hg. This results in the air being forced into the circulation. A very small amount of air in the left side of the heart can cause very serious damage to the central nervous system and to the myocardium. Divers who have died after some hours have been found to have large infarcts in the myocardium. The same kind of damage can be caused when there is bronchial obstruction producing a ball-valve effect.[7]

If these effects are not understood, the finding of cardiac infarcts in the myocardium of an apparently drowned swimmer may result in the wrong conclusions.

The question of suicide arises when stones or other heavy articles are found in the pockets, or attached to the person, and in cases of persons who are known to have been depressed or of unsound mind.

An inmate of an asylum committed suicide by drowning himself in a basin of water. When the discovery was made, the upper part of the chest was resting against the front of the basin, the head was sunk just under the level of the brim of the basin, the legs were bent under the body, but the knees did not rest on the floor.

The question of homicide is raised under such circumstances as the following:

In cases where, upon the banks of the water in which the body has been found, there are evidences of a struggle, and especially when articles belonging to other than the deceased person are found on the banks associated with those known to have belonged to the deceased; or where, grasped in the hand of the drowned person, there are fragments of clothing or hair, not corresponding to his own.

In cases where, on post-mortem examination, the usual internal signs of death by drowning are absent, and lesions due to violence are found on the body. It is necessary, however, to remember that suicides who have determined to end their lives may have attempted this by one method, but having failed to achieve their purpose, have completed the act by drowning. For example, in one of our cases an elderly man tried to commit suicide by cutting his throat with a razor. From the back room in the house where the razor had been used blood-stains were traced to a swing-bridge over a stream, a distance of about 200 yards, and in a shallow part of the water the body was found.

Although homicidal drowning by pushing the victim into the water may be comparatively easy, it is very uncommon, but occurs occasionally in the case of children or of helpless persons.

In those cases in which marks of violence are found upon a body taken from water, it is necessary for the medical examiner to give careful attention to detail, since he will probably be asked to express an opinion as to whether or not the lesions were produced during life, and, if so produced, whether they alone account for the death.   The differentiation between ante-mortem and post-mortem wounds is discussed under the heading of wounds and their characters (pp. 246 and 256).   The question as to whether wounds upon a body are of suicidal, accidental, or homicidal origin may sometimes be determined by local circumstances referable to the water itself.   In navigable rivers or canals, bodies may sustain injuries, not only extensive in character but peculiar in kind, from the propellers of passing ships (Fig. 50).

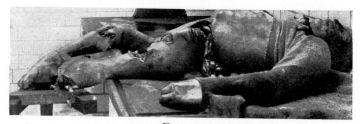

FIG. 50

A body showing extensive injuries caused by the propeller of a ship

Such injuries may cause almost complete evisceration, and fractures with complete or partial removal of a limb or limbs are of frequent occurrence.

In contrast to such cases there are those in which, in consequence of the nature of the injuries found, one can only come to the conclusion that death was due to violence by assault.

When decomposition of a body is far advanced, it will probably be impossible to give any opinion as to whether the lesions were produced before or after death.   In every case, when injuries are present, the whole circumstances must be fully considered and weighed before an opinion is given that they are homicidal in origin.   The examiner must satisfy himself that the lesion could not have been produced in any other way or accounted for in the light of other evidence.

The flotation of the body of a person who has died from drowning depends upon the process of putrefaction.   After a body has sunk, it again comes to the surface and floats after a variable period.   Putrefactive gases play a very important part in flotation, which will therefore be hastened in summer and delayed in winter.   If the water contains putrescent material, putrefaction will be hastened and so will flotation. Putrefaction is slower in onset when the body lies in a running stream than when in still water. In winter, a body will probably come to the surface in about a fortnight's time, and this period will be diminished by about a week in summer. Many circumstances may modify this, for example, heavily clothed bodies and lean bodies will take longer to reach the surface than lightly clothed or fat bodies.

SUFFOCATION

The term suffocation embraces the causes by which death is produced by impediment to respiration, not due to pressure externally and immediately applied to the windpipe. It does not, therefore, include deaths by hanging, strangulation, or throttling, but comprises deaths by smothering or overlaying, those due to foreign bodies in the larynx,

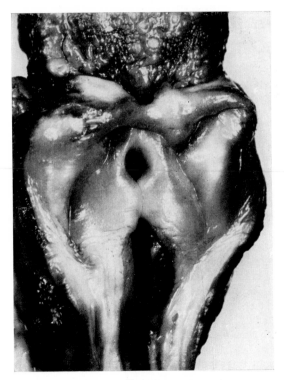

FIG. 51

Oedema of the glottis—angioneurotic—in a girl aged twenty. Death occurred within twelve hours after extraction of four teeth. (By courtesy of the late Dr Robert Richards, Aberdeen University)

trachea, and bronchi, and those due to irrespirable gases. Suffocation may, therefore, result from natural disease, accident, or violence suicidally or homicidally applied. Death by suffocation may be caused:

By prevention of the action of the muscles of respiration.
By obstruction to the entrance of air through the mouth and nostrils.
By obstruction of the larynx, trachea, or bronchi.
By inhalation of irrespirable gases.

It may arise from:

Tumours in the throat or larynx.
Bursting of a pharyngeal or tonsillar abscess.
Exudations affecting the mucous membrane of the air-passages, including acute oedema of the glottis.
Accumulation of bronchial secretion, especially in bronchitis of young children or elderly persons.
Rapidly accumulating pleural effusions, especially if bilateral.
Pulmonary oedema.
Severe haemorrhage in phthisical cases.
Bursting of aneurysms into air passages or lungs.
Convulsions, especially in young children.

It may likewise result from such accidents as:

Pressure on the chest with fixation of the thoracic walls, as in cases of overlaying, in falls of material in mines, quarries, collieries and buildings, pit-cage accidents, and lift accidents.
Impaction of bodies in the larynx, trachea, or bronchi. This is by no means uncommon in intoxicated persons. In choking, the impacted material may consist of imperfectly masticated food, bones, partial dentures, and a variety of other things. Objects, such as rubber balloons, may be inhaled by children during play or accidental inclusion of the head in a plastic bag may cause death. Regurgitation of fluids into the air-passages may occur in a variety of cases, especially infants, and produce fatal asphyxia. In adults, regurgitation may occur during a state of unconsciousness and, not infrequently, in cases of intoxication. In these cases, regurgitated stomach contents, readily recognisable as such, may be found in the pharynx, larynx, trachea, bronchi, and in the bronchioles. Most frequently there is also evidence of regurgitated material around the mouth and nostrils. We have seen many cases of people put to bed in a drunken condition and found dead in the morning due to inhalation of vomitus. Just as in the case of unconscious patients, all those seriously under the influence of alcohol should be transported and managed in the semi-prone position. Post mortem

examination shows external signs of asphyxia, and the pharynx, larynx, trachea, and bronchi contain a quantity of vinous smelling frothy fluid.

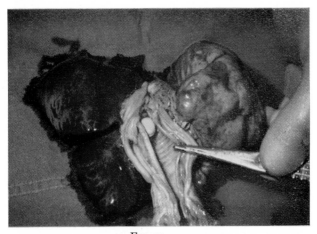

FIG. 52
Showing bean in trachea

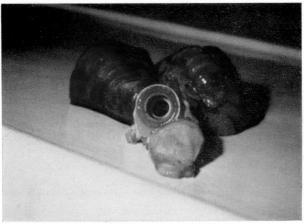

FIG. 53
Showing teat impacted in larynx

Inhalation of fluid, or food particles, especially against the epiglottis, may be responsible for fatal laryngeal spasm.

Gardner[8] has made investigations into the aspiration of food and vomit. His experiments showed that when barium sulphate was introduced through a gastric tube into the stomachs of ten patients immediately after death, subsequent radiographs of the lungs disclosed that in seven out of the ten cases, barium had entered the lungs, reaching the alveoli in several.   He is of the opinion, therefore, that unless the trachea is blocked as soon as the patient dies, necropsy evidence of ante-mortem aspiration cannot of itself be considered conclusive.

Pressure of the mouth and face of an unconscious person against a yielding surface, such as a cushion, mattress, or thick rug.

Inhalation of irrespirable gases, such as sulphuretted hydrogen, sulphur dioxide, chlorine, carbon monoxide, smoke in burning buildings, in coal-pits, and other confined spaces; the vapours of iodine, bromine, and ammonia; and the acrid fumes of mineral acids.

Direct deprivation of oxygen has become recently a fairly common course of suffocation.   These cases occur in caravans and poorly ventilated confined spaces where paraffin and other heaters are used.   Deaths also occur in children who, during play, confine themselves in disused refrigerators.   Suffocation can occur rapidly when children place their heads within polythene bags.   Acute oxygen lack occurs in the holds of ships where the oxygen has

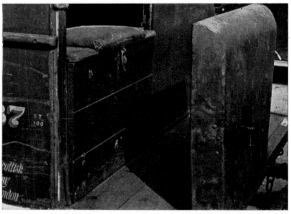

Fig. 54

A unique case of suffocation of two small boys in the driver's box of a disused delivery van.   The box, or locker, measuring 29½ inches long, 13 inches wide, and 20 inches deep, was beneath the driving seat.   It appears that the boys climbed into it in play, and that the lid came down and held firm. Experiments with the fastening on the locker showed that when the lid was dropped sharply the hasp failed to connect, but it slipped easily over the staple when the lid was let down lightly. (By courtesy of H.M. Coroner for the City of Leicester)

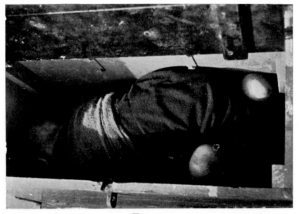

FIG. 55

The driver's box, or locker, on the disused delivery van, showing fastening (Fig. 54). (By courtesy of H.M. Coroner for the City of Leicester)

been used up by materials stored in the hold and by rusting metal. In the latter case multiple deaths sometimes result from rescuers failing to realise the danger.

Suffocation may also be caused homicidally in many ways, including the following:

When pressure is applied over the mouth and nostrils with fixation of the lower jaw, at the same time as fixation of the chest walls by the weight of the body of the assailant.

By placing foreign bodies, such as paper, dough, or other plastic substance into the mouth and larynx of newly born infants.

By covering the face with a pillow, or applying the hand over the mouth and occluding the nostrils with the fingers.

Post-mortem appearances

Since the proximate cause of death in suffocation is asphyxia, the reader is referred to a former chapter for the signs of death from this cause (p. 135). There are, however, certain points to which special attention should be directed, and it must be emphasised that there is no uniformity in the external appearances. Although frequently, in asphyxia, the face is more or less livid in colour and congested in appearance, the conjunctivae are injected, and the lips and ears are of dark colour, it should be clearly appreciated that these conditions are found only in some cases of death by suffocation. In many cases, the face is pale or only slightly dusky in colour, and there may be an absence of congestion either of the eyes or of the lips. As a rule,

M*

however, lividity is well marked in the lips, ears, and finger-nails. In children who have died from asphyxial causes, the livid tint of the nails of the fingers and toes is almost constant.

In certain cases of asphyxia, not only are the conjunctivae congested, but small petechial haemorrhages are present. The variation in the

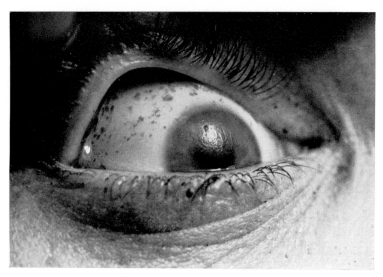

FIG. 56

Subconjunctival petechial haemorrhages

external manifestations is due in large measure to the rapidity with which the asphyxial process is initiated and completed.

In addition to the principal signs of death by asphyxia already discussed in a former chapter, some light may be thrown upon the cause of death by noting particularly the following points:

In deaths caused by inhalation of carbon monoxide, due to the formation of a stable compound between the gas and the haemoglobin, carboxyhaemoglobin, the colour of the blood is bright red. This is noted not only in the principal blood-vessels, but in all the organs of the body (Fig. 225).

In most cases of suffocation in children, and in certain of those in adults, small petechial haemorrhages may be seen on the serous surfaces of the heart and lungs (p. 135).

Suicidal suffocation by the insertion of foreign bodies into the back of the throat has occurred in a number of cases, and portions of clothing and other materials have been used for this purpose.

ILLUSTRATIVE CASES

Renton[9] has recorded the following case. A man was brought to a workhouse with a history of delusions. In the evening he suddenly became violent and was placed in a padded room. He quietened down and went to sleep. Twenty minutes later, it was observed that his bedclothing had been thrown off, and on closer examination he was found to be dead. Inside the mouth was a piece of flannel, about 1 foot long by 1 inch broad, and behind it were two strips similar in length. The last of these was so firmly packed over the epiglottis that it was withdrawn with difficulty. He had obtained the cloth by tearing his blanket.

Other instances of placing foreign bodies in the throat show homicidal motive, and include such acts as forcing mud or dough into the throats of newly born children, or a handkerchief in the case of adults. In one of our cases, the murder of a young woman, a tightly compressed pocket-handkerchief was found impacted in the pharynx. There were also some wounds on the head and face, but death had resulted from asphyxia due to suffocation. The wounds were not of a character to cause death, but were sufficient to have stunned the deceased.

Occasionally deaths result from rupture of the larynx and trachea following relatively trivial injury to the front of the neck with resultant bilateral pneumothorax.[10]

Suffocation by the inhalation of coal-gas is a common form of suicide. This may be caused by turning on the gas in a room, putting the head in a gas oven, or by placing a gas tube in the mouth. Accidental death also may result readily from the inhalation of coal-gas under a great variety of circumstances (p. 565).

TRAUMATIC ASPHYXIA

There is a form of suffocation to which the term 'traumatic asphyxia' has been applied. It is brought about by compression of the chest and abdomen as the result of the victim being crushed between heavy bodies, for example, by a pit-cage, by a fall of coal, or by being crushed in a crowd.

The leading features are:

A deep red or violet discoloration of the face, neck and upper parts of the body.

Very injected conjunctivae with perhaps a varying degree of extravasation of blood.

A well-defined demarcating line between the discoloured upper portion of the body and the lower normally coloured part of the body, which in some cases may be as high as the clavicles or neck.

Other features which may be present are:

Extensive petechiae of the skin.

Proptosis of the eyes.

Fundal haemorrhages.

Gordon and Thompson[11] have described five cases and are of the opinion that the causation of the skin discoloration is due to sudden over-distention of the veins with consequent paralysis of the walls. They are of the further opinion that the occurrences of haemorrhages into the optic nerve or sheath and damage to the retina by venous back

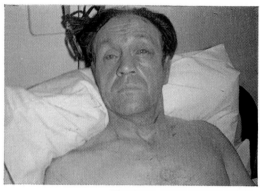

FIG. 57.

Traumatic asphyxia. This man was injured when a crush barrier collapsed at a football match. Petechial haemorrhages can be seen on his upper chest and his conjunctivae are intensely congested. (Photograph by courtesy of Mr W. Sillar, Southern General Hospital, Glasgow.)

pressure are responsible for the ocular complications. The amount of lividity differs in various cases owing to the period of time, short of producing death by suffocation, in which the mechanical chest pressure is in operation.

Early in 1943, 173 persons died from asphyxia due to suffocation by compression in a crowd. Briefly, the accident resulted from someone falling on a stair leading to a London tube air-raid shelter, with the resultant piling up of persons from behind and above. The victims were pressed together, with restriction of chest movement. It was found that some of the persons on the top had died and some at the bottom were brought out alive. Almost the last person removed from the bottom was a girl of seven who walked without assistance to the first-aid post. There was not a case in which the ribs were broken, and there were only a few cases in which bones were fractured.

In 1971 a similar accident occurred near the end of a football match at Ibrox Park, Glasgow. Again probably as a result of one person stumbling a mass of bodies built up in the comparatively confined space of a stairway leading down from the terracing. Of the 66 who died nearly all exhibited classical signs of traumatic asphyxia. Apart from minor abrasions, the only other injuries found were a few fractured limbs.

A striking feature of traumatic asphyxia is the way in which recovery can take place even in cases showing very marked signs.

HANGING

Hanging may be defined as that form of death which is caused by suspension of the body by a ligature which encircles the neck, the constricting force being the weight of the body. A frequent method is the use of a running noose. The proximate cause of death is asphyxia or comato-asphyxia.

The time occupied in the process of death depends chiefly upon two factors, the severity of the constricting force and the point of application of that force.

The amount of the constricting force depends upon whether or not the body is completely suspended. Complete suspension is not essential since the partial weight of the body is adequate for the purpose. Persons have succeeded in hanging themselves although their feet were in contact with the floor. Only a slight degree of constriction of the neck is required to cause eventual death. When, however, the entire body is suspended, greater weight is thrown upon the ligature and a greater constricting force results. When such a degree of force is applied to the neck, death supervenes more rapidly than in the case of partial suspension with a diminished degree of constrictive force. When the ligature is not tight, death may ensue slowly, chiefly from the effects of coma induced by disturbance of the cerebral circulation as the result of pressure on the vessels in the neck. The point of application of the force is an important factor not only in the time occupied in dying, but in the subsequent post-mortem appearances.

Experiments have proved that the degree and rapidity of the onset of asphyxial symptoms are greatly influenced by the situation of the ligature on the neck. When the ligature is placed between the lower jaw and the hyoid bone and is moderately tightened, the effect is to disturb breathing, which, however, continues, but at the end of two minutes the subject has to be disengaged from the noose. When the ligature is placed over the larynx, the experiment has to cease at the end of one and a half minutes. When placed over the cricoid cartilage, the experiment cannot be continued for even a few seconds because of embarrassment to respiration. The pull required to occlude the air-passages and vessels of the neck varies with the musculature. It is usually less than one would expect. Polson gives a figure of 7 lb for occlusion of the carotid arteries and quotes figures of 33 lb for closing the trachea and $36\frac{1}{2}$ lb for the vertebral arteries.[12]

The effect of a ligature constricting the neck is primarily the partial or complete occlusion of the air-passages, which obstructs air entry to the lungs. As the result of this compression, the cerebral circulation is also impeded. The amount of compression exercised on the phrenic and vagus nerves is yet another factor in the causation of death. Apart from implication of respiration a person may die from the effects of suspension. This is well illustrated in the case of a man upon whom tracheotomy had been performed for malignant disease of the throat, and who suspended himself by the neck, the line of ligature being above the site of the cannula. At post-mortem examination signs of asphyxia were absent, but the blood-vessels at the base of the brain, and in the substance of the pons and medulla, were found engorged. In the majority of cases of suicidal suspension the ligature is placed either between the thyroid cartilage and the hyoid bone, or between the hyoid bone and the lower jaw. The constricting force of the ligature causes the tongue, soft palate, and larynx to be pushed upwards and backwards, thus cutting off the passage of air.

Pressure on the vagus nerves may cause cardiac inhibition and sudden death before asphyxial manifestations are established. This possibility should not be overlooked at the post-mortem examination of bodies of persons found hanged.

As in other forms of death from asphyxia, the heart continues to beat for a few minutes after the cessation of respiration, and, therefore, artificial respiration on a suspended person may prove successful if the body is cut down within five or six minutes after the commencement of suspension. After this period, there is little chance of success in the re-establishment of breathing.

External post-mortem appearances

The face is usually pale, but may be dusky in hue. The lips are bluish in colour, and the tongue and mucous membrane of the mouth may share in this coloration. The position of the tongue varies from normality to protrusion slightly beyond the line of the teeth. Tongue injury is unusual. Saliva may be seen trickling from the corner of the mouth as the result of increased salivation prior to death, due to stimulation of the salivary glands produced by the ligature. Petechial haemorrhages may be found under the conjunctivae and, more rarely, on the eyelids and forehead. The conjunctivae are frequently congested.

Very early putrefactive discoloration is often seen on the lower abdominal wall. This is caused by the accumulation of blood in the lower parts of the body.

Turgescence of the penis, in varying degree, with or without evidence of seminal or prostatic fluid may occasionally be seen, but when present, has no specific bearing on death by hanging. Fluid at the tip of the penis is sometimes present in deaths due to a variety of causes. We have seen it in the case of a man fatally stabbed in the chest, and in several other cases. In some of these, the fluid contained spermatoza. Only in two instances was marked turgescence of the penis observed. It is most probable that engorgement of the penis may be the result of hypostasis, and that seminal or prostatic fluid may be found by reason of gravitation, or possibly of rigor mortis. The voidance of urine or faeces is merely indicative of the loss of power of the sphincters which may occur in all deaths.

Local conditions of the neck. The incidence and character of the marks on the neck will probably indicate the mode of application of the ligature. All marks on the neck should be critically examined to determine whether death is attributable to suspension, or to throttling, followed by suspension to cloak the commission of crime. Should scratches be present, they must be carefully considered in relation to whether or not they could have been produced by the ligature. Scratches on the neck or face in the presence of a soft pliable ligature should evoke suspicion, although it must not be forgotten that the dying person, in vain attempt to loosen the ligature, may have produced scratches with his finger-nails.

The line of the ligature must be carefully examined. In suicidal suspension, it usually follows the line of the lower jaw, then passes obliquely upwards behind the ears, where it is commonly lost. The situation of the mark will, however, be largely influenced by the method used in the application of the ligature, for example, whether in the form of a loop or a running noose. In the former method, the mark will be most prominent on the part of the neck to which the head has inclined, and less marked over the region of the open angle of the loop. When a running noose has been employed, the mark more or less encircles the surface of the neck, and is most prominent at the point underlying the knot. The reason for the ligature line being close to the lower jaw in the bulk of cases, in which a running noose is used, is that as the body sinks in the act of suspension the ligature gradually slides up the neck until it is fixed by the line of the lower jaw. The relation of the body to the point of suspension and to the ground must also be taken into account, since a variety of angles will be produced and may affect the incidence of the point of constriction. In some cases, the mark may pass over the thyroid cartilage and in others the hyoid bone, but in the bulk of cases it is situated between the hyoid bone and the line of the lower jaw.

A suicide may pass the ligature twice round the neck before he suspends himself, and a double mark, one more or less circular, and the other, oblique, may be seen. A composite ligature, consisting of a series of strands of rope or cord, may be used. A suicide is not particular as to the kind of ligature he employs, and will probably use what is at hand for the purpose. Ropes, handkerchiefs, braces, leather straps, belts, bed-sheets, and scarves, among others, are frequently employed. All of these factors will produce modifications in the character of the mark or marks found upon the neck. Occasionally, unusual features are found. In the case of a man who hanged himself by a chain, the contour of the individual links was discernible on the skin.

Another case was that of a man who had suspended himself from the knob of a window-shutter about 4 feet above the ground. On the left side of the neck there was a single ligature mark, but on the right side there were three separate furrows, with small intervening ridges of skin of livid colour. The explanation was that the man had used, as a ligature, a series of strands of ordinary ham-string.

In cases of suspected infanticide when a mark is found on the neck of an infant, the possibility that it may have been due to constriction by the umbilical cord during birth must not be overlooked. Since however, the umbilical cord is a soft structure and is unlikely to produce other than limited constriction when situated around the neck, the mark is not usually deep, and does not show the typical appearance of the ordinary ligature mark.

There may be indications in the vicinity of a ligature mark, such as scratches or small bruises, which are suggestive of the nature of the ligature used, although the ligature may not be available for inspection. These may have been produced by a ligature of coarse texture, or alternatively, by the finger-nails of the victim, or those of an assailant in throttling, prior to suspension of the body to simulate suicide by hanging. In doubtful cases, to eliminate the possibility of the body having been suspended after death, a piece of tissue from the ligature mark should be excised so that histological examination may determine the presence or absence of vital reaction. When available, the ligature should always be retained for detailed examination.

The colour of a ligature mark may show wide variation and may range from a parchment shade to a purplish hue. Frequently a bluish-red colour may be evident, but sometimes the site of the ligature may be almost devoid of colour. Quite frequently, at first a pale colour may be present, but this subsequently assumes a brownish, dried appearance. The line of application of the ligature is usually depressed, and the degree of depth depends upon the nature of the ligature, the amount of pressure on the tissues, and the duration of the suspension.

When bruising is found associated with the mark, its presence indicates that the violence responsible was operative either during life, or was applied immediately after death while there was continuance of molecular life of the tissues. When suspension has occurred during life, there is usually some degree of bruising of the tissues associated with the site of constriction, but this may be very slight.

Internal post-mortem appearances

The appearances are those of asphyxia. The brain and cranial sinuses show marked congestion. As in death by suffocation, subpleural punctiform haemorrhages may be found, in addition to the signs already described under asphyxia.

A detailed dissection of the tissues of the neck should be made to detect injury of the deeper structures. In a great many cases of hanging, however, the most striking feature is the absence of lesions in the neck. Occasionally the following may be found: tearing of the platysma, injury to the sterno-mastoid muscles, damage to the thyrohyoid ligament, and fractures of the thyroid cartilage and hyoid bone.

Petechial haemorrhages may be found on the epiglottis, in the larynx, and trachea. The trachea will usually show a varying degree of congestion in which the epiglottis is frequently involved.

Accident, suicide or homicide

When it has been established that death has resulted from hanging, the next question is, whether it was suicidal, accidental, or homicidal?

It is a statistical fact that death by hanging is a common form of suicide and there is, therefore, a strong presumption in favour of suicide.

In many undoubted cases of suicide some portion of the body is found in contact with the ground. The amount of the body so resting may vary in extent from the major portion of the trunk to merely the tips of the toes. In one of our cases the point at which the rope was attached was only 3 feet from the ground, and the lower part of the body from the hips downwards was resting on the floor. In another, the legs from the knees downwards, were resting.

At the same time, it must not be forgotten that a suicide may give himself a drop. In one case, the suicide tied a piece of rope to the banister railing of a stairway, placed his neck within the noose, then jumped into the well of the stairway. The drop was ten feet, and examination showed that the neck had been dislocated.

The question becomes more complicated, however, when wounds produced by blunt or sharp weapons are found upon the body of the suspended person. Such are sometimes found in suicidal cases. They are well illustrated in the case of a man who tried to suspend himself but the ligature broke. He next butted his head against the walls and wounded himself. He tried again to hang himself from the ceiling with a bed-sheet fixed to a strap round his neck. This attempt was successful. A suicide may first attempt to cut his throat and then hang himself. Sometimes the attendant circumstances, apart from mere suspension, indicate suicidal action.

Cases of hanging occur which have the appearance of being suicidal,

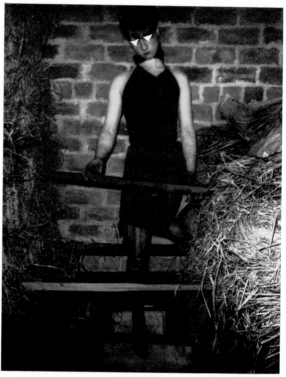

FIG. 58
Case of accidental hanging resulting from
sexual aberration

but are now usually considered to be accidental. The victims suffer from sexual aberration and sexual satisfaction is obtained from the act of partial suspension, very often in female clothing. Although death frequently occurs this does not appear to be intended. The aim of the sexual deviant is to increase sexual sensation through partial asphyxia. In addition to suspension, the partial asphyxia is sometimes obtained by the use of plastic bags or coal-gas. The majority of these cases occur in young males (Figs. 58 and 59).

Accidental hanging sometimes occurs. A case is recorded of a boy who went into a cowshed in which was a swing attached to a beam. He climbed up to this beam, with the intention of sliding down one of the ropes of the swing, but in his descent a woollen scarf round his neck

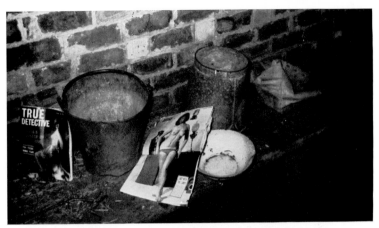

FIG. 59

View seen by boy from position of hanging

caught on a long nail fastened in the beam, and he became suspended. He was found in this position, and cut down. His face was very cyanosed and he was unconscious, but was resuscitated.

Homicidal hanging is rare. Except in cases of weakness from senility or other enfeebling cause, or under very unusual circumstances, the act cannot readily be perpetrated by one assailant. Usually more than one are involved in its commission. When resistance has been offered, marks of violence are likely to be found.

Hanging is sometimes used to conceal murder. The most famous case of this was the Emmet Dunne murder where the victim was found suspended and thought to be a case of suicidal hanging. Subsequently it was found, after exhumation of the body, that death was due to homicidal trauma to the neck structures and Emmet Dunne was convicted of murder.

STRANGULATION

Strangulation may be defined as that form of death which is caused by a constricting force applied around the neck by means of a ligature without suspension of the body. Throttling, or manual strangulation, is that form of death which is caused by compression of the throat, the constricting force being the fingers and the hand or hands of the assailant.

Ordinary strangulation may be caused accidentally, suicidally, or homicidally. The most common, however, is homicidal, and the majority of these are associated with sexual assaults on females. The constricting mark is usually found at a lower level on the neck than in hanging, but may be found at any level, and frequently direct pressure is exerted upon the larynx. The mark more or less completely encircles the neck transversely. In some cases it may be continuous, but in others it may be invisible at some part of the neck. The nature of the

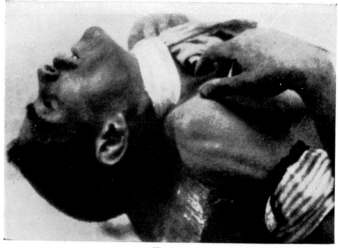

FIG. 60

Suicidal strangulation. The ligature used was a piece of fabric torn from the man's clothing and folded several times. It was retained in position by means of a half-knot

ligature employed plays a prominent part in this respect. The degree and character of injury to the deeper tissues of the neck are dependent on the amount of violence used in the application of the ligature. The underlying muscles frequently show some degree of extravasation, due to rupture of the capillary vessels. The laryngeal cartilages and trachea are usually intact, but in some cases, especially homicidal cases, fractures of these structures are present. Fracture of the hyoid bone is unusual. The injuries in homicidal strangulation are usually more extensive than in accidental or suicidal cases, due to the fact that an assailant frequently uses more force than is necessary to cause the death of his victim. It is in such cases that extensive deep-seated injury is likely to be found. When a ligature is suddenly placed around the neck of a person and pulled tightly, the assaulted person is rendered unconscious very quickly and is unable to offer much resistance.

There is no doubt that suicidal strangulation does occur but it is a diagnosis which should be accepted by the forensic pathologist with some reluctance.   It is usually effected by tying the ligature.   When only a half-knot is employed the nature of the material composing the ligature will be the determining factor as to whether the ligature will maintain constriction of the neck or loosen after consciousness of the individual is lost.   In some cases, the ligature is fastened with a double knot.   Sometimes a ligature is passed round the neck several times.   In differentiating between suicidal and homicidal strangulation, significance cannot be placed either upon the nature of the knot or its position on the neck.   Strangulation may occur under the most unexpected circumstances.   In one case, a woman laid herself on a bed, attached the running noose of a rope round her neck, and tied the other end of the

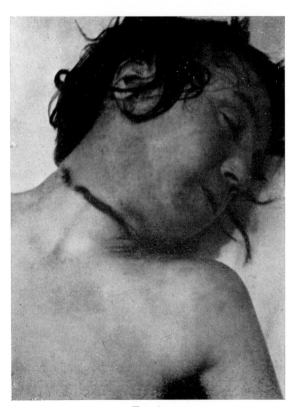

Fig. 61

Ligature mark, caused by rope, in a case of strangulation

rope to a heavy piece of metal which she threw over the iron bar of the bed-frame.

Accidental strangulation occasionally occurs and may happen in a variety of ways, for example, a boy climbed an apple tree and slipped between the branches, his jacket, which was buttoned at the neck, turned up round his neck and strangled him.   A boy was strangled by his scarf while playing with a dog.

Strangulation being an asphyxial death, the external and internal signs of asphyxia will be apparent, and what has already been described under this subject applies.   The extent and character of the signs will depend in large measure upon the rate of the asphyxial process.   When the constricting force has been considerable they will be well marked. It must not be forgotten, however, that in certain cases signs of asphyxia may be very slight if death has supervened quickly from cardiac inhibition, due to pressure on the carotid nerve plexus.

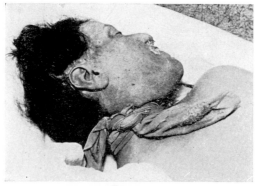

Fig. 62

Case of homicidal strangulation.   Note small quantity of foam at nostrils and corner of mouth.   (By courtesy of the Commissioner of the Metropolis, Scotland Yard)

MANUAL STRANGULATION

This is invariably homicidal.   There is always some damage to the tissues of the neck but the extent of the bruised areas will depend upon the relative positions of the assailant and victim, the manner of grasping the neck, and the degree of pressure exercised upon the throat.   Whatever the pattern, the medico-legal examiner should suspect manual strangulation if he finds circular bruises on the neck and if these are associated with small crescentic abrasions he should be hesitant to accept any other diagnosis.   The marks are usually found over the lateral aspects of the larynx or trachea, and most frequently correspond

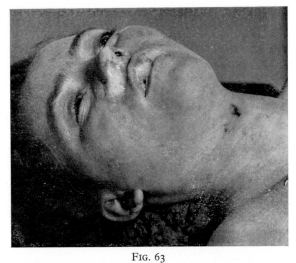

FIG. 63

Homicidal throttling.   Note foam at nostrils and mouth, also
marks in front of neck

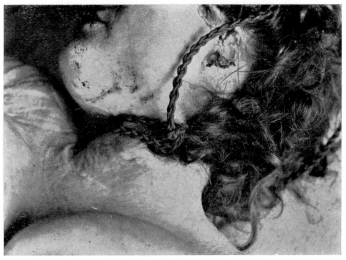

FIG. 64

Homicidal strangulation with telephone wire cord (Fig. 65)

to a thumb mark on one side, and a larger mark, or series of marks, on the other, due to compression by the fingers. When the hands of the assailant operate from behind the victim, the compression will be applied practically all round the neck, but certain areas of bruising will be more prominent than others due to the pressure of the finger-tips.

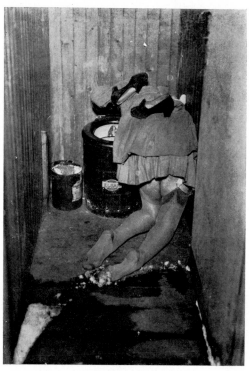

FIG. 65
Homicidal strangulation. Position of body as found
(Fig. 64)

As a rule there is extensive bruising of the tissues, which is frequently accompanied by fracture of the laryngeal structures, and, commonly, the hyoid bone. Further, there may be bruising or laceration of the tongue as the result of it having been pressed against, or caught between the teeth. In some cases, there may be practically no evidence of bruising on the surface of the neck, although fairly extensive bruising of the deeper tissues may be found, together with fracture of the hyoid bone. The bruising of the deeper tissues is usually discrete in character and frequently the muscular tissues are involved. The extent will naturally depend upon the degree of pressure used. Occasionally bruising of muscle may be very slight. For this reason an individual dissection of the muscles of the neck *in situ* should be made in cases where strangulation is suspected.

Fracture of the hyoid bone is a common occurrence, and when it is present indicates that considerable violence has been applied to the neck. It negatives suicide and provides strong indication of homicide. It was at one time considered to be absolutely diagnostic of homicidal throttling. With the increase in the variety of accidental injuries associated with modern machines and especially the automobile, it has come to be recognised that fracture of the hyoid bone can occur quite often as a result of accident. Forbes[13] reports a case of fracture of the hyoid bone as the result of pressure and counter-pressure, but unrelated to throttling by the hand. It involved a motor-tractor driver, whose machine had an attached scraper which was controlled by a wire rope, half an inch in diameter. Accidentally, a loop of the rope had got round the driver's neck, which had been pulled up to the winch, thus compressing the tissues of the neck. When ossification between the body and the horns of this bone has occurred, in subjects of middle age and over, fracture occurs more easily. There may also be fracture of the laryngeal cartilages or of the trachea when considerable violence has been used.

Occasionally a medical witness may be asked in a given case whether the hyoid bone might not have been fractured by artefact. This bone, as a rule, is not easily fractured post-mortem, and such a possibility can be eliminated when extravasation has been found at the site of fracture. He may also be asked to demonstrate how the throat might have been grasped by the assailant. In relation to this point it should not be forgotten that certain marks upon the surface of the neck may not bear an exact and corresponding relationship to underlying deep-seated bruising. This can readily be accounted for by the fact that the mobility of the skin may alter the relationship which normally exists between it and the underlying structures when certain forms of pressure are applied.

The absence of bruising upon the skin, when deep-seated bruising is present, can be accounted for by the maintenance of pressure until death has supervened, since compression of the skin will empty the vessels in it during life, and the heart may have ceased to beat before the pressure has been removed.

Bruising of the tongue, the floor of the mouth, the mucous lining of the larynx, and the epiglottis are common findings in cases of throttling. The areas involved vary from small petechial haemorrhages to bruises of appreciable size. The skin and underlying tissues at the back of the neck should always be examined carefully for evidence of bruising, the result of counter-pressure exerted by an assailant.

Since asphyxia is the cause of death, the external and internal signs associated with it will be present, usually in accentuated form, since the asphyxial process is rapid. It must be remembered, however, that if pressure has been applied over the carotid sinus there may be an immediate vaso-vagal inhibition and a carotid sinus reflex arrest of respiration and circulation. In such cases the asphyxial signs may be either slight or practically absent due to the sudden onset of death. In one of our cases of manual strangulation, although there were surface bruises on the neck, deep bruising was absent, apart from a small, localised haemorrhage in the tissue clothing the joint between the body of the hyoid bone

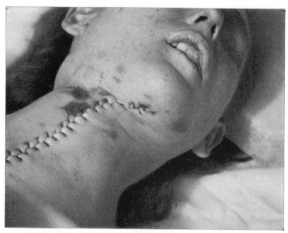

FIG. 66

Abrasions on neck in a case of manual strangulation

and its left cornu. There was an abnormal degree of mobility at the left synchondrosis. X-ray examination did not disclose fracture. Although there were certain asphyxial manifestations, it seemed clear that cardiac inhibition, due to pressure over the carotid sinus, had brought life to a close. The victim of the assault was pregnant, and had been in sub-average health.

In throttling there are three impediments to the normal functioning of the body, namely, obstruction of respiration, interference with the blood supply to the brain, and pressure on the carotid nerve plexuses which are composed of fibres from the vagus, sympathetic, and glosso-pharyngeal nerves.

The possible effects of trauma in the region of the carotid sinus may be far-reaching, and are thus worthy of note. Jokl[14] describes fatalities in the boxing ring due to trauma of the lateral regions of the neck with total absence of pathological findings at the autopsy to explain the catastrophe. Another author, whom he cites, has observed a case of sudden death due to a blow over the lateral part of the neck. Jokl also

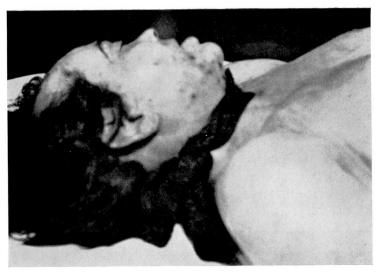

FIG. 67

Homicidal strangulation with a tie (see Figs. 68 and 69)

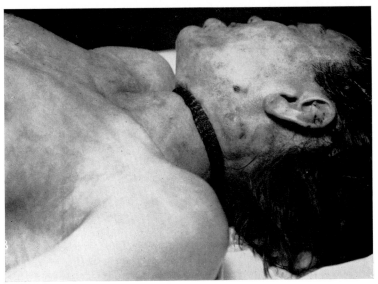

FIG. 68

Homicidal strangulation with a tie (see Figs. 67 and 69)

records the case of a knock-out in a fencer caused by a blow to the carotid sinus.

When definite local evidence of violence, such as has been described, is found and asphyxial signs coexist, death has been produced by throttling.

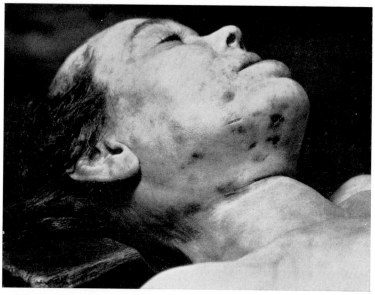

FIG. 69

Appearance of neck after removal of ligature (see Figs. 67 and 68)

ILLUSTRATIVE CASES

The following case is given at some length, since it is illustrative of most of the injuries commonly found present in death by homicidal throttling:

The body of a woman, aged fifty-two, was found floating in a canal a short time after death. Post-mortem examination showed that death had not been caused by drowning but from the effects of compression of the throat which had brought about cardiac inhibition during the process of asphyxia. The lips were bluish in colour and a small quantity of fine bubbled foam was present at their margins. The tongue was pressed against the edges of the teeth that remained in the lower jaw and those in the upper denture. There were a few minor injuries on the body, including the face, but the principal injuries were confined to the tissues of the neck. The skin covering the front and sides of the neck was wrinkled and lax and was of an irregular faint bluish hue, but no discrete bruises were visible. The tongue was slightly swollen and the middle third of the anterior margin showed two slightly raised nodular protrusions which were faintly blue in colour. On section, these areas showed extensive haemorrhage throughout the substance of the muscle. There were also two additional areas, of similar but less pronounced character, on the right of the midline of the tongue. The most marked of these haemorrhagic areas corresponded in position to a gap left by the lateral incisor and canine teeth on the right side of the lower jaw. The epiglottis showed twelve scattered punctate haemorrhages in the mucosa. The larynx showed similar haemorrhages immediately below the vocal cords. There was some scanty fine foam at the base of the epiglottis, and a thin film of foam covered the lining of the trachea. The muscles of the neck showed multiple haemorrhages as follows:

Diffuse haemorrhagic staining in the left platysma muscle, 2 inches by 1 inch;

Blood-clot over the middle of the outer surface of the left sterno-mastoid muscle;

Two areas of bruising extending throughout the left sterno-mastoid muscle. One area measured 1 inch by $\frac{1}{2}$ inch and was situated on the anterior margin close to the middle of the muscle. The other measured 2 inches by 1 inch and was situated at the lower end of the muscle;

A bruise in the right sterno-mastoid muscle at the level of the larynx, extending throughout the muscle substance in the region of its anterior border and measuring $1\frac{1}{2}$ inches by 1 inch. There was a similar area, showing evidence of clot, at the lower end of the muscle;

Bruising at the lower ends of both sterno-hyoid muscles and in the same regions of both sterno-thyroid muscles;

Two areas of bruising, each the size of a pea, in the muscles at the root of the tongue immediately to the right of the midline;

A small bruise over the lower border of the right submaxillary gland;

A bruise in the thyro-hyoid membrane at the point of junction of the left greater cornu with the body of the hyoid bone;

A bruise in the middle line of the neck immediately above the hyoid bone.

The hyoid bone was fractured through the right greater cornu at a point 1·3 centimetres from the tip of the tubercle. The line of fracture, which was oblique in character, ran from above downwards and forwards. The periosteum in the region of the fracture showed a slight degree of extravasation.

Tissue from the bruised areas was examined microscopically, and

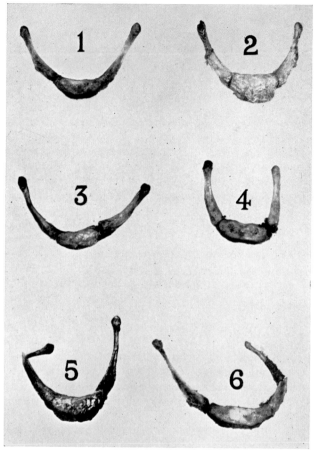

FIG. 70

Hyoid bones.

1 and 2, normal.   3 and 4 show subluxation at left synchondrosis.
5 and 6 show fracture of the right and left cornu respectively

from the character of the extravasation and infiltration of blood, it was evident that the lesions had been produced during life.

When all the circumstances of the case were fully considered, it seemed clear that either the woman had been dead when her body entered the water or that death had occurred almost as soon as she had entered the water or within a very short time thereafter, and that it could not have been a case of accident or of suicide.

In another case, pressure had been applied to the upper part of the throat and floor of the mouth.   The deceased man was fifty-eight, and at the time of the fatal assault was under the influence of alcohol. The blood alcohol content was 228 milligrams per 100 millilitres and the urine alcohol content was 340 milligrams per 100 millilitres. The face showed a large number of petechial haemorrhages which covered an area extending from the upper part of the forehead to the under surface of the chin (see Fig. 74). The lining of the eyelids of both eyes showed pin-point haemorrhages and there were also bilateral subconjunctival haemorrhages. There was no external evidence of bruising on the surfaces of the neck or under surface of the chin. The tongue was congested and showed diffuse extravasation almost throughout its entire substance. The greater part of the lateral margins showed bruising and the front of the tongue was similarly affected apart from a small portion at the tip. The back of the tongue was the seat of blackish blue dis-coloration which extended backwards to the anterior surface of the epiglottis, which was slightly oedematous, as were the structures of the upper part of the larynx. The structures, including muscle, in the sublingual and submaxillary regions on both sides showed marked extravasation, but this was more extensive on the left side. The tissues in the left submaxillary region were oedematous. The hyoid bone, laryngeal structures, and trachea were uninjured and there was no extravasation of blood into the tissues surrounding them.

One of our cases of throttling was of rather an unusual nature since the victim of the attack survived for about three-quarters of an hour, and was able to return to his home both by bus and by walking. Post-mortem dissection showed marked extravasation in the deeper tissues of the floor of the mouth, more marked on the right side. On the right side of the neck, the tissues around the hyoid bone were bruised, and to a lesser extent on the left side. From the top of the thyroid cartilage down to the upper border of the breast-bone and extending laterally to the deeper tissues on both sides of the neck, there was massive bruising. The bruising extended to the posterior wall of the pharynx and to the adjacent wall of the oesophagus. It travelled laterally from the posterior border of the thyroid cartilage to the opening of the larynx. The epiglottis was congested, the left anterior part was oedematous and on the right anterior part there was bruising. Bruising was also present on the right lateral and anterior walls of the upper part of the larynx. The right vocal cord was bruised and oedematous with a markedly diminished air channel. Further bruising affected the lining membrane of the oesophagus. The right superior cornu of the thyroid cartilage was fractured together with the left cornu of the hyoid bone. The right cornu was more mobile at its synchondrosis than its neighbour. Death resulted from oedema glottidis.

The following case is one of strangulation by a ligature applied to the neck. The deceased female was aged twenty-three. The finger-nails, toe-nails, and lips showed some lividity and scanty pinkish-coloured

fluid exuded from the nostrils and mouth.   A small group of punctate
subconjunctival haemorrhages was present over the upper outer
quadrant of the right eye and a few smaller haemorrhages were situated
on the outer corners of the rims of the eyelids.   A similar condition
affected the left eye.   Both conjunctivae were slightly congested.   An
artificial silk scarf formed a single ligature around the neck and was held
fairly tightly by a reef-knot which was firmly tied.   The following marks
were present on the neck: Over the front were two principal marks.

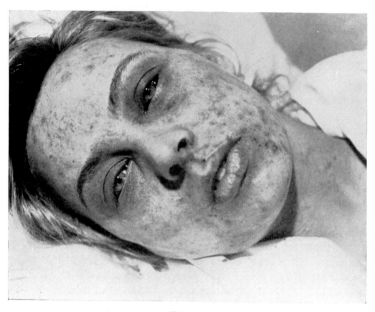

FIG. 71

Petechial haemorrhages on face in a case of attempted murder by strangulation
(By courtesy of Professor Gilbert Forbes, Glasgow University)

The mid-point of the lower mark was at a level of $1\frac{3}{4}$ inches above the
upper border of the sternum.   The mark then passed slightly upwards
over the right of the front of the neck, the highest point being 2 inches
above the sterno-clavicular joint.   The mark also passed slightly upwards over the left of the front of the neck, the highest level being
$1\frac{1}{2}$ inches above the clavicle.   The maximum level on the right side of
the neck was at a point 3 inches below the lobe of the ear, behind which
a slightly forked formation of the mark was seen.   Close to the midline
of the back of the neck, these forks united and the mark continued round
the back and left side of the neck.   The average breadth of the mark was
$\frac{1}{3}$ inch.   Over the front of the neck and above the ligature mark

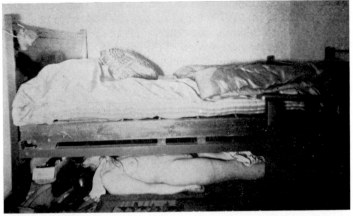

Fig. 72

Strangulation caused by a scarf held in position by a complete knot

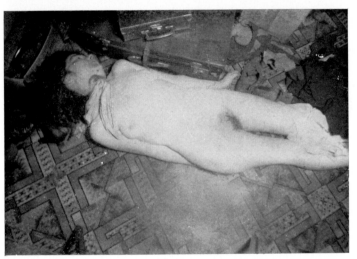

Fig. 73

The same case as in Fig. 72

described, there were several interrupted and less defined pressure marks, due to the ligature, which ran horizontally in relation to the mark which encircled the neck. Running from the immediate left of the middle line of the neck to a point 1 inch below the angle of the right lower jaw was an irregular, curved, parchment-like area which measured $3\frac{1}{2}$ inches by 1 inch. It was of curved contour with convexity towards the jaw. This mark corresponded to the position of the ligature knot and adjacent parts of the ligature when the head was flexed and directed slightly to the right. All the marks upon the neck were of dark red colour and were leathery to the touch. Two punctate abrasions were present, one on the under surface of the left side of the lower jaw and the other on the right side of the chin. Three similar abrasions were present on the right side of the neck. On dissection of the tissues of the neck, two small areas of extravasation associated with the ligature

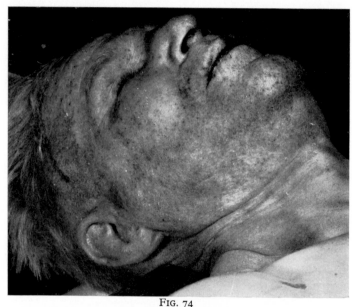

FIG. 74

Multiple petechiae extending from the upper part of neck and covering the face can be seen

mark were seen. Both were superficial. The laryngeal structures, the trachea, and hyoid bone were intact. The tongue showed a slight indentation on the under surface of the tip corresponding to the position of the left lower incisor tooth. Incision into this area did not show evidence of extravasation. The epiglottis was slightly congested.

This case illustrates well the difficulties which can arise in cases of strangulation, as even after a lengthy investigation there was some doubt as to whether death was homicidal or suicidal.

References

1. MILES, S. Br. med. J., 3, 597, 1968.
2. MUELLER, B. Dt. Z. ges. gericht. Med., 54, 267, 1963.
3. TIMPERMAN, J. J. forens. Med., 16, 45 1969.

4. BURGER, E.   *Dt. Z. ges. gericht. Med.*, **64,** 21, 1968.
5. MODELL, J.H. & DAVIS, J.H.   *Anesthesiology*, **30,** 414, 1969.
6. CRAIG, A.B.   *J. Am. med. Ass.*, **176,** 255, 1961.
7. COOPERMAN, E.M., HOGG, J., & THURLBECK, W.M.   *Can. med. Ass. J.*, **99,** 1128, 1968.
8. GARDNER, A.M.   *Q. Jl Med.*, **27,** 227, 1958.
9. RENTON, J.M.   *Br. med. J.*, **1,** 493, 1908.
10. POLSON, C.J. & HORNBAK, H.   *Med.-leg. J.*, *Lond.*, **28,** 88, 1960.
11. GORDON, W.I. & THOMSON, A.M.W.   *Glasg. med. J.*, **130,** 180, 1938.
12. POLSON, C.J.   *The Essentials of Forensic Medicine*, 2nd ed.   Oxford: Pergamon, 1965.
13. FORBES, G.   *Police J.*, **18,** 27, 1945.
14. JOKL, E.   *The Medical Aspects of Boxing*, pp. 67–8.   Pretoria: Van Schaick.

Chapter 7

DEATH FROM LIGHTNING, ELECTRICITY, AND BURNING

Death and injuries from lightning

IN Great Britain the annual number of deaths caused by lightning is very small, but such deaths are much more frequent in tropical and sub-tropical countries.

The medical jurist is likely to be consulted in relation to bodies which bear the marks of injury of which lightning may be the probable cause in contradistinction to other forms of violent death.

Lightning results from an electrical discharge between a negatively charged cloud bank and a positively charged object on the earth.[1]

Jex-Blake[2] states that the lightning flash is a rush of protons and electrons through the air with a liberation of a great amount of energy along a path of two kilometres. The current is direct and of about 1,000 million volts and probably in the region of 20,000 amperes. The duration of a single stroke is about one-thousandth of a second. The flash takes meandering channels with secondary flashes branching off. The diameter of the channel down which the lightning travels is estimated as at least eighteen feet. When it hits the earth, objects a hundred feet or more apart may all be struck.

Spencer[3] describes four elements in a flash:

1. The direct effect of the current.
2. Burning by superheated air.
3. Effects of expanded and repelled air around the flash.
4. The 'sledge-hammer blow' given by compressed air pushed before the current.

Spencer holds the view that the shock produces instantaneous anaemia of the brain, due to sudden spasmodic contraction of all the cerebral arteries, the muscular fibres in their coats being firmly contracted. The heart suddenly and forcibly contracts and remains in that state until death supervenes or until stimulated by the return of some blood into it. Cessation of respiration results from sudden anaemia of the medulla and spinal cord. When a person is brought into contact with a flash of lightning, death is usually immediate.

Even when an individual is more remote from the flash, concussion may result. A flash causes very considerable air-pressure, and its effects are not infrequently responsible for severe injuries to the body.

Lightning-stroke usually causes immediate unconsciousness. The intense disturbance of the air in the immediate vicinity of the flash may either remove the clothing from a body or tear it very extensively.

The most trivial lesions found after lightning-stroke are streaky surface burns which only involve the epidermal layer of the skin. These are frequently characteristic in pattern and have been called 'lightning prints' or 'arborescent markings' from their tree-like character. They

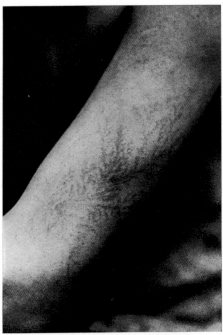

FIG. 75

Arborescent markings on arm. The photograph was taken four hours after accident. Eleven hours after accident, markings had entirely disappeared

have been likened also to frost designs. They may be found on various parts of the body.

The lesions most frequently seen following lightning-stroke may be summed up as follows: (1) Wounds of almost any description; (2) fractures, simple, compound, comminuted, single or multiple; (3) burns of almost any shape, linear, streak, patch, or of arborescent form; (4) ecchymoses; (5) singeing of the hair of scalp, face, or body; (6) impressions of metallic articles upon skin, due to their high temperature.

The view that the electric lesion is not a true burn, but is painless and without inflammatory reaction, is expressed by Jex-Blake. Vasoconstriction and vaso-paralysis with subsequent thrombosis account for the pathological effects.

In addition, such conditions as blindness, deafness, paralysis, loss of memory, delirium, and convulsions may result.

A very significant indication of lightning-stroke is the magnetisation of metallic articles found on the person, or of articles carried by the individual, when struck.

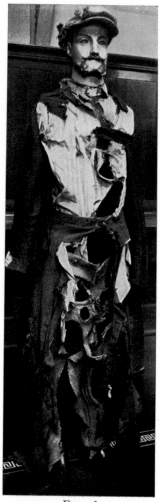

FIG. 76
Effects of lightning-stroke on clothing, which is fitted on lay figure

The internal post-mortem findings are in many cases remarkably negative. The surfaces of the lungs and pericardium frequently show petechial haemorrhages. Congestion of the brain, lungs, kidneys, suprarenals and spleen may be found, and haemorrhage into the pancreas and necrosis of this organ are described. Gangrene of the caecum after lightning-stroke is recorded.

Critchley[4] has described the histology of the lesions found in the central nervous system following the effects of lightning and electricity. These include focal petechial haemorrhages scattered throughout the brain, especially in the medulla. When the cranium has been directly hit by lightning, large vascular tears may be found in the cerebrum, or the entire brain may be swollen, softened, and almost diffluent. Chromatolysis of the pyramidal cells and the nerve cells of the medullary nuclei may occur, and the damaged cells show a dark, shrunken and uniformly stained nucleus often eccentric in position.

When a dead body is found after a thunderstorm, and there is an absence of marks upon it, death may not have resulted from lightning-stroke but from syncope due to sudden fright, since many persons are greatly alarmed by a thunderstorm.

Dill[5] reports the case of a man who was killed by lightning while sheltering under an aeroplane during a thunderstorm. A lightning discharge occurred close by. The man's body was found under the wing and close to the body of the plane. Under the body there were camouflage netting and a piece of metal tubing. Some 6 to 8 feet away was a wire earthing, attaching an aerial to a metal rod. There was a small hole in the victim's cloth cap and a small hairless spot, corresponding to the position of the hole in the cap, on the right parietal region of the head. On each buttock was a circular area, $1\frac{1}{2}$ inches in diameter, having the appearance of a recent burn. The deceased was wearing boots with iron heels and toes.

Lightning fatally injured two soldiers while playing in an Army Football Cup Final replay at Aldershot in April 1948. Two flashes of lightning, unaccompanied by rain, occurred. One of the flashes was to the right of, and another immediately above, the players. The referee and seven others, including three players, were taken to hospital where two of the players died. Several of the spectators had to receive attention for minor injuries. An incident took place at the Ascot Race Meeting in 1955. Forty-five people were injured by lightning flash and two died.

Death and injuries from electricity

The use of electricity is so general, both for industrial and domestic purposes, that accident is almost inevitable. This may occur in a variety of circumstances and frequently causes instantaneous death either from respiratory paralysis or from ventricular fibrillation.

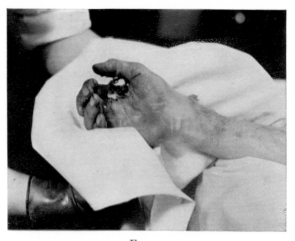

FIG. 77

Electrical burn due to grasping conductor of a pylon carrying 20,000 volts.   (By courtesy of Dr J. A. Imrie)

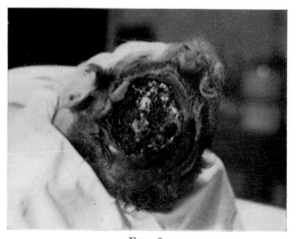

FIG. 78

Same case as Fig. 77.   The man fell back and his head con-
tacted the pylon while his hand still grasped the conductor.
Note extensive burn.   (By courtesy of Dr J. A. Imrie)

When accidents from electricity occur there are a number of composite factors responsible; these include voltage, amperage, resistance,
and earthing.   Amperage, on account of tissue resistance, is of greater
importance than voltage in the production of electrical shock.

The work of Langworthy and Kouwenhoven[6] has contributed

important information.   They have found that the principal conductors of electrical current in the body are the fluids and that most of the current travels along the blood-vessels.   The resistance offered by the various organs differs, since it bears a certain relationship to the morphological and chemical composition of the organs.   In their animal experiments it was shown that when a low-tension current was passed through the heart, complete inhibition occurred and fibrillation was produced by the direct action of the current on the muscle fibres and ganglion cells of the heart.   With high-tension current, the heart stopped immediately, but when the current was broken the ventricles started to beat rapidly and strongly and the arterial pressure rose. With high voltages, the brain and spinal cord were more often injured, but with low voltages fibrillation of the heart occurred.

The cardiac and respiratory centres in the medulla are very vulnerable to electrical current.

That voltage alone is not the sole factor in producing death is shown by the fact that death has frequently resulted from 110 volts up to 250 volts and that recovery has followed exposure to 2,500 volts.   In a communication sent by courtesy of Dr A. P. Millar, Dorchester on Thames, Oxford, a case of recovery following exposure estimated at 11,000 volts is described.   One important factor in the likelihood of a fatal accident by electricity is the condition of the hands, feet, and clothing of the person exposed to the electrical discharge.   When these are wet or damp, the effects are more serious since the resistance of the skin is lowered by moisture.   Weber's personal experiments indicated that there is danger in grasping the conductors of two alternate currents when the difference between their intensity exceeds 100 volts.   He believes that the reason why electrical engineers seem to have an apparent immunity from higher voltage is that they are constantly on their guard from this knowledge and are insulated by dry shoes, whereas workmen are more careless and may be working in damp shoes.

The part played by moisture is responsible for the occasional death from electricity which occurs in bathrooms through defective electrical fitments.   If a person in a bath switches on an electrical appliance which is defective, through the unearthed wire touching it, he may probably be electrocuted from the current passing through the water and piping, since the remaining wire is earthed, and he becomes a link in the faulty circuit.

Burns caused by electricity

A burn is frequently present at the point of contact and is caused by the generation of heat due to the resistance of the skin.   The site of exit by the current may also show an area of burning.   High-tension currents produce considerable localised burning, and in the case of the hands the appearance is blackish brown and often resembles a dark-coloured glove.   Such burns are usually 4th or 5th degree lesions. Wakely suggests the term 'electrical necrosis' rather than 'electrical burns'.   Uncomplicated specific electrical skin lesions will only be present when a small amount of heat is generated by a low-voltage current with a short duration of contact.   He explains that the skin, especially if dry, is a highly resistant barrier, and is by contact the place of entry and exit of the current with resultant liberation of considerable heat.   High-voltage currents generate much greater heat and produce injuries in which the characteristics of the primary electric lesion are overshadowed by the ordinary burning which is caused by the high temperature, sometimes accompanied by a flash or flame.   He states that the electric arc, which may generate up to 7,000°C, is commonly responsible for this type of lesion.   In some cases of death caused by electricity, external signs are minimal or absent.

ILLUSTRATIVE CASES

The following cases may be taken as typical of the effects of electricity:

A man was admitted unconscious to an infirmary, his arms and head being severely burned.   He was employed in a power station, and had accidentally fallen on the 'bus bars' connected with the switchboard which had a 6,500 voltage.   The following burns were found upon the body: (1) On right arm: (a) a burn of 6th degree running from lower ends of radius and ulna on dorsal surface to lower ends of three outer metacarpal bones; (b) a burn of 5th degree all round forearm from wrist to 4 inches up the forearm; and (c) a burn of 5th degree in front of elbow-joint.   (2) On left arm: (a) a burn of 6th degree over whole of palm of hand and palmar surfaces of fingers and thumb; (b) a burn of 5th degree along the whole anterior aspect of forearm and in front of elbow-joint; (c) a burn of 3rd degree extending for $3\frac{1}{2}$ inches from wrist up the back of forearm; and (d) a patch of burning of 2nd degree on the left axilla.   On the head, there was an area of burning of 6th degree above and behind the left ear, measuring $4\frac{1}{2}$ inches by $3\frac{1}{2}$ inches.   The breathing was of Cheyne-Stokes type.   He died eight hours after admission, without regaining consciousness.

A young man died from an electric shock under the following circumstances.   Two boys, employed in the same works as the deceased, thought to play a trick on him, and attached a wire from an electric light switch in a room to the handle of the door.   The deceased on trying to turn the handle fell to the ground.   When picked up almost at once, he was still breathing, though unconscious, and artificial respiration was employed, but without success.   One of H.M. Divisional Electrical Inspectors of Factories said that, from the evidence, the deceased had sustained the full shock of the discharge, about 230–250 volts, in view of the fact that he had been standing on damp soil. There was a wound ½ inch long on the right palm at the base of the little finger.

A lady, aged sixty-one, died of shock from a current said to be alternating, of 50 cycles per second at 240 volts. The deceased was

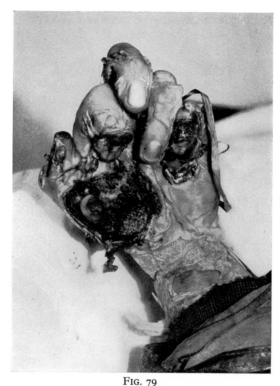

FIG. 79

Electrocution

Site of entrance of current—11,000 volts—with charring to bone

(By courtesy of the late Dr Robert Richards, Aberdeen University)

found in bed with wireless headphones still in position, and electric sparks were playing at the points of contact of her metal-rimmed spectacles. Examination showed the deceased was grasping a brass standard electric lamp. Burns were found between the index finger and thumb of the left hand and, of smaller size, on the face and scalp, corresponding to points of contact of spectacles and headphones. Electrical experts found an exposed wire in the flex of the standard lamp which proved to be the cause of the short circuit. Another bared wire was present in the telephone circuit of the wireless set, causing a second short circuit through the metal body and headbands.   It was believed that deceased received the full voltage.

A woman, aged thirty-one, was found dead in her house one morning. A chromium electric table-lamp was lying on the floor close to her right hand.   She had been in the act of rolling the flex when one of the wires became detached from the base and came into contact with the metal, thus electrocuting her.   There were marks of scorching on the metal

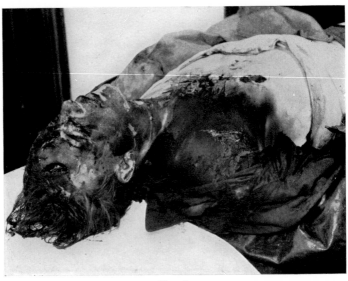

FIG. 80

Electrocution

Same case as Fig. 79 showing site of current exit on right side of neck where it caused a large excavated wound with charring of chest tissues and flash burns of face.   (By courtesy of the late Dr Robert Richards, Aberdeen University)

at the base of the lamp.   The voltage was 250, alternating current.   On the skin over the lower part of the upper third of the right forearm there were three small, brown abraded areas.   The superficial vessels of the brain and the cranial sinuses were congested.   The brain, which showed multiple petechial haemorrhages, was oedematous.   A few similar haemorrhages were present over the surfaces of the basal lobes of the lungs.   The chambers on the right side of the heart were dilated and the dilatation was more marked in the instance of the right auricle. The right auricle and ventricle, together with the associated great vessels, were very congested.   The organs of the body were also congested.

An unusual fatal case resulting from electrical contact has been reported. A training aircraft dropped a strip of tinfoil in a garden. A woman ran to collect it and was electrocuted.   The tinfoil in falling had become entangled with overhead electric cables.

In death from electricity, the post-mortem signs will naturally depend upon whether the fatality has occurred primarily from respiratory or cardiac paralysis.   When due to the former cause, asphyxial signs will form the predominant features.

Various changes may be observed in the central nervous system, including haemorrhages in the brain which vary in size, when there has been contact with high voltages.   The nerve cells may show various abnormal manifestations.   These have been dealt with in relation to the effects of lightning (see p. 197).

Accident and suicide are the commonest causes of death from electricity.

Capital punishment by electrocution

In America this is quite a common method of inflicting the last penalty of the law.   The person is strapped to a chair and metal electrodes are placed over the head and around one leg.   An alternating current of about 1,700 volts and 7 amperes current strength is passed through the body for about sixty seconds.   The current is passed through the body a second time and is continued for a similar period to ensure that life is extinct.   It has been recorded that in death from electrocution, the brain is heated to 140°F and that vacuolation around the vessels has been noted.

DEATH FROM BURNING

A burn may be defined as a lesion which is caused by the application of heat or of chemical substances to the external or internal surfaces of the body, the effect of which is a more or less marked destruction of tissue.   This definition, therefore, includes all lesions whether produced by fire, water, or chemical action.

A scald may be defined as a lesion which results from the application of liquid at or near boiling-point, or from steam.

Deaths from burning are not uncommon and burns may be produced in the following ways:

Solid bodies at a highly elevated temperature;
Liquids at or near boiling-point;
Current or pressure steam;
Corrosives;
Friction;

Lightning and electricity;
X-rays and ultra-violet rays.

Lesions found upon the body present a variety of appearances. On a body which has been subjected to the influence of fire, the lesions may be graduated from the simplest erythematous blush, through the different surgical degrees of burning, to charring of a greater or lesser portion of the body.

The old surgical classification of burns is as follows:

Burns of the first degree.
   Erythema, transitory swelling, and subsequent desquamation of the surface layers of epidermis.
Burns of the second degree.
   Vesication.
Burns of the third degree.
   Partial destruction of the true skin.
Burns of the fourth degree.
   Total destruction of the true skin.
Burns of the fifth degree.
   Destruction of the subcutaneous tissue and involvement of muscular tissue.
Burns of the sixth degree.
   Extension in depth with involvement of large blood-vessels, nerve trunks, serous cavities, and bone.

It may be simpler to regard burns as:

1. Erythema of skin.
2. Destruction of epidermis.
3. Destruction of whole skin.
4. Destruction of deep tissues, e.g. muscles, bones, organs.

The law does not differentiate between the causes of the lesions, and terms them all as burns. Frequently, bodies taken from a burning building present some appearances of the effects of burning, but it must not be supposed that in all cases death is attributable to this cause. Some persons may have died from asphyxiation, some from shock or fear, and others from injury, either through falling from a height or from debris falling upon them. In such cases, therefore, although the external appearances may show the effects of burning, the internal appearances may point to another cause of death.

In one of our cases, fire broke out during the night in a lodging-house. The number of the victims was thirty-nine, and most of them bore evidences of contact with fire. The character of the burns, in several instances, showed that some of the lesions were produced before, and some after, death. In certain cases, the area of burning was very extensive. In seven cases there were marked signs of asphyxia, and in all of these the tongue was protruded to varying distances beyond the line of the teeth, and in each it was blackish in colour, partly from lividity and partly from deposited soot.

The medico-legal points which demand consideration in connection with bodies exposed to burning are the following:

Are the lesions found due to burning?
Were they produced before or after death?
Do they account for death?
Are there lesions, other than those due to burning, which might alone account for death?
Are the burns accidental, suicidal, or homicidal?

Are the lesions found due to burning?

The lesions and appearances caused by fire may be summarised as follows:

Vesicles, more or less widespread.
Roasted patches of skin, or of deeper parts of the body.
Singeing or burning of the hair of the body or of the clothing.
Deposits of carbonaceous material on the body.

Those caused by scalding are:

Erythema.
Vesication.

Those caused by corrosives are:

Inflammatory redness of skin.
Ulcerated patches of skin.
Discoloration and staining of skin and clothing.
It should be noted that vesicles are rarely found when corrosive acids or alkalis have been used. When phosphorus, dissolved in carbon disulphide, has been employed, vesication will probably be found, because the phosphorus becomes oxidised by the air and is ignited when the carbon disulphide evaporates.

The diagnosis, therefore, between burning by fire and by scalding may be established by the presence or absence of certain lesions upon the body. Wherever singeing of the hair or clothing, deposition of carbonaceous material on the skin or clothing, and charring of tissue are found, fire has been the cause of the lesions. In such cases, some degree of vesication will also be found. If vesication is extensively present and the other signs are absent, it may be affirmed that the injuries have resulted from scalding.

The lesions found on a body when corrosives have been applied are characteristic. The differentiation between lesions due to corrosives and those due to fire or heated fluid or steam, may be established by the following points:

The absence of vesication.
The presence of coloured stains on the skin or clothing.
The presence of chemical substances in the stains (see p. 218).

Marks of burning may be found upon a body and on the clothing which may not have been caused by fire, but by friction, as is shown in the following case.

A man employed in a saw-mill disappeared from his usual place during working hours. The workmen employed in the neighbourhood of the shaft, in which the driving-belt of the machinery revolved, had their attention attracted by the odour of burning which came from this shaft. The body of the man was found at the bottom of the shaft, between the wall and the driving-belt. Extensive marks of burning were found both upon the body and the clothing.

Were the lesions produced before or after death?

The answer to this question depends upon the presence or absence of vital reaction in the lesion. The presence of vesication, the character of the fluid in the vesicles, and the inflammatory changes in and around

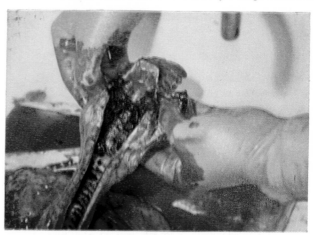

Fig. 81
Carbonaceous material in air passages

the vesicles are highly important. If the vesicles show the following characters, vital reaction has occurred:

Serous fluid which contains both albumin and chlorides;
An inflammatory areola around the vesicle;

Inflammation of the base of the vesicle;

The presence of pus.

When pus is present it indicates that the person has lived for at least thirty-six hours after the injury. On the other hand, it may be affirmed that the vesicle was of post-mortem origin if the following characteristics are present:

If the vesicle is limited in size, and its contents are scanty;

If it contains air, or only a small quantity of non-albuminous fluid with an absence of chlorides;

If inflammatory reaction is absent.

Vesicles may be produced shortly after death, when molecular life of the tissues is still present, but in this event the vesicles do not contain albumin.

As a general principle it may be stated that a vesicle which shows marked evidence of vital reaction has been produced during life, but that a vesicle which contains air, and which shows no evidence of vital reaction, has been produced after death.

On making a dissection of a body which may have been exposed to fire, attention should be specially directed to the air passages where carbonaceous material may be present. A sample of blood should also be examined for carboxyhaemoglobin. These lines of examination may afford important evidence as to whether the person was alive or dead when the fire originated.

Do the lesions account for death?

This question raises several points, including the age and general health of the deceased person together with the area of the body involved by the burns. In broad terms, it may be stated that children succumb quickly to the primary effects of shock due to burning, and to the secondary effects from inflammation of the serous membranes, such

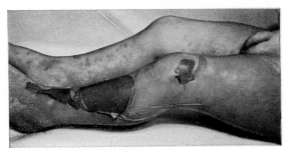

FIG. 82

Extensive burns

as pleurisy, peritonitis and meningitis, from perforating ulcer of the duodenum, and from septic absorption.   The primary effects are due to the increased fear response, the thinner skin, the greater skin sensitivity, and the greater heat loss during the shock phase.

The danger to adult life from burning is usually in direct proportion to the extent of the body surface involved rather than to the severity of

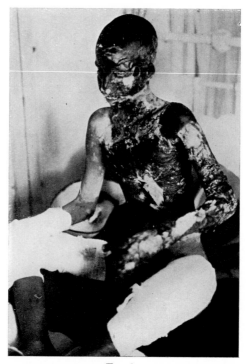

FIG. 83

A case of recovery from burning affecting an extensive area of body surface

the burn itself, when limited in area.   Burns, although comparatively superficial, which involve one-third to one-half of the surface of the body, are generally fatal.   As the result of many observations, we have noted that death has usually ensued in cases in which one-third of the body surface has been implicated.

In individual cases, however, recovery may follow even when large areas have been affected.   Involvement of approximately 10 per cent of the body surface, or even a smaller area, has caused death in young children.   Rosenthal[7] states that the conception of the pathogenesis in burns is that there is a local accumulation of fluid which begins immediately or shortly after the injury and an increase in the blood concentration. When this process becomes too severe, the blood-pressure falls and death results from cardiac failure or secondary shock. Autopsy findings in thirty fatal cases showed that eleven deaths occurred after shock had been overcome. In five of these, death was attributed to 'sepsis, hypoproteinaemia, and anaemia'.

There have been few problems in medicine which have produced such a variety of theories and explanations as that of the lethal effects of burns. The fact that inevitable death can result from the destruction of a relatively small area of the most superficial part of the body has always been a mystery to doctors.

Sevitt has made an extensive study of the causes of death after burning.[8] He found that in a large series of burns non-bacterial complications accounted for 37 per cent of cases. In the remainder, septicaemia and bronchopneumonia were the commonest causes. He did not consider non-bacterial toxaemia to be a valid explanation of death after burning.

Recently in America, after a long period of experimental work, fairly convincing evidence that burnt skin produces a toxin which induces neurological disturbances and eventually death, has been found[9, 10, 11]. If this work can be confirmed and antitoxins produced the long-standing mystery of burn toxicity and its treatment might be solved.

There is no doubt that an important factor is also the protein loss. Protein is lost in the exudate from the burned areas and further loss occurs from excess catabolism.

Occasionally acute renal failure occurs and in these cases survival is rare.[12, 13]

Are there lesions, other than those due to burning, which might alone account for death?

This question arises when there is a suspicion that fire has been used to conceal crime, and it will depend entirely upon the condition of the body, together with the attendant circumstances, whether a definite answer can be given.

It must be remembered in this connection that fissure fractures of the skull, fractures of long bones and fissures of the muscles are often found following exposure to fierce heat and that extradural haemorrhage sometimes accompanies heat fractures. Extradural haemorrhages caused by heat are usually easily recognised. They have a pink spongy appearance which is very different from the blood in the ordinary extradural haemorrhage. Occasionally, where there is great destruction, the diagnosis may be difficult. We have, unfortunately, no record of the appearance of a traumatically induced extradural haemorrhage in a body which has subsequently been involved in a conflagration. We have had experience of an unusual case where death occurred from a combination of slow excessive heat and anoxia. The entire body was baked and dehydrated (Fig. 85). The condition of the brain is shown in Fig. 86. X-ray examination of charred bodies may prove of importance in detecting or eliminating the presence of a bullet or bullets.

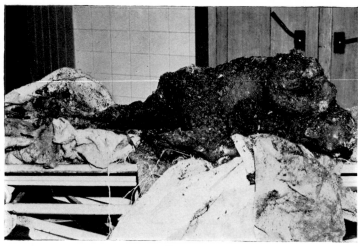

FIG. 84

This photograph of charred human remains suggests the difficulties of identification and determination of the cause of death in a conflagration

Are the burns accidental, suicidal, or homicidal?

The majority of deaths from burning and scalding occur by accident. In this country, deaths are rarely suicidal or homicidal.

The following are examples of the variety of accidents resulting in death from burning:

Persons falling into the fire due, for example, to age, disability, intoxication, or epileptic seizure.
Children falling into vessels of scalding water.
Adults falling into vats of scalding fluids or molten metal.
Children upsetting vessels containing boiling liquids.
Children playing with matches, fireworks, or interfering with fires.
Conflagrations.
Bursting of boilers.
Explosions in mines, or of gas or gunpowder.

With regard to legislative precaution against the exposure of children to risks of burning, the Children and Young Persons (Scotland) Act,

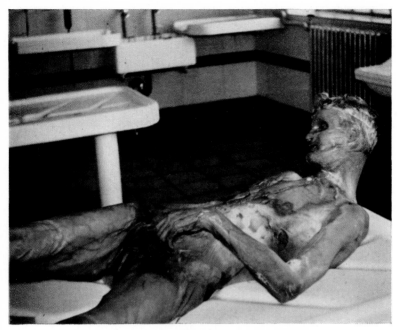

FIG. 85

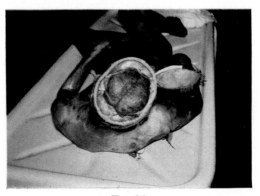

FIG. 86

1937, enacts that: if any person who has attained the age of sixteen years has custody, charge, or care of any child under the age of seven years, and allows that child to be in any room containing an open fire-grate not sufficiently protected to guard against the risk of the child being burned or scalded, without taking reasonable precautions against that risk, and by reason thereof the child is killed, or suffers serious injury, he is liable

G M J—P

on summary conviction to a fine not exceeding ten pounds. This provision does not affect such person's liability to be proceeded against by way of indictment.

The Children and Young Persons (Amendment) Act, 1952, applicable to England, makes similar provisions with regard to the case of children

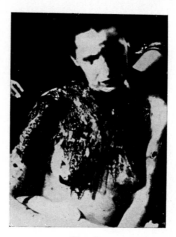

FIG. 87

Effects of nitric acid throwing. Severe burning of upper part of body, and loss of vision of right eye

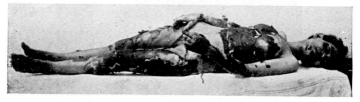

FIG. 88

Fatal case of burning due to clothing having been set on fire

under the age of twelve years exposed to the risk of burning by an open fire or any heating appliance.

Homicidal burning or scalding is not common, but from time to time deaths are caused by the wilful application of fire. It has been accomplished by throwing a lighted paraffin lamp, by saturating the clothing of the victim with inflammable liquid and setting it alight, by a violent attack with a red-hot implement, by throwing boiling water, and by other methods.

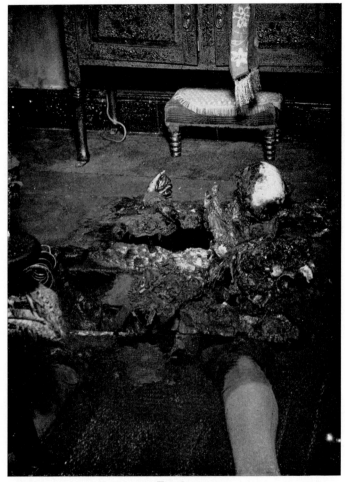

FIG. 89

Almost complete destruction of body with relatively slight surrounding damage. The fuel was supplied by the natural body fat (Fig. 90). [By courtesy of Dr J. B. Firth, formerly Director North Western Forensic Science Laboratory (Home Office).]

ILLUSTRATIVE CASES

An elderly woman was charged with having assaulted and caused the death of two children, aged three and four years respectively, by putting them on a fire. Post-mortem examination showed that the children had died from shock consequent upon extensive burns.

A mother was charged with having, while she was in an intoxicated condition, put her infant of four months into a scalding bath. Both legs were scalded. On the left leg, extending from the knee to the little toe, was an area devoid of epidermis, and on the right cheek, an oval-shaped vesicle ½ inch in diameter. The cause of death was shock.

Of the many fatal cases of burning and scalding which we have seen,

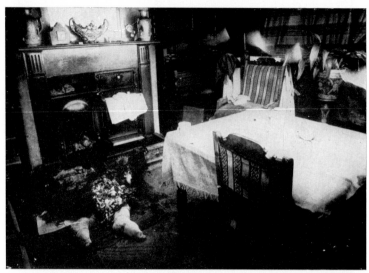

FIG. 90

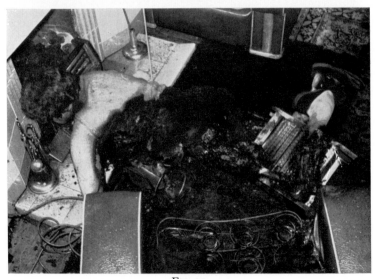

FIG. 91
Localised destruction of tissue by heat with minimal
damage to surroundings

some were of unusual character. In one case, for example, a man fell into a cauldron of boiling maize in a distillery, and when the body was recovered it was in a condition of heat-stiffening, and had assumed the 'pugilistic attitude' frequently seen in such cases. The arms were extended from the shoulders, and the forearms partially flexed. The legs also were partly flexed at the knees. Heat-stiffening occurs in bodies exposed to intense heat by burning or immersion in hot liquids and is due to coagulation of the albuminates in the muscles. Rigor mortis does not supervene in such cases and the primary rigidity persists until the onset of putrefaction. From the position assumed by the limbs, which simulates the general attitude of a boxer, the term 'pugilistic attitude' has been applied to this condition (Fig. 92).

From an analysis of our cases we find that some of the causes of burning were, by gunpowder, by molten metal, by boiling porridge, by heated metal, by a red-hot poker, by scalding fluid, by falling into a tub of boiling water, by setting bedclothes or personal clothing on fire, by accidental incineration of a motor car, by fires attributable to different causes, by steam, by scalding in a railway carriage, and by accidents with lamps.

The facts of an unusual case of burning due to accident are worthy of record:

The deceased man had been a passenger in a motor car which was involved in a collision with another car. At the time, he occupied the near rear seat. After the impact, the car, out of control, mounted the pavement, where it struck an electricity section box, before falling over on its near side. Petrol flowing from the tank at the rear of the car became ignited by sparks from the electric cables in the section box, and within a few minutes the car was ablaze. Four of the occupants, including the driver, were released, but it was found impossible to extricate the deceased, as the rescuers had to retreat on account of the intense heat. When the fire brigade had extinguished the blaze, the body of the trapped man was removed from the burnt-out car.

Post-mortem examination showed that the body was in a condition of heat-stiffening, and the 'pugilistic attitude' of burning was well demonstrated. The entire head, face, and upper part of neck were charred. The chest and abdomen showed 3rd and 4th degree burns, and the back, together with parts of both buttocks, showed 3rd degree burns. The arms and hands were burned, the lesions varying from 2nd to 6th degree. The pubic hair was singed, and the penis and scrotum were charred. The legs showed 1st to 5th degree burns, but both feet were practically unaffected, having been protected by footwear (Fig. 92).

The pharynx, larynx, trachea and main bronchi showed the presence of carbonaceous material. The blood did not show the presence of carboxyhaemoglobin.

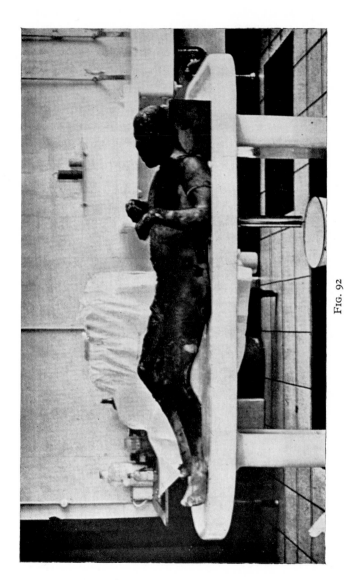

FIG. 92

The effects of burning caused by accidental incineration of a motor car. The 'pugilistic attitude' is shown

In cases where a body has been exposed to fierce heat, lesions which suggest infliction by a sharp instrument may sometimes be found. These are due to the bursting open of the tissues, and on close examination can be differentiated from incised wounds produced by a knife (pp. 234 and 422).

Suicide by burning is rare in this country, but cases are on record of persons who have thrown themselves into baths, vats, or cauldrons of boiling fluid or molten metal.

In the East, suicidal cases occur in which persons have saturated their clothing with petrol and set it alight.   In recent years this has been used as a method of political protest in Europe.

Post-mortem appearances

While the external appearances of burning have been described, something remains to be said regarding the internal appearances. These will depend upon whether death has resulted from shock or asphyxia or whether the individual has survived the immediate effects of burning and has died from subsequent complications such as inflammation of the serous surfaces, septicaemia, pneumonia, or nephritis. Occasionally duodenal ulceration may develop following burning and it

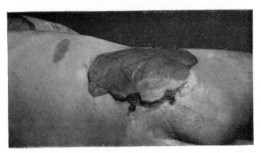

FIG. 93
Burning, first to third degree

has been suggested that changes in the blood may lead to occlusion of the small vessels.

In asphyxial cases, blood taken from the heart should be examined for the presence of carboxyhaemoglobin.   The nasal passages, pharynx, larynx, trachea, and bronchi should be carefully inspected for the presence of carbon particles.   When these are found, there is indication of smoke inhalation (Fig. 81).

In delayed death from burning, a toxaemic condition develops probably due to combined causes, including septic absorption, and is indicated, post-mortem, by the presence of cloudy swelling and other changes in certain of the organs, including the liver. This condition has already been described (p. 209).

Burning by corrosives

Cases which involve the throwing of corrosive fluids occasionally occur, and the chemicals often used are either acids or alkalis. These fluids are usually thrown upon the face, with the object of destroying vision or causing facial disfigurement.

In Scotland, it is a crime for any person wilfully, maliciously, and unlawfully to throw at, or otherwise to apply to, any other person any sulphuric acid or other corrosive substance, calculated by external application to burn, injure, murder, maim, disfigure, disable, or with intent to do some other grievous bodily harm.

The law of England on this subject is embraced in the Offences Against the Person Act, 1861, where it is enacted that: Whosoever shall unlawfully and maliciously . . . put or lay at any place or cast or throw at or upon or otherwise apply to any person, any corrosive fluid or any destructive or explosive substance, with intent . . . to burn, maim, disfigure, or disable any person, or to do some grievous bodily harm to any person, shall, whether any bodily injury be effected or not, be guilty of felony.

The diagnosis of lesions due to burning by corrosives depends upon the following points:

1. Character of the lesions.
2. Marks of staining due to chemical action.
3. Absence of signs produced by fire or scalding liquids.
4. Identity by analysis of the corrosive used.

The lesions do not present the same variation in appearance as those by fire, or the characteristic vesication of scalding. The colour of the stains upon the skin or clothing may afford a guide to the nature of the corrosive. Nitric acid produces a yellowish stain, sulphuric acid and caustic alkalis leave reddish-brown or dirty-brown stains, while hydrochloric acid and carbolic acid cause whitish or greyish-yellow stains on the skin and mucous membrane. In some cases the colour of the stain upon the clothing may be vitiated by the colour of the fabric. Sulphuric acid, or oil of vitriol, is probably the most commonly employed acid, but other acids and alkalis are also used.

The soiling fluid may be extracted from contaminated clothing or removed from the surface of the stained skin. Removal of corrosive substances from the skin may be effected, in most cases, by the use of pledgets of cotton-wool moistened with distilled water.

ILLUSTRATIVE CASE

The following case is illustrative of serious injury produced by the use of nitric acid. The neck and chest, which were involved extensively, showed yellow discoloration of the skin, superficial corrosion, and necrotic areas.

Discrete yellow spots were scattered over the face, the corneae were opaque, and the conjunctivae markedly congested and oedematous. The acid had run down both arms and the front of chest on to the upper half of abdomen. Twelve days after the assault, the burned areas had sloughed and many deep sloughs were separating, chiefly from the regions of the left shoulder and side of chest. The temperature fluctuated between 102° and 104°F. Five days later all the sloughs had separated, and the temperature was normal. Vision of the right eye was lost, there being necrosis of the lower half of the upper eyelid, while the tissues of the eye were destroyed. Three months after the sloughs had separated, the burns had healed (Fig. 87).

BURNING BY X-RAYS

Repeated exposure to X-rays continued over long periods may produce lesions, both extensive and serious, which prove refractory to treatment. Radiologists and others who have been so exposed have suffered from severe dermatitis, affecting the hands, especially the region of the finger-nails, which has caused degenerative changes including warty growths. Ulceration is not infrequent in such cases, in which there is always the possibility of the development of epithelioma. The chronicity of the lesions, together with the possible risk of malignancy, has led to amputation of the fingers or portions of them in a number of cases. The nature of the lesions produced as the result of a single exposure in excessive dose depends upon the extent of over-exposure, and may vary from slight erythema to ulceration and necrosis of tissue which is difficult to heal and which may take many years to do so. When blistering results from overdosage, the skin is very friable and ulceration is a frequent advent. The difficulty in the healing of these lesions probably results from a condition of endarteritis obliterans in the smaller vessels, with a consequent diminution in the blood supply. The dangers from X-rays are now well recognised and these cases are rarely seen.

BURNING BY ULTRA-VIOLET RAYS

The local effects of over-exposure of the skin to sunlight usually vary from erythema, mild or severe, to vesication which may be of limited or extensive character.   The use of artificial sun baths has now become fairly general, but overdosage, particularly in those unaccustomed to them, may produce severe erythema.

References

1. ARDEN, G.P., HARRISON, S.H., LISTER, J., & MAUDSLEY, R.   *Br. med. J.*, **1**, 1450, 1956.
2. JEX-BLAKE, A.J.   *Lancet*, **1**, 351, 1946.
3. SPENCER, H.   *Lightning, Lightning Stroke and its Treatment.*   London: Baillière, Tindall, & Cox, 1932.
4. CRITCHLEY, M.   *Lancet*, **1**, 68, 1934.
5. DILL, A.V.   *Br. med. J.*, **2**, 426, 1942.
6. LANGWORTHY, O.R. & KOUWENHOVEN, W.B.   *J. ind. Hyg. Toxicol.*, **13**, 31, 1930.
7. ROSENTHAL, S.R.   *Ann. Surg.*, **106**, 111, 1937.
8. SEVITT, S.   *Medicine Sci. Law*, **6**, 36, 1966.
9. *Annals of the New York Academy of Sciences*, **150**, 792, 1968.
10. *Annals of the New York Academy of Sciences*, **150**, 807, 1968.
11. *Annals of the New York Academy of Sciences*, **150**, 816, 1968.
12. CASON, J.S.   *II Int. Congr. Res. Burns*, p. 12.   Edinburgh: Livingstone, 1966.
13. CAMERON, J.S.   *Proc. R. Soc. Med.*, **62**, 49, 1969.

Chapter 8

DEATH FROM STARVATION AND NEGLECT AND FROM COLD AND EXPOSURE

CASES of death from starvation occur in one or other of the following circumstances: (1) famine; (2) entombment in pits, mines, or landslides; (3) neglect on the part of parents or guardians; (4) wilful withholding of food; (5) wilful refusal to take food.

The law takes cognisance of those cases which are due to wilful neglect and unintentional neglect. In addition to wilful starvation being an offence at common law, it falls, especially in the case of children, under statute law, which shows close similarity in both England and Scotland. The Children and Young Persons (Scotland) Act, 1937, consolidates in its application to Scotland certain enactments relating to persons under the age of eighteen years. It contains provisions which are of importance in connection with the prevention of criminal neglect and starvation.

Part I of the Act, which deals with Child Life Protection, contains certain provisions for preventing objectionable traffic in child life and for the protection of children under nine years whose custody has been undertaken for reward.

If a person undertakes for reward the nursing and maintenance of a child under nine years, apart from its parents or having no parents, he must give notice in writing thereof to the local authority, and should the child die or be removed from his care he must within twenty-four hours thereof give notice in writing of the death or removal to the local authority and to the person from whom the child was received. In the case of death he must within a like period give similar notice to the Procurator-Fiscal of the district within which the body lies. On receipt of such notice the Procurator-Fiscal must hold an inquiry into the cause of death, unless there is produced to him a certificate by a duly qualified medical practitioner certifying that he personally attended the child during its last illness and specifying the cause of death, and the Procurator-Fiscal is satisfied that there is no ground for holding an inquiry. Failure to give any of these notices is an offence.

Power is also given to the local authority to fix the number of children under nine years who may be kept in any dwelling, and to order the removal of any child kept in unsuitable premises or by unsuitable persons.

Part II enacts certain provisions for the prevention of cruelty to and exposure to moral and physical danger of, children and young persons. It makes it an offence for a person who has attained the age of sixteen and has the custody, charge, or care of a child or young person under that age wilfully to assault, ill-treat, neglect, abandon, or expose him in a manner likely to cause him unnecessary suffering or injury to his health, or to fail to provide adequate food, clothing, medical aid or lodging for him, or to take steps to procure such under the Acts relating to the relief of the poor where he is unable to provide this himself.

If a person goes to bed under the influence of drink and a child under three years of age in bed with him is suffocated, such person is deemed to have neglected the child in a manner likely to cause injury to his health.

It is an offence for a person who has attained the age of sixteen years and who has the custody of any child under the age of seven years, without taking reasonable precautions, to allow the child to be exposed to the risk of burning or scalding whereby he is killed or seriously injured. This provision does not affect such person's liability to be proceeded against by way of indictment (see p. 210).

The Adoption Act, 1958, applicable to Great Britain, protects both the adopted child and the adopter. By this Act, payment for adoption is no longer permitted and no body of persons other than a registered adoption society, or local authority, may arrange for the adoption of a child. The society or local authority investigates the full particulars regarding the proposed adoption. A medical report on the state of the health of the child proposed for adoption must be obtained.

Wilful neglect and injury

Wilful neglect of children is accompanied by some measure of imperfect nutrition, but the degree of malnutrition usually stops short of starvation. The Children and Young Persons Act, however, definitely lays down what derelictions of duty on the part of parents or guardians come within the category of neglect or cruelty to children. These are:

Failure to provide adequate food,
                     adequate clothing,
                     medical aid,
                     lodging.

If he cannot provide these himself he must apply to the authorities to make provision.

Evidence of neglect depends usually on the state of cleanliness and clothing of the child and the state of nutrition.

Dirty, unkempt, imperfectly clad children offer clear indications of the absence of proper parental care, and a filthy condition of skin and clothing, a verminous state of body and hair, with marks of scratching or ulceration, or even disease of the skin, assist in the completion of the picture. These conditions, when found, may be taken as sufficient evidence of general neglect.

Malnutrition is usually obvious but the evidence of it should always be definitely established by accurate description of the amount of body fat and weight comparison made with average children of similar ages. When the malnutrition has been established it must then be decided whether or not it is due to neglect or to the various other factors which can cause children to be undersized and undernourished. The most important of these are tuberculosis, malabsorption syndromes, diabetes

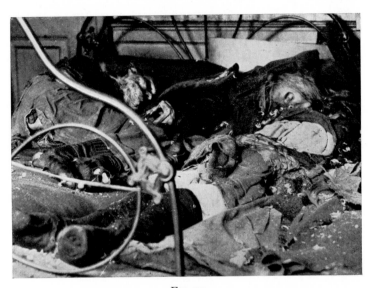

FIG. 94

The bodies of two aged persons who were found dead, the result of starvation
(By courtesy of the late Dr Robert Richards, Aberdeen University)

mellitus, congenital heart disease, psychological disturbance, pyloric stenosis, facial deformities interfering with sucking, rickets, and malignancy. The use of steroids can produce severe stunting in children.

When malnutrition is due to one of these causes it is the duty of the parents to provide medical attention.

In post-mortem dissection, therefore, all evidences of disease, if present, must be noted with relation to their effect upon production of emaciation. In the absence of disease, there would be grounds for inferring that death was due to inadequate nourishment. It must not be overlooked that diminished nutrition may be a determining factor in the causation of certain diseases, and the difficult question of cause and effect may arise occasionally.

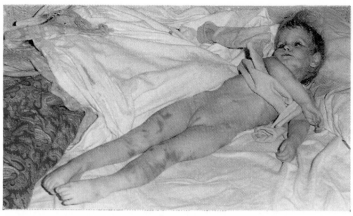

FIG. 95
Body of child showing multiple surface injuries

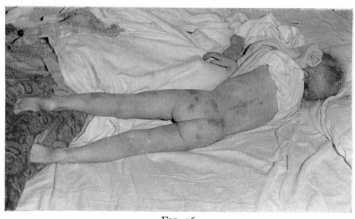

FIG. 96
Same case as in Fig. 95

In all cases, and especially those of children, the examiner should make inquiry regarding the mental condition of the person.

Battered children[1, 2]

The fact that infants and young children are frequently ill-treated by their parents has long been known to experienced medico-legal examiners. Over the years the authors have seen a considerable number of children who have died as a result of parental violence. Recently more attention has been directed to these cases, partly as a result of the finding of unexplained fractures of bone in children who were being examined for some other condition, and there has been a tendency to consider them as something completely separate from the violence which human beings are constantly inflicting on one another.

We have always avoided using the term 'battered baby syndrome' and we think that it is a pity that this term was ever used to describe what really amounts to brutal violence to children. The tendency to regard violence to children as some kind of medical or sociological curiosity can only do harm, at any rate to the children. Violence to children will be found to increase with the general increase in violence in a community. It is not a universal phenomenon and there are communities where it is almost unknown. Personal observation and the records of the authorities indicate a very low incidence in Spain.

It is considered by some that these injuries to children are always inflicted during sudden isolated fits of temper. This has not been our experience. Trube-Becker, in Germany, has described thirteen cases of deliberate starvation of infants ranging from sixteen days to one year, for which there were ten convictions.[3] He suggests that this is more common than battering.

Medico-legal examiners, who spend a large part of their lives in close contact with human violence, have no built-in reluctance to accept the possibility of criminal trauma to children, but this is often not true in the cases of physicians and surgeons and ordinary members of the public who cannot believe that these things are done to children. It is important that when doctors find marks of violence on children they should recognise the possibilities and if they think that there is any doubt about their causation they should report the case to the Procurator-Fiscal. In hospitals, these cases should always be reported to a senior member of the staff who should take the appropriate action. We have seen cases where subsequent death could have been prevented by doctors taking action when earlier evidence of violence was available to them. This is certainly one occasion when the strict adherence to the principles of professional secrecy is wrong (*see* p. 52).

Cameron, Johnson, and Camps[4] have studied in retrospect the history of twenty-nine cases and provide a very interesting table comparing the original story with the probable truth in each of these cases. This paper should be read by anyone who has any doubts about the possibilities of parental violence to children.

The usual story in our cases is that a child has been found dead in its cot and that it had been ailing for a short period prior to death.

Post-mortem dissection reveals such injuries as fractures of the skull, subdural haemorrhages, multiple rib fractures, or ruptures of liver or spleen. At this stage, one of the parents usually reports that he or she remembers the child having had a recent fall. When this explanation is not accepted, one of the parents may confess that the child was continuously troublesome and that they applied the violence to end this intolerable situation.

Some of these cases show minimal external signs of injury and unless a detailed post-mortem dissection is made, the true cause of death is missed. We include photographs showing the more obvious kinds of external injury which occur in battered children (Figs. 95, 96).

One reason for the absence of external signs of injury may be that these children are often shaken violently rather than struck causing subdural haematoma.[5]

We have encountered more frequently in the recent cases which we have investigated the explanation that the internal injuries which we

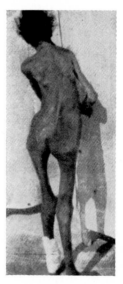

FIG. 97
Subject showing general
effects of advanced mal-
nutrition

have found were due to attempts at resuscitation. There are occasions when this is manifestly false but there are others when it can cause great difficulty in arriving at the facts. Even after the most detailed investigations there will remain cases where the forensic pathologist is in doubt about the mechanism of death.

In estimating the amount of violence which has been applied to a child the possibility of blood disorders causing abnormal bleeding into the tissues or abnormal reaction to minor trauma, should be considered. These conditions are rare and nearly always there will be some history of their occurrence before the incident which is being investigated (see p. 246).

Signs of starvation

The following clinical pictures are based on observations of prisoners-of-war returning to this country during the spring of 1945, of Dutch persons shortly after liberation, and of the inhabitants of Belsen concentration camp. The author acknowledges reference to the monograph of Dr Janet Vaughan.[6] Cases of starvation may be divided into two groups, namely, dry cases and wet cases. In the first of these groups there was extreme emaciation, the body weight deviating from

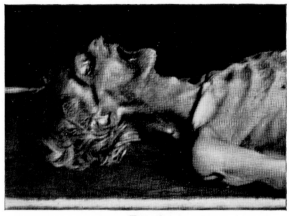

FIG. 98
Emaciation

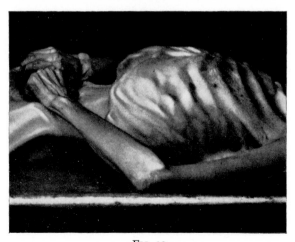

FIG. 99
Same case as in Fig. 98

the normal by 39 to 50 per cent. In severe cases, the blood-pressure was not obtainable and the pulse was impalpable. Gross cyanosis was evident and the feet showed slight oedema. In the second group, oedema involved the face, arms, legs, and feet in marked degree. Frequently there were ascites and pleural effusions. Pyrexia was common and watery diarrhoea was the rule. In Belsen, the men were eunuchoid and the women acquired male characters. Anaemia was usually present.

In concentration camps in Holland, living skeletons were seen in whom the weight of the bones, usually 15 per cent of an adult's body weight, accounted for 50 per cent of the four to five stones that these people weighed.

It has been shown that the limited amount of protein, which would suffice if the calories are adequate, is devoted to the production of energy. The plasma thus becomes deficient in proteins, its osmotic pressure falls, and the fluid leaks into the tissues. Children do not develop typical oedema, but are pale and doughy-looking.

Post-mortem appearances. The body shows an absence of fat and the skeletal muscles gross wasting. The organs are frequently pale, and the heart, liver, kidneys, and spleen are atrophied. The omental and mesenteric tissues are lacking in fat and are atrophied. The intestines are also atrophied and a non-specific ulceration may affect the large bowel. The gall-bladder usually contains dark-coloured bile, gall-stones may be present, and the urinary bladder is practically empty.

An adult may survive complete privation of food and fluid for a period of from seven to ten days. If water is taken, this period will be greatly lengthened and the person may survive for many days. Cases have been reported in which survival continued for as long as fifty-eight and sixty-one days. Special regard must be paid to the age and state of the particular person. Young subjects usually succumb more readily than adults, and healthy young adults will probably survive much older persons.

DEATH FROM COLD AND EXPOSURE

Death from cold and exposure in this country is infrequent. In recent years, however, there have been a few cases reported every winter of old people, living alone, dying from hypothermia. In such cases, the primary cause of death is attributed to a decreased dissociation of oxygen from the haemoglobin to the tissues which have a diminished capacity for utilising it. The liability to this form of death is less in robust persons than in newly born infants, young children, and aged or debilitated subjects. The factor of intoxication plays an important part in many cases, since in drunkenness the body temperature readily becomes subnormal due to surface loss of heat from dilated capillaries. The symptom of drowsiness, which is often experienced by persons who have been exposed for considerable periods to rigorous weather, is probably attributable to the effects of a progressive oxygen starvation of the brain.

Cases do occur in healthy young adults taking part in sporting activities in the Scottish mountains during winter. This is due to the special conditions. Individuals suffer exceptionally rapid heat loss owing to the unusual combination of low temperatures and very high winds. Deaths have occurred in well-equipped experienced mountaineers who have been isolated for considerable periods. They have also occurred in skiers and climbers, who have been exposed for relatively short periods, because they have failed to appreciate the risks and have been inadequately clothed.

Post-mortem appearances

External. Irregularly shaped red patches are present over limited areas of the exposed surfaces of the body (p. 155). The situation of these is determined by the areas of the skin exposed to the air, since they are not found upon covered portions of the body. They must not be confused with hypostasis which is found only on the dependent parts, or with the bright red coloration of the skin in carbon monoxide poisoning, which is found equally upon parts exposed to, and covered from, the air. The coloured areas, due to cold and exposure, are usually well marked on the cheeks and on the mucous membrane of the lips. These areas may be attributed to the marked degree of oxygenation of the haemoglobin in the blood within the capillary vessels which has occurred directly through the skin and mucous membrane.

In some cases quite marked oedema is present. This can affect the whole body, but is usually most marked in the face where it can give the appearance of myxoedema.[7]

Internal. The blood generally has a bright red colour in bodies seen within a comparatively short time after death, due to the lack of dissociation of oxygen from the haemoglobin, the result of the cold temperature to which the body has been exposed.

The internal organs and the large vessels show a marked degree of congestion. The brain and meningeal vessels are also congested. There may be submucosal haemorrhages in the stomach and areas of fat necrosis in the region of the pancreas. Sludging of the blood appears to be responsible for the lesions.[8, 9] The post-mortem signs may not be distinctive in character, and in arriving at a conclusion in any given case that death was due to exposure and cold, it is essential that all the circumstances must be investigated with care.   In view of the similarity of the coloured marks on the skin to those in carbon monoxide poisoning, a spectroscopic examination of the blood should be made when there is any element of doubt (p. 346).

Sometimes evidence of freezing will be found upon the body.   We have seen cases of death from cold and exposure in which there was audible crackling on flexing the knee joints, apparently due to the fragmentation of frozen synovial fluid.   It is not inconceivable that the body of a murdered person might have been carried from a house and laid in the open in order to divert suspicion.   Should the body have become frozen, some indication of the time of exposure, following death, may be afforded by observing whether or not rigor mortis supervenes after thawing of the body.   In such a case, the place where the body was found should be carefully examined, especially when wounds are present upon the body, before the balance of evidence is finally adjusted in the determination of the cause of death (p. 261).

Gardner[10] quotes a personal communication from Rabinowitch, McGill University, regarding several deaths which the latter ascribes to the action of intense cold on the carotid sinus.   In winter, when the temperature was many degrees below zero, babies placed out-of-doors to sleep were sometimes found with nothing to account for death at the post-mortem examination.   In these cases it was discovered that there was a gap between the head covering and the blankets.   Experimentally, Rabinowitch has been able to produce sudden death on laboratory animals by allowing a stream of cold air to play on their necks over the position of the carotid sinus.   In the children and animals, post-mortem examination showed similar findings, namely, congestion of the organs and no diminution of the blood volume in the right side of the heart or in the veins leading to it.

Cold injury in the newborn with fatalities has been described in Britain.[11]

References

1. CAFFEY, J.   *Br. J. Radiol.*, **30**, 225, 1957.
2. FAIRBURN, A.C. & Hunt, A.C.   *Medicine Sci. Law*, **4**, 93, 1968.
3. TRUBE-BECKER, E.   *Dt. Z. ges. gericht. Med.*, **64**, 93, 1968.
4. CAMERON, J.M., JOHNSON, H.R.M., & CAMPS, F.E.   *Medicine Sci. Law*, **6**, 2, 1966.
5. GUTHKELCH, A. N., *Br. med. J.*, **2**, 430, 1971.
6. VAUGHAN, J.   *Med. A.*, p. 326, 1946.
7. MANT, A.K.   *J. forens. Med.*, **16**, 126, 1969.
8. MANT, A.K.   *Medicine Sci. Law*, **4**, 44, 1964.
9. READ, A.E., EMSLIE-SMITH, D., GOUGH, K.R., & HOLMES, R.   *Lancet*, **2**, 1219, 1961.
10. GARDNER, E.   *Clin. J.*, **62**, 56, 1943.
11. BOWER, B.D., JONES, L.F., & WEEKS, M.M.   *Br. med. J.*, **1**, 303, 1960.

Chapter 9

THE MEDICO-LEGAL ASPECTS OF WOUNDS

ALL lesions of the body, external or internal, caused by the application of violence may be designated as wounds.

A wound is therefore a solution of continuity of any of the tissues of the body caused by injury.

By the Offences Against the Person Act, 1861, which applies to England, provision is made for the punishment of those who inflict injury upon others. The sections of special importance in regard to wounding are:

Wounding or causing any grievous bodily harm to any person by any means whatsoever with intent to murder is a felony.

Wounding unlawfully and maliciously by any means whatsoever or causing any grievous bodily harm to any person or shooting at any person or attempting to discharge any kind of loaded arms at any person with intent in any of these cases to maim, disfigure, or disable any person, or doing some other grievous bodily harm to any person is a felony.

Wounding unlawfully and maliciously or inflicting any grievous bodily harm upon any person either with or without any weapon or instrument is a misdemeanour.

The practical effect of the distinction between felonies and misdemeanours has been removed by the Criminal Law Act, 1967.

The terms 'bodily harm', 'injury', and 'grievous bodily harm' are not defined in the Act.

In Scotland there is no Act corresponding to the Offences Against the Person Act, but such offences are criminal at common law.

The Prevention of Crimes Act, 1953, prohibits the carrying of offensive weapons in public places without lawful authority or reasonable excuse.

WOUNDS IN RELATION TO DANGER TO LIFE

In order to convey some meaning to the minds of others with respect to the relative gravity of wounds, certain descriptive terms have been applied to them, and medical practitioners should have clear and definite conceptions of what are meant by these terms.

A slight wound means one in which the lesion is neither extensive nor serious, which heals rapidly, and which leaves no deformity behind it.   A dangerous wound is one that is either extensive or serious with relation to the organ or part wounded, which presents surgical difficulty in its cure, but which is not attended usually by fatal consequences.   A mortal wound is one which almost immediately after its causation or within a short time thereafter causes death by interfering with the function of a vital organ, or with the general functions of the body.

Wounds involving the following structures are the cause of many deaths within short periods after their infliction:

> The heart and large blood-vessels.
> The brain and upper part of the spinal cord.
> The lungs.
> The stomach, liver, spleen, and intestines.

From time to time unexpected recoveries occur, for example, Singleton[1] records a case of wounding which involved the interventricular septum of the heart with survival for forty-five days after operation.   He also describes further cases in which recovery followed the suture of a wound in the wall of the left ventricle, wounding of the pericardium, without operation, and the lodgment of a bullet in the right ventricle, the patient remaining well after a period of two years. In another of his cases, a bullet had perforated the wall of the left ventricle, and without operation the patient lived for eleven days.

In recent years with improvements in anaesthetics and surgical intra-thoracic techniques, recovery from penetrating wounds of the chest has become much commoner.

Frequently, we have seen homicidal deaths which were caused either by penetration of one of the cavities of the heart, the aorta, the pulmonary artery, the common carotid artery, the jugular vein, or the femoral vein.   In these cases death followed almost immediately.

A wound is dangerous to life only when the danger is imminent. The term should not be employed to designate a wound which, originally simple in character, becomes dangerous from unexpected complication such as infection, even although the wounded person may die as the result of the complication.   Grievous bodily harm is inflicted when the injury causes some measure of pain or inconvenience to the assaulted or injured person, and so affects the health of that person.   It would appear that shock falls within the term 'bodily harm'.[2]

Doctors giving evidence in court about the seriousness of wounds should describe to the court the condition of the wound prior to treatment.   We have frequently had complaints from Judges and Advocates that particularly young doctors tend to suggest that because a wound has been successfully treated it was not serious; for example, a slash across the face involving the facial artery and the insertion of 20 sutures.

WOUNDS IN RELATION TO CULPABILITY

Homicide is the killing of a self-existent human being by another human being. The destruction of an unborn child or a partially born child is not homicide (p. 401).

The death must not be too remote from the injury, otherwise the presumption is in favour of another cause of death.

Justifiable homicide is the term applied to homicide which is justified by the circumstances which led to the killing of a person, for example:

A woman who kills a person who attempts to rape her:

A person who kills another in self-defence, provided that the force or means used is not more than is necessary for the purpose of self-defence, that there is reasonable apprehension that the attacker intends to inflict serious injury or to kill, and that there is no opportunity for the person attacked to apply to the public authorities for protection or to make his escape.

To constitute the crime of murder, there must be wilful and malicious intent to kill, or a wicked recklessness as to the consequences. In Scotland, the term 'culpable homicide' is applied to the act of one who kills another while doing an unlawful act, or by his gross and wicked negligence, without any wilful and malicious intent to kill, or by a wicked recklessness as to the consequences.

There are three groups into which culpable homicide may be classified:

1. Where there is intent to kill, and the homicide is neither murder nor justifiable homicide, for example, when there is gross provocation.
2. Where there is no intent to kill, but death results from unlawful conduct by the person responsible.
3. Where homicide is caused by negligence or rashness in the performance of a lawful act, for example, driving a motor car.

In England, the analogous term for this crime is manslaughter.

In the crime of murder, the accused must accept the risk of the state of health, age, and sex of the deceased when the injury was inflicted. While this is correct in theory, the courts in Scotland in practice do make allowances for subnormal weaknesses in the victim, for example, deaths resulting from assaults causing skull fractures in individuals with abnormally thin skulls. In England, if the injured person survives the injury for a year and a day, and death supervenes thereafter, the crime committed ceases to be one of murder.[3]

When skilful surgical operative procedure is required, following the infliction of a wound, and after it the injured person dies, the person who caused the wound is chargeable either with the crime of murder, or culpable homicide, or manslaughter. In such circumstances, however, it would be competent for counsel on behalf of the accused to lead evidence to prove that the treatment was not skilfully applied. If the person who applied the treatment is a registered medical practitioner and if it has been applied for the purpose of cure and in good faith, the assaulted person would be considered to have been skilfully treated, unless it is proved that the original injury was not in itself dangerous to life, or that improper treatment caused death.

In November 1938, at Denbigh Assizes, during the trial of a man on a charge of manslaughter, it was stated that the death of the deceased was not the result of the injury inflicted by the accused, but on account of the prolonged period of anaesthesia resulting from the surgeon's stool having slipped when the located bullet had been about to be removed. This accident had caused delay, and when the operation had been resumed, the location of the bullet had changed. The patient died under the influence of the anaesthetic. Post-mortem examination showed the presence of an enlarged thymus gland. Medical evidence was led to the effect that if the surgeon had not sustained this accident, the bullet would have been removed and recovery would have resulted. Death was due to chloroform poisoning. The accused was found not guilty.[4]

CHARACTERS OF WOUNDS

In cases of wounding, it is important that the character of the wound, in relation to the class of weapon by which it was produced, should be properly designated. For this purpose we classify wounds as follows:

Incised wounds.
Lacerated wounds.
Contusions or bruises.
Abrasions or scratches.
Firearm wounds.

Incised wounds

An incised wound may be defined as a solution of continuity without loss of substance. Such a wound is produced by a sharp-edged instrument, such as a knife, scissors, glass, the sharp edge of a metal vessel, or earthenware, among others. Such instruments may be used either to cut or stab.

The form of an incised wound depends upon the method of using the instrument. When it is used as in stabbing, the form of the wound is fusiform or spindle-shaped, due to the greater gaping of the tissues in the central part of the wound, but when it is used for cutting, the wound

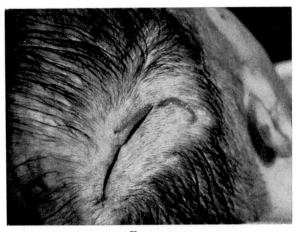

FIG. 100

Incised wound of scalp. Note curved abrasion close to anterior angle of wound

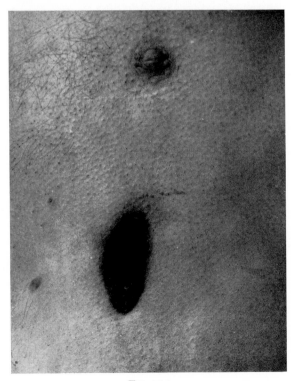

FIG. 101

Stab wound of the chest

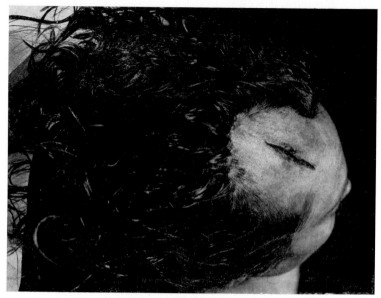

FIG. 102

A lacerated wound of the scalp

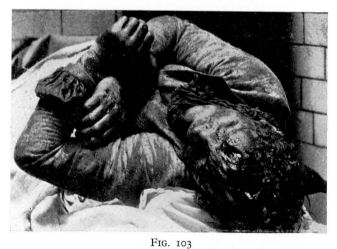

FIG. 103

Homicidal injuries.   Note lacerated wounds on head and right hand.
The wrists are tied together

will show a more or less linear contour. The degree of gaping or retraction depends upon the amount of elasticity of the tissues severed, and upon the direction of the wound. A wound made in the direction of the muscle fibres will gape less than one made at right angles to them.

The edges of an incised wound are clean-cut, regular, and well defined, begin abruptly, show maximum retraction in the centre, and terminate gradually.   An incised wound usually causes copious bleeding.

With relation to the class of weapon which produces stab wounds, the wounds are broader than the thickness of the blade which causes them, and their length is usually somewhat less than the breadth of the instrument.   This is caused by gaping of the edges with a resultant slight decrease in the length of the wound.   When an incised wound has

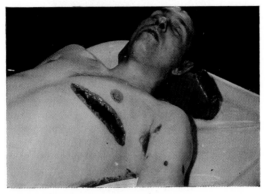

FIG. 104
Incised wound of chest made for the purpose of performing cardiac massage

passed through a limb, the wound of exit is likely to be smaller than that of entrance, because of the common tapering character of instruments capable of producing wounds of such depth.   It may happen, however, that by reason of uniformity of breadth of blade, exit and entrance wounds are practically indistinguishable in size.   The question frequently arises as to the degree of force which has been used in penetrating wounds of the body.   It should be remembered in making an estimate of this, that the main force is required to pass through the clothes and skin.   Once these have been penetrated a sharp knife passes onwards through other tissues and internal organs with relatively little force.   Where of course bone has been cut, for example ribs, this is entirely different.

Under certain circumstances, and in certain situations on the body, wounds produced by a blunt instrument may simulate the appearances of an incised wound.   These wounds are usually found over bone which is thinly covered with tissue, in the regions of the head, forehead, eyebrow, cheek, and lower jaw, among others. When such a wound exposes hair-bulbs at its edges, it is possible by examining these carefully to decide whether they have been cut or crushed and thus establish whether the wound was caused by a sharp or blunt instrument. As a rule, especially in the living subject, a wound produced by a blunt instrument will disclose some degree of bruising and swelling of the edges and the deeper tissues will be less cleanly severed than when divided by a sharp-cutting instrument.

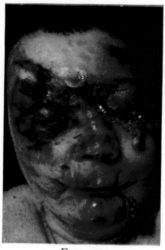

FIG. 105

Multiple lacerated wounds caused
by kicking

Lacerated wounds

These wounds are caused by forcible contact with blunt instruments, and their edges are irregular, with a varying degree of tearing. As a rule, there is an absence of correspondence between their shape and that of the instrument which produced them. If the violence has not severed the tissues completely, on separation of the edges, small irregular bridges of connective tissue will probably be seen stretching across the gap. Oblique impact with a blunt instrument may produce a flap-like tear and when caused by automobiles and occasionally by other machines can result in large degloving injuries (p. 328).

Lacerated wounds are usually accompanied by a varying degree of contusion at the edges, and when death has not been immediate, the margins frequently show a degree of swelling. The extent of contusion and swelling found will depend upon the degree and incidence of the

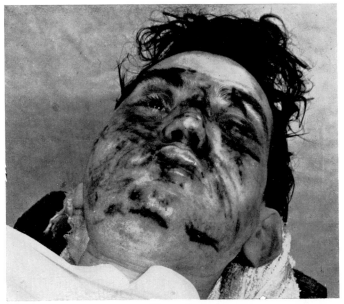

FIG. 106

Multiple lacerated wounds of the face due to kicking

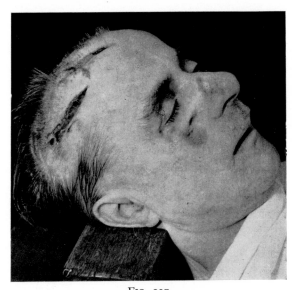

FIG. 107

Multiple lacerated wounds of the scalp produced by two
blows with shovel. Contusions are present on the face

concussive force, and the resistance of the tissues. When the site of injury involves tissue overlying bone, as on the scalp and face, bruising may be marked. Lacerated wounds may or may not bleed much. This depends upon whether the smaller blood-vessels are wholly or only partially severed; in the latter case, because of the inability of the vessels to retract, bleeding may be profuse, but in the former, the severed ends may retract and seal with clot and, consequently, there

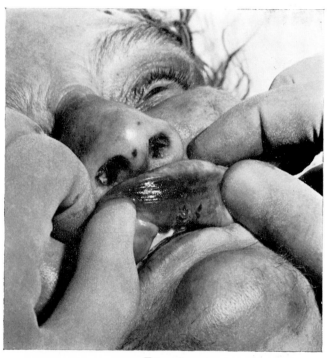

FIG. 108

Bruising and lacerations of lip in case of homicide. These injuries tend to be missed in the descriptions of external and internal injuries

may be relatively little haemorrhage. Lacerated wounds usually show some loss of substance, the process of healing is slow, and an extensive scar may result. It must not be forgotten that in certain instances the edges of a lacerated wound may appear quite regular when examined by the naked eye, and the use of a magnifying glass may be necessary to disclose the existing irregularities.

Incised and lacerated wounds may puncture the tissues, penetrate a cavity of the body, or perforate or transfix a limb. More usually such wounds are incised, but comparatively blunt-pointed, thin

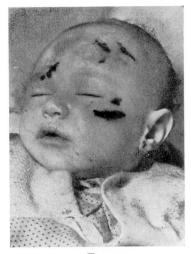

FIG. 109

Lacerated wounds of the head and face caused by repeated blows against the wall of a room

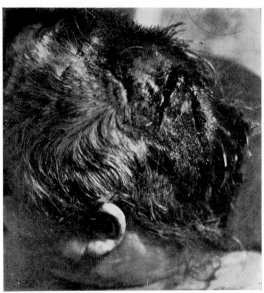

FIG. 110

Multiple lacerated wounds of the scalp

weapons may also produce them.   An element of bruising of the edges may be present, depending upon the nature of the weapon used.   A punctured wound is one that pierces the tissues.   The term 'penetrating' should be used to designate a wound which, passing through the tissues, enters a cavity of the body, such as the thorax or abdomen. A perforating wound is one which transfixes the tissues, for example, by passing through a limb.   The depth of such wounds is greater than the length or breadth.   To indicate the general character of the instrument which inflicted such wounds, the terms 'incised' or 'lacerated'

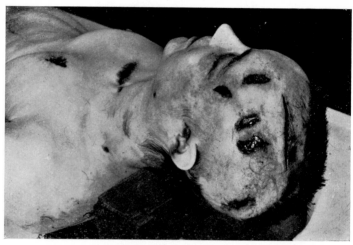

FIG. III

Multiple lacerated wounds of the head due to blows by an iron bar

should be included in the designation of the wounds, for example, punctured-incised, punctured-lacerated, perforating-incised, and penetrating-lacerated.

Contusions or bruises

A contusion may be defined as a breach of continuity of the structure of the true skin or subjacent tissues without loss of external continuity, caused by the application of a blunt instrument.   Some degree of contusion is frequently found in or around the edges of lacerated wounds, and firearm wounds.   The term contused wound should be abolished, since wounds are either caused by sharp or blunt instruments   If the edges of an incised or a lacerated wound show contusion, the fact ought to be noted, but the nature of the wound will determine the group to which it belongs, and indicate the class of weapon which has produced

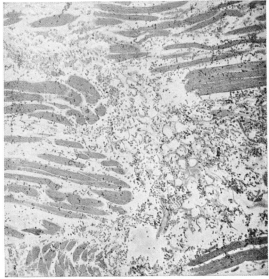

FIG. 112

Bruising.   Extravasation of blood and infiltration of the
muscular tissue by corpuscles.   × 65

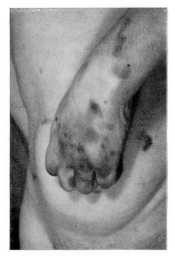

FIG. 113
Bruising

it.   The term 'incised' ought to be used only to signify a wound caused by a cutting instrument, and the term 'lacerated' to a wound caused by a blunt instrument.   The element of contusion, when present, should be treated only as an incidental fact, suggestive of the probable amount of violence used, and the likely type of weapon employed with relation to the injured part.

As the result of the injury, blood extravasates from the damaged vessels and infiltrates the surrounding tissues, thus giving rise to the condition sometimes termed ecchymosis.   Contusions or bruises vary in size from a small discoloration to an extensive swelling, as in haematoma.   The extent of rupture of the subcutaneous vessels depends, under normal circumstances, upon two principal factors, namely, the severity of the concussive force and the vascularity of the part struck. The extent of a bruise may increase considerably after infliction, due to continued extravasation of blood and infiltration of the tissues.   This may also be seen after death as the result of the diffusion of blood pigment and the changes which occur in the pigment.   When bruising is deep-seated, the surface appearance may prove to be misleading, since the colour change may be slight in comparison with the amount of blood which has collected in the deeper tissues.   Lax tissue frequently bruises more readily than firm tissue, for example, the eyelid as opposed to the palm of the hand.   The time of onset of discoloration varies in different circumstances, and the colour depends upon the amount of blood extravasated together with its distance from the surface of the skin.   After bruising has commenced, the bruising tends to deepen in colour until the blood ceases to be effused.   The part shows some swelling.   Later, the blood separates into serum and coagulum, and as the serum is absorbed the swelling becomes reduced.   Gradually the clot also becomes absorbed, and during this process the bruise undergoes changes in colour—from violet to blue, from blue to green, from green to yellow, until, at last, the skin assumes its normal hue.   Haemoglobin in an enclosed space or cavity is acted upon by tissue enzymes. These are responsible for the formation of haematoidin which produces a chocolate colour.   The infiltrated blood cells, through the action of histiocytes, ultimately produce bilirubin which imparts a yellow colour to the bruised area.

Only in a very general way, and after consideration of all the circumstances, can the period at which the original violence was applied be inferred from the colour-tone of the contusion.   Usually in a bruise of average size the dark-blue colour appears about the third day, the greenish, from the fifth to the seventh day, the yellowish, from the eighth to the tenth day, and the normal tint will probably be restored to the part between the thirteenth and eighteenth day.

When bruising is extensive and deep-seated, the colour takes a longer time to appear externally.   It should also be remembered that the part

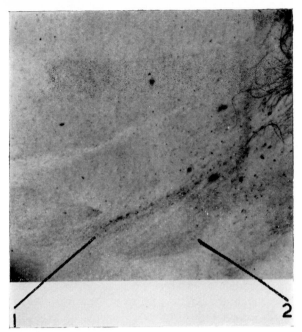

FIG. 114A

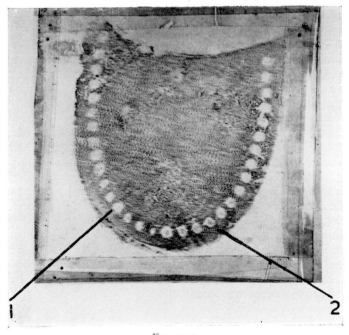

FIG. 114B

The imprint of a heel can be seen on the skin of the victim's abdominal wall (A). When compared with a photograph of the heel of the assailant's shoe (B), nails designated 1 and 2 show as discrete smaller bruises on the skin where the external discoloration appears does not in the case of deep-seated extravasations necessarily indicate the exact point of application of the violence. Owing to the disposition of the planes of areolar tissue and muscles in the limbs and other parts of the body, the discoloration, due to infiltration of blood, may show itself either above or below the part struck.

Severe internal injury may result from the forcible application of a blunt instrument without any apparent surface bruising. This occurs most frequently in automobile running over accidents when the body may show no signs of external injury and internally there may be multiple severe lacerations in the abdominal viscera.

In scorbutic, purpuric, and haemophilic subjects the amount of discoloration present in bruising may be out of all proportion to the amount of violence used, and if the presence of such a factor is not recognised, very erroneous opinions may be formed.

Under certain circumstances, ecchymosis may result from causes other than application of external violence. In cases of whooping-cough, on account of the explosive nature of the cough, ecchymoses are quite commonly found in the conjunctivae, and, less frequently, in the face and neck. When through embarrassment of breathing there is increased blood-pressure, small and spontaneous extravasations of blood may result, as, for example, in asphyxial cases.

Ante-mortem and post-mortem bruises. The signs which are indicative of ante-mortem production of bruises are swelling of the tissues, discoloration of the skin, extravasation of blood into the true skin and subcutaneous tissues, with infiltration. When a bruise is well developed, an examiner is justified in assuming the view that it was produced during life. Nevertheless, for medico-legal purposes, a microscopical examination should be made to verify the presence of infiltrated blood. Since infiltration is possible only while the heart is beating, this sign is conclusive that the injury was produced during life (Fig. 112). While molecular life remains in the tissues, considerable violence applied to a dead body with a blunt instrument will produce a slight degree of blood extravasation, but never to the same extent as during life, and infiltration of the tissues will be absent.

Suspected areas of bruising should always be incised to differentiate them from colour marks due to hypostasis, since both conditions may coexist in the same region of the body. In bruising, extravasated blood is present, but in hypostasis the severed small vessels are filled with blood and extravasation is absent.

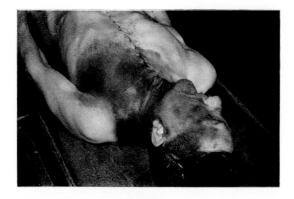

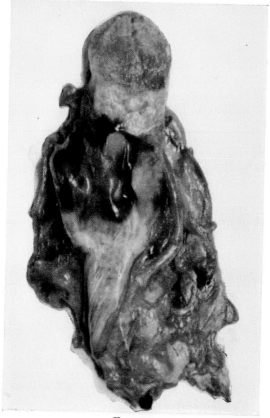

FIG. 115

Massive bruising of tissues of neck and thorax caused
by kicking with rubber-soled shoe and resulting in
death from asphyxia

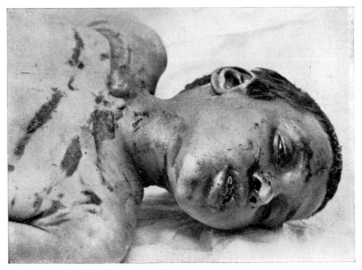

FIG. 116
Multiple abrasions and contusions

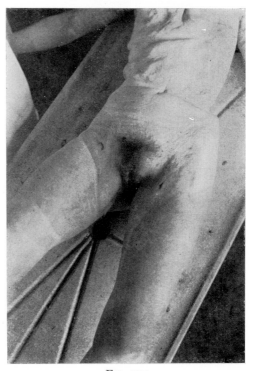

FIG. 117
Abrasions on thighs due to finger-nails

Abrasions or scratches

An abrasion is the most trivial form of wound, being restricted to skin injury.   Such injuries may provide very significant indications in certain cases.   The causative agent is frequently a finger-nail, and the scratches so produced may be found on many parts of the body.   The face, neck, arms, thighs, and female genitals are fairly common sites. They may be associated in minor degree with ligature marks upon the neck and with cases of throttling.   The regions of the inner sides of the

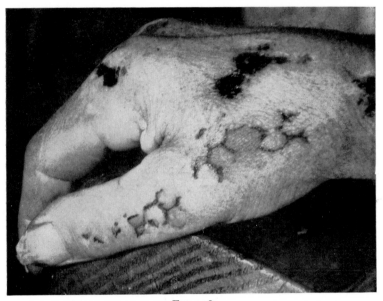

FIG. 118

Abrasions showing pattern of motor car radiator.   The subject was run down by a motor car and died from head injuries

(By courtesy of the late Dr Robert Richards, Aberdeen University)

thighs and genitals may be abraded in rape cases where there has been considerable resistance.   Their form, extent, and location will depend on the circumstances of each case.   They are commonly found in vehicular accidents, more particularly when the body has been dragged over a rough surface.   With abrasions the effusion of blood is scanty, and where the lesion is uninfected, healing is rapid.   Abrasions of post-mortem origin present a brownish-yellow, dried, parchmented appearance, and there is no evidence of bleeding.   A similar condition may occasionally be found on certain areas of a dead body due to the obliteration of fine capillary vessels.   Those inflicted some time before death will show some evidence of vital reaction, including congestion of the vessels in the dermis under the site of injury.

General data upon which the kind of instrument used may be inferred from the nature of the wound

The forms of wounds are very variable, and frequently their shape bears no relationship to the weapon which has produced them. At the same time, there are certain features which may assist in arriving at a conclusion.

Wounds which show sharply defined edges are, in practically all cases, the result of injury caused by a sharp instrument. The rare exceptions are wounds which have been produced over bony ridges or

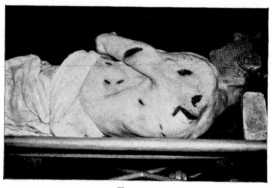

FIG. 119
Multiple knife injuries—homicidal

prominences by forcible contact with a blunt instrument. Differential diagnosis between the use of a sharp or blunt weapon in these cases can be established by careful examination of the condition of the hair-bulbs at the wound edges with a hand-lens and by the fact that a wound caused by a blunt instrument will probably show some evidence of bruising and swelling at the edges and a less clean severance of the deeper tissues.

When a sharp-pointed, edged instrument, used perpendicularly, enters the body, the wound is less in length than the breadth of the instrument, and broader than the thickness of the blade.

When the same instrument enters the body obliquely, the edges of the wound may appear unequal, one edge being straight and the other curved, and, not infrequently, owing to the bevelled shape of the wound, beads of subcutaneous fat may appear between the edges.

Injuries caused by glass and earthenware present different appearances. Some closely simulate wounds by an instrument of the dagger type, others by instruments used as in cutting.

In wounds of the scalp caused by pieces of glass or crockery, small fragments of these substances may be found either in the tissues, or embedded in the bone itself, from which the nature of the weapon used can be determined. We have found this in several cases.

Injuries by glass very frequently show a parallelism of the edges of the wound with a sudden tapering at one end, to form a superficial scratch or abrasion.

Wounds with ill-defined, irregular, or ragged edges, which may be linked by small bridges of connective tissue, are always caused by forcible contact with a blunt instrument. When found on the scalp, whole or crushed hair-bulbs may be picked out of the edges of the wound.

Wounds of mixed character may be found upon the body, most commonly the head, when a bottle has been the weapon. In these cases co-existent bruises, lacerated wounds, and incised wounds may be found and the general appearance of the lesions may suggest that different types of weapons have been used. The explanation lies in the fact that the unbroken bottle has been the cause of the contusions and lacerations, and that while these injuries were being inflicted the bottle has broken, with the result that incised wounds are added to the seat of injury. When a sharp-bladed knife strikes a convex surface of the body obliquely, for example, the arm or leg, the wound produced will be curved in shape.

Contusions or bruises found upon the body are the result of forcible application of a blunt instrument. In most cases they do not afford any further clue to the character of the instrument used, but occasionally from their defined nature and from the presence of more than one mark of similar shape, a reliable opinion may be possible. A series of contusions in the form of stripes, the breadths of which closely correspond to one another, would be indicative of the application of a stick, a leather strap, or similar weapon. In bruising, the amount of extravasated blood is not always a reliable indication of the severity of the violence used, since certain parts of the body, because of their vascular character, for example, the genitals, may bruise readily. Extensive bruising may result from the application of a very moderate degree of violence in persons of purpuric, haemophilic, or scorbutic tendency. It must also be noted that under rare and exceptional circumstances ecchymoses may develop spontaneously. In offering an opinion as to the amount of violence used from the extent of the extravasation present, the preceding factors must receive due consideration.

Wounds which are cruciform, stellate, circular, or oval in shape, and to which on other parts of the body in a more or less direct line other wounds correspond, are produced either by traversing weapons or missiles. Single wounds of this character may either be due to a missile which has entered the body and is retained or to sharp-pointed

instruments. Usually the history of the case will determine the difference, and in dead bodies dissection will clear up any difficulty. The
recognition of firearm wounds becomes obvious, when around the
wound there is evidence of scorching or engraining of the skin with
particles of carbon, or with the products of smokeless powder.

Description of wounds

In dealing with wounds which form the subject of medico-legal
inquiry, great accuracy in their description must be observed. The
following points should be noted:

> Situation.
> Shape.
> Surface dimensions.
> Estimate of the depth.
> Condition of the edges.
> Presence or absence of ridges of tisssue.
> Condition of the base.
> Presence of foreign bodies.
> Age of the wound.

Situation of the wound

The description of the situation of wounds will in many cases
eventually be presented to laymen, and for this reason, whenever possible
it should relate to well-known points of the body, recognisable by
them. Where, however, this could cause confusion strict anatomical
terms should be used.

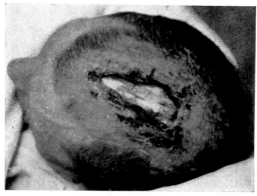

FIG. 120
Self-inflicted wound of scalp caused by an axe

Sometimes from the position of a wound upon the body considerable light may be thrown upon the likely mode of its production. Certain parts of the body are chosen sites for suicidal wounds, as, for example, the throat, chest, forearm, groin, and thigh. Wounds on certain other parts oppose, if they do not absolutely negative, the suggestion of suicide, by reason of their inaccessibility, for example, wounds on the back. Not only do wounds on the vertex frequently negative suicidal production, but also accidental production, since it is rare to injure the vertex by a fall from the standing position (Fig. 185). Nevertheless, an opinion in such cases must not be lightly given, as the following case, for which we are indebted to Dr W. McWilliam, will clearly demonstrate. A patient in a mental hospital attempted to commit suicide by using an axe. He seized the shaft with both hands and brought the

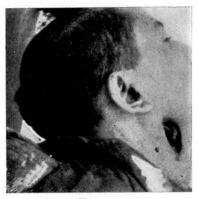

FIG. 121

Homicidal stab wound of the neck

cutting edge up towards his head, thus inflicting a scalp wound which also destroyed the periosteum and scored the outer table of the parietal bones in three places, to a depth of $\frac{1}{16}$ inch. He did this without rendering himself unconscious. If the patient had succeeded in his attempt, and if he had been found dead, it is highly probable that the injury might have been regarded as the result of a homicidal act (Fig. 120). In cases where wounds are found upon the throat of a dead body, it is advisable always to examine the hands carefully. In this way it may sometimes be possible to distinguish between homicidal and suicidal cut-throat wounds, for in the former class of case, unless the victim is taken unawares from behind, or is otherwise unable to offer resistance, the hands when used in defence are liable to be injured (Figs. 129 and 132). Homicidal wounds are usually inflicted over some vital region of the body, either on the front of the chest near the region of the heart, on the neck, on the head, or on the back between the shoulders.

Shape of the wound

This may afford important information in relation to the class and type of weapon which may have caused the injury. The subject has already been discussed (see p. 250).

In particular it should be remembered that especially in stab wounds the shape is very much affected by the direction of the underlying muscle fibres.

With regard to the expression of an opinion as to whether a specific instrument has caused a particular wound, the opinion should be limited to the statement that the wound could, or could not, have been inflicted with such an instrument, and that the appearances of the wound are consistent or inconsistent with its infliction by such an instrument or class of instrument.

Surface dimensions and depth of the wound

Not only must the recorded measurements of the wound or wounds be accurate, but the relative positions between the sites of the wounds, when there are more than one, must be carefully noted. The direction and extent of the depth of wounds also demand close attention and detailed description. Any incisions made post-mortem should avoid interference with the site of previous injury.

Should it prove necessary to insert a probe, care must be taken to select one with a blunt end and force must not be used. Unless these precautions have been adopted, it may subsequently be alleged by the defence that at least part of the injury was produced by the investigation. Broadly speaking, it is better to defer the use of a probe until dissection has reached a stage when its passage can be seen and controlled.

When wounds are found upon a clothed part of the body, it is important to examine the different superimposed garments both together and separately. All evidences of the passage of instruments through the fabrics must be carefully noted and measured, together with their relation to the situation of the lesions on the body. In this way a lead may be given as to the position of the assaulted person at the moment of the assault, a point of considerable importance, especially in penetrating wounds of the chest. Occasionally it happens that on examining a loose undergarment, more marks of perforation are discovered upon it than there are wounds on the part of the body corresponding to the position of the garment, or on the outer clothing. This is due to wrinkling or folding of the underwear.

In the examination of a dead body upon which there are several wounds, it is necessary to assess their individual importance in relation to the fatal issue.

It should be remembered that the colour of bruises can alter greatly during a period after death. Where they are important factors in the reconstruction of a case, they should be photographed at four-hourly intervals until stabilisation has occurred.

It must not be forgotten that death may result from a comparatively small wound.

We recall a case in which a boy of between seven and eight was stabbed on the back of the neck by another boy. The wound proved fatal, and post-mortem examination disclosed a partial severance of the spinal cord. The knife used had a narrow, thin blade which had insinuated itself between the third and fourth cervical vertebrae, leaving an almost imperceptible wound at the site of entry (p. 269).

Condition of the edges, sides, and base of the wound

A hand-lens should be used for this examination and probably the most important point is to determine whether the wound has been caused by a blunt or sharp instrument. The facts to be noted are the presence or absence of bruising at the edges, the condition of hair-bulbs, the presence of bridges of tissue between the walls, the presence of fragmented bone, and the condition of blood-vessels and nerves in the base of the wound.

The condition of the tissues surrounding the wound should also be examined. Deep bruising may be present and there may even be commencing inflammatory changes.

Presence of foreign bodies

Wounds should always be carefully examined for these. The most likely to be present are bullets, pieces of glass, fragments of knife blades, particles of paint, and pieces of metal resulting from explosions or electrical accidents. They may be important not only for the purpose of understanding the cause of the injury but also for identifying an assailant.

Age of the wound

The question as to the age of a wound may arise under a variety of circumstances.

Ojala, Lempinen and Hirvonen[5] have studied the vital reaction of the tissues to incised wounds. Using human tissues taken from subjects at operations, they found that leucocytes were present in the skin connective tissue after one hour and in the fat of the wound after 30 minutes. Macrophages appeared within two hours. Previous work done on animals to some extent confirms these findings. They are important in connection with medico-legal problems as examiners may have to make decisions concerning the relation of injuries found on a body to known traumatic incidents, for example, the finding of neck bruising in the body of a woman discovered in a house after a fire where there was strong suspicion that she had been attacked and rendered unconscious for the purpose of committing murder by burning, but there was also a possibility that the neck injuries had been caused by previous traumatic incidents.

In connection with longer periods the following have been found:

Cellular infiltration well marked microscopically in 12 to 18 hours after the injury.

During the first 24 hours the margins of the wound temporarily adherent by blood and serum, and vascular congestion; swelling and leucocytosis are present.

New capillaries probably formed in about 36 hours.

In 48 to 72 hours, spindle-shaped cells which run at right angles to the vessels present.

Pus may be seen in septic wounds after 48 to 72 hours, or sometimes earlier.

In five to six days, fibrils which run parallel to the vessels have become established.

When a wound heals by granulation, as it always does if there is loss of substance and the edges cannot be brought into apposition, the stage of granulation exists for so variable a period, and depends on so many factors that an accurate estimation cannot be given.

Granulation tissue is subsequently transformed into young scar tissue, its cellular elements disappearing as the fibrous tissue increases in amount.   While these changes are occurring, the surface is being covered by epidermis which grows from the margins of the wound, and, by proliferation, gradually covers the granulations with a thin pink pellicle.   As it increases in thickness, it assumes a bluish hue and when cornified becomes whitish in colour (p. 88).

Conclusions

After taking into account all these factors the examiner should direct his attention to the reconstruction of the cause of the injuries. He should first decide the instrument, then the degree of violence, the possibility of accident, the direction of the wound, and the relative position of the parties.

Ante-mortem and post-mortem wounds

In medico-legal practice the differentiation between wounds inflicted before and after death is most important.   In arriving at an opinion, a detailed examination is necessary.   If signs of vital reaction are present, the injury has been produced during life.

The signs of vital reaction will naturally depend on the period of survival following injury, and these may be swelling, effusion of lymph, pus formation, or evidence of repair. When inflammatory signs in any degree are found, they constitute definite evidence of infliction of the injury during life. When there is an element of doubt, microscopical examination of tissue sections must be made before arriving at an opinion as to whether the wound was of ante-mortem or post mortem origin. Even if the victim has survived the injury only for a period of

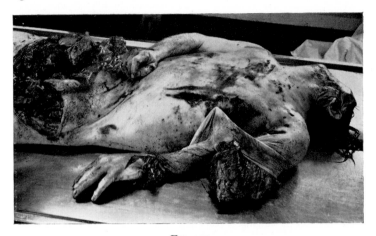

FIG. 122

Body of a man after being 5 minutes on a busy motorway. The intestines collected from the roadway are enclosed in the plastic bag

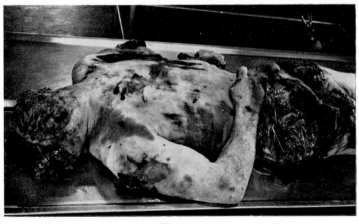

FIG. 123

Same case as in Fig. 122

some hours, leucocytic infiltration will probably be evident on microscopical examination.

It should not be forgotten that, so long as molecular life remains in the tissues, some retraction of the edges of a wound inflicted after death may occur.

A word of caution is appropriate in connection with haemorrhage and the inferences to be drawn as to whether it is significant of ante-mortem or post-mortem origin. As a rule, profuse haemorrhage is indicative of the injury having been produced during life, but, on the other hand, absence of copious blood cannot always be regarded as a sign of post-mortem injury since shock or rapid death following an extensive or mortal wound may readily account for its absence. When gross post-mortem injury occurs a considerable quantity of blood may collect as the result of oozing from dilated vessels. Such factors should receive careful consideration.

When there are multiple massive blunt instrument injuries, even with the most detailed examination it may be impossible to decide which wounds are ante-mortem and which post-mortem or indeed if any of them are ante-mortem. We have seen a body jammed between the undercarriage of an electric train and the track having been carried along for the better part of a mile with resultant progressive disintegration of the body. The same kind of effects can be produced when a body is left on a busy motorway at night. We have seen a case in which the victim, during a period of five minutes on a motorway at night, was run over eight times by cars and heavy lorries, producing a state of disintegration which made it impossible to make a decision about the timing of many of the wounds. (Figs 122, 123).

Is the wound accidental, suicidal, or homicidal?

This question is bound to arise in every case in which a dead body, with marks of violence upon it, is found. The nature and distribution of wounds may settle this issue without any further investigation, for example, multiple gun-shot wounds in an inaccessible part of the body would give a certain indication of homicide, whereas a single revolver wound in a site of choice, for example within the mouth, would be fairly conclusive evidence of suicide. There are of course many cases where we have to deal with the estimation of probabilities much more finely balanced than these.

We have experienced difficulties in arriving at a decision between accident and homicide, when we have had to examine bodies with blunt instrument injuries. Often these bodies are lying with their injured heads close to corners of stone fenders or projecting pieces of furniture and there is a history of intoxication. It is really professional experience which enables an examiner to know the kind and extent of the injuries which are liable to occur in a drunken fall and to be able to make a mental comparison with probable homicidal injuries. It is important that this judgment should be accurate as it will alter the whole course of the subsequent investigation (Figs. 125, 126).

Further assistance can be obtained from a consideration of the

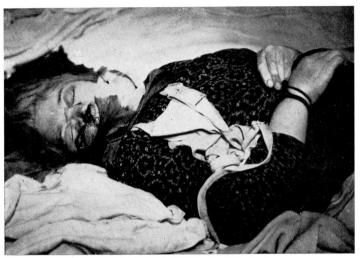

FIG. 124

Case of murder. In addition to multiple wounds of the head, the body showed the application of a gag and wrist ligatures

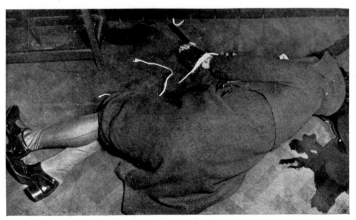

FIG. 125

Photograph showing scene of murder. Note the many details which should be recorded prior to disturbance of body

G M J—S

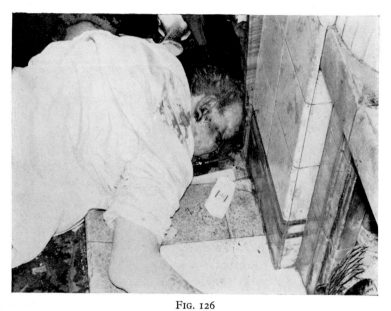

FIG. 126

Case initially considered to be accidental but the injuries were later shown to have been caused in the furtherance of theft

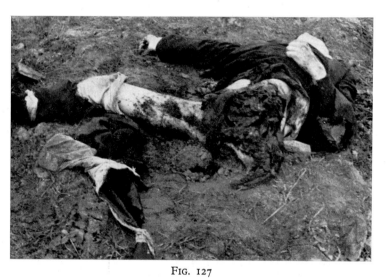

FIG. 127

The effects of an explosion of a small bomb which the boy had placed in his trouser pocket

position of the body and its surroundings and in particular the position and direction of blood-stains and blood splashes (p. 341).

The direction and dimensions of the wound have an important bearing on the relative positions of the assailant and the assaulted person when the wound was inflicted. Such information is of special importance in cases of wounding by firearms, but the direction of the wounding is also of importance in many other cases, for example in cases of stabbing. When the relative positions of the assailant and assaulted person are in question by reason of absence of direct evidence as to the manner of the infliction of the wound, the medical examiners may be expected to offer some opinion on the point from the characters of the wound or wounds.

The hands should be inspected for blood-staining, weapons, hairs, pieces of torn clothing, and other objects. The suspect weapon, when present, should be scrutinised for blood-staining and its applicability for the infliction of the injuries found should receive detailed consideration. This examination, so far as handling is concerned, should be deferred until the finger-print experts have concluded their investigation (see p. 64).

ILLUSTRATIVE CASE

In a case of culpable homicide in which an old man, who was brutally attacked by a man of twenty, died as the result of the violence, an examination of the locus made it clear that the assault had been a prolonged one. It had commenced at the entrance to a cottage and had been continued along the passage and in the kitchen. The instruments of attack were pieces of a wooden curtain pole. Human tissue was present on the floor of the passage, on the leaf of a kitchen table, on the walls, and on a gilt frame of a picture. Several of the pieces of the pole showed attached hair and hairs were also adherent to different articles. A comparison between these specimens and the hair on the head of the victim showed that all were generally consistent with a common source. Blood-staining, which was copious and diffuse, was present on the front door of the cottage (Fig. 196), in the passage, and in the kitchen. The assaulted man survived for some twenty-eight hours. His injuries, which for the greater part involved the posterior half of the scalp, over an area of $7\frac{1}{2}$ by 6 inches, were lacerated in character. Multiple wounds were present, and the majority which extended to bone had caused separation of the scalp from the skull. Several flaps, in irregular form, were attached to the posterior margin of the front half of the scalp. Considerable areas of scalp tissue were missing from points where the skull had been completely denuded of tissue. Other lacerated wounds were present on the face, and there was fracture of the bone of the nose and the left malar bone, together with two linear fractures of the skull.   The irregular surface of one end of a piece of curtain pole, thought to have been used, was considered responsible for the scattering of the small portions of tissue during the attack.

Cut-throat wounds

Homicidal incised wounds of the throat are of frequent occurrence. The wounds may be found on the throat at any level, and their direction is dependent upon the relative positions of the assailant and his victim. For this reason, these wounds may assume a variety of directions in different cases, more especially when a struggle has taken place and the

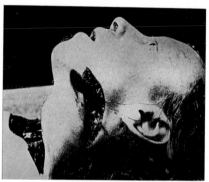

FIG. 128
Case of homicidal cut-throat.   The lower wound,   on   slightly   higher   level   than clavicles,   severed   muscles,   blood-vessels, and trachea

ultimate wounding has been inflicted by the assailant in a frenzied state.   It is unwise to attempt differentiation between homicidal and suicidal cut-throat solely on the grounds that the former shows a more gross appearance and shows greater severance of tissues than the latter. It is true that in a number of suicidal cases the wound may have a rather less pronounced character, that there may be tentative and trivial wounds on the neck, and that the severance of tissues may not be so extensive as in homicidal cases, but in others the injuries may be very extensive.   In one of our cases, the suicide, who was insane, inflicted a wound which was 8 inches long and severed completely all the tissues of the neck down to the vertebral column, the anterior aspect of which showed a surface cut caused by the razor used.   In homicidal cases there may be multiple deep wounds inflicted in different directions, and their multiplicity, together with the injuries produced, may clearly indicate

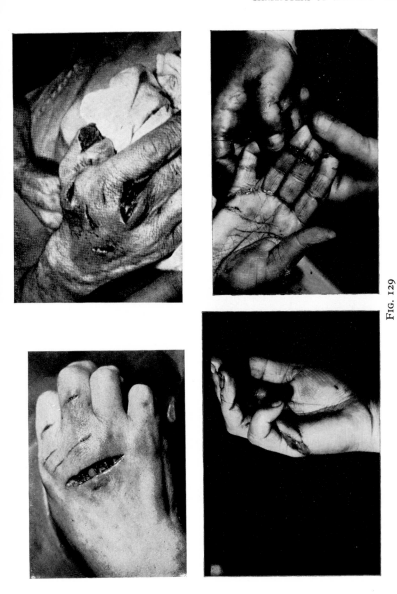

FIG. 129

Defensive wounds of the hand

that the wounding has been continued after volitional movements of the victim had ceased.

All the circumstances must be placed under strict review in certain cases, before a differential diagnosis between homicidal and suicidal cut-throat can finally be made. Defensive incised wounds upon the hand or hands of the victim are reliable indications of the hands having been interposed between the weapon and the victim's body, and are

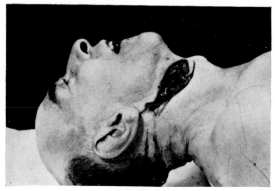

FIG. 130

Suicidal cut-throat, also Fig. 131

(By courtesy of Dr J. A. Imrie)

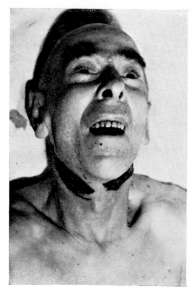

FIG. 131

thus presumptive of homicidal attack (Fig. 132).   Such wounds should not be confused with wounds made over the wrist in a previous attempt at suicide by severance of arteries.

In suicidal cases, when a right-handed person cuts his throat, the wound is inflicted from left to right and, as he makes the wound, considerable pressure is applied to the cutting instrument.   When the wound has been well established, the pressure is decreased until finally the blade is withdrawn from the surface of the neck.   As a result, the part of the wound which has been inflicted initially is of greater depth than the terminal part, made during the gradual withdrawal of the blade, which becomes progressively more shallow in character until the extremity of the wound is reached.   The tailing of the wound is therefore indicative of the site of the withdrawal of the blade.   The line of the wound is usually from left to right and usually from slightly

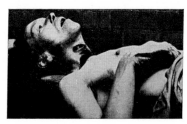

FIG. 132

Case of homicidal cut-throat.   Multiple wounds on neck.   Wound on right hand caused by the victim attempting to shield herself

above downwards and across the neck.   If, however, the instrument is held in the left hand there will be a reversal of most of these features. While in some cases of suicide, tentative wounds may be present on the neck, they are by no means common to all.   Since a suicide usually extends the head preparatory to inflicting the wound, its line may be more or less transverse, and the great vessels of the neck may escape serious injury as the result of the protection which is afforded by the sterno-mastoid muscles and the prominence of the larynx.   The air-passages are frequently injured.   In order of frequency, the sites of injury are over the thyroid cartilage or the thyro-hyoid membrane, over the cricoid cartilage, above the hyoid bone, or over the upper part of the trachea.

In cut-throat injuries, when death results, the cause of death is haemorrhage, air embolism, or septic pneumonia brought about by aspiration, or the effects of local infection.   Aphonia is a frequent manifestation due to injury of the recurrent laryngeal nerve or nerves, or of the vocal cords.

In certain cases of cut-throat wounds, the body of the wounded person may be found either close to the spot where the wound was inflicted or at some distance from it.   In the latter event, there will probably be a trail of blood leading to the place where the body is found.   The distance between these points will vary very greatly in different cases.

In one case a man, after inflicting a wound on his throat, walked a distance of 200 yards before he finally ended his life by drowning.

In another, where a young man killed his sweetheart on the public road by cutting her throat, it was evident from the commencement of the blood-marks on the footpath to the point where her body was found that she had travelled a distance of 105 yards.

The possible distance which a person may walk after receiving the wound will largely depend upon the rapidity of the loss of blood.   In those cases of suicidally inflicted throat wounds in which the suicide has ended his life in some other way, it is usually found that the injuries to the throat are not extensive and that important vessels have not been cut.   When the large blood-vessels have been severed, the rapid and extensive loss of blood will quickly induce collapse, and therefore the distance travelled after the infliction of the wound will probably be short. When the question of distance traversed becomes one of some importance, the answer must be obtained from a careful examination of the wound or wounds on the throat and consideration of the general vigour during life of the person wounded.

Illustrative case of homicidal cut-throat

On the front of the neck there was a large, gaping wound, which extended from ear to ear.   The right extremity was $1\frac{1}{4}$ inches below the level of the lobe of the right ear and $1\frac{1}{2}$ inches behind it.   The left extremity was situated $2\frac{1}{2}$ inches below the level of the lobe of left ear

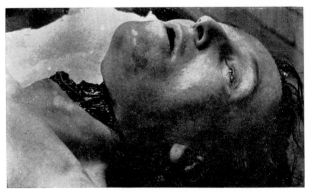

FIG. 133
Homicidal cut-throat

and directly below it.   At each extremity there were three distinct tails or gashes.   The wound measured 8 inches in length, and its gape was 3 inches.   All the muscles in front of the neck, the important blood-vessels and nerves, together with other structures, were severed down to the cervical spine, and the bodies of the third, fourth, fifth, and sixth vertebrae showed surface injury by the weapon.   Lying in front of the vertebral column there was a sharp-pointed, sharp-edged piece of steel, measuring $\frac{1}{4}$ inch long and $\frac{1}{8}$ inch broad, which filled, accurately, a gap in the razor which was found.   Between the under surface of the point of the chin and the principal wound were numerous superficial scratches running at different angles.   On the back of the right, middle, and ring fingers there were superficial wounds caused by the weapon.

Stab wounds

Homicidal stab wounds are most frequently found on the neck, chest, back, and abdomen.   The commonest are on the left side of the chest.   Suicidal wounds as the result of stabbing, are comparatively rare.   Figure 134 shows a case of suicide due to multiple stab wounds

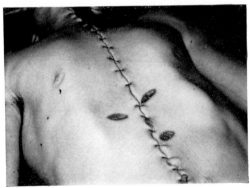

FIG. 134

Case of suicide due to multiple stab wounds of the abdomen

of the abdomen.   Haemothorax is a frequent complication of pene-trating wounds of the chest, and the effusion of blood varies widely in quantity.   The amount may be relatively small, but in some cases the pleural cavity may contain 2 or 3 pints of blood.   Injury of the intercostal vessels or of the lung, or both, is usually the source of the bleeding.   Pneumothorax, haemo-pneumothorax, or subcutaneous emphysema, are conditions which often result from such injuries of the chest.   Stab wounds of the chest frequently pierce the heart or large vessels. The aorta is often injured at some point situated close to the heart. In many cases of homicide, the wounds are multiple and their number will often give a clear indication of the determined character of the attack (Fig. 136). When the weapon has been directed to the abdomen, a variety of injuries may result, and almost any of the abdominal organs may be implicated, although the liver, stomach, and intestinal tract are commonly involved. Occasionally there may be a

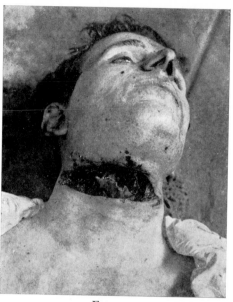

FIG. 135

Case of suicidal cut-throat. Thyroid cartilage was divided, together with all the structures down to the deep vessels on both sides. The left internal jugular vein was the only one of these vessels injured

protrusion of bowel through the wound (Fig. 137). Stab wounds of the neck commonly result in injury to the carotid vessels and jugular veins. Certain stab wounds may be almost imperceptible on the body surface if fine weapons have been employed, for example, narrow-bladed knives, needles, hat-pins, etc. When exploring wounds produced by stabbing, it is sometimes noted that disparity exists between the length of the peccant weapon and the depth of the wound track. This is due to the impact of the weapon compressing the tissues struck (p. 273 and Fig. 140). Volitional movements, following serious injury, may be retained for some time (see p. 296). In one of our cases a vigorous young man ran after his assailants for a distance of between 40 and 50 yards before collapsing, despite the fact that post-mortem examination showed an incised wound which passed through the wall of the left ventricle and measured $\frac{1}{4}$ inch in length.

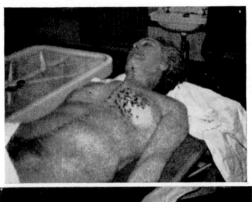
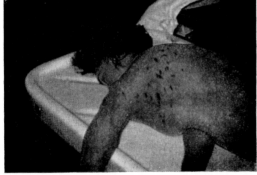

FIG. 136

Multiple homicidal stab wounds, ninety in number, on front, side, and back of chest

ILLUSTRATIVE CASES OF STAB WOUNDS

Suicidal stab wounds by hat-pin

One night a woman arrived by train at a town near Glasgow; she was obviously ill and the police were called. On being taken to the police station, a long hat-pin was found sticking through her neck from front to back. After medical attention she was conveyed to hospital, but died soon afterwards.

On the left side of the neck, $2\frac{1}{2}$ inches below the lower jaw, and $\frac{1}{2}$ inch to left side of midline of the neck, was a small punctured wound. On the back of the neck to right side of spine was a dark reddish point which, on being incised, exuded some blood. One and a half inches

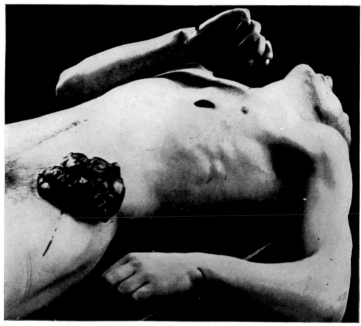

FIG. 137

Stab wounds on chest and abdomen.   Note incised, defensive
wounds on wrists

below the left nipple, and $\frac{3}{4}$ inch to inner side, was a small punctured wound, and $\frac{1}{2}$ inch above it were two superficial puncture marks.

On dissection of the tissues of the neck, it was found that the perforating wound had not entered any important blood-vessel or seriously injured any important structure.   The puncture wound on the left breast had entered the intercostal muscles between the fifth and sixth ribs, the pericardial sac, and the left ventricle.   The left pleural cavity contained 550 ml of fluid blood.

Homicidal stab wound of left eye

The upper lid of the left eye was bruised and swollen.   An incised wound, measuring $1\frac{1}{2}$ inches, was present on the upper eyelid close to eyebrow and perforated the eyelid.   Examination of the interior of the skull showed a considerable amount of clotted blood covering the left half of cerebrum.   At the base of the brain and in a line with the back of the left orbit was a wound which had severed the pons for about two-thirds of its breadth.   Further examination showed that the weapon had passed between the upper part of the eyeball and the roof of the

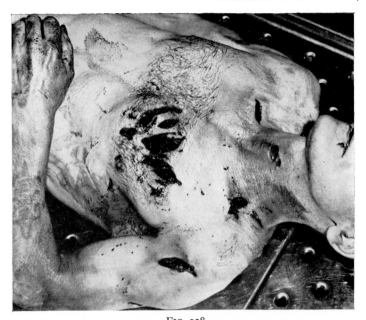

FIG. 138

Multiple stab wounds. With multiple wounds in this target area there
is no doubt about the purpose of the assault

orbit in a backward, inward, and slightly upward direction, had slightly
injured bone at the back of the orbit, and had severed the internal
carotid artery within the skull cavity. The entire length of the wound
from the eyelid inwards was almost 4 inches. The weapon, on which
were found blood-stains, was an ordinary table-knife. The blade
measured $5\frac{1}{2}$ inches, and its breadth, which was uniform, was $\frac{7}{8}$ inch.

Homicidal stab wound of neck

A punctured incised wound, $\frac{5}{8}$ by $\frac{3}{16}$ inch, was situated $1\frac{1}{2}$ inches
below the lobe of left ear, and almost parallel to lower surface of the
lobe. The wound penetrated the internal jugular vein and pharynx.

Homicidal stab wound of neck with broken bottle

An incised wound, $2\frac{1}{2}$ inches long, was situated on the left side of the
neck. It commenced at the base of the anterior attachment of the ear
and extended downwards on to the neck. The upper part of the wound
involved the lobe of the ear from which a partially severed portion was
still attached to the side of the face by a slender strip of skin. The

wound on the neck increased in depth from above downwards and attained a maximum depth of $1\frac{3}{4}$ inches. The internal jugular vein had been penetrated.

Homicidal stab wound of back

A spindle-shaped, incised wound, measuring $\frac{1}{2}$ by $\frac{1}{8}$ inch, was situated at a point $1\frac{1}{4}$ inches to right of middle line of vertebral column and over tenth interspace. A second wound was present on the immediate right of the vertebral column and 3 inches above the first wound. It measured $\frac{3}{8}$ by $\frac{1}{8}$ inch and presented similar characters to the first wound. There were also incised, defensive wounds on the right index and middle fingers, and on the left thumb, together with a linear wound of the epidermis covering the front of the right wrist. The

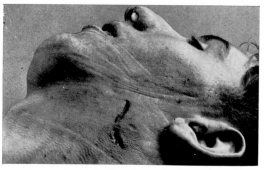

FIG. 139
Stab wounds on neck

right pleural cavity contained 4 pints of blood, and there was an incised wound on the lateral aspect of the right lung, 2 inches above its basal margin. The injury to the lung, which measured $\frac{1}{2}$ inch in length and $\frac{5}{8}$ inch in depth, had been caused by the entry of a knife through the lower of the two wounds on the back.

Homicidal stab wound of chest

A wound was situated over the sterno-clavicular articulation of the left clavicle, measured $\frac{3}{4}$ inch in length, and entered the common carotid artery. Death was practically instantaneous.

Unusual fatal stabbing

The wound was on the front of the chest, $\frac{1}{2}$ inch below the level of the left nipple and $\frac{1}{4}$ inch to the left of the midline. It penetrated the sternum opposite the inner end of the fourth left costal cartilage. The broken end of a pointed pen-knife blade was embedded and projected through the inner surface of the bone for $\frac{5}{16}$ inch. The blade had been sheared on the outer surface of the bone with which it was flush. The anterior mediastinal tissues showed extravasation, oedema, and emphysema. The wound pierced the pericardium and also the underlying anterior wall of the heart, just below the right auriculoventricular border which showed a very irregular, excavated lacerated wound $\frac{3}{4}$ inch long. Although the wound passed deeply into muscle it had failed to effect entry through the endocardial surface. The character of the wound was due to repeated contact between the heart wall and

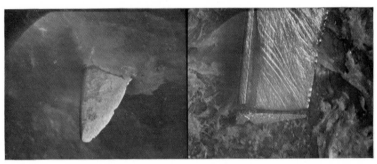

FIG. 140	FIG. 141
Posterior surface of sternum showing projection of embedded portion of blade which passed inwards for a distance of $\frac{5}{16}$ inch, causing laceration of anterior wall of heart (see Fig. 141)	Broken end of pocket-knife blade embedded in sternum. Photograph of anterior surface of the bone. Note base of broken part of blade of suspect knife placed almost in contact with embedded portion of blade (see Fig. 140)

the point of the embedded broken blade caused by combined action of the heart and breathing prior to death. A suspect's knife was submitted for examination when it was found that the larger blade had been broken. Comparison between the embedded portion of the blade and the remaining part of the blade in the knife was fully consistent with the two pieces having been part of one blade (Figs. 140, 141).

References

1. SINGLETON, A.D.   *Am. J. Surg.*, **20** (N.S.), 515, 1933.
2. R. v. Miller [1954] 2 W.L.R., 138.
3. KENNY, C.S.   In *Outlines of Criminal Law*, 15th ed., p. 16, ed. Turner, J.W., Cambridge University Press, 1944.
4. *Medico-legal Review*, **7**, 78, 1939.
5. OJALA, K., LEMPINEN, M., & HIRVONEN, J.   *J. forens. Med.*, **16**, 29, 1969.

Chapter 10

FIREARM WOUNDS

The great majority of firearm wounds are caused by one of the following:

> The revolver.
> The automatic pistol.
> The rifle.
> The shotgun.

The first three of these are rifled and fire single projectiles. The last is a smooth-bore weapon and fires multiple small projectiles from a cartridge. The term rifling is used to describe spiral grooves and ridges usually called lands running the length of the barrel. These impart a spinning motion to the projectile.

The calibre of revolvers, automatic pistols and rifles is usually given as the diameter in decimal parts of an inch, for example, ·38, ·45. A shot gun is usually described as being of a certain bore. This is calculated by finding the number of lead balls which exactly fit the barrel, and which can be made from a pound of lead.

The revolver

This has been so designated on account of the fact that the weapon has a cylindrical magazine situated at the rear of the barrel which is capable of a revolving motion, and which has accommodation for five or six cartridges, each of which is housed in a separate chamber. After a shot has been fired, the circular magazine is rotated by the cocking of the hammer, and in this way the next cartridge is brought into proper position for firing. The cartridge (Fig. 156) of a revolver bullet has a projecting rim around the edge of the base, and the bullet is composed of lead or lead mixed with an alloy. Revolver ammunition is sometimes charged with black powder, although smokeless powder is usual. This type of weapon has a muzzle velocity of about 600 feet per second or less, and is termed a low-velocity weapon.

When a revolver is fired at very close range, almost in contact with the body surface, the wound of entrance is not circular in contour, but is cruciform or stellate with lacerated edges. This results from laceration of the tissues with some excavation due to expansion of the liberated gases. When the site of the injury is hair-covered, the hairs will show evidence of singeing, and when the ammunition has been charged with black powder there will be burning, in varying degree, around the entrance wound, together with an irregular ring of carbon deposit, usually about a quarter of an inch or more in diameter. In addition, the skin will show tattooing with powder particles driven into the skin. At distances beyond 6 inches the effect is different. The gases no longer enter the tissues and the wound is approximately circular and corresponds to the size of the projectile. Such wounds show marginal bruising and some inversion of the edges. There may also be an area of tissue bruising around the wound. The edges may show a grease

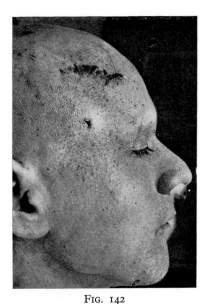

FIG. 142

Entrance wound of revolver bullet which lodged in brain. Tattooing by powder particles is seen around wound. The darkened area above is due to scorching

collar. Bruising tends to disappear at about 6 inches, although there will probably be some evidence of bruising and of powder marks. At a range of about 12 inches and over, the skin around the wound does not, as a rule, show evidence of powder marks.

When the weapon has been fired at very close range, almost in contact with the surface of the body, the wound of exit is usually of smaller size than the wound of entrance. With increased range this finding is usually reversed and the exit wound is frequently larger than the wound of entrance, due to laceration of tissue by the bullet being deviated in its passage through the body as a result of deflection in varying degree. When the projectile encounters bone the extent of deflection may be very great and the behaviour of the bullet may display many vagaries in the terminal part of its course. Should splintered bone be carried before it the tissues are lacerated, and the resultant wound is frequently very large. Except in contact shots, the wounds

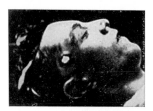

FIG. 143

Entrance wound of revolver bullet which passed through head. Size of wound is indicated by circular disc of paper

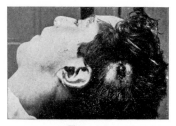

FIG. 144

Exit wound, in same case, larger than entrance. The edges are everted

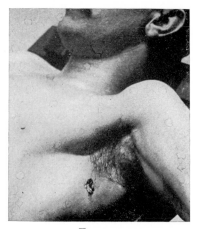

FIG. 145

Exit wound of revolver bullet. Note underlying haematoma

of entrance and exit may be of similar size when obstruction has not been encountered by the bullet.

Occasionally medium-range gunshot wounds can be confused with penetrating stab wounds. If the possibility is kept in mind, the examiner, by careful inspection with a hand lens, can nearly always make the distinction.

At close range the velocity of the bullet sets up great destructive forces within the body and these affect tissues at considerable distances from the track of the projectile.   It is unwise to dogmatise on the characters of revolver wounds, especially in regard to wounds of entry, since so much depends upon the pattern, calibre and condition of the

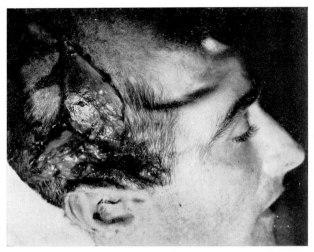

FIG. 146

Suicidal wounding by service rifle bullet at contact range.   Note extensive laceration around entrance wound and depression of frontal bone due to fracture

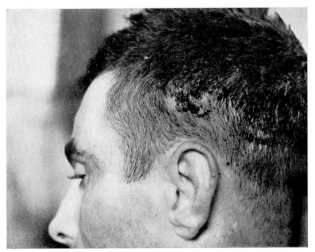

FIG. 147

Exit wound in case illustrated in Fig. 146

weapons which may produce them; there are also many other factors which must be taken into consideration.   With a view to determining the likely range at which a wound was inflicted, firing experiments with the suspect weapon should be made and the results of the tests carefully examined in relation to the known ranges.   Microscopical comparisons

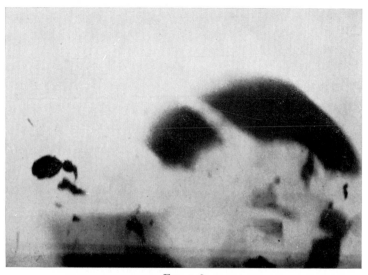

Fig. 148

X-ray study of calibre ·22 bullet passing through bone

(Exposure time 1 microsecond)

Radiograph showing the destructive action of a bullet passing through a piece of beef shin-bone.   The pressure has forced the marrow out of the bone and the splintering of the bone and broken particles of the bullet may be seen

(By courtesy of *Life* magazine, New York, and the Westinghouse Laboratories, Bloomfield, N.J.)

can also be made between the particles of carbon removed from the region of the entrance wound and from the various experimental targets.

The automatic pistol

This type of firearm is so named because when a cartridge is fired, the empty cartridge case is ejected, and a new cartridge slips into the breech automatically, as the result of the recoil.   The cartridges are contained in a vertical magazine in the stock of the weapon, which usually holds six or seven cartridges.   This class of firearm is better

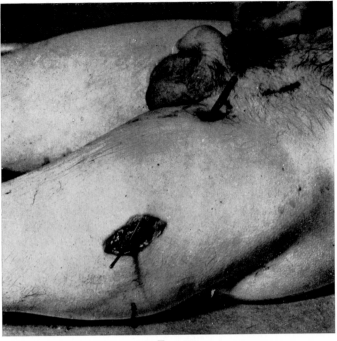

FIG. 149

Entrance and exit wounds by service rifle bullet. Abrasion in pubic region caused by impact of bullet with stem of button on great-coat. The femur was fractured

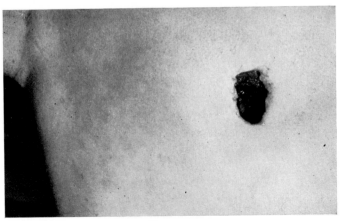

FIG. 150

Exit wound of service rifle bullet

G M J—T**

termed 'self-loading' than automatic, since, as Burrard points out, an automatic firearm is one which will continue to fire, and go on firing, so long as the trigger is held back, whereas in all 'self-loaders' the trigger must be pressed for every shot that is fired. The cartridge case, which is almost rimless, contains smokeless powder. Since this type of weapon fires a bullet with a muzzle velocity up to 1,200 or more feet per second, the outer casing of the projectile is composed of hard metal such as nickel, steel, or cupro-nickel, although the inner core is composed of lead. The wounds produced have the characters of those already described under revolver wounds.

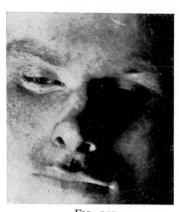

FIG. 151

Entrance wound on upper lip produced by bullet from military rifle. Note tattooing of face with powder particles

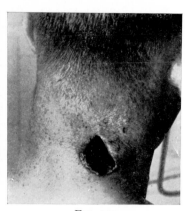

FIG. 152

Exit wound produced by the same bullet as in Fig. 151, and by splintering of bone

Propellant powders

Black powder, or gunpowder, is composed of potassium nitrate, sulphur, and charcoal, and grey, or smokeless powder, of nitrocellulose, or of a combination of nitrocellulose and nitroglycerine, gelatinised, to retard the rapidity of the explosion and to maintain a uniform pressure on the projectile. Smokeless powder is grained into solid cylindrical patterns. The combustion of smokeless powder produces much less flame and smoke than combustion of black powder, since the process is more efficiently performed with the former than with the latter. The powder deposit around the wound, even at close range, is much less when smokeless powder is used, and around wounds inflicted at a range of a few inches, burning and tattooing are much less marked.

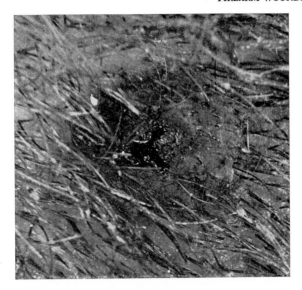

FIG. 153

Infra-red photograph of entrance wound on back of head.
Bullet was of ·22 calibre. Note cross-shaped contour of
wound due to close range

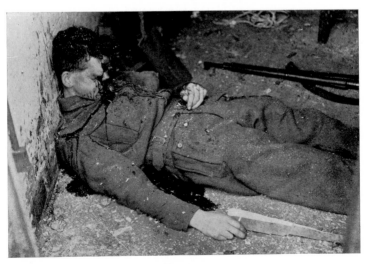

FIG. 154

Suicide with a military rifle. The butt end of the weapon was rested on the
ground, the forehead applied to the muzzle, and the trigger released by means
of a piece of wood

The rifle

Common examples of this weapon are the military rifle and the miniature rifle. The service rifle formerly used by the British army has a magazine and bolt action and a muzzle velocity of about 2,500 feet per second. Even at 3,000 yards it has a velocity of over 300 feet per second. The pressure in the firing chamber is about 20 tons per square inch. As the bullet leaves the barrel it rotates at about 3,000 revolutions per second. With such a high initial velocity the bullets frequently pass through the body, and if no resistance to their passage has been encountered, the size and shape of the entrance and exit wounds may be very similar except, perhaps, for some inversion of the edges in the former and eversion of the edges in the latter. The tissues through which the projectile has passed are usually the seat of bruising in varying degree. This is due to what has been called 'tissue quake'. This is the destruction of tissue in the area surrounding the path of a high-velocity bullet. The entrance wound, as a rule, is approximately the size of the bullet which has produced it. If, however, bone is encountered by the missile in its passage through the body, there may be considerable deflection, or splintering of bone or both. When the bullet thus deviated from its path ploughs through the tissues to force an exit, or when fragments of splintered bone are forced out through the tissues, the wound of emergence will be large and of lacerated character. It may measure several inches in diameter (Figs. 147, 149, 150, 152). When the head is the seat of wounding, at, or near, contact range, the entrance wound may be of large size due to extensive laceration of tissue which is frequently accompanied by diffuse fracture of underlying bone (Fig. 146). It has been noted that, at short ranges, when a rifle bullet has passed through more than one limb—for example, the thighs—although the entrance wound of the limb first struck is frequently fully consistent with expected characters, the exit wound is lacerated and large, despite the absence of bone damage. The entrance wound on the second limb may show very extensive laceration, several inches in diameter, due to alteration in the path of the flight of the bullet experienced by traversing the first limb.

It was found that the destructive effect in the body could be increased by using small bullets at very high velocity and with a rate of twist close to instability. These principles were applied in the development of the 7·62 mm N.A.T.O. cartridge, which has now been adopted by the British army. The Americans use a smaller very high-velocity bullet which is reputed to turn end over end after contact, thus causing very severe tissue destruction.[1]

Attempts have been made to estimate the distance of discharge of rifled weapons by studying the lead pattern deposited round the entrance wound. Cimino and Debney[2] have made experimental firings with a number of different weapons and state that the lead patterns found clearly distinguished between weapons discharged at

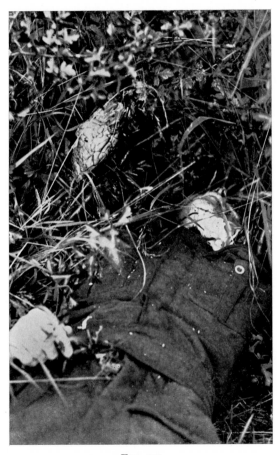

FIG. 155

Suicide with a military rifle. The skull was comminuted and the brain, seen suspended in the undergrowth, was forcibly ejected from the cranial cavity

(By courtesy of Dr J. A. Imrie)

two feet and three feet. This might be a valuable investigation in shooting deaths. The test is done by spraying saturated aqueous sodium rhodizonate solution on the suspect surface which has been previously acidified. Lead gives a blue reaction.

Shotguns

These weapons have for their projectile collections of small shot which vary in size, depending upon the type of cartridge employed. They are extensively used for shooting game. They are also the reserve weapon of many police forces throughout the world.

The cartridge (Fig. 156) is a cylinder made either of impregnated paper or plastic usually 2½ inches in length and closed at the end by a brass cap with a projecting rim and at the other end either by a cardboard wad or by crimping in the walls of the cylinder.

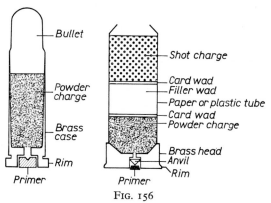

Fig. 156

Respective diagrams of the cartridge for a revolver and shotgun

In the centre of the brass cap there is a percussion device which when struck with the hammer explodes the powder. The contents of the cartridge progressing from the base to the crimped end are:

A base wad.
The powder.
The over powder wad.
The main wad.
The under shot card.
The shot.
The over shot wad.

The shot vary in size from what is called dust shot, where the cartridge contains a very large number of small particles of lead to buckshot where there may only be six or eight large lead pellets filling the cartridge. The importance of this is that dust shot is lethal at very short range only, whereas the large types of shot are lethal at sixty yards or more.

The importance of understanding the construction of a cartridge to the medical examiner is that it helps him to understand the effects which are produced by its discharge and also the damage which can be caused by constructional defects.

The muzzle velocity of a twelve-bore shotgun, which is the commonest gun in use, and has a barrel dimension of 0·729 of an inch, has a muzzle velocity of about 1,100 feet per second. This velocity remains almost constant for three yards and thereafter falls fairly rapidly.[3, 4, 5]

After firing, the pellets disperse soon after their exit from the barrel, and this dispersion increases with the range. The degree of dispersion

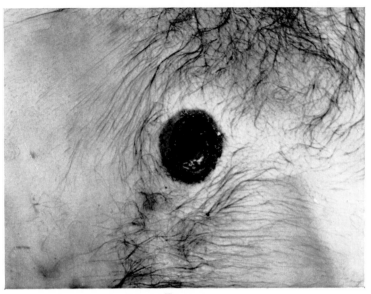

FIG. 157

Contact shotgun wound showing bruising caused by muzzle and bruising on chest wall produced by internal damage

can be controlled to some extent by a 'choking' device near the termination of the barrel. This takes the form of a slight constriction which varies in degree in different weapons. To describe this, such terms as 'full choke' and 'half choke' are used. In certain weapons there is no 'choke' device.

If a shot is fired close to the body surface, up to a few inches, the shot enters as a mass, and in addition the liberated gases and flame lacerate the tissues, which show evidence of burning, carbon deposit, and powder tattooing. The wads may be forced into the wound, and this may prove an important clue to the class of cartridge used. When the gun has been fired at from 1 to 3 feet from the body, a more or less irregularly circular wound about $1\frac{1}{2}$ to 2 inches in diameter will be produced (see Fig. 157). There will be evidence of some degree of scorching, carbon deposit and tattooing. So far as dispersion is concerned, with a 'half-choke' gun the pellets will show a spread of about 5 inches in diameter at a range of 5 yards, about 12 inches in diameter at 10 yards, about 16 inches in diameter at 15 yards, and about 20 inches in diameter at 20 yards. To determine the dispersion at the same ranges with a gun of 'full choke', an approximate method is to deduct a quarter from the measurements of these diameters of spread. At a range of over a yard and up to about 3 yards, evidence of burning disappears and probably only faint tattooing will be found. Beyond a yard, the entering shot produces an irregular wound, and, at 9 feet

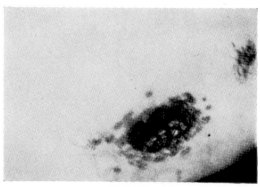

FIG. 158
Homicidal wound on left side of chest caused by
shotgun

there will be dispersion of the pellets and individual pellet holes may be detected.

Commercial cartridges nearly always have smokeless powder. Some loaders sometimes use black powder and this causes increased blackening and tattooing.

Walker[6] recommends the use of infra-red photography for the determination of powder marks on clothing and finds it of considerable assistance in the estimation of range. Smokeless powder residues do not give a dense black pattern of individual spots when photographed with infra-red light, but black powder residues do. By this method a permanent graphic representation of the powder residue pattern is produced without destruction or alteration in the fabric. Blood-stains do not greatly interfere.

Accurate estimations of the pellet patterns at different ranges are not possible, since so much depends upon the idiosyncrasies of individual cartridges. This is due to the fact that the cardboard wad is so frequently dislodged in an oblique fashion that turbulence of the shot occurs within the barrel and thus affects the pellet patterns at other than close ranges. With regard to the size of the area of wounding produced by a sporting gun, almost irrespective of choke, an approximate estimate, at different ranges, may be obtained by using this simple formula:

If X = range in yards, then the diameter of the wound = $(X + 1)$ inches.

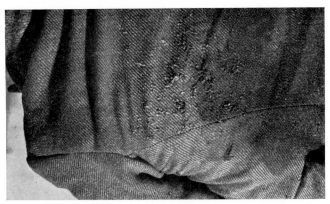

FIG. 159

Multiple perforations of clothing by pellets from sporting gun
(see Fig. 160)

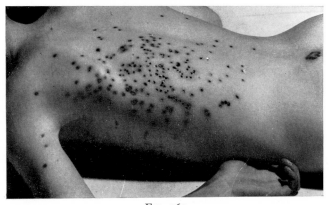

FIG. 160

(See Fig. 159)

Wounds produced by pellets from sporting gun fired at about 10 yards. Some 207 pellet wounds present, covering maximum spread of about 12 inches. Injury on left buttock is a bruise. (Figs. 159 and 160 by courtesy of Chief Constable of West Riding of Yorkshire, Wakefield)

It should be clearly understood, however, that the dimension of the area of wounding, as calculated in the foregoing, is that of the cone of the shot spread, measured on a plane perpendicular to the line of fire and upon a relatively flat surface.

When a suspect weapon is being investigated, trial shot patterns from the gun should be studied at various ranges.

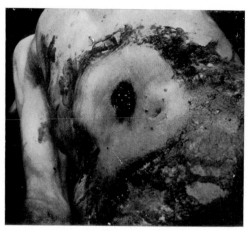

FIG. 161
Abdominal wound by shotgun

Injuries caused by industrial guns firing various fixing devices

These guns are being much more frequently used and accidental deaths and a few cases of assault have occurred.

The commonest type of gun fires studs.[7] Stud guns are used to fire metal studs into steel, wood, or concrete. They have a muzzle velocity of up to 1,400 feet per second. The studs are made of steel and are usually of ·22 or ·38 calibre. They have tremendous penetrating power[8] but tend to be unstable, causing great tissue destruction. They are usually discharged at close range and produce powder marking and laceration of the tissues. Occasionally, due to the instability of the projectile, the wound may be the exact shape of the profile of the stud.

It has been suggested that there should be further legislative control of the use of these 'weapons'.[9]

Identification of firearms

Since the revolver, the self-loading pistol, and the rifle, fire a single bullet, it is necessary to make provision to maintain the bullet in a state of stability during its passage through the barrel of the weapon and

during its flight. This is effected by the rifling on the inside of the
barrel caused by the lands and grooves previously described (p. 274).
As the bullet passes along the barrel of the weapon at high speed its
surface comes into intimate contact with these lands, forcing it into a
spin which, when the bullet emerges from the muzzle, exerts a type of
gyroscopic action. A fired bullet will thus show indentations of a series
of slanting parallel grooves, varying in number from four to seven,
made by the lands. The pattern of the rifling in weapons of different
manufacture varies both in number of grooves and direction of the
riflings. The markings upon fired bullets thus become of high value
in the identification of the weapon from which they have been fired.

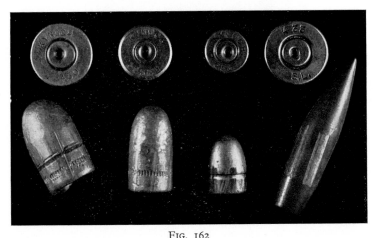

FIG. 162

Top—Striker pin impressions on fired cartridge cases.
Foot—Rifling marks on fired bullets

Fired cartridge cases also may be identified with the firearm from
which they were ejected. Such investigation is based on the facts
that an individual firearm will impart to the cartridges which it fires,
its specific markings on the breech face and striker. In self-loading
and automatic weapons, the ejector mark upon a fired cartridge may be
compared with the characters of the metal block of the firearm which
causes the ejection of the cartridge. For comparison purposes, test
rounds should be fired from the suspect weapon and the cartridges
compared in detail with those under examination. It is more difficult
to establish identity by means of a fired bullet than by means of a fired
cartridge case, since there is more chance of a static pressure mark on
the latter than sliding pressure on the former. Cartridge case markings
are also more easy to interpret. The greatest care must be exercised
in removing a bullet from a body so that marks due to artefact, such as

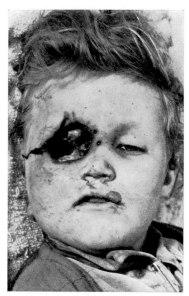

FIG. 163
Entrance wound caused by sporting
gun at close range (Fig. 164)

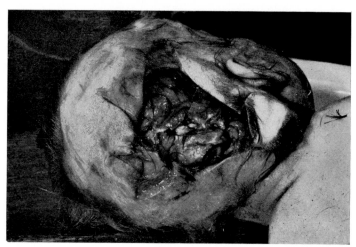

FIG. 164
Exit wound in the same case (Fig. 163)

scratches, are not produced on the bullet. Such markings may vitiate subsequent identification of the projectile. When necessary, the use of forceps, the gripping arms of which have been covered with rubber tubing, is recommended. When the bullet has been extracted an identification mark should be engraved upon its base.

Since the identification of firearms and their projectiles should always be undertaken by firearm experts, the necessary technique has

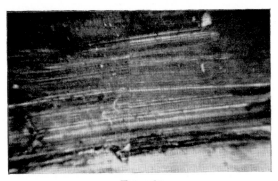

FIG. 165

Comparison photomicrograph. Matching of land engraving marks on crime and test bullets

(By courtesy of the City of Glasgow Police)

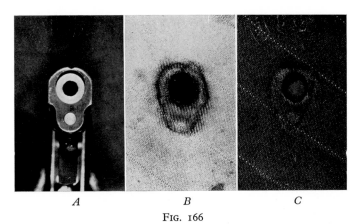

| *A* | *B* | *C* |

FIG. 166

A, Muzzle of self-loading pistol. B, Infra-red photograph of scorched area on clothing showing contour of *A*. *C*, Ordinary photograph of scorched area on clothing. The outline showed that strong pressure must have been applied to the surface at the moment of firing. Such contours are of importance in the reconstruction of crime.

(By courtesy of the City of Glasgow Police)

been omitted. The reader who desires such information should consult standard works on the subject.[10, 11, 12, 13]

Bullet wounds of the head

When a bullet enters the skull and emerges, an examination of the entrance wound will show that the aperture in the bone differs in relation to the outer and inner tables; more bone is splintered from the inner than from the outer table. The converse is found in the exit wound in which a greater amount of bone is removed from the outer

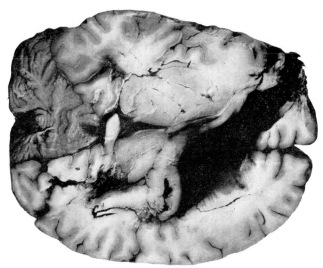

Fig. 167
Bullet track through cerebral hemispheres.
Note laceration of brain tissue

than from the inner table. The reason lies in the fact that there is an expanding impulse transmitted through the bone. The exit aperture is as a rule larger than that of the entrance. In certain cases, the possibility of a bullet ricocheting after entering the cranial cavity must not be overlooked, and in the odd case in which it occurs the deviation in direction of travel may be such that the point of emergence may occur in the most unexpected place. A rifle bullet on encountering the skull may, on account of its high velocity, probably cause an extensive fracture of bone due to sudden liberation of energy. When a bullet strikes the head at a very narrow angle to the surface, and glances from it, a gutter wound of the scalp and skull will result. When the skull is involved, there may be severe splintering of the inner table.

Bullet wounds on other parts of the body

In performing a post-mortem examination in a case of shooting, certain precautions must be adopted.   If there is a single wound upon the body, it must be a wound of entrance, and therefore the bullet must be recovered.   Should the entrance wound be soiled with blood, great care must be exercised in sponging it away so that any tattooing of the skin may not be disturbed.   When the bullet has been fired through the palate, unless it has emerged from the skull, no wound will be visible on the exterior of the body.   Exit wounds never show evidence of carbon deposit, burning, or powder tattooing.   It is frequently found that the track of the bullet is a devious one due to its deflection by bone, and the projectile may ultimately be found in a most unexpected situation.   This point is of practical significance, when the question arises in the case of two wounds being found on the body not corresponding to the likely line of traject, as to whether they have been produced by one or two bullets.   The bullet may take a straight path through the body, and in this event the relative positions of the entrance and exit wounds will indicate the direction of fire. When a cavity has been penetrated and a quantity of blood has collected, a careful search for a bullet in the effused blood should be made.   The possibility of the bullet being overlooked in such a case might result through its removal in a measuring vessel with the blood.

An X-ray examination to identify the position of the bullet or fragments should always be made where possible.   Without this it may be extremely difficult to locate the bullet at the post-mortem dissection. We have made long searches for small bullets embedded in the body of the sphenoid bone, the spinal canal, and the hip joint.

When the bullet penetrates the skin obliquely, the contusion collar is more pronounced on the aspect of the wound corresponding to the direction of entry of the missile, and thus indication of the direction may be given.   Sometimes the bullet strikes the body at a tangent, and instead of penetrating the tissues merely grazes them, producing a furrow of varying depth.   The fact that a single bullet may cause several wounds on the body, for example, perforation of the arm followed by entrance into, and exit from, the chest, must not be overlooked.   Disintegration of a portion of the projectile, fragmentation of bone, or the emergence of foreign bodies, such as pieces of metal button, may be responsible for multiple wounding.

A spent bullet may cause surface injury only, in the form of bruising or laceration, and it may be very difficult to arrive at an opinion as to cause and effect unless the history of the case is clear.

It is unwise to express an opinion regarding the nature and course of firearm missiles until all the facts of the case have been considered.

The following cases will illustrate many of the points which have been touched upon.

ILLUSTRATIVE CASES

Fatal wounding by bullets fired from revolvers and automatic pistols

Revolver bullet.   We examined the body of a man alleged to have been accidentally shot in a private shooting club.   An ovate wound, measuring $\frac{5}{8}$ by $\frac{3}{8}$ inch, was situated on the left temporal region.   The eyelids were deeply bruised.   The scalp tissues, over an area 6 inches in diameter around the wound, contained extravasated blood.   In the left temporal bone was an ovate aperture of the same size as the wound of entry.   Over the surface of the brain was a thin layer of blood.   On the outer surface of the left frontal lobe was an area of laceration.   The bullet had passed through the substance of both frontal lobes, been deflected backwards through the right half of the cerebrum, and had

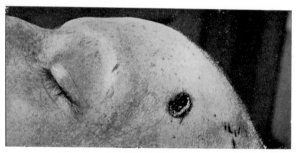

FIG. 168

Entrance wound of bullet, extracted from the brain.   Bullet
entered head sideways due to ricochet

finally lodged in the right occipital lobe.   The roof of each orbital cavity was the seat of fracture.   The bullet, which was distorted, measured $\frac{9}{16}$ by $\frac{5}{16}$ inch.

It appeared that both accused and deceased were members of the club, and that both were expert shots.   The deceased in friendly rivalry challenged the accused to hit a clay pipe which the deceased man was to hold in his mouth, and it was during the act of shooting at the pipe that the deceased was killed.   The bullet had struck the pipe, been deflected at an angle, and had entered the head of the victim (Fig. 168).

Multiple revolver bullets.   This case is illustrative of the occasional multiplicity of small-calibre revolver bullet wounds in suicide.

Over the third and fourth intercostal spaces, covering an area of 3 inches in diameter and at a distance of $1\frac{1}{2}$ inches from middle line of chest, was an area of scorching (see Fig. 169).   Within this area were five punctured wounds, the edges of which were black. Each wound was $\frac{1}{5}$ inch in diamerer. Multiple firearm wounds suggest homicide rather than suicide, but in a number of suicidal cases such wounds may be found. In these suicidal cases, bullets of small calibre, ·22 or ·25, are usually employed. A number of instances have been met with where several bullets of this type have penetrated the heart.

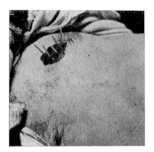

FIG. 169

Suicidally inflicted revolver bullet wounds of chest, five in number

Automatic pistol bullet. A circular entrance wound, situated on the left side of chest, $1\frac{1}{4}$ inches external to, and in line with nipple, measured $\frac{1}{8}$ inch in diameter. The edges showed a grease collar and underlying bruising which measured $\frac{3}{8}$ inch in diameter. On right side of chest, 3 inches external to nipple, and in line with it, was a faintly bruised area $\frac{1}{2}$ inch in diameter. In the centre a small ill-defined linear abrasion was situated, and palpation over this area disclosed the presence of the bullet. On the inner surface of middle-third of right upper arm, corresponding in position to the abrasion on side of chest, was a faint bruise, approximately $\frac{1}{2}$ inch in diameter. Dissection of the body showed that the bullet had passed through the tissues of the chest wall, had fractured the fourth rib, and penetrated the left lateral surface of pericardium, and interior surface of the heart, immediately to the left of the interventricular septum, at a point $1\frac{1}{2}$ inches above apex of heart. It emerged from the heart on the right side, 1 inch below auriculo-ventricular border, passed through the right lateral surface of pericardium, the inner surface of the lower portion of the middle lobe of right lung, and into right chest wall, in fourth interspace, where it lodged immediately beneath the skin. Both pleural cavities contained blood-clot, which amounted to 3 pints in the left cavity and $2\frac{1}{2}$ pints in the right.

Service rifle bullet. The entrance wound, which was situated 5 inches above the anterior superior spine of left ilium and $2\frac{1}{2}$ inches external to it, penetrated the abdominal cavity between eleventh and twelfth ribs. There was no scorching or tattooing. The exit wound, which was lacerated and measured 5 by 2 inches, was situated on the back, immediately to the left of the middle line of lumbar region of vertebral column. There was marked loss of muscle tissue and laceration. The cavity formed barely admitted the closed fist, and at its base the upper pole of left kidney could easily be palpated. There was a quantity of free blood in both flanks and the tissues around left kidney were bruised and lacerated. The kidney was severely lacerated, and its lower pole had almost been severed. The left transverse processes of third and fourth lumbar vertebrae were comminuted.

Shotgun injury. The body was found on a farm road with a large wound in the abdomen, and the shotgun of the deceased man lay by his side. On the front of abdomen there was an almost circular wound, measuring $1\frac{5}{8}$ by $1\frac{3}{8}$ inches, through which a small mass of intestine protruded. The wound was immediately above, and to right of, the umbilicus. There were no marks of tattooing around the wound, but the edges were scorched. The abdominal cavity contained 600 ml of blood. On the inner surface of the abdominal wall the wound measured $3\frac{1}{2}$ by $2\frac{3}{4}$ inches. In the wall of the intestines there were many small shot. In the lower part of lumbar portion of vertebral column the bodies of the vertebrae were peppered with shot, and the surrounding tissues, including the main abdominal vessels, were severely injured. Lying in blood in the left side of the pelvis were the entire wad of a cartridge and fragments of clothing, in which were several pellets of shot (see Fig. 161).

Unusual case of volitional movement following automatic pistol wound of brain.

Kerr[14] records a most unusual case. The facts put briefly were that an elderly man shot himself with a ·45 Colt automatic pistol. The wound of entry was situated under chin, 2 inches from point, and immediately to left of midline. The wound passed into skull, just behind roof of left orbit, passed through frontal and temporal lobes of brain, which were lacerated and pulped, then passed through skull on left side of frontal bone making an exit, $1\frac{1}{2}$ inches in diameter, and severely lacerating scalp, $3\frac{1}{2}$ inches directly above left eye. Following the injury, the man walked from a garden shelter, near a hotel where he lodged, to the grass in front of the shelter and continued in a circle for about 165 yards. He returned to the shelter, where he rested upon a seat and finally returned to his hotel. On his arrival there, he rang the bell, spoke to the servant, hung up his umbrella in the hall, took off his overcoat, and walked upstairs to the bathroom where he collapsed and lost consciousness. The brain showed considerable laceration and haemorrhage. Portions of brain had been blown through the top of the skull on to the roof of the shelter. The man lived for three hours after his injury.

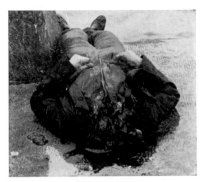

FIG. 170

Decapitation due to firing an explosive charge placed in the mouth. This was a case of suicide, and a detonator was employed to fire the charge

References

1. GREENWOOD, C. *J. forens. Sci. Soc.*, **6**, 124, 1966.
2. CIMINO, A.M. & DEBNEY, J.E. *J. forens, Sci. Soc.*, **8**, 8, 1968.
3. GREENWOOD, C. *J. Forens, Sci. Soc.*, **6**, 125, 1966.
4. DRAKE, V. *J. forens. Sci. Soc.*, **2**, 85, 1962.
5. DRAKE, V. *J. forens. Sci. Soc.*, **3**, 22, 1962.
6. WALKER, J.T. *New Engl. J. Med.*, **216**, 1024, 1937.
7. SPITZ, W.U. & WILHELM, R.M. *J. forens. Med.*, **17**, 5, 1970.
8. MAGE, S. & SYE, K.C. *New Engl. J. Med.*, **267**, 1020, 1962.
9. *British Medical Journal*, **1**, 460, 1968.
10. McCAFFERTY, J. *J. forens. Sci. Soc.*, **5**, 11, 1965.
11. BARNES, F.C. *Cartridges of the World*. Gun Digest Co., 1965.
12. MATTHEWS, J.H. *Firearms Identification*. University of Wisconsin Press, 1962.
13. SMITH, W.H.B. *Small Arms of the World*. Stackpole, 1966.
14. KERR, D.J.A. *Lancet*, **1**, 467, 1945.

Chapter 11

HEAD AND OTHER INJURIES

HEAD INJURIES

We shall discuss:

> Injuries to the scalp.
> Concussion.
> Gun-shot wounds.
> Fractures of the skull vault and base.
> Extradural haemorrhage.
> Subdural haemorrhage.
> Subarachnoid haemorrhage.
> Intracerebral haemorrhage.
> Contusion and laceration of the brain.
> Amnesia.
> Post-contusional syndrome.

Injuries to the scalp

Bruising. Bruising of the scalp occurs in every case of head injury with the exception of incised wounds. The bruising may be very extensive but sometimes it is localised and in situations which tend to be missed with the ordinary post-mortem reflection of the scalp. Bruises are frequently found in the deep tissues of the scalp just above the orbital ridges and in the posterior part of the scalp below the occipital protuberance. The finding of these may completely alter the assessment of the case. It is surprising how much bruising there can be in the deep tissues of the scalp without showing on the external surface. The finding of deep bruising in the scalp may be the first evidence found in the investigation of battered children. Localised bruising is nearly always found in the temporal region when there is an underlying extradural haemorrhage. Very large thick haemotomata may conceal the presence of vault fractures.

Lacerations. The commonest cause of laceration of the scalp is the motor vehicle. The second most common in the West of Scotland is criminal assault with a blunt instrument. A very few are self-inflicted, mostly in the mentally deranged.

The first thing to decide when examining a scalp laceration is that it has in fact been caused by a blunt instrument. It is in this situation that there is the greatest difficulty in differentiating wounds made by blunt and sharp instruments (p. 250). The next consideration is whether the lacerations are accidental, homicidal, or suicidal. Multiple severe lacerations widely scattered over the scalp are almost always homicidal. The difficult cases are where one or two lacerations are found on the head of a man known to have been in a state of intoxication. If the lacerations are about or below the level of the occipital protuberance

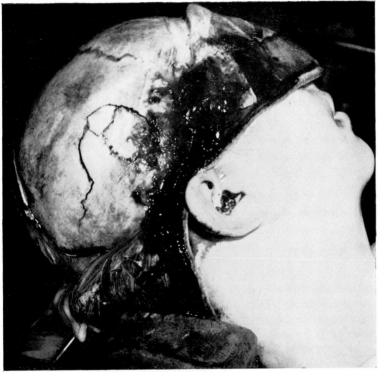

FIG. 171

Blunt injury of the skull showing extensive scalp bruising and comminuted fracture of skull in case of homicide

the probability is in favour of accident. If the lacerations are on the sides or top of the head the cause is probably homicidal.

Incised wounds. These are uncommon on the head, but when they occur are usually criminal and associated with incised wounds of the face due to razor slashing. The only commonly occurring incised wounds of the scalp are caused by flying glass usually the result of automobile accidents or explosions.

Concussion

All head injuries of any severity are accompanied by some degree of concussion.   This is really a term to describe symptoms rather than a pathological entity.   It is usually used to describe a cessation of cerebral function resulting from trauma to the head.   It may be part of and the initial stage in much more serious head injuries but it is usually used to describe a transient period of unconsciousness from which the patient recovers without residual cerebral damage.   The mechanism of the condition is doubtful, and many theories have been propounded. These are for surgeons and neuropathologists and we do not propose to discuss them.   In any case the latest theory will probably be out of date by the time this book is published.

Gun-shot wounds

Gun-shot wounds of the head in civilian practice are usually suicidal. Accidental and homicidal cases in our experience occur about equally. The lesions found vary from single-pellet injuries to almost complete destruction of the skull.   The decision of homicide, suicide, or accident will depend on the detailed findings described in the section on firearm wounds (p. 274), in particular the range of discharge and the accessibility of the site.

Fractures of the skull

Such fractures may implicate either the vault or base of the skull, or both, and may be caused either by direct or indirect violence.   When direct violence is applied to the vault, as, for example, by a blow, the lines of fracture radiate from the point of impact and, speaking generally fractures of the skull usually occur at the point or points at which the greatest force has been applied.   The views of Rowbotham[1] are that the precise manner in which the bone breaks is determined by the fact that its tensile strength is less than its power to resist compression and therefore whichever table of the skull happens to be on the convexity of a bend, and thus subjected to stretch, will be the one to fracture first.   A counter force must act on the skull at the same time as the injuring force, if a fracture is to occur, and the rigid support which the skull receives at its occipital condyles is one of the most important anatomical features concerned in the mechanisms of fracture of the skull and injury to the brain.   Fractures of the vault often result also from the effects of indirect violence transmitted from the base, or as the result of compression of the skull which has exceeded the degree of its temporary expansion.   When the vault has been the seat of injury, the fracture may be simple or compound, linear, or comminuted, with or without depression.

The degree of compression, when present, will naturally vary and it may be slight in degree or extreme, as, for example, when fragmented bone is driven inwards, perhaps into the substance of the brain. In rarer cases, the fractured area may show some elevation. Fractures of

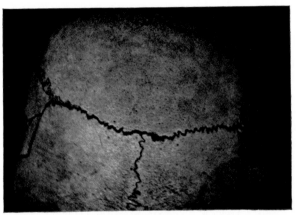

FIG. 172

Comminuted fracture of skull with slight separation of fronto-parietal suture

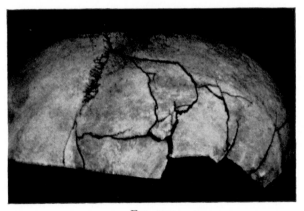

FIG. 173

Comminuted fracture of skull

the skull may be extensive yet unaccompanied by gross injury of the brain, but it must not be forgotten that serious intracranial injury may result from a simple fracture, or perhaps without fracture, as the result of contrecoup and consequent extradural and subdural haemorrhages or laceration of the brain substance.

With regard to fractures of the base, here again these may follow either direct or indirect violence. Direct violence is not commonly a cause, but one must not overlook the type of case in which there has been the passage of an instrument through the orbital cavity or where a firearm wound has perforated the palate (see p. 310). Indirect violence is the common cause of basal fractures which are frequently produced by falls from a height when the feet or buttocks of the injured person strike the ground first. Fractures of the vault often extend to the base. When compression of the base is the cause of fracture, the line follows the path of least resistance and is deflected from the thicker and more resistant portions of bone. Apart from penetrating wounds of the skull, the brain may also receive injury by distortions of the skull, or by movements of the brain within the cranial cavity.

In all medico-legal post-mortem examinations, the membranes should be stripped thoroughly from the base so that the presence of fracture may be verified or excluded. Occasionally fractures run across the base of the skull from one side to the other at the anterior or posterior margins of the middle fossae. These are difficult to see and unless gentle traction is applied to the frontal and occipital bones they may be missed. When, however, this traction is applied, it may be found that the whole base of the skull is split in two.

When violence is applied to the skull, certain factors play a part in the determination of the type and character of the resultant fracture. These include the position of the head when struck, the degree and nature of the violence applied, the area affected, whether the force applied is general or localised, and the thickness of the bone, which varies considerably in different individuals. Depressed fractures of the vault produced by a blow with a heavy instrument of limited striking surface, or by a lighter instrument of similar area used with considerable force, show a shape of depression in the bone resembling approximately the shape of the striking area of the weapon used. Further, the inner table of the bone will be more extensively splintered than the outer table. Comminuted fractures are produced by violence from heavy objects with a fairly large striking surface or as the result of repeated blows, more or less over the same area, by an instrument of limited striking head. Surrounding the area of comminution, linear fractures, radiating in different directions, will usually be observed.

Extradural haemorrhage

This is always traumatic in origin. It results from a rupture of one of the branches of the middle meningeal artery and is nearly always associated with a fracture of the squamous part of the temporal bone. These fractures may be very small and difficult to see and they may not show on X-ray examination. They are, however, nearly always present. Occasionally rupture of a venous sinus may cause extradural haemorrhage. The haemorrhage separates the dura from the skull and produces marked depression of the brain.

The early diagnosis and treatment of this condition is one of the most successful surgical procedures. Failure to make the diagnosis still occurs fairly frequently even in the presence of the characteristic history and results in inevitable death due to compression of the brain. Sometimes even with early diagnosis and operation it may be impossible to remove the clot and relieve the pressure on the brain.

Probably the greatest difficulty in making the correct diagnosis results from the minor degree of trauma. We have recently seen a case where the blow was caused by a small weight on a fishing line being cast by a child.

The examiner should keep in mind the possibility of post-mortem extradural haemorrhage caused by heat (p. 209).

Subdural haemorrhage

This is usually traumatic in origin and in young healthy adults is invariably so. The bleeding comes from the cerebral venous system and is usually caused by rupture of a communicating vein or a venous sinus with resulting compression of the brain. The actual site of haemorrhage is rarely found. In our experience it nearly always occurs in the contrecoup position. The chief exception to this is in cases where there are extensive fractures and severe laceration of the brain. This subdural haemorrhage is frequently associated with contusion of the grey matter. There is usually considerable swelling of the brain and if the victim has lived for some time there may be serious obstruction of the posterior cerebral arteries causing large infarcts.

Subarachnoid haemorrhage

This occurs most frequently in young adults and in the elderly. The bleeding comes from the cerebral arterial system and is usually caused by rupture of a vessel in the circle of Willis. Sometimes the haemorrhage comes from one of the anterior cerebral arteries and occasionally from a posterior cerebral artery. In the young the haemorrhage usually comes from a ruptured congenital aneurysm or other arterial defect. In the elderly the haemorrhage usually results from arterial degenerative changes and hypertension.

Subarachnoid haemorrhage has always been a somewhat controversial subject amongst medico-legal examiners. Most forensic pathologists have been reluctant to accept trauma as a major factor in the production of subarachnoid haemorrhage and even when there has been some associated trauma have tended to report these deaths to the authorities as being due to natural causes. Simonsen[2] however has made a retrospective review of a large series of cases of subarachnoid haemorrhage in which there was evidence of trauma. In 88 per cent of these cases the injury was sustained during fights and in 87 per cent there was definite evidence that the deceased had been under the influence of alcohol. He concludes that it is likely, though not proven, that minor head injuries may give rise to rupture of a normal basilar artery, that alcoholic intoxication increases this possibility, that the trauma need not be particularly great, and that injuries striking at a level of the base of the skull are particularly apt to induce these haemorrhages. Simonsen's paper is a very important one and should be read by everyone who has to deal with this problem. It may be that we shall have to modify our views somewhat on the causation of subarachnoid haemorrhage.

Forensic pathologists investigating subarachnoid haemorrhage as a cause of sudden death see a different picture from that seen by pathologists dissecting bodies who have died in hospital from subarachnoid haemorrhage. The haemorrhage seen by the forensic pathologist is usually a massive haemorrhage covering the whole base of the brain and brain stem. The hospital deaths result from more gradual bleeding and the haemorrhage found at the post-mortem dissection is very much smaller and thinner.

Intracerebral haemorrhage

Intracerebral haemorrhage occurs most frequently in the elderly and in middle-aged hypertensives. It is usually spontaneous and does not often present a medico-legal problem.

There are however two situations where medico-legal difficulties do arise.

Where cerebral haemorrhages occur slowly from small vessels the victims can remain mobile and quite frequently injure themselves fairly severely in the pre-comatose state. Externally they may look very like the victims of multiple trauma.

Occasionally people have cerebral haemorrhages in situations where they are likely to receive cerebral trauma as a result of attacks of unconsciousness, for example, driving cars or riding bicycles. In the subsequent post-mortem examination it may be very difficult to decide the priority of the lesions. It can be difficult to differentiate between multiple small haemorrhages due to trauma and those caused by anoxia resulting from cerebral swelling and oedema.

Cerebral haemorrhages occur occasionally in cases under treatment with anticoagulants, for example, warfarin. The first sign of haemorrhage is usually haematuria but this may be missed, and attempts may be made to relate the haemorrhage to accidental trauma.

Contusion and laceration of the brain

Contusion of the brain varies from tiny punctate haemorrhages in the grey matter to large areas sometimes involving a whole lobe. When the skull is fractured there are frequently areas of bruising at the site of fracture and these may be associated with lacerations. When there is no skull fracture the main area of contusion is nearly always in the area of the brain directly opposite the area of impact, that is, the contrecoup position. The reason for the damage occurring in the contrecoup position is obscure. The simplest explanation is that the brain is bounced within the rigid bony cage of the skull and the maximum impact of the bounce is directly opposite the point of application of force. It may also be caused by shearing forces set up by sudden rotation and deceleration of the skull.

At post-mortem dissection occasionally it is found that patients who have shown serious effects of head injury and even decerebrate rigidity have very little apparent brain damage. Strich[3] has examined these cases and found that they had tears in the corpus callosum and histology showed retraction balls where axons had been torn. If these patients live for some time, demyelination of nerve fibre tracts can be demonstrated in the brain stem and spinal cord.

Some patients appear to die as a result of progressive swelling of the brain tissues and at post-mortem dissection the principal finding is a large swollen brain with very tense dura and flattened convolutions.[4] The reason for the swelling is not known but the probable cause of death is anoxia due to interference with the blood supply.

We have recently seen a case where a young man died suddenly shortly after admission to hospital with multiple injuries. He did not appear to have severe head injuries but showed cerebral symptoms immediately before death. At post-mortem dissection no definite trauma was found in the brain but there were widespread punctate haemorrhages indicative of fat embolism (see p. 325).

Sometimes where there have been head injuries there may not be much brain damage and the cause of death may not be apparent. In these cases the answer can occasionally be found by careful examination of the neck and removal of the spinal cord where severe contusion may be found. There is usually some bruising of the para-vertebral muscles but this may be obscured by the results of carotid injections for angiography.

Lindenberg and Freytag[5] have described a special type of cerebral damage resulting from trauma in infants. They state that in children of five months old or younger it is rare to find cerebral contusions and the typical lesions in these cases are tears in the white matter of the temporal and frontal lobes of the brain. These can be seen on naked-eye examination but are difficult to distinguish from artefacts. Microscopic examination shows tears in the cerebral cortex at the crest of the convolutions. These findings are based on the examination of sixteen cases and if they are confirmed over a larger series they will be important for medico-legal examiners, as they may be the main evidence of the cause of death in injured children. Unless specially looked for these lesions may be missed.

Severe lacerations of the brain are usually caused by vehicular

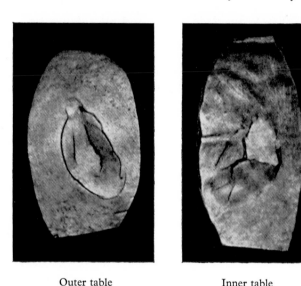

Outer table   Inner table

FIG. 174

Depressed fracture of skull, showing outer and inner tables

accidents or falls from heights. The effect depends mainly on the part of the brain affected and the amount of haemorrhage. The causation is usually evident and they do not as a rule present medico-legal problems. When they are found in homicidal cases they provide evidence of a great degree of violence.

In all cases of head injuries when there are skull fractures, even hair-line fractures of the anterior fossae, there is always a risk of meningitis.

A further complication of head injury, where unconsciousness occurs, is Klebsiella infection of the trachea and bronchi via the tracheostomy used for ventilation purposes in intensive care units.

It is interesting to note that out of forty-three boxing fatalities submitted to post-mortem dissection in only one instance was subarach-noid haemorrhage found.

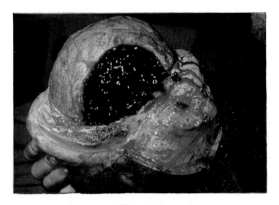

FIG. 175

Extradural haematoma

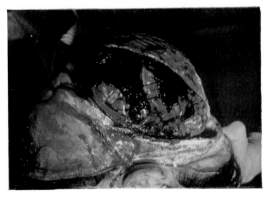

FIG. 176

After removal of dura, subdural haema-toma is visible (same case as in Fig. 175)

Intracerebral haemorrhage is usually due to disease of cerebral vessels. When close to the surface, it may be the result of laceration.

A review of necropsy records comprising 461 cases of fatal intracranial haemorrhage has shown that roughly half of these were due to hyper-tension and almost a third to aneurysms and other vascular malfor-mations.[6]

G M J—X

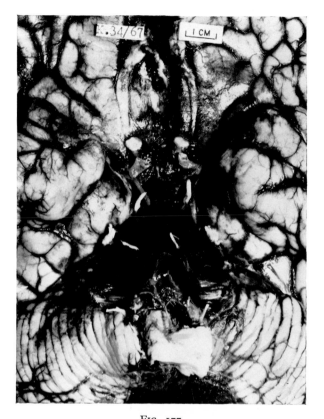

FIG. 177

Spontaneous subarachnoid haemorrhage from aneurysm. (By courtesy of Professor Hume Adams, Institute of Neurological Sciences, Glasgow)

Amnesia following head injuries

Amnesia, or loss of memory, following head injuries is quite common and is usually associated with concussion. Russell,[7] who investigated several hundred cases, states that after head injuries, accompanied by immediate loss of consciousness, certain disturbances of memory occur, that on full recovery there is little or no recollection of events during the period of confusion following injury, and that after recovery there is no memory of the moment of injury. 'Permanent' retrograde amnesia may vary from a period of seconds up to seven days, the latter being the longest period found in the investigation of over two hundred cases. He adds that, in over five hundred cases, he has never known a 'permanent' retrograde amnesia to cover a period of more than a week before the injury, and that in his view it seems probable that cases in which it appears to last for years are really cases of hysteria. He stresses the further point that a retrograde amnesia of several years' duration may appear to be present before consciousness has fully recovered, because the memory for distant events tends to return before the memory of more recent occurrences. In cases recovering from concussion, events which occurred immediately before the injury are occasionally remem-

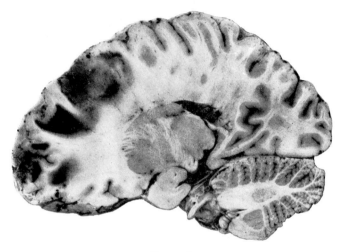

FIG. 178

Contusion of cerebral hemisphere showing multiple
areas of extravasation

bered indistinctly during the period of confusion, even though there will be complete amnesia for these events after consciousness has return-ed in full. This may result in the patient making false accusations. McConnell[8] states that prolonged amnesia, in certain cases, after cranial injury is due to the presence of subdural fluid associated with reduction in the volume of the brain.

Amnesia has been used unsuccessfully by the defence as rendering the accused unfit to plead to the charge in a murder case.

Post-contusional syndrome

Somewhere between 20 per cent and 60 per cent of all those who suffer head injury show after effects which are probably partly organic and partly psychogenic. There has been a tendency amongst many observers to suggest that most of the symptoms complained of are not genuine and are due either to malingering or compensation claims. O'Connell[9] thinks that the malingering aspect has been exaggerated and is less than one per cent. The commonest symptoms are headache, dizziness, insomnia, and impairment of concentration and memory.

ILLUSTRATIVE CASES

The following cases of head injury illustrate some of the different types of lesion which may be found.

Caused by poker with rounded head. Twelve lacerated wounds were present on the scalp. An extensive compound comminuted fracture involved the right fronto-parietal region of the skull. Many pieces of bone, mixed with lacerated brain tissue, were present in the site of injury.

Caused by a sharp-pointed poker. Both eyes were bruised. In the left lower eyelid, towards inner canthus, was a lacerated wound, $\frac{7}{8}$ inch in length, which passed through tissues of lid, penetrated tissues on inner side of orbit, and fractured orbital plates of upper maxillary and ethmoid bones. The surface of right lobe of cerebrum was covered by a thin layer of extravasated blood, which was more marked on front and under surfaces of right frontal pole. A laceration of brain-substance, which admitted tip of little finger, was situated on under surface of right frontal pole into which the crista galli of ethmoid bone had been driven. The assaulted man lived for five days. These injuries were caused by a violent thrust of the instrument.

Caused by a fall on kerb of pavement following assault. A fracture involved the base of skull, extended to the vault, and measured $3\frac{1}{2}$ inches in length. A subdural haemorrhage was present. In addition, on vault of skull was a depressed fracture composed of irregular bone, which had been partially rounded off, thus indicating that it had been present for at least several years. It was ascertained that twenty-one years before, the deceased had been struck on the head with the pointed end of a slater's hammer (Fig. 179).

Caused by corner of axe. Two and a half inches above upper level of lobe of left ear was a clean-cut wound, measuring $1\frac{1}{2}$ inches, which passed to bone. Immediately beneath the wound was a depressed fracture of skull, $\frac{7}{8}$ inch in length. This involved inner table of parietal bone, which was broken into four pieces, over an area of $3\frac{1}{2}$ by 4 inches. There was an extensive extradural haemorrhage. The brain tissue was contused over an area of 2 by $1\frac{1}{4}$ inches.

Following the injury, the deceased left his house, proceeded to the police station to get his injury dressed, but left because he would not await the arrival of the surgeon. He continued drinking during the course of the afternoon and evening, and late at night went to sleep in an empty house, with a companion, where in the morning he was found dead.

Homicidal injuries caused by unknown weapon. The following wounds and fractures, among others, were present: A crescent-shaped, incised wound, $1\frac{1}{2}$ inches, exposing frontal bone 2 inches above level of

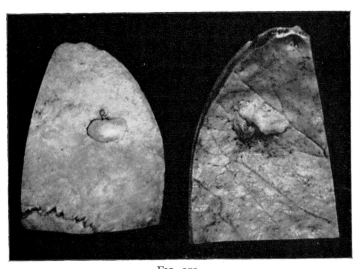

FIG. 179

Localised, depressed fracture of skull, outer and inner tables, showing evidence of repair

right eyebrow. The frontal bone was fractured at base of wound. On the scalp, $1\frac{1}{2}$ inches behind wound described and 4 inches above lobe of right ear, was a second incised wound, 1 inch long, which penetrated to bone. Farther back on the scalp was a third incised wound, gaping in character, from which brain-tissue emerged, and which measured 3 inches. In addition, there were two incised wounds of small size which penetrated to bone. There had been bleeding from left ear.

The deep tissues on right side of head showed extravasation over an area, 9 by 4 inches. The bones forming right side of skull were comminuted, and detached portions of bone varied in size from the finger-nail to the palm of the hand. Lacerated brain-tissue mixed with bony debris protruded from the skull opening.

On the surfaces of both lobes of cerebrum was an extensive subdural haemorrhage.   There was also a fracture of base of skull on right side of anterior fossa over roof of right orbital cavity.   The suture between occipital and parietal bones was separated.   This was more marked on right side.

Unusual injury by broken bumper of motor car.   The victim, while at a distance of 30 feet from a collision between two motor lorries, was struck on the head with a piece of metal, weighing half a pound, which, having been broken off the front bumper of one of the vehicles, shot in the direction of the fatally injured man.   The piece was impacted in the right frontal region of skull.   The bone was comminuted over an area of 3 by 4 inches.   Extending backwards from posterior margin of this area was a linear fracture, almost parallel to middle line

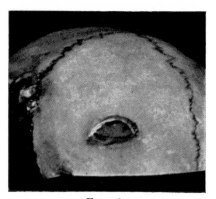

FIG. 180
Localised, depressed fracture of skull

of vault and at $1\frac{1}{4}$ inches to right of it, which terminated at anterior border of occipital bone.   Two further linear fractures forked downwards from the first.   The area of comminution of frontal bone was continuous with a wedge-shaped, and almost completely detached, portion of bone which had its apex in the central part of anterior fossa of skull.   There was fracture of both orbital plates and of cribriform plate.   The sides of the wedge measured $2\frac{1}{4}$ inches, and the base, which was directed upwards, measured 2 inches.   An extensive subdural haemorrhage was present.   The superior articular process of seventh cervical vertebra was also fractured and there was partial separation of sixth and seventh cervical vertebrae with exposure of intervertebral disc and surrounding bruising.

Caused by kick on face.   The nose was slightly flattened with some deviation to right, and there was bruising of both upper eyelids over the inner halves. Entire lower lids were similarly involved. Bruising affected bridge of nose. Other minor facial and body injuries were also present. Examination of the brain showed generalised purulent meningitis. There was fracture of fronto-nasal junction, basal fracture of crista galli of ethmoid and two fractures of the cribriform plate. Fracture of the cribriform plate is often associated with laceration of the dura and thus the risk of meningitis is introduced since the fracture communicates with the nasal passage.

Alleged fist blow on face and fall on stone floor. Death occurred in an aged man eight days after the injury. There was a small localised extradural haemorrhage, at base of brain, on floor of posterior fossa to the left of, and just behind, foramen magnum. A small localised subdural haemorrhage was situated over right orbital plate and was related to an area of surface laceration on under surface of frontal pole of right cerebral lobe. The laceration continued backwards over the under surface of the lobe for a distance of $4\frac{1}{2}$ inches. There was also a laceration on under surface of left lobe of cerebellum. A smeared, subdural haemorrhage was present over surfaces of brain, together with a similar haemorrhage on under surface of cerebellum.

Severe head injury with recovery. A man of thirty-one was attacked with a hammer. Three lacerated wounds were present on left side of head. They were roughly parallel, horizontal in direction and 1, 2, and 3 inches, respectively, above the external auditory meatus. The uppermost wound was 2 inches long and the lower wounds 1 inch. The surrounding tissues were pulped and fragments of bone and brain were evident on the surface between the wounds. On removal to hospital, the wounds were cleaned, excised, and stitched. Some bone fragments were removed. Patient remained unconscious for five days. A right-sided facial paralysis developed two days after the injury and persisted for twelve days. He was fed by nasal catheter. He was able to say such words as 'yes' and 'no' and to write legibly twelve days after the attack. He also appeared to understand all that was said to him and was able to feed himself. His condition had improved sufficiently thirty days after sustaining the injuries to allow adequate exploration of the damaged brain. A scalp flap was turned down and many indriven fragments of bone with pulped brain tissue were washed out. About a cubic inch of brain tissue seemed to be missing. The dura was too damaged to allow suture. During the latter half of the operation a blood transfusion was maintained. The patient made satisfactory progress but aphasia persisted. He was discharged eight weeks after admission, walking quite normally. On the morning of the assault we inspected the scene of crime. The blows had been struck while the victim lay in bed. The pillow, densely stained with blood which had soaked through to the bolster beneath, showed two small pieces of brain tissue adherent to its surface. The wall at the head of the bed was considerably bespattered with small blood-stains, also the back wall and ceiling. Adherent to the ceiling were what appeared to be small pieces of brain tissue. We also examined a blood-stained joiner's claw hammer which had been found in the house. Following discharge from hospital, the man reported at intervals. At first the bone gap was very pulsatile, but gradually developed a dense fibrous protective layer. When seen two years later, he had been back at his former work for some months. He was instructed to report occasionally in case a 'dural cyst' should develop. The writer is indebted to the late Professor J. A. G. Burton for the clinical notes.

Causation of injuries

On the general question of wounding in relation to accidental, suicidal, or homicidal causation the field is too wide, both as to the types of wounds and their attendant circumstances, to permit of a dogmatic statement of guiding principles which would be of absolute value to the student. It is in this matter that experience, powers of observation and interpretation are brought into operation, more especially when the evidence is of a purely circumstantial nature. An examiner will be well advised to form conclusions with caution, since circumstances may prove deceptive. In many cases, however, there is no reasonable doubt that the wounds have been caused by homicidal infliction.

Should circumstantial evidence lead to the apprehension and trial of a suspected person, while there may be no doubt regarding the wounds on the body of the deceased, there may be, and frequently is, doubt regarding the manner in which they were produced, or the type of weapon used.

One of our cases illustrates the point. A woman was found dead, lying on her back in a bedroom with a number of bruises and some abrasions on the body, scalp, forehead, left eye, arms, and legs. Among several blood-stains upon the carpet, the principal one, which had saturated the material, was some inches to the right of the head. Two upper teeth in a denture were broken, pressure had been applied to the tissues of the neck, and some of the abrasions had the appearance of having been caused by finger-nails. Her husband was charged with murder. The evidence, on behalf of the Crown, was to the effect that death was due to cardiac arrest during the process of asphyxia, and that the character and distribution of the injuries were inconsistent with self-infliction, although some were consistent with accident. The woman had taken a large quantity of alcohol, and analysis of the blood showed that the quantity was equivalent to almost a bottle of whisky.

Evidence for the prosecution was that this amount might have rendered the woman liable to sudden cardiac collapse, that the pressure to the neck had been applied by human hands, and that the injuries might have been caused by a person endeavouring to restrain the woman, although the amount of alcohol consumed would probably have caused a condition of coma rather than one of violence. Evidence regarding the broken teeth was that the fracture was consistent with violence, and that if they had been broken by striking the edge of the kerb around the fireplace, they would have been more shattered. Medical evidence, on behalf of the defence, was that the woman might have died from the effects of alcohol, suffocation might have been caused by regurgitation

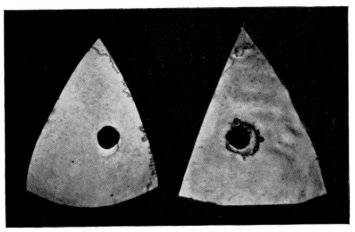

FIG. 181
Localised, depressed fracture of skull produced by the
tooth of a rake

of stomach contents into the larynx and trachea, that the bruising could have been caused by a fall, and that the scratches might have been caused by an attempt to lift the limp body, which would be heavy. The charge of murder was reduced to one of culpable homicide. The jury returned a unanimous verdict of not guilty.[10]

Sometimes there are strange vagaries in the manner of suicidal wounding, and when a suicide is suffering from insanity, well developed in form, the wounds are often very extensive in character.

With regard to injuries in general, all that can be said is that the whole circumstances of the wounding, and the environment of the body when found, must be completely observed, considered, and weighed before an opinion is expressed regarding accidental, suicidal, or homicidal causation.

Photographs are shown on pages 318–320 of a case which is of considerable interest in connection with the problem of homicide or suicide.   This case was seen by Dr J. A. Imrie and Dr Edgar Rentoul and was at first thought to be murder, but after detailed examination and consideration was recognised as a suicide.

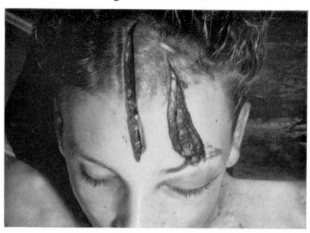

FIG. 182
Homicidal injuries caused by an axe

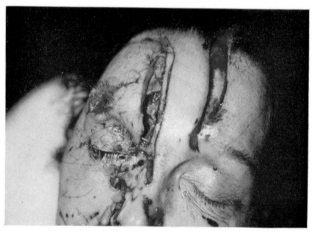

FIG. 183
Accidental injuries caused by a motor car

The important points in arriving at this decision were: the extent and wide distribution of the blood-staining, together with the absence of disturbance of articles in the kitchen indicating volitional movement of deceased with absence of struggle; the multiplicity of blows restricted to a relatively small target area of the scalp; the circumscribed under-lying injury in the skull unaccompanied by underlying brain damage, but with fragmentation of the actual damaged part of the skull. The aperture in the bone measured 2 by $1\frac{1}{2}$ inches, and twenty-seven fragments of bone were collected, varying in size from $\frac{1}{4}$ inch in diameter to $\frac{3}{4}$ by $\frac{3}{8}$ inch (*see* p. 320).

Homicidal injuries

The two cases which follow are illustrative of typical homicidal injuries:

A woman was found dead in her shop. The wrists had been firmly bound together by strong, cord-like material, and beneath the body was an axe, with its wooden shaft broken into two pieces. Lying on the floor was an empty glass siphon-bottle.

The forehead and top of head showed multiple wounds. No other marks of violence were present on any other part of the body. The vault of the skull was severely comminuted and pieces of broken bone lay in the scalp tissues. Some of these fractures extended into base of skull. The frontal lobes of brain were severely lacerated, and the surface and base of brain were covered with effused blood. From the appearances of the wounds it seemed likely that they had been caused by the weapon found, the head of which showed both axe and hammer-head formations.

In the second case, the face, trunk, arms, and thighs of the woman's body were covered with dirt mixed with blood. There were several wounds on the left side of face, all lacerated in character, the left ear was almost completely torn from the head, and the cartilage split in several directions. The wounds on the right side of the face were fewer in number, but the upper half of the right ear was also torn from the scalp. The upper lip on its inner surface was pulped, and protruding from between the lips was a fractured portion of the upper jaw to which some teeth were attached. Most of the wounds, almost uniform in size and shape, measured $1\frac{3}{4}$ inches in length, and were crescentic in form. The front of the chest and neck were extensively bruised, and on the left side there was a crescentic-shaped wound of the same length as the wounds on the face. The thighs and arms also were extensively bruised.

Dissection of scalp showed a pulpy condition of left temporal muscle with extensive extravasation and similar, but less marked, bruising of right temporal muscle. Dissection of the face showed extensive bruising of tissues, especially on left side, together with the following compound fractures: (*a*) floor of left orbit, (*b*) zygomatic process (comminuted), (*c*) upper maxilla (comminuted), (*d*) mandible, on right and left sides (comminuted), and (*e*) nasal bone.   There were fractures of second, third, and fourth ribs on right side, each rib in two places, and of second and third ribs on left side.   The appearances, together with the uniform size and shape of the wounds and bruises, were consistent with their infliction by a booted foot.

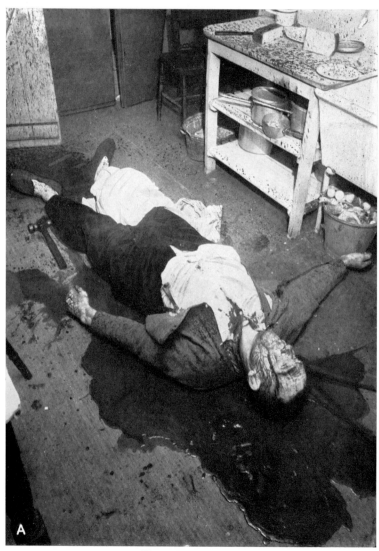

Fig. 184A   (p. 315)

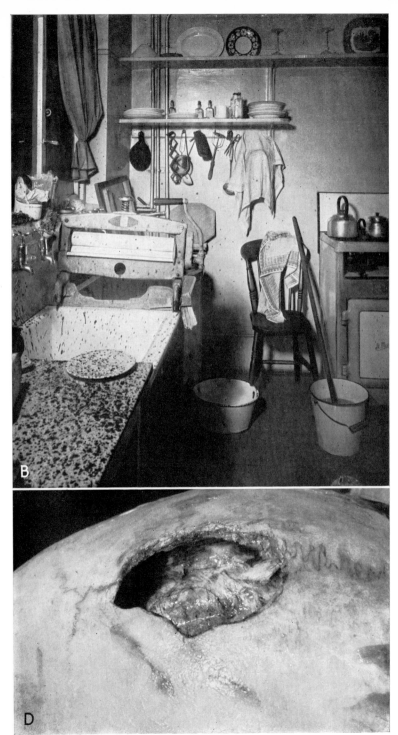

FIGS. 184B and 184D (p. 315)

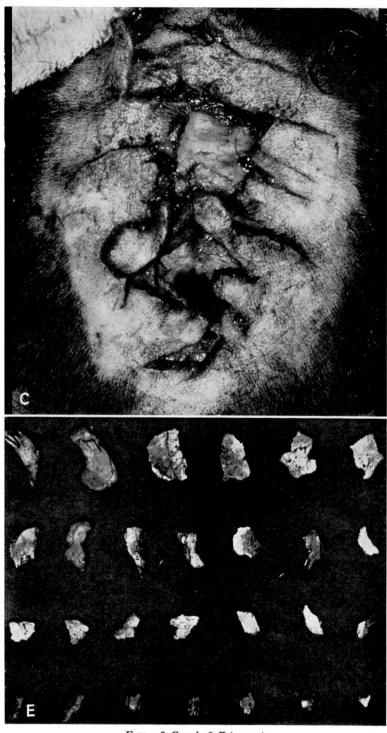

FIGS. 184C and 184E (p. 317)

Unusual fatal accident

A girl, aged thirteen, was found lying on the road. It was raining and becoming dark. Later she died in hospital from the effects of a comminuted, depressed fracture of the skull. The principal external injury was a lacerated wound of stellate shape, with three limbs measuring $1\frac{1}{4}$, $\frac{1}{2}$, and $\frac{3}{4}$ inches, situated immediately to the right of the midline of the crown of the head. The wound communicated with the interior of the skull, and the surface of the brain was exposed. The comminuted, depressed fracture, from which eight small bone fragments

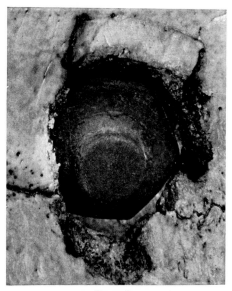

FIG. 185

Comminuted, depressed fracture of vault of skull. Nut of wheel is shown *in situ*

had been removed by operation, measured $1\frac{1}{4}$ by 1 inch. The inner surface, which showed the same measurement, had two small pieces of bone still partially attached to the edges, and four similar pieces had been completely detached. Underlying this area was a surface laceration of brain. Subsequently a request was made to examine the wheel of a motor bus in relation to the injury. A specimen of hair was removed from the edge of the scalp wound. On a solid disc of the wheel, ten six-sided nuts were mounted, and on one of them some staining was observed, together with a few adherent hairs.

The approximate measurements of this nut were as follows:

Transverse measurement between angular points of sides = $\frac{7}{8}$ inch.

Measurement between parallel edges of sides $=\frac{7}{8}$ inch.
Length of side of nut and projecting bolt $=1\frac{1}{2}$ inches.

Certain surfaces of the nut, when impinged on plasticine, produced a stellate impression similar to the shape of the wound on the head of the girl.   The stained material on the nut could not be identified either as mammalian or human blood, although presumptive tests for blood were positive.   The staining was scanty and had the appearance of having been diluted with moisture.

The hairs, when compared with those from the head of the girl, showed characters which were fully consistent with a common source.

Examination of the footwear of the girl gave clear indication of marked and irregular wear of both soles and heels.   These areas had been reinforced with material in a very amateurish fashion and would readily have caused the girl to stumble forward, more especially if she had been running with wet shoes and had tried to stop quickly.   The injury upon the head was fully consistent with infliction by the wheel which had been examined, and could have been produced by the head falling forward and striking the nut while the wheel was in motion (Fig 185).

OTHER INJURIES

Spinal injuries and fractures

The frequent sites of injury are the upper or lower part of the cervical, and the lower part of the dorsal or upper part of the lumbar, regions of the vertebral column.   When direct violence has been applied, however, any portion of the spine may be the seat of fracture.   The principal factors in the production of these fractures include direct crushing, compression due to a fall from a height, either the feet or buttocks striking the ground first, and overflexion or extension.   The act of judicial hanging produces fracture of the upper part of the cervical region, and the atlas or axis may be involved in this type of injury. When fracture occurs in the upper part of the cervical region and the cord is injured, death ensures rapidly (Fig. 186), but when the lower regions are implicated, death may not result, although paralysis of the parts of the body below the site of fracture supervenes rapidly, especially when displacement of the fragments occurs.   The extent and character of the paralysis will obviously depend upon the position of the fracture.   When the cord is seriously injured there is an initial period of flaccid paralysis.   When the injury is not permanent, that is, the cord is not severed, there may be recovery from this condition of spinal shock.   When, however, the cord is severed, after a period of time the paralysis becomes spastic and permanent.

Fractures of the thoracic and lumbar spine are relatively stable and unless very severe tend not to cause spinal damage.   Shearing forces

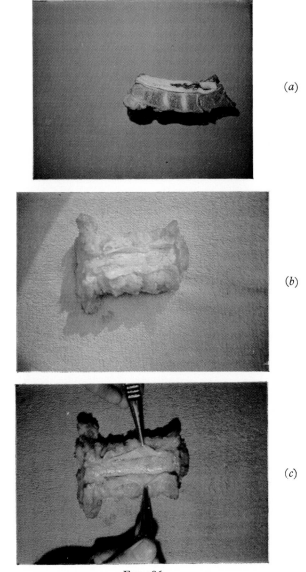

(a)

(b)

(c)

FIG. 186

Spinal cord damage in relation to fracture dislocation of cervical spine (C4,5). Note that there is complete transection of the cord, although in view from the outside the cord appeared intact. The dissection of the spinal cord is shown in reverse order. (By courtesy of Mr W. Sillar, Southern General Hospital, Glasgow)

in the cervical region are, however, very likely to cause rupture of the ligaments, instability, and severe cord damage. Even if the initial impact does not cause damage, this may very easily be produced during transport of the victim.[11] When the fracture is complete, due to either direct or indirect violence, separation usually takes place through an intervertebral disc to which is attached a piece of the body of the vertebra situated immediately below the site of separation. We have seen this type of lesion in a number of cases. Fractures which are incomplete assume many forms and include compression of the vertebral body, separation of the transverse process or spine, together with linear fracture of the vertebral body. In wounding by firearms, marked fragmentation of one or more of the vertebrae is sometimes found. In a case of fatal wounding by a rifle bullet, both the third and fourth cervical vertebrae were severely comminuted and fragments of bone had been extruded through the wound of exit.

Fracture of other bones

Fractures of other bones of the osseous frame may cause death on account of their situation, extent, or complications. Fractures of the ribs are of considerable importance in certain medico-legal cases, more especially when due to crushing, since adjacent and important structures are readily injured, including frequently the lungs and less often the heart. Laceration of the lung is often associated with fracture of one or more ribs, and haemothorax, pneumothorax, interstitial emphysema, intrapulmonic and intrapleural haemorrhage, pleurisy, pneumonia, pulmonary abscess, or air embolism are complications to be considered. Injury to lung, for example bruising or laceration, may result from crushing or impact without rib fracture. We have examined the bodies of many persons, especially of those run over by vehicles, in which such injuries have been found. Rib injury sometimes occurs in the course of restraining violent insane persons, and occasionally a suspicion may arise that greater physical force than necessary may have been employed with ensuing fatal results. In the investigation of such cases, the fact that certain asylum patients, especially those suffering from general paralysis of the insane, may be affected by excessive fragility of bone should not be forgotten. In these cases the ribs are readily fractured, and the examiner making the post-mortem examination should test the frangibility of the unbroken ribs and, if thought necessary, retain a specimen for pathological investigation. When bones are fragile, forcible movements of a body after death are occasionally responsible for fracture. Occasionally rough handling by mortuary attendants can cause fractures. We have seen a very bad fracture of the cervical spine caused in this way. Rough handling of this kind is unfortunately most likely to occur when bodies are in an advanced state of putrefaction and it is then difficult to know whether injuries are ante- or post-mortem.

Possible fractures of the pelvis in accidental injuries due to falls from a height, crushing, and vehicular accidents, should always be looked for.

Fat embolism

This occurs after fractures of long bones and widespread soft tissue trauma. These injuries release globules of fat into the circulation and

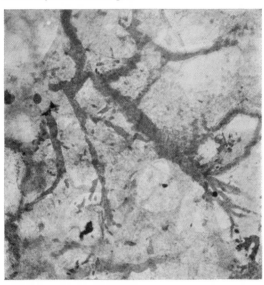

FIG. 187

Fat embolism of the lung following multiple fractures.
× 50 diameters

into the lungs. The Birmingham Accident Hospital has reported evidence of fat embolism in 1 to 2 per cent of long bone fractures and 12 per cent of cases with multiple injuries. Severe oedema results and the tissues are affected by hypoxia.[12] This is probably the cause of the multiple punctate haemorrhages found in the brain in these cases. We have come to regard these haemorrhages as diagnostic of fat embolism in deaths after severe injuries even although very little fat is found in the brain tissue. It may be in some cases that the damage to the brain is caused by the sudden release of large quantities of fat into the cerebrovascular system.[13]

Clinically the onset of symptoms can occur a few hours after the injury. At this time their significance is infrequently recognised, as the picture is confused by the general effects of trauma (p. 328). Usually symptoms occur 48 hours after the injury and they may provide evidence of damage to the lungs, brain, and myocardium. It is at this stage that the petechial haemorrhages begin to appear on the skin.[14]

The exact mechanism causing the severe effects of fat embolism remains obscure but it should be kept in mind when any case of severe trauma is not progressing as expected and cerebral symptoms develop.

Post-mortem examination of tissue microscopically, with haemalum and Sudan III staining, will show fat globules in the vessels of the lungs, brain, or renal glomeruli (see Fig. 187).

Visceral injuries

Penetrating wounds of the abdomen may be homicidal, suicidal, or accidental. Danger to life arises from three principal causes, namely, shock, haemorrhage, and sepsis. The application of violence by a blunt instrument may readily produce rupture of the internal organs without leaving any visible external mark of violence. Similarly crushing of the abdominal wall with resultant visceral injury may leave practically no evidence on the surface, especially when death has been almost instantaneous. Most of these injuries are caused by road traffic accidents (p. 246). The organs which may be injured by blows include the liver, spleen, small intestine, and the urinary bladder. The bladder in a distended condition, not uncommon in intoxicated persons, may be ruptured by a kick. We have seen cases of this character, in one of which the tear, situated on the upper surface, measured 2 inches. Rupture of the bladder may also occur from penetrating wounds or as the result of fracture of the pelvis. An interesting case of rupture of the liver, which resulted from external violence by a forcible blow from the head of a second person, was examined by us. There was no evidence of external injury. The deceased man, who had been able to return to his home, survived the injury for some hours. Post-mortem examination disclosed a rupture of the liver at the junction of the right and left lobes. The abdominal cavity contained 875 ml of blood. Kicks and falling on hard objects, together with crushing, are responsible factors in the production of liver rupture. The right lobe is the common site of injury.

In another case a boy of fifteen, who was standing on a bunker in order to reach a shelf, fell on account of collapse of the bunker. He soon became ill. The abdomen became tender and distended, and the abdominal respiratory movements were restricted. There was dullness in the left flank which extended up to the left costal margin. Pain was referred to the left shoulder. Operation disclosed rupture of the spleen accompanied by a large internal haemorrhage. The boy died while under the anaesthetic.

Spontaneous rupture of the spleen sometimes occurs in malarial cases.

Weston[15] describes the case of a girl, aged nine, who was running along a garden when she tripped and fell, striking her left costal margin and epigastrium on the edge of a step. Operation disclosed that the spleen was almost completely divided. Recovery took place.

Rupture of the stomach by external violence is uncommon. Kidney injury usually results from crushing, but sharp blows or forcible kicks may be responsible factors.

Rupture of the mesentery of the small bowel is a fairly common result of crush injuries and we have frequently seen it in cases where kicking or stamping on the abdomen has occurred. It is sometimes found in battered children (p. 225).

Vehicular injuries

The commonest vehicular injuries are caused by vehicles being suddenly decelerated. The occupants proceed at the speed at which the vehicle was travelling until their bodies are decelerated by striking parts of the car or by landing on the road or on top of the vehicle or

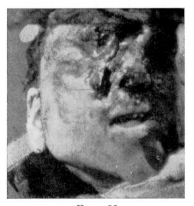

Fig. 188

Multiple lacerated wounds of the face,
with fracture of underlying bones, due
to crushing by an electric train

object causing the original deceleration, after they have been projected through the windscreen. If the person remains in the vehicle the usual areas of initial severe impact are the feet and legs causing Pott's fractures, fractures of the tibia and femur, and dislocation of the hip. The head hits the windscreen or roof and the sternum comes into contact with the steering wheel or the top margin of the scuttle in the case of the passenger.

These impacts produce severe scalp and facial lacerations, skull and facial fractures, brain damage and chest injuries, including fracture of the sternum, multiple rib fractures, and rupture of the aorta and heart.

The facial and head injuries very frequently result in extensive bleeding into the air-passages and this may cause death from inhalation. We have seen cases where there would have been probable survival if this danger had been recognised and the patient transported in the semi-prone or coma position.

Both passenger and driver may sustain very serious abdominal injuries, including rupture of the liver and spleen. Liver injuries occur more frequently in drivers than passengers.[16]

In addition to these injuries the movements of the body can produce sudden severe flexion and extension injuries of the neck, known as whiplash injuries These can cause damage to the nerve roots and the spine and occasionally result in quadriplegia (p. 322).

The violence of the impact when vehicles are travelling at speed can produce explosive-like effects and if the passengers are not strapped in they can be projected from the vehicle through the bursting doors. When this happens they usually sustain extremely severe injuries.

Pedestrians struck by vehicles show a great variety of blunt instrument injuries and occasionally their wounds may look like incised wounds (p. 237). A characteristic injury is that of degloving where the skin and superficial tissues are stripped from the underlying tissues over large areas of the limbs or lower abdomen. By far the commonest serious injury to pedestrians is fracture of the lower limb.[17] These fractures are caused by bumpers and when bodies are found on roads apparently the victims of hit-and-run accidents these fractures should always be looked for, as they provide some evidence that the pedestrian was erect at the time of the incident and was not either run over on the road or deposited there for the purpose of concealing homicide. This possibility should always be kept in mind when investigating apparent vehicular trauma and an attempt should be made to relate the injuries to the reconstruction of the incident. The finding of a discrepancy between these has led to the detection of homicide. In the case of H.M. Advocate v. Robertson, a man was convicted of the murder of a woman by running her over after previously rendering her unconscious.[18]

Accidents to pedestrians usually occur in urban areas and after the initial impact the victims are usually thrown on to the bonnet of the car and if the speed is greater on to the roof. If this is not recognised examiners may have difficulty in understanding the injuries found on pedestrians. The majority of vehicular injuries to pedestrians occur in children and the elderly. When young adult and middle-aged pedestrians suffer vehicular injuries in urban areas there is a high probability that they are under the influence of alcohol. The blood of the victim should always be tested for alcohol and barbiturates in all adult motoring deaths.

We examined the body of a man who had been killed through being wedged between a motor vehicle and a stone wall. The injuries included crushing of the chest wall, with multiple fractures of ribs on both sides, fracture of sternum, and severance of vertebral column in mid-dorsal region, with marked over-riding at the site of fracture. The visceral injuries included laceration of right lung with irregular separation of the three lobes, laceration of left lung, diaphragm,

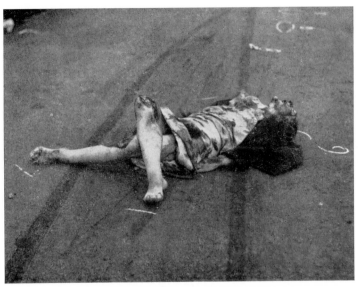

FIG. 189

A case of murder originally suggestive of accident. The woman had been run over twice. On the body were wounds of ante-mortem and post-mortem origin

pericardium, and apical portion of heart which was detached. The thoracic aorta was severed at the atrium. The greater part of the right lobe of liver was extensively lacerated. Although there were a number of abrasions present on the surfaces of the body, there was no evidence of bruising externally.

Fractures of the mandible are commonly found and are often associated with extensive injury of the skull. In one of our cases the mandible was fractured in three places, the posterior part of the body of the sphenoid bone was detached, and there was rupture of the contiguous cavernous sinuses. In addition, there was an almost complete transverse severance of the medulla and pons. The fracture of the sphenoid bone extended laterally in different directions across the middle fossa to the temporal and the parietal bones on the right side, and to the basal portion of the temporal bone on the left side. A further fracture extended forwards from the sphenoid bone and led to an area of fragmentation of the roof of the right orbital cavity before passing upwards on to the frontal bone. The right occipito-parietal suture was mobile.

In many cases a varying degree of protrusion of brain substance, the result of comminution, is present. Extradural, subdural, and subarachnoid haemorrhages may be found together or alone, depending upon the nature and extent of the head injury (see p. 302). Especially when the head is involved, the hair and scalp should be examined carefully for glass particles, and any found should be retained for subsequent comparison with glass from a suspect vehicle. A specimen of hair close to the site of wounding on the scalp should also be preserved for comparative examination with any hairs subsequently found adherent to the car thought responsible for the injury. In one of our cases, material taken from an offside door of a suspect car consisted of fourteen small pieces of tissue which varied in size from an ordinary pinhead to that of a glass-headed pin; histological examination established the fact that the fragments consisted of muscular, connective, and epidermal tissue. Serological examination showed that the tissue was of human origin.

The blood of the victim should be grouped to facilitate subsequent comparison with suspect staining.

The clothes and skin should always be examined for the presence of offprints from tyres which may identify the vehicle.

Crush injury and renal function

This condition may follow injury due to the pinning of a limb or limbs beneath heavy material for a period of several hours.[19] The first signs are erythema or blisters of the compressed part with loss of sensation and paralysis. Swelling of the underlying necrotic muscle follows, due to the plasma leaking through the injured capillaries, and haemoconcentration results. Renal damage due to the substances absorbed from the necrotic muscle is probably produced as soon as the circulation to the damaged part is re-established, although often not noticeable clinically until some days later. The urine which may either be of a reddish or smoky hue, is acid in reaction and contains albumin. The damaged limb, or limbs, becomes progressively swollen and tense for four to five days. There may be vomiting and abdominal rigidity. The first week is the critical period. Skin and muscle may slough away and sepsis may supervene. Death may be sudden in those affected by this syndrome. Usually after a few days oliguria develops due to either mechanical or physiological blockage of the renal tubules due to the presence of myohaemoglobin from the necrotic muscle. The incidence of the condition is related to the period of crushing. The post-mortem findings are desquamation and necrosis of the cells of the ascending loop of Henle and the distal convoluted tubule with pigmented casts in the lumen of the tubules.[20]

Injuries of genitals and genito-urinary and intestinal tracts

Crane and Moody[21] describe the case of a boy who fell from a roof and landed astride a fence. He sustained a lacerated wound on inner aspect of upper part of left thigh. Two weeks later pus was present in

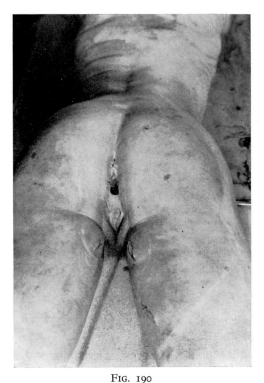

FIG. 190

Body shown in Fig. 65. Marked dilatation of anal orifice and rectum due to the insertion of a blunt object following death

the urine. A month after the accident he suffered from pain and difficult micturition which were accompanied by swelling of the penis. A piece of wood, 3·5 by 0·5 centimetres, was removed from pendulous part of the urethra. Six days later cystoscopic examination showed a larger fragment in the bladder and, on left lateral wall, the site of entrance was observable. This fragment measured 6 by 0·5 centimetres. The splinter of wood had been driven up the inner aspect of thigh, through the obturator foramen, and into the bladder, where the fragment had split. Evidence of extravasation of urine or haemorrhage was absent.

Injuries of the urethra in the male, including rupture, with extravasation of urine, may follow a kick or blow on the perineum or a fracture of the pelvis. The male genitals may be the seat of trauma by blows, kicks, machinery or vehicular accidents, and those of the female, more commonly by the first two factors.

Vernon and Kelly[22] describe the case of a man aged twenty-five, a

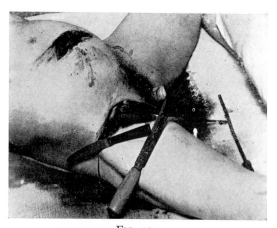

FIG. 191

A case of murder with mutilation of vulva, and wounding of abdomen and right groin. (By courtesy of the Commissioner of Police of the Metropolis, Scotland Yard)

steward, who, while lying in his bunk, became involved in an argument with a stronger man. In the scuffle that followed he was pulled by the penis. The skin was torn through at a level $\frac{1}{2}$ inch from the junction of the penis with the pubic region, the tear involving nearly the whole circumference of the organ, less than 1 inch of skin being left intact on the posterior surface. The suspensory ligament of the penis was exposed, but had escaped injury. We were recently involved in a case where a mother cut the genitalia from her infant. The baby survived (p. 71).

Delprat[23] records the case of a tractor-driver whose tractor bumped into a ditch and whose clothing became entangled in the mechanism. The man's penis was torn out in the gears.

Harden[24] reports a case of mutilation of the external genitalia by an angry paramour. There was a large pear-shaped avulsion of pubic region, extending from line of hair on mons veneris, including clitoris and upper third of vulva. In the lower part of right hypogastrium was a deep cut with a protrusion of several inches of omentum. Recovery followed operative treatment.

Fox and Barrett[25] report three similar cases of vacuum cleaner injuries of the penis, resulting from masturbation by the insertion of the penis into the tube of a vacuum cleaner and the operation of the suction mechanism.

Psychopathic states, in which there is sexual perversion, have sometimes led to self-mutilation of the genitals. Such cases are usually found among male subjects. Injuries to the sexual parts are not infrequently homicidal, and it is more than probable that many of these are the result of insanity.

Apart from mental derangement of the perpetrator, vulvar injuries are sometimes the result of brutal assault by responsible persons. We have seen a few cases of women who have died as the result of severe haemorrhage following vulvar injuries by kicking. In these cases the wounds were situated either within the labia minora or on the under surface of the symphysis pubis. In all cases of vulvar woundings, caused by sharp instruments, there is a grave danger of severe haemorrhage owing to the great vascularity of the parts.

Intestinal trauma is most commonly produced by penetrating injury, although a kick upon the lower part of the abdomen may be responsible. In one of our cases, a kick on the abdomen caused rupture of the ileum, which is the commonest site of injury from this cause.

James[26] describes the case of a young farmer who jumped backwards from a waggon and received an impalement wound of the rectum from the handle of a pitchfork stuck in the ground. Laparotomy showed an irregular, peritoneal tear in the retrovesical pouch, and two hay seeds were found lying on the anterior surface of the stomach. A left iliac colostomy was performed, was closed a month later, and recovery followed.

Hambly[27] reports details of a boy of fifteen who dropped from a beam and, as he dropped, one of his companions made a move at him with a 5-foot steel rod which pierced the perineum. The rod was pulled out and a piece of string was tied round it to mark the depth of entry. Operation showed that the wound passed under rectal mucosa, through the pelvic mesocolon, abraded the transverse colon at its lower border, completely transfixed a portion of the small intestine, and made an aperture in the great omentum at the lower border of the stomach. The wound was closed, without drainage, and uninterrupted recovery followed.

Baumgarten and Cantor[28] report the case of a woman who fell on a small table supported by an iron rod. The top of the table broke and the woman became impaled upon this rod, which passed through the vagina and bladder and entered the peritoneal cavity, where it penetrated a loop of ileum and almost completely cut the mesentery free from its attachment. The patient recovered and was discharged from hospital on the fourteenth day.

Animal bites

It must not be forgotten that certain injuries found upon bodies may have been caused, post-mortem, by carnivora, such as rats, mice, dogs, and other animals. In these cases, it is most important to differentiate these injuries from ante-mortem wounds (see pp. 246, 256).

Cases Illustrative of Unusual Injury

Removal of head from body by dog

A man of sixty-three had not been seen by any of his friends for four days. The police broke into the locked house and found the fully clothed but headless body lying in front of the fireplace. A collie

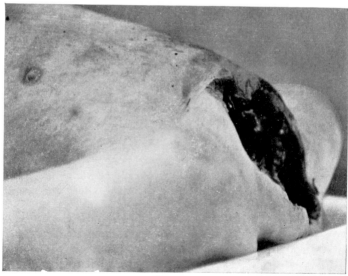

Fig. 192
Decapitation, by a collie dog, following death

dog also in the room was most hostile and had to be shot. Examination of the body showed that death had been due to coronary disease. The head had been severed close to the level of the upper borders of the sternum and clavicles, in front, and the line of severance had been continued to the back, at a fairly uniform level. The wound of severance, which showed serrations, was of the lacerated type (see Fig. 192). The cervical vertebrae, with the exception of the seventh, which showed irregular damage, were missing. The arch of the aorta, part of the trachea, most of the oesophagus, and the upper lobe of the left lung had been removed. The condition of the body was consistent with death having occurred some four or five days prior to examination,

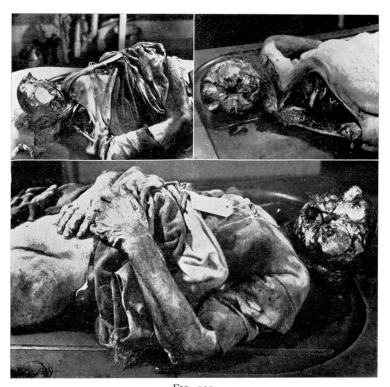

FIG. 193

Post-mortem injuries caused by a Scots terrier dog

(By courtesy of the late Dr Robert Richards, Aberdeen University)

and the injuries were consistent with having been caused by the teeth of a dog. All the injuries had been made after death. A post-mortem examination of the dog showed that the stomach contained portions of skin, subcutaneous tissue, muscle, bone, lung, brain, trachea, and aorta. A piece of scalp tissue, with greyish-white hair, and three bundles of greyish-white hair, were also found. In all, twenty-seven pieces of bone were recovered. Vomited matter, on the floor of the room, contained fourteen pieces of lung tissue, the largest measuring 5 by 3 inches. On the floor of the room, the greater part of the denuded vault of the skull was found. The lower half of the occipital bone, the entire base of the skull, and bones of the face, except the mandible, were missing. The major part of the mandible was found near the dog. The edges of severance of the skull were very irregular. The dog, driven to desperation by hunger and thirst, had attacked the exposed part of the body.

Foreign bodies in the stomach, rectum, and bladder

Foreign bodies, of very varied character, are often found in the stomach. Not only are children prone to swallow such things but adults are by no means exempt and may do so either accidentally or deliberately. Intentional swallowing of objects is not uncommon among inmates of mental hospitals. Wheeler[29] relates the case of a male patient in an asylum from whose stomach, by gastrotomy performed on three occasions within a period of some six years, 1,300 foreign bodies were removed. These consisted of staples, pieces of glass, a nail file in three portions, and a host of miscellaneous metallic foreign bodies. Radiological examination also disclosed foreign bodies in the ileum, colon, and rectum. On one occasion two nails, two staples, and two pieces of glass were removed from the intestine by enema. As the result of his habits, the patient suffered from subacute and acute haemorrhagic gastritis. The submucosa was diffusely haemorrhagic, oedematous, and moderately inflamed. He survived.

Foreign bodies are occasionally found in the rectum, urethra, and bladder, commonly as the result of perverted sexual practices. Miscellaneous articles have been found in the rectum, as the result of erotomania, and these have included small bottles, and in one case, a cold cream jar with a lemon inserted into its open end.

Kraker[30] describes the case of a youth, aged eighteen, who was mentally retarded. He was admitted to hospital complaining of pain over the lower abdomen, dysuria, and frequency of micturition of some five weeks' duration. There was suprapubic tenderness and the prostate was enlarged, soft, and tender. A pencil was removed from the bladder by the suprapubic route. It measured $1\frac{3}{4}$ by $\frac{5}{16}$ inches and was covered with phosphates. The boy first stated that he had swallowed the pencil but later admitted that he had pushed it along the urethra, some five weeks before, and that he had taken twenty minutes to accomplish the act.

Death from air-pressure

A man was accused of having discharged a pneumatic air-pressure pipe at a boy. A blast of air which entered his mouth caused almost instantaneous death. Post-mortem examination showed that the face was markedly swollen, the tongue was protruded, and the upper lip was bruised. The whole surface of the body, with the exception of the feet and ankles, was emphysematous and crepitant. The lungs were collapsed.

Brown and Dwinelle[31] record three examples of rupture of the colon, with gaseous distension of the abdomen, due to the application of a compressed-air jet to the anus. In one of these, the jet was merely thrust inside the clothes through a tear in the leg of the trousers. It has been reported that more than half of sixty-five cases on record have died.

In one of our own cases, two young garage mechanics held down a boy, who was visiting the garage, and placed the nozzle of an air compressor under his clothes in the region of the anus. He was admitted to hospital collapsed and with a greatly distended abdomen. When a needle was introduced through the abdominal wall, a large quantity of air escaped under pressure. The boy died in a few hours. At necropsy, the principal feature was massive necrosis of the bowel with multiple perforations.

Effects of blast

In air. Blast is the result of the abrupt release of a large volume of gas formed by detonation of a high explosive, usually trinitrotoluene (see p. 703).

Three definite waves are recognised:

1. Wave of positive pressure.
2. Wave of mass movement of air (displacement).
3. Wave of negative pressure.

The pressure and air displacement are the causal factors in injury. The positive pressure is followed by a negative one which initiates marked suction effects. The results on the surroundings and persons in the vicinity of the explosion may be uniform. Often, however, freak effects of force, distribution, and direction are observed, probably due to such causes as uneven rupture of the bomb casing and to reflection and deflection of the blast from oblique and irregular surfaces.

In addition to the trauma caused by the impact of primary and secondary missiles, together with the effects of forcible propulsion of the subject against solid objects, injury may also result from an abrupt change in pressure upon the soft tissues, which most frequently affects the chest and abdomen.

Pulmonary concussion, varying in degree, is almost invariably present in those who have received injuries when in buildings which have sustained damage through a direct hit by a bomb or parachute mine. This condition is not so frequently present when bombing has occurred in the open.   Mechanical factors are present in enclosed spaces, since pressure increases until the walls and roof of the building give way. Contusion and rupture of both hollow and solid viscera are frequently found, without any accompanying bone injury under such conditions. Secondary injuries may be superimposed by falling debris.

When injury from blast has been sustained, haemorrhage into the air-passages and a consequent blood-stained froth at the mouth are common.   Should the victim survive for a sufficiently long period, signs of pneumonia appear.   At post-mortem examination, rib markings may be found on the surface of a lung or lungs.   There may be signs of pneumonia with haemorrhage into the substance of the lung, liver, spleen, kidneys, adrenals, bladder, and sometimes the brain.   Fat embolism may also be present.

When death takes place immediately, the lesion in the chest is mainly haemorrhage from the alveolar capillaries.   There is no massive external haemorrhage, although bleeding into large portions of lung, usually in the costo-phrenic region, is often found.

Multiple petechial haemorrhages of the lining of the auditory passages, and sometimes also of the tympanic membrane, are of frequent occurrence due to the effect of near blast.   The condition may be accompanied by rupture of one or both ear drums.

In water (immersion blast).   The explosion under water of mines, bombs, depth charges, and torpedoes gives rise to somewhat similar lesions, and although the destructive waves of mass movement and suction are absent, the primary impact is conveyed over a wide area of surrounding water.

The effects are most marked on tissues or viscera containing air. The large intestine, with its contained gas, thin walls, and scanty muscle is frequently injured.   The small intestine is less commonly affected. The muscular, elastic stomach suffers least.   Retroperitoneal haemorrhages are almost constant, and laceration and rupture of bowel walls common.   Internal damage is more severe when the abdomen is facing the explosion.

As with blast in air, solid viscera are affected in degree varying from contusion to multiple rupture.   Spinal concussion, often transient in character, is frequently observed.   Death may result with little or no external evidence of violence.

Traumata which can be caused by medical procedures

Over the years we have seen a great variety of injuries caused by doctors in the treatment of patients.   We list some of these:

Fractures of ribs and sternum during resuscitative procedures.

Rupture of abdominal organs during resuscitative procedures (p. 226).

Penetration of the aorta during sternal marrow biopsies.

Intra-abdominal haemorrhage from liver biopsy.

Retroperitoneal haemotomata after kidney biopsy.

Fractures of bones during electro-convulsive therapy.

Rupture of the oesophagus or air-passage due to endoscopic examination.

Damage to the cervical tissues from carotid angiography.

Injury and malignancy

There has long been controversy about the relationship of trauma to the production of various forms of cancer.[32, 33]

The balance of opinion appears to be that a single traumatic incident is very unlikely to be the cause of subsequent malignancy unless there has been some chronic complication, for example, osteomyelitis.

Where however there has been repeated trauma of tissues over a long period the balance of opinion is probably in favour of this being a possible cause of malignant changes.

The problem is important in connection with compensation cases, especially in America, and when these cases occur reference is usually made to Ewing's Postulates. Ewing gave the criteria which he thought must be present before malignant change could be related to trauma.

He stated that the site of injury must correspond to the region in which the tumour develops.

The trauma must be severe with tissue damage.

There must be evidence that there was no pre-existing disease.

The time interval should be at least three months and in most instances should be much longer.

Cases where the relationship has been accepted:

Tumours developing in burn scars.

Squamous-cell carcinoma following osteomyelitis.

Oesophageal cancer following strictures of the oesophagus.

References

1. ROWBOTHAM, G.F. *Acute Injuries of the Head.* Edinburgh: Livingstone, 4th ed. 1964.
2. SIMONSEN, J. *J. Forens. Med.* **14,** 146, 1967.
3. STRICH, S.J. *Lancet,* **2,** 443, 1961.
4. JENNETT, W.B. *Medicine Sci. Law,* **10,** 35, 1970.
5. LINDENBERG, R. & FREYTAG, E. *Archs Path.,* **87,** 298, 1969.
6. RUSSELL, D.S., FALCONER, M.A., BECK, D.J.K., & MCMENEMEY, W.H. *Proc. R. Soc. Med.,* **47,** 689, 1954.

7. RUSSELL, W.R. *Lancet*, **2**, 762, 1935.
8. McCONNELL A.A. *Lancet*, **1**, 273, 1944.
9. O'CONNELL, B. *J. forens. Med.*, **8**, 122, 1961.
10. H.M. Advocate v. Watson, *Med.-leg. crim. Rev.*, **9**, 128 and 176, 1941.
11. ASHWORTH, J. *Br. med. J.*, **4**, 414, 1969.
12. ROSS, A.P.J. *Ann. R. Coll. Surg.*, **46**, 159, 1970.
13. GEE, D.J. *J. forens. Med.*, **4**, 60, 1967.
14. *British Medical Journal*, **3**, 476, 1970.
15. WESTON, A. *Br. med. J.*, **2**, 1142, 1932.
16. BOWEN, J.A.L. *J. forens. Med.*, **17**, 12, 1970.
17. MACKAY, G.M. *Br. med. J.*, **4**, 799, 1969.
18. High Court of Justiciary, Nov. 1950.
19. BYWATERS, E.G.L. & BEALL, D. *Br. med. J.*, **1**, 427, 1941.
20. BENTLEY, G. & JEFFREYS, T.E. *J. Bone Jt Surg.*, **50-B**, 588, 1968.
21. CRANE, J.J. & MOODY, A.A. *J. Am. med. Ass.*, **104**, 1702, 1935.
22. VERNON, H.R. & KELLY, R. *Br. med. J.*, **1**, 925, 1935.
23. DELPRAT, G.D. *J. Am. med. Ass.*, **125**, 274, 1944.
24. HARDEN, A.S. *Am. J. Surg.*, **29**, (N.S.), 453, 1935.
25. FOX, M. & BARRETT, E.L. *Br. med. J.*, **1**, 1942, 1960.
26. JAMES, T.A. *Lancet*, **1**, 326, 1939.
27. HAMBLY, E.H. *Lancet*, **2**, 672, 1938.
28. BAUMGARTEN, E.C. & CANTOR, M.D. *Am. J. Surg.*, **25**, (N.S.), 343, 1934.
29. WHEELER, P.H. *Med.-leg. crim. Rev.*, **9**, 109, 1941.
30. KRAKER, D.A. *Am. J. Surg.*, **29**, (N.S.), 449, 1935.
31. BROWN, R.K. & DWINELLE, J.H. *Ann. Surg.*, **115**, 13, 1942.
32. SHAPIRO, H.A. *J. forens. Med.*, **12**, 89, 1965.
33. GOWING, N.F.C. *J. forens. Med.*, **8**, 116, 1961.

Chapter 12

EXAMINATION OF BLOOD AND BLOOD-STAINS

THE examination of blood-stains is made:

At the site of crime.
On the body and clothes of a victim of injury.
On the body and clothes of a suspected person.
On suspect weapons.

In all these situations the examiner will be concerned with proving the presence of human blood and if possible finding the group to which it belongs.

The examination of whole blood is made in the following situations:

Blood group of victim of an assault.
Blood group of assailant.
Blood groups of parties concerned in a charge under the Criminal Law Amendment Act, 1885, section 5.
Blood groups of the parties where it is alleged that mothers, after delivery in hospital, have been given the wrong babies.
Occasionally to attempt to find the father when two men are claiming to be the father.
For the proof of adultery in divorce proceedings.
Investigation of transfusion reactions.
Elimination of blood dyscrasias in cases showing bruising, for example, battered children.

Samples of blood are of course used for a large number of toxicological purposes.

Blood-stains at the site of crime

The examiner must first make a general appraisal of the distribution of the blood-stains, noting not only the areas where blood is present but also those areas where it is absent, as both these findings may play an important part in the reconstruction of the crime.

A detailed examination should then be made of the blood-stains, including their sizes, shapes, colour, and condition. While the examiner is making this examination he should be attempting a provisional reconstruction of the positions of the parties and the shape of the assault.

Blood which falls vertically on a surface produces a circular stain with crenated edges. As the angle of impact decreases the stains become elongated and when the angle is very acute the stains take the shape of an elongated indian club. The blood always comes from the direction of the thick end of the club.

It is sometimes necessary to find how far blood-stains have penetrated

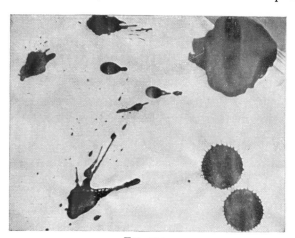

FIG. 194
Blood-stains of various shapes

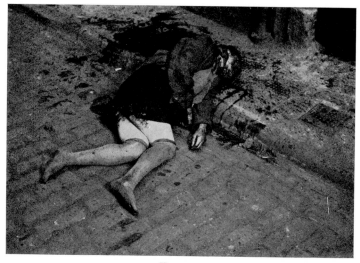

FIG. 195
Blood-stained scene of murder

through fabrics, for example a pillow, as this may provide information about the length of time the source of bleeding has been in contact with the material.

It should be remembered that blood-stains may show finger- or foot-prints. If this possibility is not kept in mind from the very

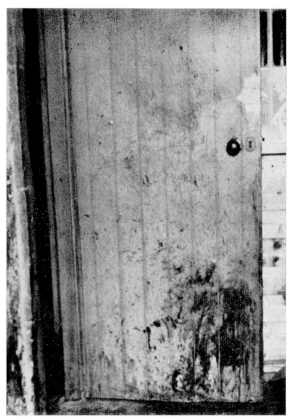

FIG. 196

Blood-staining on a door at the scene of crime

beginning of the investigation this evidence may be lost. We have recently been concerned in the investigation of two murder cases in which the murderer was detected only as a result of the observation and examination by the police of prints in blood-stains. One of these was a foot-print on oil cloth which showed many stains and might very easily have been lost or obliterated during the investigation.

Blood-stains on the victim and his clothes

The examination of these is rarely as important as that at other sites. These stains should however always be recorded. They may be of value where an accused person attempts to explain the presence of blood-stains on his clothing or body by suggesting that these were caused by his attempts to rescue the victim or some other form of innocent contact.

The nails of females who are the victims of sexual assaults and those dying from strangulation should always be examined for the presence of blood-staining or skin particles, as their finding may provide valuable corroborative evidence.

Blood-stains on a suspect

Staining is rarely found on a suspect unless beneath the finger-nails. It is however frequently found on his clothes and may be extremely important corroborative evidence. Most assailants are nowadays well aware of the significance of blood-stains on their clothes and they tend to take appropriate action. It is therefore necessary to look for stains in places which they are likely to have missed, for example behind buttons, inside the turn-up of trousers and on the welts and in the stitching of shoes.[1]

Blood-stains on suspect weapons

The importance of finding blood-stains on weapons is usually related to their being found in the possession of the accused. Occasionally however they may show the finger-prints of an accused person as well as the blood-stains. The exposed parts of weapons are frequently cleaned but staining may still be found in recessed areas. We have found significant blood-staining after removing the rivets and dismantling the handle of a knife and beneath the head of an axe which had been withdrawn with hub extractors.

Examination of the stains

It is usual to employ some kind of sorting test to eliminate stains which may look like blood but are not.

We have over a great many years used for this purpose the benzidine test. This is an extremely sensitive test, it is easy to use and the reagents were readily available and easily carried. Unfortunately however benzidine has been found to be strongly carcinogenic, and restrictions have been placed on its supply. It is unwise to continue using this test.   Probably the best sorting test now available is the amidopyrine test.   The reagents are:

Saturated solution of amidopyrine in 95 per cent ethanol.
10 volumes solution of hydrogen peroxide.

The suspect stain is touched with a piece of filter paper.   Four drops of amidopyrine reagent are added, followed by two drops of hydrogen peroxide solution.   If the reaction is positive a purple colour appears within a few seconds.   The test works better with very much stronger solutions of hydrogen peroxide but these are caustic to the skin.

It is customary to discuss the fallacies for the various blood-sorting tests, but if these are regarded purely as sorting tests the detailed investigation of fallacies is irrelevant.

Proof of the presence of blood

The simplest way to do this is to demonstrate the presence of haemochromogen, which is reduced alkaline haematin.   We use two methods:

1. Scrape a small quantity from the surface of the stain on to a microscope slide and add a drop of Takayama's solution:

Sodium hydroxide (10 per cent) .	.	3 ml
Pyridine	.	3 ml
Glucose (saturated solution)	.	3 ml
Distilled water	.	7 ml

   Within a few minutes pink feathery crystals develop (Fig. 197).
   Produced in this way these crystals are proof of the presence of

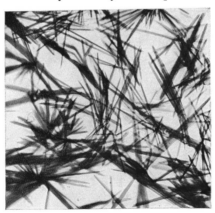

FIG. 197
Haemochromogen crystals.   ×75

blood.   If the crystals are examined by a microspectroscope the characteristic absorption bands of haemochromogen are seen (Fig. 199).

2. Make a solution of the suspect stain in normal saline.   Place a few drops of the solution in a short narrow-bore glass tube.   Add four drops of Stokes' reagent which is made by using a particle of ferrous sulphate, a particle of Rochelle salt (sodium potassium tartrate), and a few drops of ammonia.   If the solution contains blood the characteristic absorption bands of reduced alkaline haematin will be seen in the microspectroscope when transmitted light is passed through the solution (Fig. 199).

Various changes can take place in haemoglobin as a result of age and atmospheric conditions.   If oxyhaemoglobin is exposed to a vitiated atmosphere it will become deoxidised haemoglobin or reduced haemoglobin.   In a very impure atmosphere, after a lapse of time, due to

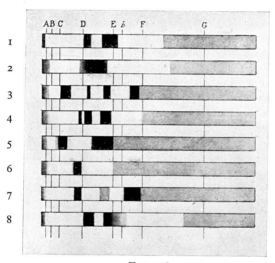

FIG. 198

Blood spectra

1. Oxidised haemoglobin or oxyhaemoglobin.	5. Acid haematin.
2. Reduced haemoglobin.	6. Alkaline haematin.
3. Methaemoglobin.	7. Sodium-fluoride haemoglobin.
4. Alkaline methaemoglobin.	8. Carboxyhaemoglobin.

oxidisation, methaemoglobin will probably be formed.   By examining a solution of the stain spectroscopically, the form of the haemoglobin will be indicated by the spectrum shown, since haemoglobin and its derivatives have the capacity of absorbing certain light-rays after they have passed through a prism. The following spectra are characteristic of the various states in which haemoglobin may be found:

Oxyhaemoglobin. Two distinct bands are present between the Fraunhofer lines D and E, the one nearer D being about half the breadth of the other and more defined.

Reduced haemoglobin. One broad band between D and E is visible.

By adding a few drops of Stokes' reagent, or a few drops of ammonium sulphide, to a solution of oxyhaemoglobin, the spectrum of reduced haemoglobin will be seen on spectroscopic examination.

Methaemoglobin. Four absorption bands are seen. Two of these resemble the bands in oxyhaemoglobin, the third is situated in the red between the C and D lines, and the fourth, which is placed between the E and F lines, is more indistinct (Fig. 198).

Haematin. Haematin is found in old blood-stains. The spectra of both acid and alkaline haematin are of little diagnostic value on account of lack of definition. These are seen in Figure 198. When alkaline haematin is treated with ammonium sulphide, haemochromogen is produced.

Haemochromogen or reduced alkaline haematin. This spectrum consists of two bands. The first is a dense narrow band in the yellow part of the spectrum, almost midway between the D and E lines, the second is broader and less dense, and lies in the green part of the spectrum. Part of the purple is also absorbed.

After the presence of blood has been proved the next step is to determine its origin and usually we are concerned with whether or not it is human. This depends on demonstrating the reaction between the antigen contained in the blood and the antibodies contained in a prepared rabbit anti-human blood serum. The solutions which have already been prepared to prove blood may be used for this purpose. These solutions should be diluted until they show a faint pink colour.

A small quantity of anti-human serum is placed in a narrow-bore test tube and the solution is run on to the surface of the serum. At the interface of the fluids, if the blood is human, there appears a white line resulting from the precipitin reaction between the anti-human serum and the human protein. The white line should appear within five minutes. These anti-sera are not absolutely specific and reading the test within a short time removes the possibility of error.

A similar reaction can be obtained between the blood of other animals and their appropriately prepared anti-sera. Very reliable commercial

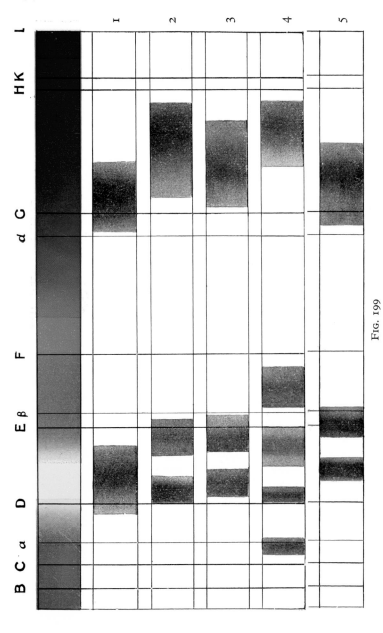

FIG. 199

1. Reduced haemoglobin.   2. Oxyhaemoglobin.   3. Carboxyhaemoglobin.   4. Methaemoglobin (neutral)
5. Haemochromogen.

anti-sera are now available for a large variety of animals. It is customary to set up the blood solution in question not only against antihuman serum but against several other anti-sera as controls. A sample of a solution of unstained material whenever possible should be put up also. Usually the blood solutions become sufficiently clear by sedimentation. They may however have to be centrifuged. Occasionally the solutions cannot be cleared and the precipitin reaction should then be allowed to take place in agar.

The simplest way to do this is:

Mix 4 g purified agar with 300 ml of distilled water. Add a small quantity of merthiolate as a preservative. Heat at 100 degrees Centigrade until clear. Spread the agar solution in a Petri dish and allow to solidify. Cut a small hole at the centre and three or four similarly sized holes round the circumference of a circle about 1 inch in diameter and cover the bases of the holes with a thin layer of agar. Place the unknown blood solution in the centre hole and the anti-sera in the other holes. After about 48 hours a positive reaction can be seen as a curved white line occurring between the unknown blood solution and the related anti-serum.[2]

In the British Isles a positive precipitin reaction following the demonstration of the presence of haemochromogen can be accepted as proof of the presence of human blood. In countries however where there is a possibility of the presence of blood of the higher monkeys the method of testing which we have described would be inadequate. When there is this risk a titration method must be used when it will be found that human blood will react with serum in much higher dilution than monkey blood.

Other medico-legal tests based upon the precipitin reaction

Since precipitins are produced for almost any soluble animal or vegetative protein, this fact has been utilised not only for the identification of the source of blood serum, but for other medico-legal determinations, for example, the identification of the source of seminal fluid, bone fragments, and portions of flesh.

Anti-human globulin test for human blood

The anti-human globulin test has been used to determine the presence of human blood.[3] It is known that red cells, sensitised by incomplete anti-Rh antibodies and washed free of serum, are agglutinated by serum of a rabbit previously immunised against human globulin. When this rabbit serum is previously mixed with human serum, then agglutination is inhibited. If, therefore, anti-human globulin serum is mixed with an extract of a human blood-stain and subsequently tested against sensitised red cells, the agglutination reaction will be inhibited. This inhibition is not produced, with the possible exception of the apes, by other than human blood and thus forms the basis for a test for blood of human origin.

There is no available test for the differentiation of male from female blood-stains. The examination of cellular nuclei may sometimes establish the question of sex.

GROUPING OF BLOOD-STAINS

Having established that a blood-stain is human it may be necessary to attempt to find its group. Average figures for the ABO group percentages in Great Britain are:

O	.	.	.	.	46 per cent
A	.	.	.	.	42 ,, ,,
B	.	.	.	.	9 ,, ,,
AB	.	.	.	.	3 ,, ,,

The value as evidence therefore of grouping the blood in a stain will depend very much on the group of the individual who shed the blood.

It is very rare when we are dealing with stains to be able to find cells in a condition which will enable grouping to be done by the direct methods used for the grouping of whole blood. Indirect techniques therefore have to be employed and they detect either the agglutinins or the agglutinogens. Most laboratories concentrate on the agglutinogens but the use of the agglutinins can be valuable either as corroboration of the result obtained from the agglutinogens or by themselves, especially when it may be necessary to obtain a rapid result.

Detection of agglutinins

A small quantity of the dried blood is scraped from the stain, or a portion of the stained material, about $\frac{1}{2}$ square centimetre, is removed. The blood is dissolved in normal saline, 5 cubic millimetres for each milligram of blood. At a minimum, 15 cubic millimetres are required for the test. The tube in which the dilution is being made should be corked, left at laboratory temperature for an hour, then placed in a refrigerator overnight. The solution may now be tested with A, B, and O cell suspensions. One per cent and 20 per cent suspensions are recommended. The results of the tests should be examined many times during several hours, if necessary, until decisive readings are possible.[4] Frequently this test is unsuccessful owing to the weakness of the antibodies and it becomes increasingly unreliable as the age of the stains increases. Weiner[5] has introduced a modification which increases greatly the effective range of the test. After the initial reading, two drops of gum acacia solution are added to each test tube. The mixtures are allowed to stand at room temperature for two hours and a second reading taken. The tubes are then centrifuged at 500 r.p.m. for a minute and then a final reading is taken. The gum acacia solution is prepared by dissolving 10 grams of gum acacia and 1 gram of dibasic sodium phosphate in 90 millilitres of distilled water and sterilising in an autoclave at 10 lb of pressure for 10 minutes.

By this method Weiner has successfully grouped stains which were more than a year old.

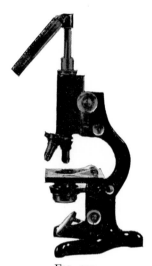

FIG. 200

A simple form of micro-spectroscope

Detection of agglutinogens

Agglutinogens cannot be detected by direct agglutination, since the blood cells lose this power on drying, but their presence may be shown by their ability to absorb agglutinins a and b and their power to inhibit the action of the sera containing these agglutinins. If the blood in the stain contains agglutinogens A and B it will absorb a and b agglutinins from the test sera, and when these are subsequently tested against known test corpuscles, the absorption which has taken place will become apparent. Corresponding absorption will result if only agglutinogen A or B is present in the stain. The portion of stained material should be mixed with Group O serum, about 10 cubic millimetres of extract being required for the test. The mixture, in a corked tube, should be left for an hour at laboratory temperature and then placed in a refrigerator overnight. Two sets of serum and saline dilutions, 1–2, 1–4, 1–8, etc., are prepared on a slide. To each of the sets, a 1 per cent suspension of A and B cells is added and the results are recorded, after an hour in a moist chamber. When the stain is on fabric a control, using the unstained cloth, should be utilised.[6]

The foregoing is the classical method of grouping blood-stains and it has proved a reliable method over many years. It does, however, present difficulties. The greatest of these is that it cannot be used on very small stains. This classical method has been described as a substractive method because it measures the diminution of activity in the anti-sera after they have been in contact with the stain. In recent years several workers have grouped stains by what has been described as an additive method.[7, 8] This depends on the fact that antibody is absorbed by the stained material and this can be demonstrated by subsequently adding suspensions of A and B cells and noting the agglutination which is produced by the absorbed antibodies. The simplest and most useful application of this technique is the following which was described by Nickolls and Pereira.[9]

Small pieces of blood-stained material are placed on two cavity slides. A drop of anti-A serum is added to one and a drop of anti-B serum to the other and the separate fibres of the material are teased out. After an hour, the anti-serum is pipetted off and the fibres are very carefully washed three times with saline. A drop of a 0·5 per cent suspension of the appropriate red cells in a 1 per cent solution of bovine albumen in saline is then added to each slide. The slides are placed in a moist chamber in a 50 degree Centigrade oven for ten minutes. They are then cooled and left in a moist chamber for two to five hours. After two hours, the slides are examined periodically under a microscope. Agglutination of the A cells indicates that the stain on the material belongs to Group A. Agglutination of the B cells indicates that the stain on the material belongs to Group B. No agglutination indicates that the stain belongs to Group O. Controls of unstained material should be run simultaneously.

We have found this to be a very useful technique. Stains which would be far too small to be grouped by the classical method can be accurately grouped in this way. We think, however, that when blood-stains are old the classical method gives more reliable results.

The grouping of blood-stains when the stains are large, fresh, and uncontaminated is easy. If, however, the stains are very small, old, and contaminated it may be extremely difficult and in a considerable percentage of stains submitted to medico-legal laboratories it may be impossible. We think that the grouping of stains should always be done by those who have no knowledge of the possible group to which the stain may belong.

Reports have been published of methods to determine the MN and Rh subgroups of stains. We have not found any method which gives sufficiently reliable results for these groups for presentation as evidence in courts of law. Some years ago we thought that we had devised a method for establishing the MN groups for stains. We finally tested the method by examining a large number of completely unknown stains prepared in another laboratory. We did not produce an accuracy of more than 70 per cent and this is of course valueless as evidence for presentation in court. It is a useful exercise for those engaged in grouping blood-stains for medico-legal purposes to subject themselves to this test.

Grouping of whole blood for medico-legal purposes

We have detailed most of the situations where this is required at the beginning of this chapter.

Many blood group systems have been found since Landsteiner's original discovery of the ABO system and some of these are now used in cases of disputed paternity and in the other types of cases where whole blood is available.

The following are the blood group systems used in specialised serological laboratories in this country together with the cumulative exclusion rate for putative non-fathers in Great Britain.

System	Approximate percentage cumulative exclusion
ABO	17·6
MNS	37
Rh subgroup: D, C, and E .	53
Kell	55·8
Lutheran	56
Duffy	58
Kidd	59

It should be clear however that the figures given are averages: they do not represent the chances of exclusion in individual cases and it is very unlikely that any single individual would have the chance of exclusion shown in the table. His chance might in fact be much greater or much less.

All these groups are based on factors present in the red cells of the blood. Their value for determining paternity is based on the fact that they are passed from parents to offspring in accordance with the rules of heredity first worked out by Mendel. These rules have not only been proved theoretically but have been demonstrated in practice by the study of the blood groups of a very large number of families.

A textbook of medical jurisprudence is not the place for a discussion of the principles of genetics but it may be of value to non-medical readers to see examples and note the basic ideas involved. We show two examples of the transmission of the MN factors (Fig. 201).

Serum proteins are now known to have the same type of hereditary

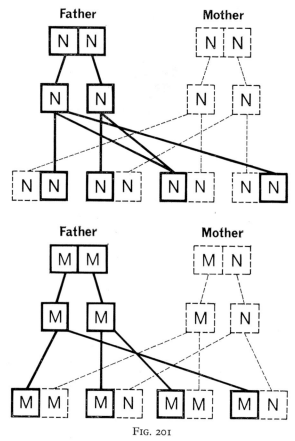

FIG. 201

Examples of transmission of the MN factors

transmission as the red cell factors and they have been used for determination of parentage. A great deal of experimental work has been done on these and it is probable that a large number of substances will be found to have a hereditary transmission.

Two of these have been used fairly extensively. These are the haptoglobin groups and the Gc groups. Every person belongs to one of three haptoglobin groups 1–1, 1–2, and 2–2. In Western Europe, 15 per cent of the population belong to 1–1, 47 per cent to 1–2, and 36 per cent to 2–2. These groups can exclude 18 per cent of non-fathers. As these groups do not depend on the reactions of red cells they cannot be determined by an agglutination reaction. They are isolated by studying their migration through appropriate media. The usual method of doing this is by starch gel electrophoresis. A constant current is passed through the starch gel and the haptoglobins migrate towards the anode: the rate of migration produces the separation and the various haptoglobins can be identified by staining techniques.

The Gc groups are also 1–1, 1–2, and 2–2, and are distinguished by electrophoresis in the same way as the haptoglobins. They exclude 15 per cent of non-fathers in Western Europe.

The Law Commission Report on Blood Tests and the Proof of Paternity in Civil Proceedings discusses the possibility of using Gm groups, blood tissue enzymes and lipo-proteins, but we have no knowledge of their having been accepted in this country, although the Gm groups have been accepted in Norway.

We think that all judges who are involved in the decision of paternity cases in courts in which blood groups are used would be well advised to read a volume such as *Human Blood and Serum Groups* by O. Prokop and G. Uhlenbruck, 1969, published by McLaren & Sons, so that they may have some idea of the complexity of the subject.

The principal types of civil proceedings in which blood tests are relevant are divorce, nullity, and declarations of legitimacy and affiliation.

There has been doubt about the right of courts to order the taking of blood tests in these cases. The problem is due to a conflict between the interests of the child and the interests of justice.

Lord Sumner in Russell v. Russell [1924] A.C., p. 748, stated: In the administration of justice nothing is of higher importance than that all the relevant evidence should be admissible and should be heard by the tribunal that is charged with deciding according to the truth. To ordain that a court should decide upon the relevant facts and at the same time that it should not hear some of those relevant facts from the person who best knows them and can prove them at first hand, seems to me to be a contradiction in terms. It is best that truth should out and that truth should prevail.'

Lord Denning stated recently: 'Should it come to the crunch the interests of justice must take first place.' Lord Sachs on the other hand has said that since applications for blood tests invariably had some motive of self-interest, they who sought to place the stamp of illegitimacy on small children must bear the onus of showing that it was to the child's advantage or at least not to the child's disadvantage.

The House of Lords giving judgment in two recent cases[10,11] has to some extent settled the issue. They ordered that tests should be taken in two cases where there appeared to have been conflicting judgments by the Appeal Court.   Lord Reid stated: 'The court must protect the child, but it is not really protecting the child to ban a blood test on some vague and shadowy conjecture that it may turn out to be to its advantage.'   Lord Hudson stated: 'The interests of justice in the abstract are best served by the ascertainment of the truth and there must be few cases where the interests of the child can be shown to be best served by the suppression of the truth.'

While these statements are all very well in general their Lordships may find themselves with cases where the taking of a test is certainly not in the interests of a child and they may have considerable doubt whether or not to make an order.

Part III of the Family Law Reform Act, 1969, deals with the use of blood tests in determining paternity.

Section 20 provides that, 'In any civil proceedings in which the paternity of any person falls to be determined by the court hearing the proceedings, the court may on an application by any party to the proceedings, give a direction for the use of blood tests to ascertain whether such tests show that a party to the proceedings is or is not thereby excluded from being the father of that person and for the taking within a period to be specified in the direction of blood samples from that person, the mother of that person and any party alleged to be the father of that person or from any, or any two of those persons.'

Section 23 states that where a person fails to comply with instructions of the court to provide a blood sample, the court may draw such inferences from this fact as appear proper in the circumstances.

The various provisions of the Act are to be brought into force by Statutory Instruments.

In Scotland the position is different.   The subject was considered in a divorce action, the case of Whitehall.[12]   The Second Division refused to order tests stating that according to Scots practice the court will not compel a party to furnish material to support his opponent's case.

There is a very detailed discussion of the Scottish court's views in the case of Imre v. Mitchell's Tutors and Curators and Another.[13]   This case was appealed to the First Division of the Court of Session and the decisions of the Lord President and Lord Carmont should be read by all who are interested in this problem.   They particularly dealt with the necessity that those giving consent to the taking of blood should understand in full the possible legal results.   Lord Clyde stated that the advisers of a party called on to provide a blood sample should ensure that the consequences were appreciated, and where a child is concerned should hesitate before allowing a course to be taken which might have a devastating and lasting effect on the child's whole life, especially when the law will not compel such a step.[14]

We were involved in the Imre case in connection with the performance of the blood tests and were very interested in these judgments.

We personally prefer the Scots Law Lords' interpretation of the law to the English decisions.

References

1. WHITEWAY, R.V. & MANT, A.K.   *J. forens. Med.*, **1**, 260, 1954.
2. CULLIFORD, B.J.   *Nature, Lond.*, **201**, 1092, 1964.
3. ANDERSON, J.R.   *Br. J. exp. Path.*, **33**, 468, 1952.
4. HARLEY, D.   *Medico-legal Blood Group Determination.* Heinemann, 1943.
5. WEINER, A.S.   *J. forens. Med.*, **10**, 130, 1964.
6. HARLEY, D.   *Medico-legal Blood Group Determination.* Heinemann. 1943.
7. KIND, S.S.   *Nature, Lond.*, **187**, 789, 1960.
8. COOMBS, R.A. & DODD, B.E.   *Medicine Sci. Law*, **1**, 359, 1961.
9. NICKOLLS, L.C. & PEREIRA, M.   *Medicine Sci. Law*, **2**, 172, 1962.
10. *The Times*, 23 July, 1970.
11. [1970] 3 W.L.R., 366.
12. 1958, S.C., 252.
13. 1958, S.C., 439.
14. BROWNLIE, A.R.   *J. Forens. Sci. Soc.*, **5**, 171, 1965.

Chapter 13

MEDICO-LEGAL ASPECTS OF SEXUAL FUNCTIONS AND CRIMINAL ABORTION

THE following subjects which relate to the sexual functions are treated in this chapter:

> Impotence and sterility in the male.
> Impotence and sterility in the female.
> Intersex and hermaphroditism.
> Surgical sterilisation.
> Nullity of marriage on the ground of impotence.
> Artificial insemination.
> Pregnancy and criminal abortion.

Impotence and sterility in the male

The question of impotence in the male arises frequently in nullity of marriage cases, and less frequently in disputed paternity cases, and in cases of rape. Impotence is the inability to have sexual intercourse, whereas sterility is the inability to impregnate.

Below the age of puberty, the male is presumed to be sexually impotent. Puberty is generally held to be attained at the age of fourteen years, and by the term 'puberty' ought to be meant the attainment of virility, not merely the power of coitus, for the latter power often commences earlier than puberty or virility, and continues for some time after procreative power has ceased. Fairfield[1] reports a case in which a girl aged thirteen was reputed to have been pregnant by a boy of the same age. Absolute certainty was lacking, but the boy himself had no doubt. She points out that the boy's feat was, according to English law, impossible, since it is an 'irrebuttable presumption' that a boy under fourteen cannot procreate a child (see p. 427). Although the law fixes the age of attainment of virility, it places no limit upon the period of age above puberty when a male ceases to be sexually potent. Cases of virile power in elderly men are well known and authenticated. This point was raised in the famous Banbury peerage case, where the putative father was eighty years of age at the date of the birth of the claimant, but the judge ruled that there was no legal limit to the age when procreative power ceased.

That procreative power in old men is possible is demonstrated by the fact that spermatozoa have been found in a man of ninety-six.

Certain conditions of the central nervous system, such as hemiplegia, paraplegia, locomotor ataxia, disseminated sclerosis, syringomyelia, and fracture of vertebrae with cord injury may cause impotence, but this is not always so.   In locomotor ataxia, although the pro-creative power becomes weakened and, latterly, is destroyed, there are well-authenticated cases in which, in the earlier stages at least, pro-creative power has continued.   Impotence may also be produced by premature ejaculation, endocrine dysfunction, the abuse of alcohol and drugs, but most frequently by psychical causes.   The physical causes of impotence afford the safest basis upon which to found an opinion, but psychical causes are more common as the basis of declarators of nullity.   Relative impotence is sometimes present and may be due, among other causes, to neurasthenia, frigidity, or sexual perversion.

Absence of the penis constitutes absolute impotence, since there is no organ for intromission, and in cases of partial amputation, per-formance of the sexual act may be rendered impossible.   Certain malformations of the male external genitals may prevent intercourse, and these include such conditions as intersexuality, hypospadias and epispadias.   In the last-named condition, the urethral orifice is situated on the upper surface of the penis, which is frequently curved upwards. In hypospadias the external meatus of the urethra is situated at some point upon the under surface of the penis or perineum.   In both hypospadias, which is fairly common, and epispadias, a more rare condition, even when sexual intercourse may be possible, the seminal ejaculate may not reach the vagina on account of the abnormal position of the urethral orifice.

Sterility, or inability to impregnate, in the male is commonly due to a variety of causes which include hypospadias, absence or atrophy of the testes, pituitary dysfunction, hypothyroidism, and the effects of gonorrhoeal infection.   Following the removal of both testicles, procreative power is progressively lost.

Impotence and sterility in the female

In the consideration of this aspect of the subject from the medico-legal point of view, it is essential that the difference between the terms impotence and sterility should be understood.   In the female, as in the male, impotence means the inability to have sexual intercourse. The term sterility, with regard to the female, means the incapacity to conceive.   The legal definition of impotence may be considered to be such physical and irremediable conformation of the sexual organs as prevents the act of coitus.

The causes of impotence in the female may be permanent or temporary.

The absence of a vagina, or one which is rudimentary in character, is often found in cases of intersexuality of which the varieties are many (p. 361).

Hodgson[2] reports a case of congenital absence of the vagina in a woman of thirty-two, who, apart from the fact that she had not menstruated, was unaware of her condition until her marriage, when coitus was found impossible. Surgical operation originated an artificial vagina, but showed that there was no trace of uterus or of any tissue representing it.

Patel[3] describes a young native woman of twenty-two, who, at her second confinement, gave birth to a living child, through the rectum. The vagina, $1\frac{1}{2}$ inches long, ended blindly. The cervix, which opened directly into the rectum, could be seen through the anal canal. The child died immediately following its birth. The first child must have been delivered also by the rectum.

Among the temporary causes of impotence are dyspareunia, excessive constriction of the vagina, hyperaesthesia of the vagina, imperforate hymen, prolapse of the uterus or bladder, and vulvar or vaginal tumours.

Turning to the question of sterility, the possibility of pregnancy must primarily depend upon the function of ovulation. Leaving on one side cases of precocious menstruation in girls under ten years, the average age at which girls in this country attain puberty is thirteen years and six months. The age of onset of menstruation is very variable and such factors as race, climate, heredity, general health, environment, diet, and hygiene play a part. While it is the rule that a woman usually becomes pregnant only after the establishment of menstruation, many cases have been recorded in which impregnation has occurred prior to the onset of the usual signs of menstruation. At the other end of female reproductive life, the time when impregnation becomes impossible through cessation of the function of ovulation is equally difficult to determine, and, although the age range may be given as between forty and sixty, an opinion on such matters must be based solely upon the circumstances of each specific case (p. 370). As it is possible for a female to conceive before the external signs of menstruation have appeared, so also must conception be reckoned as possible in a woman within a limited time after these manifestations have disappeared. We are acquainted with the case of a woman, aged forty-seven, who had ceased to menstruate for over a year and who became pregnant. Two cases have been reported, in one of which there was cessation of menstruation at the age of twenty-three, and in the other the menstrual flow continued until the age of seventy-five. Generally speaking, females who have not yet menstruated, and those who have reached the climacteric, are sterile. The only question on which menstruation may have a bearing in civil cases is that which may arise with regard to women who have ceased to menstruate at or about the usual age, and the possibility of their bearing further children, in relation to the provisions of a will. With regard to the age of fertility, in a case before the court it was held that a presumption that a woman of fifty-three was past child-bearing was a rebuttable presumption.[4] In some instances medical examination may not disclose any cause for sterility, and it has been suggested that, in a very small proportion of these, the reason may conceivably be that although the woman is menstruating normally, the menstruation may be of an anovulatory type. Another reason, in the absence of disclosure of any cause in the female, may be found by the appraisal of seminal specimens taken from the male partner.

Other causes of sterility include removal of the ovaries, certain uterine displacements and diseases, ovarian disease, and lesions

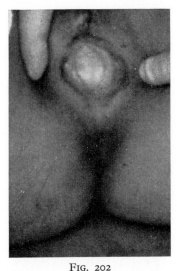

FIG. 202

Imperforate hymen. Note bulging
of hymen due to retained menses

affecting the tubes. Congenital abnormality may also produce a condition of sterility.

Andreason[5] describes a very unusual case of a Moslem woman, aged sixteen, who was sterile. On making a vaginal examination, it was found that unless the anterior wall was followed, the rectum was attained. Thus the rectum opened entirely within the vulva. The cause of the sterility probably resulted from coitus taking place in the rectum instead of the vagina.

Intersex and hermaphroditism[6, 7]

The interest in this subject has in recent years increased greatly. This has been due to a greater scientific understanding of the subject and also because of the difficulties in being certain that females competing in international athletic events are in fact females. This problem arose initially in the heavy events[8] but has now become of wider significance. In addition considerable publicity has been given to operative procedures for changing the sex characteristics.

It is common experience that there are many effeminate-looking men and masculine-looking women but usually people have no doubt about the actual sex of such cases. There are, however, a few individuals where ordinary observation leaves the matter open. The external genitalia may be of both sexes and the internal genitalia consist of both ovaries and testes or ovotestes.

The actual sex is nowadays usually determined by:

1. External anatomical characteristics.
2. Examination of the gonads, i.e. the presence of ovaries or testes.
3. Presence of nuclear sex chromatin.
4. Study of actual cell chromosomes, when the cells are undergoing mitosis, males having sex chromatin XY and females XX.

The latter two methods will establish the genetic sex of individuals. Such investigation can be done at an early age and children brought up in accordance with their true sex. In this way many of the difficulties and ambiguities which have previously been experienced ought to be prevented.

The examination for the presence of nuclear chromatin is usually done by examining microscopically cells from the buccal mucosa when the sex chromatin body (Barr body) can be clearly seen in the case of the female. It is absent in the male. The white cells of the blood also show accumulations of chromatin which protrude from the polymorph nucleus in females (Davidson body) and these cells can also be used for deciding sex.

We include some examples of cases studied by expert examiners prior to the development of modern scientific techniques for determining true sex.

Morison[9] describes the case of a person in whom there was a vagina, from the upper part of which protruded a large penis-like clitoris. Scrotum and testes were not evident, but labia were present. The enlarged clitoris did not have an urethral opening, but there was such an opening at the junction of the base of the organ and a groove which represented the vaginal orifice. On operation, an ovarian formation and testicular tissues were found in the left side of the pelvis. The subject had not experienced menstruation, sexual excitement, or desire.

Raynaud, Marill, and Xicluna[10] reported the case of a person aged eighteen, who had been brought up as a boy. There were feminine appearances—breasts, a large clitoris or small penis, and the left half of the scrotum contained a small testicle.   Every few weeks there was a slightly sanguineous urethral discharge.   There were also erections of the small penis or large clitoris and ejaculation of seminal fluid which contained active spermatozoa.   Laparotomy disclosed a left seminal vesicle, a small uterus with a Fallopian tube, and an ovary.   There was also a rudimentary vagina.   Sections of the testis showed fairly normal seminiferous tubules with spermatogonia and a few sperms.

O'Farrell[11] published an interesting series of cases of intersexuality. Five instances occurred in one family which consisted of three males and three females.

The decision of sex, in the case of the intersex, becomes important medico-legally in connection not only with questions of impotence but in those associated with sexual offences, marriage, and succession.   The question of personal identity in connection with sex has already been mentioned (p. 81).   Legally there is no definition of what constitutes male or female sex.

Surgical sterilisation

It was considered for a long time that sterilisation even with consent was legal only when it was performed to preserve the life or the mental or physical health of the patient or for well-established eugenic reasons. The basic idea seemed to have been that it was illegal to perform an operation which would enable a man to have unrestricted enjoyment of sexual intercourse without the possibility of procreation.[12]   Probably it was also thought to be against the public interest as providing a serious risk of restricting the population.   Now that the fashion amongst political leaders throughout the world favours restricting population growth, the legal attitude seems to have changed.   The risk to doctors is now not in the criminal courts for having performed an illegal sterilisation but in the civil courts for having performed an inefficient one.

In all cases of sterilisation the consent of the party concerned should be obtained after the effects and possible irreversibility of the operation have been fully explained.   If a couple are living together the consent of the spouse should also be obtained.   This is not necessary when the sterilisation is for therapeutic purposes.

It is important that there should be no mistake about the operation and it is now customary to send excised parts of the vas[13] or Fallopian tubes to a pathologist for identification.

Nullity of marriage on the ground of impotence

Every man is presumed capable of begetting, and every woman of bearing, children.   The only proof allowed, in order to rebut this presumption, is that of facts establishing that there is a permanent *de facto* incapacity with respect to the spouse.

Where there exists in one of the parties to a marriage such physical and irremediable defect or deformity as will prevent the marriage being consummated, the marriage is null, and the other party may apply to the competent court to have such nullity declared. If, after evidence, the court is satisfied that the wife or husband, as the case may be, at the time of marriage was and still is unable to consummate, it will annul the marriage unless the pursuer was aware of the incapacity before marriage. The judgment of the court is termed a Declarator of Nullity of Marriage. Divorce is the judgment of a competent court, after evidence, that a marriage which has been duly consummated is dissolved. An action of declarator will lie against a husband, if he, by reason of impotence, arising from imperfect conformation of congenital origin, or from malformation of the external genitals of an irremediable kind, is prevented from consummating the marriage; and against a wife, if she is of such congenital conformation as prevents her from permitting the consummation. Actions of declarator of nullity of marriage by wives against husbands, on the grounds of neurasthenia, psychical causes, and sexual perversion, have also been heard in the courts. It has been held that an impotent spouse has title and interest to sue for declarator of nullity.[14]

Legally, marriage is a contract between two persons of opposite sex, which presupposes on the part of each the lawful use of the body, or in other words, capability of the fulfilment of the act of physical union by coitus, and any cause, however, originating on the part of either of them which creates a barrier to coitus would, according to civil law, enable declarator of nullity of marriage. From the legal point of view, apart from statutory enactment (see p. 365), if it is satisfactorily proved that repeated endeavours of a potent husband who has tried all means short of force, have been uniformly unsuccessful, it is for the court, in the absence of any alleged or probable motive for wilful refusal, to draw the inference that the non-consummation was due to some form of incapacity on the part of the wife. From the medico-legal point of view, the primary aspect to be considered is whether there exists a physical deformity or deficiency of the body of the party against whom the action is laid which will prevent, and is likely to continue to prevent, the consummation. Erection and penetration without emission, although not constituting sexual intercourse in the full sense of the word, are sufficient in law to consummate a marriage.[15]

When an allegation is made by a wife or husband that impotence exists, it is the duty of the court to call medical evidence. Medical examiners are appointed and both parties must submit to such an examination as the medical men think necessary, in order to verify the existence, or otherwise, of the alleged impotence. If the allegation is made by a wife, in order to establish her averment, it is necessary for her to show evidence, by medical examination of her own body, that she is physically capable of having sexual intercourse.

Where the husband sues for declarator of nullity, his wife, should she defend the action, must lead medical evidence of her condition to show whether or not the allegation is true.

The examination of a husband should include the physical conformation of his genitals and microscopical examination of seminal fluid, for living spermatozoa. An opinion regarding virility must depend upon a man being like, or unlike, other men, for unless there is marked deviation from normal, an opinion implying diminished virility naturally cannot be expressed. When the male external genitals are normal, an examiner is unable to state that the virile and procreative powers do not exist, and the opinion expressed must be to the effect that no good reason exists why these should not be present. In the case of the female, however, assuming the husband is normal, the impediment is likely to be obvious, and will probably consist of such defect of the vaginal portion of the genitals as will establish the inability to permit coitus.

The development of any condition which prevents coitus, after the marriage has been consummated, will not afford legal grounds for declarator of nullity. A marriage is voidable only where the impotence has existed at and since the time of 'marriage', wholly preventing consummation.

The case of Clarke v. Clarke[16, 17] is both interesting and unusual. The parties were married in 1926, and, according to the evidence of the husband, there was never any consummation of the marriage. By the term 'consummation' penetration was presumably meant. In 1930, the wife gave birth to a son of whom the husband was unquestionably the father. The judge held that it was common ground between the parties that the birth of the child did not in itself establish consummation. It was stated in evidence that conception could occur without penetration of the vagina. Fecundation *ab extra* was an established medical fact previously noted by the courts. The judge found in favour of the husband and he was granted a decree of nullity. This case has been stated as the first of a finding of non-consummation where the husband is admittedly the father of a child of the marriage.

The case of Baxter v. Baxter[18] is of importance since from it emerged a decision by the House of Lords that the procreation of children was not the fundamental purpose of marriage. Mr Baxter's contention was that his wife's refusal to permit marital intercourse unless he used a contraceptive amounted to wilful refusal on her part to consummate the marriage, although under protest he acceded to her demand. The Lord Chancellor, Viscount Jowitt, said that he could not agree with Mr Justice Hodson and the Court of Appeal that the husband's acquiescence in the conditions imposed by his wife barred him from obtaining a decree.   On that view of the matter it was necessary to consider whether the case of Cowen v. Cowen[19] was rightly decided in 1945.   In that case the Court of Appeal held that sexual intercourse meant ordinary and complete intercourse and did not mean partial and imperfect intercourse.   They further declared that the use of contraceptives frustrated one of the principal ends, if not the principal end of marriage.   Lord Jowitt said that the institution of marriage generally was not necessarily for the procreation of children, nor did it appear to be a principal end of marriage as understood in Christendom, which, as Lord Penzance said years ago, might be defined as 'the voluntary union for life of one man and one woman to the exclusion of all others'. His Lordship was unable to believe that Parliament in passing the Matrimonial Causes Act, 1937, intended the courts to be involved in inquiries as to the merits and effects of various contraceptive precautions.   He took the view that in this legislation Parliament used the word 'consummate' as that word was understood in common parlance and in the light of social conditions known to exist.   There was, in his opinion, no warrant for the decision in Cowen v. Cowen and the present appeal should be dismissed.   Lord Wright, Lord Merriman, Lord Simonds, and Lord Normand concurred and the appeal was unanimously dismissed.

There is no statutory definition of what consummation means. In the case of White v. White[20] it was held that coitus interruptus did not constitute wilful refusal to consummate.

Mr Justice Ormrod has the distinction of being the only medically qualified High Court judge.   In 1970,[21] he had before him a petition for declaration of nullity involving important questions of law and medicine.   The facts were that C, a male, went through a ceremony of marriage with A, knowing that A had been registered at birth as a male, but had undergone an operation involving removal of testes and scrotum with the formation of an artificial vagina.   Only two months after marriage, C petitioned for a decree that the marriage was null and void or that it be declared null for non-consummation.   A crosspetitioned for a decree of nullity for C's wilful refusal to consummate. The judge found A to be of male chromosomal sex, of male gonadal and genital sex, but psychologically a transsexual.   He held (1) that, A being biologically male, the marriage was void; (2) that use of the artificial vagina could never constitute true intercourse.

Some medico-legal aspects of artificial insemination

Artificial human insemination may be defined as the deposit of semen in the vagina, the cervical canal, or the uterus by instruments to bring about pregnancy unattained or unattainable by sexual intercourse.

The seminal fluid used for this purpose may either have been obtained from the woman's husband or from a donor. Certain recommendations have been made when a donor is used for this procedure,[22, 23] and these include that:

1. The donor must not be a relative of either spouse, he should be potent, should be of age, his age should not exceed forty, and he should have had children of his own.
2. His race and characteristics should resemble as closely as possible those of the husband of the woman to be inseminated, his mental and physical history, together with his personal, familial, and general health must have proved satisfactory, and such examination should include the Wasserman reaction and Rh grouping, and should exclude such diseases as tuberculosis, diabetes, epilepsy, endocrine dysfunction, and psychosis.
3. He must be willing to donate his seminal fluid for the purpose, his wife must agree that he may do so, and both he and his wife must accept that the donation will result from an act of masturbation.
4. He should be unaware of the destination of the donated seminal fluid and of the result of the insemination.
5. The woman to be inseminated, and her husband, must desire in written form that a donor, preferably unknown, should be used.
6. The physician in charge of the case should keep the relevant documents in his possession, with instructions that, in the event of his death, they should be destroyed unread. He should never undertake the procedure without the knowledge and full consent of both spouses, and a nurse should be present when the insemination is undertaken.
7. For practical purposes, a semen bank might be established.

Possible legal issues arising from artificial insemination. There is, at the present time, little settled law in connection with this subject applicable to Britain, thus when either the semen of a donor, or a specimen from a semen bank, is used, a number of important issues may arise for solution. Among many, the following may be mentioned:

1. What would be the legal position of a mother in relation to the registration of the birth of her child born as the result of artificial insemination, or of the woman's husband in similar connection? It would seem that the proper course would be to state that the child was fatherless. If the mother registers the child as that of her husband, or the husband registers it as his own, it would constitute the making of a false declaration.
2. Could the donor be cited as co-respondent in divorce proceedings?
3. What of possible incest between offspring from the same seminal

donor ?　It has been estimated that a fecund donor, submitting two specimens weekly, could produce some four hundred children weekly, or some twenty thousand annually, and it has been pointed out that thus a considerable risk of the mating of the children of the same father could arise.

4. What might be the attitude of the General Medical Council toward a practitioner who undertook the procedure of artificial insemination ?

A summary of some of the findings of the Departmental Committee on Human Artificial Insemination published in 1960 states:

1. The fact that a live child has been born as a result of artificial insemination of a woman with seed of her husband should be a bar to proceedings by either spouse for nullity of marriage on the ground of impotence.
2. Acceptance by a wife of artificial insemination with the seed of a donor without the consent of her husband should be made a new ground for divorce or judicial separation.
3. The fact that a live child has been born as a result of artificial insemination of a woman with seed of a donor, to which the parties of the marriage consented, should be a bar to proceedings by either spouse for nullity of marriage on the ground of impotence.
4. There should be no amendment of the laws relating to legitimacy or registration of birth.
5. While the practice of artificial insemination by a donor is strongly to be discouraged, it should not be declared criminal or be regulated by law.

It would appear that few of these aspects have so far come before the courts in Britain, but it seems clear that if the practice becomes prevalent, some form of legislation will become imperative.

In February 1957, the question as to whether a wife who has had a child by artificial insemination from a donor could be held in Scottish law to be guilty of adultery came before the Court of Session. The Outer House held that for adultery to be committed there had to be two parties physically present and engaging in the sexual act at the same time and that artificial insemination did not satisfy this test.[24] It follows that a child conceived following artificial insemination from a donor in a married woman is presumably legitimate.

Pregnancy in its medico-legal aspects

The question of pregnancy may come before a medico-legal examiner in various ways and for diverse reasons. The following are the principal:

As a reason why a woman should be excused attendance as a witness at a trial.

In a case of slander in which it has been said of an unmarried woman, a widow, or a wife living apart from her husband, that she is pregnant.

To declare whether or not a woman, who has raised an action of damages for breach of promise of marriage and seduction, is pregnant, or has been delivered of a child.

To say whether or not a woman is with child, the possible heir to an estate, her husband having but shortly before died, in order that in the disposition of the estate the law of succession may be duly satisfied.

In cases of supposed imposture of pregnancy, to say whether or not the woman has been pregnant, and has been recently delivered of a child.

To form an opinion whether or not a woman, at or about the age of the climacteric, is likely to become pregnant either for the first time, or in continuation of a series of pregnancies, with relation to the question of succession to real or personal estate.

To declare in cases of alleged criminal abortion whether or not the woman has actually been pregnant.

In cases of alleged concealment of birth or pregnancy and infanticide or child-murder, to determine whether the woman has or has not been pregnant, and, if she has been pregnant, to say whether or not she has been recently delivered of a child.

With relation to pregnancy as an excuse for the attendance of a woman as a witness, it should be clearly understood that pregnancy in itself is not an excuse, except when it is so far advanced that delivery is imminent. At the same time, a valid excuse for non-attendance may be offered, and will probably be accepted, if, owing to any intercurrent condition arising out of the pregnant state, she would suffer risk or prejudice the child by such attendance (see p. 29).

Imposture of pregnancy is rare, but such cases occasionally occur.

For the methods of establishing the existence of pregnancy, textbooks on the subject should be consulted.

Signs of pregnancy in the dead body

From the external appearances of the body alone the chief signs will be those present at the stage of the pregnancy at which the woman died, but no special importance need be attached to these, since by opening the uterus both the existence of pregnancy and the stage which it has reached can be determined.

The ovaries, especially in cases of abortion, should be examined to

detect the presence of a corpus luteum (see Fig. 203). The significance of its presence lies in the fact that when the ovum is discharged
from the ovary, the follicle becomes a corpus luteum and forms progesterone. It prepares the subject for pregnancy, and if pregnancy
occurs, the placenta liberates a luteinising substance which causes the
corpus luteum to persist and to continue to form progesterone. If
pregnancy does not occur the corpus luteum atrophies and the hypertrophied uterine mucous membrane is discharged. This is accompanied by loss of blood. If pregnancy occurs, the corpus luteum
will increase in size until about the fifth month, when it commences to
atrophy. In the absence of pregnancy it will atrophy in about ten
days' time and will finally disappear, its site being marked with scar

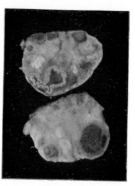

FIG. 203

Corpora lutea. Specimen
on top is a corpus luteum
of pregnancy. Specimen
below is a corpus luteum
associated with ovulation

tissue. Cases have occurred in which there has been absence of a corpus
luteum, although the subjects were pregnant. Reliance must therefore
be placed upon the condition of the uterus and its contents in the
determination of pregnancy in medico-legal autopsies.

Pregnancy with reference to female age

From time to time, young female subjects are submitted for examination to determine the existence of pregnancy, following sexual delicts.
Fairfield[25] records some interesting facts with regard to a survey of
seventy-four mothers under the age of sixteen years at the age of
confinement. Five were aged thirteen, ten were fourteen years old,
and the remaining fifty-nine were fifteen years of age. Some of the
younger girls had been the victims of incest. There were no maternal
deaths, although there were two still-births and three neonatal deaths.

Most of the labours were short and easy. Half of the babies born weighed 7 pounds or more, and one, whose mother was thirteen, weighed 8 pounds and 6 ounces. In this instance, the mother was only thirteen hours in labour, and there was no perineal tear. The youngest child in the series was thirteen years and three months at the date of confinement. Only one girl was a certified defective. There was no evidence that maternity had produced excessive nervous or mental strain in these girls, and no case of mental or nervous breakdown had been traced. Our records point in similar directions.

The case of a Peruvian child, Lina Medina, has been reported as giving birth to a live baby when she was only five years and eight months.[26]

A case of child-bearing at the precocious age of six and a half years has been recorded.[27] We have notes of a case in which a girl, aged twelve years and two months, was delivered of a child at full time. She must have conceived, therefore, at the age of eleven years and five months. Within recent years, a case of a girl of fourteen who gave birth to twins was reported in Glasgow.

Greater importance, probably, is associated with the age of certain women at the time of their delivery late in life, since important legal issues may emerge. While it is generally true that the fecundity of women lessens the nearer the age approaches the climacteric, and that impregnation does not usually occur after forty-five years of age, women have conceived and borne children when they were past fifty (p. 360).

Gilbertson[28] has recorded the case of a woman whose last child was born when she was fifty years and seven months.

Duration of pregnancy or period of gestation

The period of gestation is ten lunar months, forty weeks, or two hundred and eighty days; but in legal issues, evidence may be led to show the possible extension of this period. For practical purposes, the assessment of the date of term may be arrived at, with a fair degree of accuracy, by adding forty weeks to the date of the beginning of the last menstrual period. Since ovulation probably takes place about two weeks before the first missed period, the above estimate may be slightly excessive. So that, while it is correct to say that in a large number of cases the period of gestation is two hundred and eighty days, the menstrual cycle of many women being twenty-eight days, it must be considered as possible that the period of gestation may be longer or shorter where the individual menstrual cycle is longer or shorter.

Any data can only be founded upon cases in which, by reason of a single coitus with resulting impregnation, the duration of pregnancy may be reckoned. Even in these cases, however, coitus is not necessarily contemporaneous with conception, since a day or two may elapse between the two occurrences.   Studies have revealed that spermatozoa may survive less than two hours in the vagina, but they live as long as forty-three hours both in the cervix and the uterus where the secretions are more favourable.   It is claimed that sperms recovered after forty-three hours in the uterus can hardly be distinguished from those freshly ejaculated.[29]

Seymour's[30] investigations on the viability of spermatozoa following the introduction of seminal fluid into the cervical canal of five patients is of interest.   The spermatozoa of the donor used in the tests had marked viability.   After ninety hours, the sperms had disappeared in two cases, were found to be dead in two other instances, and were alive, but sluggish, in the fifth case.   In the last-mentioned case, after one hundred and ten hours, their condition was still the same, and pregnancy resulted.   Pregnancy occurred in three out of the five women injected.   Experimental work indicates that it is unlikely that spermatozoa retain their fecundity for more than five days after introduction to the female generative tract.[31]

Investigation has shown that fertilisation in the human subject is much more likely to occur during four to five days in each twenty-eight days and that a mating occurring at any other time in the cycle is much less likely to lead to fertilisation.   It appears that ovulation varies with the length of the menstrual cycle and ranges from the twelfth to the seventeenth day, and that fertilisation is much more likely to occur at the times in the cycle to which ovulation is restricted.

Sevitt[32] found by biopsy that ovulation can take place on any day of the first fortnight of the menstrual cycle, including the last days of menstruation.   This was ascertained by correlating the menstrual dates and the date of operation with the state of the endometrial biopsy material and the removed ovaries.   The finding supports the belief that ovulation can occur on any day of the first half of the cycle.   It follows that there is no 'safe' period in the first half of the menstrual cycle.

The following cases indicate the difficulty in determining that an abnormal period of gestation is impossible.

In the case of Gaskill v. Gaskill[33] the Court refused to grant divorce on the ground of adultery.   The husband, who was a soldier, left on service three hundred and thirty-one days before his wife gave birth to a child.   There was no evidence of adultery.   Medical evidence was led and showed that it was not impossible for the husband to be the father of the child.   Thus a period of gestation amounting to three hundred and thirty-one days has been recognised by a court of law in this country.

The case of Clark v. Clark[34] is one which involves a short gestational period.   It came before the President of the Divorce Division in 1939. The petitioner sought divorce on the ground that his wife had given birth to a child after one hundred and seventy-four days' gestation. There was no evidence of misconduct. The child weighed $2\frac{1}{2}$ pounds at birth, which it survived. His lordship stated that it was impossible to ascertain with certainty the date when conception takes place, and it was therefore possible that a child which notionally has had a gestation period of one hundred and ninety-six days or seven months, has in reality only had one of a hundred and seventy-four days. The child might therefore be comparable with any of the recorded cases whose notional fetal life had been between a hundred and ninety and two hundred days. This was a rare combination of an extremely premature child with a fixed and not a notional maximum length of fetal life, and there was no ground whatsoever for saying that the child was illegitimate.

That a period as long as three hundred and forty-nine days, although unusual, was not impossible was decided in the case of Hadlum v. Hadlum[35] while a gestational period of three hundred and forty-six days was admitted in the case of Wood v. Wood.[36] In the latter case, Lord Merriman said that 'on the information before us in this case, I absolutely decline to say that we are judicially bound to hold that the period of three hundred and forty-six days (fifteen days longer than the period with which Lord Birkenhead was dealing in 1921 (case of Gaskill v. Gaskill)) is on the wrong side of any line which can possibly be drawn, and that we are judicially bound to hold that the wife had committed adultery'. The House of Lords has held that a husband who sought divorce alleging his wife's adultery on the sole ground that she had given birth to a child three hundred and sixty days after the last act of marital intercourse was entitled to a decree.[37] A case described[38] dealing with this question is interesting. An anencephalic fetus born after a pregnancy lasting three hundred and eighty-nine days is recorded. The child although still-born made active movements until birth.

It may be taken, therefore, that while the law considers about two hundred and eighty days to be the normal period of gestation, evidence may be led to show reason why, in a given case, the period may be protracted or shortened.

McKeown and Gibson[39] from information on 15,629 births have stated that the longest confident estimates of the period of gestation in this series were three hundred and nineteen, three hundred and twenty, three hundred and twenty-one, three hundred and twenty-five, and three hundred and twenty-eight days; in two cases the duration of gestation was reliably thought to be three hundred and thirty-nine and three hundred and fifty-nine days. Their conclusion is that, for medico-legal purposes, a period of three hundred and fifty-four days from coitus to live birth is not impossible.

Signs of recent delivery in the living

This subject is closely connected with concealment of birth and concealment of pregnancy, and medical practitioners are frequently asked to examine women involved in such charges, as to whether they have been recently delivered. The following are the principal signs within eight or ten days of delivery:

Breasts. These are found to be enlarged, firm, and turgid, and a milky fluid will probably be easily expressed from the nipples. The surface veins are dilated, and there is a more or less dark coloured pigmentation around the nipples. The colour tone of the pigmentation varies; in blonde women it is usually light in colour, and in brunettes it is dark brown. Montgomery's tubercles are present.

Abdomen. In multiparae, the skin of the abdominal wall is frequently flaccid, and may be wrinkled. In primiparae, the condition of flaccidity may not be so marked, due in large measure to the better tone of the abdominal structures. There is usually evidence of striae gravidarum, slightly pink in colour, due to the stretching of the skin of the abdomen and resultant formation of scar tissue in the deeper layer of the cutis. As time elapses, the striae become white in colour as the result of diminishing vascularity of the scar tissue, and are termed lineae albicantes. Some degree of pigmentation, chiefly in the neighbourhood of the umbilicus and median abdominal line, is frequently present. On completion of labour, the fundus lies about an inch below the umbilicus, and a few hours thereafter may be slightly higher. By the tenth day, it is on a level with the brim of the pelvis. In from two to three weeks, the fundus sinks below the level of the pubis into the pelvic cavity.

Vagina, os, and cervix. The following conditions are likely to be found:

There will be a vaginal discharge, the lochia. For the first four or five days the discharge will be blood-stained; by the end of the first week it is yellowish or greenish. It then gradually loses all colour, becoming white and turbid until its final disappearance in about ten to fourteen days.

Appearance of bruising or laceration of the external genitals, usually consisting of rupture of the fourchette, swelling of the vulva, and, perhaps, some degree of tearing of the perineum.

The os uteri will be more or less patent, usually to an extent sufficient to enable one or two fingers to be passed into it for a short distance. Its lips are likely to be swollen, and one or both of them may be lacerated.

When these appearances and conditions, or most of them, are found it may safely be concluded that the woman has been recently delivered of a child.

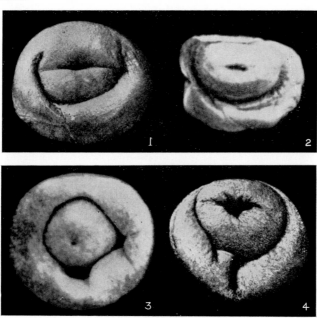

FIG. 204

External os of uterus.   (Hoffman)

1. Adolescent virgin.   Edges smooth
2. Adolescent virgin.   Edges smooth
3. In advanced age, but in virginal state.   Edges smooth
4. Multiparous woman.   More or less deeply and cicatricially notched.   May admit finger-tip

Signs of previous pregnancy

The extent and character of the signs found will depend upon whether the woman is primiparous or multiparous.   The following signs, or some of them, are likely to be found:

Lineae albicantes on the abdomen, the result of hyper-distension of the skin and resultant scar formation in the cutis.

Persistent dark areolae around the nipples.

Rupture of the fourchette or perineum, or both.

Frequently a healed cervical tear, or tears, in the region of the external os.

Absence of signs of virginity, and a non-rugose condition of the vaginal walls.

The examiner, however, must be prepared in exceptional instances to meet with cases where a woman who has borne one or more children may not exhibit on her body any of the above signs, or little evidence of them.

Superfecundation and superfetation

Superfecundation is the term applied to the fertilising of two ova, the products of the same ovulation, which are impregnated as the result of two separate acts of coitus. Superfetation refers to the fertilisation of two ova, each of which has been liberated by different ovulations. The possibility of superfecundation is generally admitted, but the proof of its occurrence is difficult in the human subject since it becomes indistinguishable from a binovular twin pregnancy. A case has been recorded, however, in which a negress has given birth to a white and a black child. Superfetation is not generally accepted as a possible occurrence, and there is divided opinion on the subject. It has been submitted that the cases cited are all explicable from the well-known facts attending the unequal growth and development of twin conceptions, where the disparity is the result of delayed delivery of the less favoured fetus. Eden has stated that if it is true that ovulation continues during early pregnancy, there is no obstacle to the fertilisation of a second ovum, and its lodgment in the uterine cavity up to the fourth month, so long as the decidual space persists. Many hold the view that ovulation discontinues after impregnation and during pregnancy. If it is possible for such cases to occur, their incidence is very rare, and each would have to be very carefully considered in the light of every circumstance before an expression of opinion as to the definite possibility of superfetation was given.

ABORTION

The law with regard to abortion has been materially altered by the Abortion Act of 1967. This however did not repeal any of the previous legislation dealing with criminal abortion and the present position can be better understood by looking at the previous law on this subject for England and Scotland and then seeing how the Act of 1967 amended and clarified it.

England. The law of England is set down in the Offences Against the Person Act, 1861, sections 58 and 59:

58. Every woman, being with child, who with intent to procure her own miscarriage, shall unlawfully administer to herself any poison, or other noxious thing, or shall unlawfully use any instrument or other means whatsoever, with like intent, and whosoever, with intent to

procure the miscarriage of any woman, whether she be, or be not with child, shall unlawfully administer to her, or cause to be taken by her, any poison or other noxious thing, or shall unlawfully use any instrument or other means whatsoever, with the like intent, shall be guilty of felony.

59. Whosoever shall unlawfully supply or procure any poison or other noxious thing, or any instrument or thing whatsoever, knowing that the same is intended to be unlawfully used, or employed, with intent to procure the miscarriage of any woman, whether she be with child or not, shall be guilty of a misdemeanour.

A noxious thing is one which will produce the effect mentioned in section 58, and if a substance given produces an abortion this will establish that it is a noxious thing.[40]   The quantity of a substance used may decide the question as to whether or not it is a noxious thing.[41]

If a woman should die as the result of criminal abortion, the charge is manslaughter.

By the Infant Life (Preservation) Act, 1929, it is enacted that:

In the trial of any person for murder or manslaughter of any child, capable of being born alive, or for infanticide, or for an offence relating to the administration of drugs or the use of instruments to procure abortion, if the jury are of the opinion that the person charged is not guilty of murder, manslaughter, or infanticide or of administration of drugs or the use of instruments to procure abortion, as the case may be, but is shown by evidence to be guilty of child destruction, such person may be so convicted and punished.

It will be observed that, under the Offences Against the Person Act, when a second party attempts to procure the abortion of a woman, the criminality or culpa of the act lies in the intent to procure abortion, and it therefore follows that the person upon whom the intentional procedure has been practised need not have been pregnant.   If, however, a woman attempts her own abortion, she is not chargeable unless pregnant.

For the provisions of this Act to apply, the abortion had to be performed with felonious intent and the law in practice recognised that the operation might be required in certain justifiable circumstances. There was never any doubt that abortion was legal to preserve the life, and physical health of the mother.   Some difficulty arose when the concept of preserving the mental health was introduced, probably not on principle, but because the idea of mental health was difficult to define.

Scotland.   By the law of Scotland anyone who feloniously causes or procures a pregnant woman to abort is guilty of a very serious crime, whether it is effected by drugs or by the use of instruments or any other means. An unsuccessful attempt is also criminal. A woman herself may be guilty, if she is aware of the purpose for which the drug is administered or the instrument used. Administration of drugs or use of instruments to procure abortion is criminal, although abortion does not follow.

It is necessary in the libel against the accused to aver that the woman was pregnant and to prove the pregnancy at the trial.

As in England, the induction of abortion as a necessary medical operation was not an offence.

If a woman should die as a result of criminal abortion, the charge is culpable homicide.

The Abortion Act, 1967

This applies to both England and Scotland and the preamble states that it is an Act to amend and clarify the law relating to termination of pregnancy by registered medical practitioners. It states that nothing in the Act shall affect the provisions of the Infant Life (Preservation) Act, 1929, and that for the purposes of the law relating to abortion, anything done with intent to procure the miscarriage of a woman is unlawfully done unless authorised by section 1 of the 1967 Act.

Section 1 states that a person is not guilty of an offence under the law relating to abortion if the pregnancy is terminated by a registered medical practitioner and two registered medical practitioners are of the opinion, formed in good faith:

(a) that the continuance of the pregnancy would involve risk to the life of the pregnant woman or injury to her physical or mental health or the physical or mental health of any existing children of her family greater than if the pregnancy were terminated. In making this decision the doctors may take into account the pregnant woman's actual or reasonably foreseeable environment.

(b) that there is a substantial risk that the child if born would suffer from such physical or mental abnormalities as to be seriously handicapped.

The treatment for the termination of the pregnancy must be carried out in a hospital vested in the Minister of Health or the Secretary of State under the Health Service Acts, or in a place approved by them for the purpose.

Where the operation is urgently necessary to save the life of or prevent grave permanent injury to the woman, the necessity for having the opinions from two registered medical practitioners and performing the operation in an approved hospital is waived.

The Act instructs the Minister of Health in England and the Secretary of State in Scotland to make regulations to provide for the forms to be

SCHEDULE 1

IN CONFIDENCE   **Certificate A**

*Not to be destroyed within three years of
the date of the operation*

ABORTION ACT 1967

CERTIFICATE TO BE COMPLETED IN RELATION TO ABORTION
UNDER SECTION 1(1) OF THE ACT

I, ...
(Name and qualifications of practitioner in block capitals)

of ....

....
(Full address of practitioner)

and I, ...
(Name and qualifications of practitioner in block capitals)

of ....

....
(Full address of practitioner)

hereby certify that we are of the opinion, formed in good faith, that in the

case of...
(Full name of pregnant woman in block capitals)

of ....

....
(Usual place of residence of pregnant woman in block capitals)

(1) the continuance of the pregnancy would involve risk to the life of the   (Ring
    pregnant woman greater than if the pregnancy were terminated;   appropriate
                                                                              number(s))

(2) the continuance of the pregnancy would involve risk of injury to the
    physical or mental health of the pregnant woman greater than if the
    pregnancy were terminated;

(3) the continuance of the pregnancy would involve risk of injury to the
    physical or mental health of the existing child(ren) of the family of the
    pregnant woman greater than if the pregnancy were terminated;

(4) there is a substantial risk that if the child were born it would suffer
    from such physical or mental abnormalities as to be seriously handi-
    capped.

This certificate of opinion is given before the commencement of the treatment
for the termination of pregnancy to which it refers.

Signed ....

Date..

Signed ....

Date..

IN CONFIDENCE   **Certificate B**

*Not to be destroyed within three years of
the date of the operation*

ABORTION ACT 1967

CERTIFICATE TO BE COMPLETED IN RELATION TO ABORTION PERFORMED
IN EMERGENCY UNDER SECTION 1(4) OF THE ACT

I, ...

(Name and qualifications of practitioner in block capitals)

of ....

....

(Full address of practitioner)

hereby certify that I *am/was of the opinion formed in good faith that it *is/was
necessary immediately to terminate the pregnancy of

....

(Full name of pregnant woman in block capitals)

of ....

....

(Usual place of residence of pregnant woman in block capitals)

(Ring
appropriate
number)

in order (1) to save the life of the pregnant woman; or

      (2) to prevent grave permanent injury to the physical or mental health
of the pregnant woman.

This certificate of opinion is given—

    A. before the commencement of the treatment for the termination of the
pregnancy to which it relates; or, if that is not reasonably practicable,
then

    B. not later than 24 hours after such termination.

Signed ....

               Date..

           * Delete as appropriate.

used by medical practitioners and the notification of terminations of
pregnancy to the Chief Medical Officers of the Ministry of Health and
the Scottish Home and Health Department.

There is a special section permitting pregnancies in members of
visiting Forces to be terminated by their own doctors in their own
hospitals on the same conditions as those stated above.

Section 4 states that no person who has a conscientious objection is
under a duty to participate in treatment authorised by this Act unless it
is necessary to save the life of or prevent grave permanent injury to the
woman.

SCHEDULE 2

IN CONFIDENCE

ABORTION ACT 1967: ABORTION (SCOTLAND) REGULATIONS 1968

NOTIFICATION OF AN ABORTION PERFORMED UNDER SECTION 1 OF THE ACT

I, ...

(Name and qualifications of practitioner)   BLOCK CAPITALS

of ....

....

(Full address of practitioner)

hereby give notice that I terminated the pregnancy of

....

(Full name of pregnant woman)

of ....

....

(Usual place of residence of pregnant woman)

The statutory grounds certified for terminating the pregnancy were:—

OTHERWISE THAN IN EMERGENCY

(1) the continuance of the pregnancy would have involved risk to the life of the pregnant woman greater than if the pregnancy were terminated;   (Ring appropriate number(s))

(2) the continuance of the pregnancy would have involved risk of injury to the physical or mental health of the pregnant woman greater than if the pregnancy were terminated;

(3) the continuance of the pregnancy would have involved risk of injury to the physical or mental health of the existing child(ren) of the family of the pregnant woman greater than if the pregnancy were terminated;

(4) there was a substantial risk that if the child had been born it would have suffered from such physical or mental abnormalities as to be seriously handicapped;

IN CASE OF EMERGENCY

(5) it was necessary to save the life of the pregnant woman; *or*

(6) it was necessary to prevent grave permanent injury to the physical or mental health of the pregnant woman.

THE PREGNANCY WAS TERMINATED AT (to be completed for all terminations)

Name of hospital/approved place/other place ....

(address) ....

....

on (date) ....

Signature of practitioner who terminated pregnancy

....

In all non-emergency cases, particulars of the practitioner(s) who joined in giving the certificate required for the purposes of section 1 should be shown below in the appropriate space(s):—

If the operating practitioner joined in giving certificate insert at A. particulars of the other certifying practitioner.
}
A. Name ....
   Address ....
   ....

If the operating practitioner did not join in giving certificate insert at A. & B. particulars of the two certifying practitioners.
}
B. Name ....
   Address ....
   ....

NOTE: This form is to be completed by the operating practitioner and sent *within seven days of the termination of the pregnancy* in a sealed envelope marked 'In confidence' to the Chief Medical Officer, Scottish Home and Health Department, St. Andrew's House, Edinburgh, 1.

Part II (ALL QUESTIONS TO BE ANSWERED
to the best of the notifying practitioner's knowledge and belief)

ADDITIONAL PARTICULARS OF PATIENT

1. Maiden surname ....
2. Date of birth ....
3. Hospital case reference number ....
4. Marital status of woman:

    1. Single   2. Married   3. Widowed
        4. Divorced/separated   5. Not known
            (Ring appropriate number)

5. Husband's occupation ....
6. Patient's occupation (if any) ....

PREVIOUS OBSTETRIC HISTORY CURRENT PREGNANCY

7. Total no. of pregnancies ....   13. Estimated duration of gestation
                          ....
8. No. of live births ....   14. Date of admission for termin-
9. No. of still births ....   ation ....
10. No. of abortions ....   15. Date of discharge (if known) ....
11. No. of surviving children ....
12. Date of last termination under Act (where applicable) ....

SPECIFIC INDICATIONS FOR TERMINATION OF PREGNANCY
(Enter reasons in appropriate section(s) below)

16. Obstetric and/or gynaecological conditions in mother ....
....

17. Other organic and/or psychiatric conditions in mother ....
....

18. Risk of abnormality of fetus ....

....

19. Medico-social reasons ....

....

20. TYPE OF TERMINATION (ring appropriate number)
    1. Dilation and evacuation   2. Abdominal hysterotomy
    3. Vaginal hysterotomy   4. Vacuum aspiration
    5. Other (specify)   ....

21. Was HYSTERECTOMY or OTHER STERILISATION carried out (specify) ....

....

22. COMPLICATIONS PRIOR TO NOTIFICATION (ring appropriate number(s))
    1. None   2. Sepsis   3. Haemorrhage
    4. Other (specify) ....

23. In Case of DEATH specify cause ....

The incidence of spontaneous and criminal abortion has never been known. Various estimates have been made but there has been very little sound evidence for these calculations. In the House of Lords' Second Reading Debate on the Abortion Bill in November 1965, Lord Silkin, for the Government, estimated that 100,000 illegal abortions were performed or attempted annually. Goodhart[42] claims this figure to be about five times too high, basing his claim on extrapolation from mortality figures. In 1964, there were 50 deaths from abortions not carried out by doctors. More information was available about therapeutic abortions, but due to inadequate statistical facilities in hospitals this information also is not very informative.

Since the passing of the Abortion Act, 1967, more accurate statistics have become available. There appears to have been a large increase in therapeutic terminations. A leading article in a recent *British Medical Journal* [43] calculated that the rate may be running at 80,000 a year. They were commenting on a report by the Royal College of Obstetricians and Gynaecologists into the First Year's Working of the 1967 Act. They stated that 90 per cent of the consultants performing operations under the Act varied sufficiently in their practice for the position to be such that members of the public in some areas were genuinely worried about the difficulty of having pregnancy terminated. Elsewhere it appeared that consultants were agreeing to terminate every pregnancy on request without serious question, not because they believed in that course but because the brevity of their decision allowed proper time for the treatment of other patients and the teaching of staff and students.

It is certainly clear that whether or not the Abortion Act, 1967, 'clarified the law relating to termination of pregnancy' it did not result in any uniformity in application of the Act by members of the medical profession.

Since the introduction of the new Act and covering the period April 1968 to December 1970 there were 160,264 notified legal abortions in England and 10,792 in Scotland. Broken down into round figures for the whole of Britain, the number of legal terminations in the first eight months after the Act became operational was 24,000, in 1969 58,000, and in 1970 92,000. There is no sign that the rate of growth is slackening.

Whereas in England the proportion of legal abortions carried out in 'approved places' as defined by the Act is about 45 per cent, in Scotland less than 0·5 per cent are carried out there.

The fastest rise in the incidence of abortion is among teenage girls, and in under sixteens there has also been a recent rise in the number of illegitimate births. In fact in 1970 there were 117 terminations for girls under the age of sixteen.

An analysis of the reasons for which abortions were authorised and carried out in the months of 1968 during which the Act was effective in England and Wales shows that by far the majority were on psychiatric grounds (18,000 out of 24,000).[44, 45, 46] Among the organic diseases recorded the most frequently given grounds were neoplastic disease, cardiac and hypertensive disease, asthma, and renal infections. A small proportion of the legal terminations was on the grounds of the fetus being defective, and here rubella was by far the commonest reason. About 4,000 cases were for non-medical reasons with the two extremes of maternal age being cited, while others referred to financial state, poor housing, and the behaviour of the husband.

CRIMINAL ABORTION

Modes of producing abortion illegally

From the terms of sections 58 and 59, Offences Against the Person Act, 1861, it will be apparent that, although the illegal employment of a poison, other noxious thing, or an instrument is condescended upon, 'other means whatsoever' will embrace any other mode which might not be comprehended under any of the named causes.

Although the actual figure is unknown, it has been estimated that about 20 per cent of pregnancies end in natural abortion, and therefore that cases of suspected criminal abortion must be investigated with great thoroughness in order to establish whether the abortion has been brought about by criminal means.

From the medico-legal point of view, the methods of inducing criminal abortion may be divided into two main classes:

> Employment of drugs.
> Employment of instruments.

Drugs

It is impossible to assert that any given drug in any given dose will produce abortion. Death may occur from poisoning without the onset of abortion.

Among quacks, the employment of drugs is a method of attempting to procure abortion, chiefly because the sale or supply may be effected under circumstances incapable of legal proof, but most of them, short of toxic dosage, have little or no effect on the uterus or fetus, since the uterus would appear to be sensitive towards them only when it is approaching term. Among the inexperienced, many drugs are employed, such as the free use of cathartic medicines. Certain other drugs are employed by those who are more enlightened, such as cantharides, diachylon, or lead plaster, made up as pills, ergot, the free use of quinine, extract of cottonwood, and several others. The practitioner who has fallen into devious ways, and who knows the comparative uselessness of drugs for this purpose, usually resorts to mechanical interference by the use of instruments.

Under disguised names, such as 'Female Remedies for Obstructions', etc., a considerable traffic in abortifacient drugs exists. By the Pharmacy and Medicines Act, 1941, no person was allowed to take any part in the publication of any advertisement referring to any article or articles of any description, in terms which are calculated to lead to the use of that article or articles of that description for procuring the miscarriage of women. This Act has been repealed by the Medicines Act, 1968, but this provision has yet to come into force.

All drugs having an abortifacient effect usually operate in one of the three following ways, namely: by acting on the body generally as a poison; by acting locally and indirectly upon the uterus through the gastro-intestinal or genito-urinary tract; by acting locally and directly upon the muscular structure of the uterus.

Little need be said about the vast number of drugs which have been used with the object of inducing abortion, but some consideration must be given to a limited number which apparently exert a definite action upon the uterus. Of these, pituitary extract, ergot, quinine, lead, and the prostaglandins are worthy of special mention.

Pituitary extract An extract of the posterior lobe of the pituitary gland exercises an oxytocic action, and stimulates the uterine muscle which is extremely sensitive to this particular substance. Pituitrin has a specific effect on uterine muscle, causing definite and strong contractions, especially near term.

Ergot. This is a true ecbolic which acts on the musculature of the uterus on account of the contained substances, ergotoxine, ergotinine, ergotamine, ergometrine and ergotaminine, in addition to histamine and tyramine. Experiments have shown that the alkaloid ergotoxine produces uterine contractions in about fifteen to thirty minutes. It is the most important factor in ergot poisoning, and causes contraction of the arterioles. Ergometrine, however, is the substance which is chiefly responsible for the action of ergot on the uterus. When given by the mouth, it produces a prolonged contraction of the uterus within about five minutes. The uterus is particularly sensitive immediately following the birth of its contents. When liquid extract of ergot is taken orally, a very marked contraction of the uterus follows after a latent period of a few minutes due to the water-soluble alkaloid ergometrine.

Quinine. It is now generally accepted that quinine definitely increases uterine contractions of a rhythmic character, raises the tone of the muscle, and that it may induce uterine contractions (see p. 687).

Lead. Diachylon, or lead plaster, which contains oleate of lead, is sometimes employed as an abortifacient. This substance is easily rolled into pills which are coated with substances of different colour. Dilling found that lead causes tonic contraction of the uterus. It is believed to have a toxic action on the trophoblastic epithelium of the ovum. For these reasons lead must be regarded as a definite abortifacient drug. Symptoms of lead poisoning have frequently shown themselves in persons who have taken diachylon for the purpose of abortion, and in some of these cases there have been fatal terminations.

In one of our cases, the pregnant woman had been given pills and had been instructed to take three of them daily until abortion resulted. The woman aborted.

Ergot and lead plaster are included in the Poisons List to which special restrictions apply (see pp. 489 and 495).

Synthetic oestrogens. There is some evidence that excessive dosages of these substances are in use as abortifacients.

Prostaglandins. Although the work on prostaglandins is in its infancy, mention of these new and powerful oxytocic hormones must be made, due to the implications of their eventual use. Prostaglandins exert an oxytocic effect on the uterus at all stages of pregnancy and at present clinical trials are in progress mainly to study their effects on the induction of labour. However, their abortifacient capabilities have been proved.[47, 48, 49, 50] Abortion on demand and at any time in pregnancy could become a practical possibility and this opens up a variety of social, ethical, and legal problems. If these chemicals become easily available, as seems probable, and are innocuous, controversy about the Abortion Act and in fact the Act itself will rapidly become irrelevant.

Reference to the study and use of these hormones is made in the list of references at the end of this chapter.[51, 52]

Instruments

Instruments may be used in the first instance or be resorted to when drugs have failed to induce abortion.

Instrumental interference, usually attempted after the second or third missed period, is brought about by the employment of a wide variety of instruments, which includes such implements as knitting or crochet needles, wooden or metal skewers, catheters, sounds, curettes, syringes, and the bark of slippery elm, among many others. Abortionists may rupture the membranes and then request the patient to report to her own doctor. A woman may induce abortion on herself, but usually this is done by a second person. Sometimes the woman may try to persuade her doctor to pass a sound on the pretext that she is suffering from a uterine displacement.

For many years, the bark of slippery elm, *Ulmus fulva*, has been employed, either in the form of a tent or as a long stem which is passed into the cervix, since it has the property of exuding mucilaginous material and of absorbing moisture, thus causing dilatation of the cervix by the resultant increase in bulk of the portion inserted. The bark is obtained from a tree which grows in Central and South America. It occurs in flat pieces of varying length and width and is about $\frac{1}{8}$ inch in thickness. The pieces are cut to the desired length and breadth prior to insertion.

The chief danger of instrumental interference is from septicaemia following wounding of the parts.

Cook[53] has recorded an interesting analysis of three hundred and fifty cases of abortion which were admitted to hospital. His conclusions were that about 40 per cent of these had probably been procured, that the commonest cause of procured abortion was probably the insertion of slippery elm bark, and that local interference was usually performed with a certain amount of mechanical skill, since it was rare to find positive evidence of injury. Uterine sepsis, accompanied by pyrexia, was present in 35 per cent of the cases, and uterine sepsis, without pyrexia, in about a further 10 per cent of the cases. Of these patients, 20 per cent were decidedly ill and 3 per cent died. With one exception, all the deaths were due to sepsis. Definite injury was present in four cases, two of which proved fatal, due to perforation of the uterus and perforation of the vaginal fornix. His analysis of the stage of pregnancy at which abortion took place was as follows:

Under two months . . . . . 46 cases
Between two and three months . . . 126 „

Between three and four months .   .   . 124 „
Between four and five months   .   .   . 44 „
Between five and six months   .   .   . 10 „

The injection of fluids into the uterus, frequently with a Higginson's syringe, for the purpose of inducing abortion is quite common.   Tepid water, soap and water or disinfectants such as carbolic acid or lysol, are often used and each is fraught with danger.   Apart from the danger of absorption of poisonous substances, in cases in which these may be employed, there is always the grave risk of sudden death from syncope or from air embolism.

Skilled interference usually leaves no traces.   When dilatation of the cervix or perforation of the membranes has been undertaken, abortion usually results in about fifty to sixty hours.   During the first three months of pregnancy, skilled interference takes the form of dilatation of the cervix under anaesthesia, and immediate evacuation of the uterus with a curette or by vacuum aspiration.   During the later months the procedure is usually abdominal hysterotomy.

The withdrawal of amniotic fluid and its replacement by the injection of strongly hypertonic solutions has been used to produce therapeutic abortions.   Cameron and Dayan[54] have described three cases in which this technique was used and death resulted from acute haemorrhagic infarction of the amygdaloid nuclei and adjacent structures in the brain. This technique is relatively simple and could well be used by criminal abortionists.

Duties of medical practitioners in relation to cases of criminal abortion

The resolutions of the Royal College of Physicians,[55] concerning the duties of medical practitioners in relation to cases of criminal abortion are:

> That a moral obligation rests upon every medical practitioner to respect the confidence of his patient, and that without her consent he is not justified in disclosing information obtained in the course of his professional attendance on her.
>
> That every medical practitioner who is convinced that criminal abortion has been practised on his patient, should urge her, especially when she is likely to die, to make a statement which may be taken as evidence against the person who has performed the operation, provided always that her chances of recovery are not thereby prejudiced.
>
> That in the event of her refusal to make such a statement, he is under no legal obligation to take further action, but he should continue to attend the patient to the best of his ability.

That before taking any action which may lead to legal proceedings, a medical practitioner will be wise to obtain the best medical and legal advice available, both to ensure that the patient's statement may have value as legal evidence, and to safeguard his own interests, since in the present state of the law there is no certainty that he will be protected against subsequent litigation.

That if the patient should die, he should refuse to give a certificate of the cause of death, and should communicate with the Coroner. (Note.—In Scotland, the Procurator-Fiscal of the area is the official to whom the communication should be made.)

The College has been advised that the medical practitioner is under no legal obligation either to urge the patient to make a statement, or, if she refuses to do so, to take any further action (see above).

(Note.—With regard to dying declarations and dying depositions, p. 46.)

Evidence of criminal abortion. Upon what must medical evidence of criminal abortion depend? The following should be taken into full and careful consideration before an opinion is offered:

The history of the woman.
The examination of her body.
The examination of the aborted material, if available.

It is important to remember that criminal abortion is most usually practised between the second and fourth months of pregnancy, although it may be induced at later periods, and that an attempt to procure abortion may be made upon a woman who is not pregnant but who merely fears that she is because her menses have temporarily ceased.

History of the woman. In many instances, this may not come within the knowledge of the medical examiner, but when there is a history of the use of drugs or instruments, all the available facts and circumstances should be carefully reviewed.

Examination of the woman's body. When opportunity offers, in living cases, the examination must be made as soon as possible, and should include a careful scrutiny of all evidence consistent with recent pregnancy together with a vaginal examination. The finger may not be able to detect small breaches of continuity, but it will probably discover changes in the 'feel' of the mucous membrane of the os, and of the patency of the os. Visual examination with a speculum is essential, since not only will the general condition of the genital tract be ascertained but, if injury is present, it will be more readily detected. In some cases of criminal abortion, haemorrhage may persist due to a retained portion of the membranes or placenta.

A suspicion of criminal abortion should be aroused when the patient shows signs and symptoms of localised sepsis or of general septicaemia. It must not be forgotten, however, that sepsis may follow natural abortion, but in such cases there is usually some preceding clinical history.

In cases of criminal abortion, death may result from shock due to internal injury, haemorrhage, sepsis, which may assume the form of peritonitis or septicaemia, or from embolism. When poisonous substances have been administered, death may supervene from their effects.

In making a post-mortem examination, the examiner should note carefully the presence or absence of the signs of pregnancy which may be visible upon the exterior of the body. The breasts should be examined and an incision on the under surface of each made to ascertain secretory activity. Having inspected the vaginal tract, dissection of the body should be proceeded with in the ordinary manner and special attention directed to the condition of the pelvic contents. The first thing to note will be the presence or absence of inflammation in this cavity, and, if present, its incidence and extent. Before removing any of the parts from the cavity, careful search must be made for the presence or absence of any penetrating wound of the peritoneum, and if present, the position and character with relation to the uterus, and the tissues penetrated must be noted. Special attention must be directed to the posterior fornix of the vagina, in the region of the pouch of Douglas, since this is a common site of injury in criminal abortion. Thereafter the pelvic viscera are removed *en masse* (p. 34). The parts are then examined, carefully and systematically, in a good light. Portions of tissue, including tissue from the placental site, for microscopic examination, should not be excised until the general examination has been completed.

The urinary tract is carefully inspected for signs of inflammation, such as might be produced by cantharides or turpentine, and the vaginal tract, for evidence of injury.

The length, breadth, and thickness of the uterus, the length of the uterine cavity, the circumference of the external os, and the length of the cervix should be recorded (p. 755). The uterus and the cervix must be examined in detail to establish or eliminate the presence of injury. When small lacerations of the cervix are detected, inquiry should be made regarding possible remedial surgical treatment in hospital prior to death, since such marks are sometimes caused when the cervix is gripped by vulsella. The ovaries are examined for the presence of a corpus luteum (see p. 370). In septic cases, any source of infection from organs other than those of the pelvis, especially the appendix, must be eliminated.

Where there are no signs of local injury, the condition of the gastro-intestinal tract must be examined very carefully for evidence of irritant poisoning, and when such evidence is found, the whole tract and its contents, together with other organs of the body, should be placed in clean jars for the purpose of subsequent analysis.

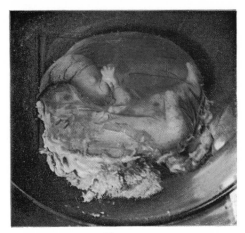

FIG. 205
Fetus lying in unruptured membranes

Examination of the aborted material.   Any available material passed by the vagina should be carefully examined, since if it can be proved that it is composed of products of conception, the fact of pregnancy will at once be established.   If a fetus has been retained, an estimation of the stage of its development should be made (p. 76).   In the dead body, portions of material found within the uterus should be the subject of detailed naked-eye and microscopic examination.   It is always advisable to remove a piece of tissue from what is thought to have been the placental site, so that the presence of chorionic villi may be identified microscopically (Figs. 206 and 207).

Has the abortion been produced criminally?

It must be kept prominently in mind that abortion may be produced accidentally, or from disease.   The commoner diseases are chronic nephritis, diabetes, acute fevers, especially of the exanthematous type, degenerative changes in the villi of the chorion or in the placenta, together with accidental haemorrhage between the uterine wall and the placenta.   Maternal syphilis causes most serious harm from the third month onwards, and in the later weeks of pregnancy may result in miscarriage and still-birth.   Diseases of the fetus are also a cause of

GMJ—CC*

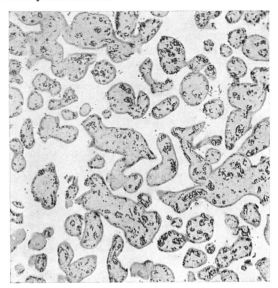

FIG. 206

Chorionic villi at earlier stage of development and vascularisation. (Section by courtesy of Dr D. McKay Hart) ×80

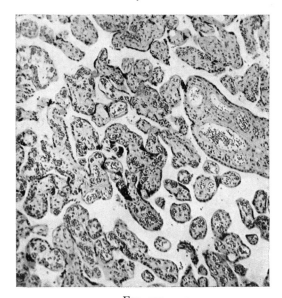

FIG. 207

Chorionic villi at later stage of development and vascularisation. (Section by courtesy of Dr D. McKay Hart) ×90

abortion. Violent emotion in certain types of women is traditionally held to be responsible.

Abortion may also be produced in some women by apparently trifling accidents, and a miscalculated step from a height, a marked and sudden jar to the body, or an accidental knock against the abdomen, may prove a precipitating cause. In other women, even serious abdominal injury may fail to precipitate the expulsion of the fetus, despite the fact that pregnancy may be approaching full-term.

The question of criminal abortion arises when there is evidence of injury to the vaginal wall, the cervix, or to the uterus.

Cases arise from time to time in which, from attendant circumstances, medical practitioners may be compromised, but in which the abortion has been brought about by the woman herself, either by the administration of drugs or by instrumental interference.

A medical practitioner may be called in after the process of abortion has been initiated by the woman herself, or by another, to save the life of the woman, and should she die without confession, and a post-mortem examination of her body should follow, it is not difficult to understand how he might be compromised in the eyes of the law, and how serious consequences to him might result. In any doubtful case he should call in a fellow-practitioner in order to safeguard himself. It is also advisable to make arrangements for a neighbour of the patient, or preferably a nurse, to be called in so that she may be able to corroborate the facts concerning the abortion, prior to admission of the patient to hospital.

ILLUSTRATIVE CASES

The following illustrative cases include many of the points which have been discussed:

General peritonitis. On the right side of the anterior fornix was a lacerated wound, $\frac{1}{2}$ inch by $\frac{1}{4}$ inch. It passed upwards and backwards for 2 inches, and penetrated the peritoneal cavity. The track admitted a No. 10 metal catheter. Two pints of pus were present in the abdomen. Around the entrance of track were five additional superficial wounds varying in length from $\frac{1}{2}$ to $\frac{1}{16}$ inch. These involved the mucosa and showed parallelism. There were also two other superficial wounds.

General peritonitis and septicaemia. Two lacerated wounds perforated the posterior wall of the uterus and entered the pelvic cavity (Fig. 208).

Slippery elm bark retained in vagina. A woman, when examined, was found to have a piece of slippery elm bark in her vagina. It

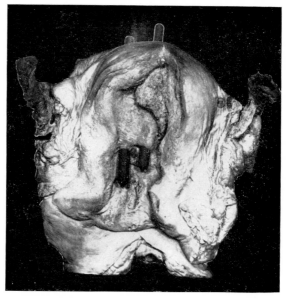

FIG. 208

Two lacerated perforations of posterior wall of uterus

measured 4 inches by $\frac{1}{2}$ inch by $\frac{1}{8}$ inch and was retained in position by a plug of cotton-wool about the size of a small walnut.   One of its ends had been cut into an arrowhead shape.   The other end had a small pledglet of cotton-wool wrapped around it.   The woman, who was four months pregnant, did not abort.   The slippery elm had not been self-inserted.   The woman had given birth to six children.

Localised peritonitis involving uterus and pouch of Douglas. The following injuries were present:

A lacerated wound, immediately to right of midline of anterior wall of vagina, 8 mm in length and in antero-posterior direction.

A similar wound 9 mm long, to right of, and just below, the first.

A similar wound, 7 mm long, on right wall of vagina, to right and slightly below the last-mentioned wound.

All three wounds were situated peripherally at points 3 cm from the external os, and pus exuded from the openings on slight pressure.   The first wound extended upwards in the posterior wall of bladder and utero-vesical tissue to the utero-vesical fold of peritoneum.   The second wound extended upwards and to the right, passing more obliquely and to a slightly higher level than the first, to terminate in cellular tissue infiltrated with pus.   The third wound terminated in septic cellular tissue at the root of the right broad ligament. In the middle of the posterior lip of cervix was a small septic opening 3 mm in diameter, and extending upwards in the posterior wall of cervix for a distance of 5 cm. A few millimetres to the right of this was a punctate wound $1\frac{1}{2}$ mm in diameter which penetrated tissue for 3 mm.

Sudden death following use of syringe. A woman was charged with inserting a syringe into the private parts of a young woman and injecting a solution of soap and water, in consequence of which she died. The woman was convicted. The victim, who was between four and five months pregnant, died suddenly from cardiac inhibition during the injection. About 350 ml of pultaceous, white, cloudy-looking material, containing many sago-like grains and with a scented odour, were found lying between the amniotic sac and the wall of the uterus. The cervical canal and both its external and internal os were dilated. The external and internal os each measured $\frac{1}{4}$ inch in diameter. The cervical canal contained some slightly blood-stained, glairy mucus. On the inner surface of the lateral wall of the cervical canal, running upwards for $\frac{1}{2}$ inch from the external os, was a surface laceration which communicated externally with a small lacerated wound on the outer surface of the os. Microscopic examination showed that the laceration had been inflicted during life, and its general appearances were consistent with recent injury and could readily have been caused by the forcible introduction of a foreign body. The extraneous substance in the uterine cavity was examined chemically and found to consist of soap. A cake of soap, similar to that used, was also analysed and the results compared with those obtained from analysis of the material found within the uterus. Both were similar in odour and chemical composition. The general development of the fetus and placenta present in uterus indicated a fourth to fifth month pregnancy.

Gordon[56] describes the case of an eighteen-year-old girl, five months pregnant, who was found lying on her back on the floor, dead, with a basin of soapy water nearby. Post-mortem examination showed air bubbles in the cerebral veins and in the external jugular veins. Frothy blood was present in the internal jugular veins, the right ventricle, right auricle, and in the pulmonary artery. A moderate amount of blood-stained fluid was in the uterine cavity. The placenta was detached from the uterine wall along its lower edge. The fetal membranes were unruptured.

Brown[57] writes of fatal air embolism after insufflation of the vagina owing to vaginal discharge, eight weeks prior to term. The substance used was 'Picragol' powder, a compound powder containing 1 per cent silver picrate in purified kaolin. Within a minute of the start of insufflation, the woman, aged twenty-five, and a primipara, complained of a feeling of being 'blown up', acute dyspnoea supervened, she had a

fit, recovered slightly, then died.   Post-mortem examination showed
dilatation of the right side of the heart.   The right ventricle contained
very little blood, frothed into large bubbles.   The right uterine plexus
contained frothy blood.   The right ovarian vein contained particles of
yellow powder.   The edge of the placenta was stripped for a depth of
about 1 to 1½ inches from the right side of the uterus.   The membranes
on this side were completely free.   Blood sinuses on the right side of
the uterus, in the vicinity of the stripped part of the placenta and
membranes, contained frothy blood, and these drained directly from
the uterine plexus already mentioned.   Insufflation of the vagina with
the cervix partly dilated had allowed the entrance of air into the blood
sinuses of the uterus, after the ballooning effect of the insufflation had
stripped the membranes and a portion of the placenta from their site.

Shapiro[58] has described the difficulties inherent in the diagnosis of
air embolism, especially where death is due to delayed air embolism.

Dodds and Mayeur[59] report a case of perforation of the posterior
vaginal wall and rectum by the hard nozzle of a Higginson's syringe.
The patient was twenty-four and pregnant.   Following suture, she
made a complete recovery and was subsequently delivered successfully
by Caesarean section.

Slippery elm bark in urethra.   Farncombe[60] describes a case of
attempted abortion by self-introduction of slippery elm into the urethra
instead of the vagina, in error.   There was a small amount of granulation tissue surrounding the urinary meatus.   Radiological examination
showed the presence of a cylindrical foreign body lying in the region of
the urethra and neck of bladder.   The woman admitted having introduced a piece of slippery elm into the womb, as she thought, during the
third month of pregnancy.   The patient, who was at full time when she
came under observation, was thirty-nine and the mother of six children,
went into labour unexpectedly before operation for removal of the
foreign body.   The labour was normal, and she was delivered of a
healthy, full-time child which weighed 7 pounds.   Considerable
damage resulted to the urinary tract.   Suprapubic cystotomy was
performed and the foreign body, projecting from the urethra into the
bladder, was removed.   It consisted of a core of slippery elm, about
10 inches long and $\frac{1}{6}$ inch in diameter.   The piece, which was doubled
on itself, had a deposit of phosphates upon it which formed a conical
mass, 4½ inches by 2½ inches.   The woman made a good recovery.

References

1.   FAIRFIELD, L.   *Lancet*, **2**, 61, 1940.
2.   HODGSON, N.   *Br. med. J.*, **2**, 61, 1940.
3.   PATEL, J.B.   *Br. med. J.*, **1**, 1159, 1937.
4.   G's Trustees v. G., 1936, S.C., 837.

5. ANDREASON, A.T. *Br. med. J.*, **2**, 211, 1935.
6. PEEL, J.H. & BRUDENELL, J.M. *Textbook of Gynaecology*, 6th ed., p. 341. Heinemann, 1969.
7. BISHOP, P.M.F. *Br. med. J.*, **1**, 1255, 1966.
8. *British Medical Journal*, **1**, 185, 1967.
9. MORISON, H. *Br. J. Surg.*, **22**, 619, 1934-35.
10. RAYNAND, MARILL, & XICLUNA. *Presse méd.*, **47**, 459, 1939.
11. O'FARRELL, J.M. *J. Am. med. Ass.*, **104**, 1968, 1935.
12. Bravery v. Bravery [1954] 3 All E.R., 59.
13. HANLEY, H.G. *Br. J. hosp. Med.*, **6**, 156, 1971.
14. F. v. F., 1945, S.C., 202.
15. R. v. R. [1952], 1 All E.R., 1194.
16. Clarke v. Clarke [1943] 2 All E.R., 540.
17. *Lancet*, **1**, 89, 1943.
18. Baxter v. Baxter [1947] 1 All E.R., 387.
19. Cowen v. Cowen [1945] 2 All E.R., 197.
20. *Lancet*, **1**, 883, 1948.
21. Corbett v. Corbett (1970) C.L.Y.B. 808; [1970] 2 W.L.R., 1306.
22. *Artificial Human Insemination*, Report held under the auspices of the Public Morality Council. Heinemann, 1947.
23. FORBES, G. *Med.-leg. crim. Rev.*, **12**, 138, 1944.
24. Maclennan v. Maclennan, 1958 S.L.T. 12.
25. FAIRFIELD, L. *Lancet*, **2**, 61, 1940.
26. *British Medical Journal*, **1**, 878, 1953.
27. McCANN. *Med.-leg. crim. Rev.*, **4**, 16, 1936.
28. GILBERTSON, J.H. *Br. med. J.*, **1**, 378, 1917.
29. FERRIS, J. *Human Fertility and Problems of the Male.* Author's Press Inc., 1950.
30. SEYMOUR, F.I. *J. Am. med. Ass.*, **104**, 1728, 1936.
31. LANE-ROBERTS, C.S., SHARMAN, A., *et al.* *Sterility and Impaired Fertility*, Hamish Hamilton, 1948.
32. SEVITT, S. *Lancet*, **2**, 448, 1946.
33. Gaskill v. Gaskill [1921], P. 425; *Lancet*, **2**, 357, 1921.
34. Clark v. Clark [1939] P. 228.
35. Hadlum v. Hadlum [1948] 2 All E.R., 412, 425.
36. Wood v. Wood [1947] P. 103.
37. Preston-Jones v. Preston-Jones [1950] 1 All E.R., 124.
38. HIGGINS, L.G. *Lancet*, **2**, 1154, 1954.
39. McKEOWN, T. & GIBSON, J.R. *Br. med. J.*, **1**, 938, 1952.
40. R. v. Hollis (1873), 28, L.T., 455.
41. R. v. Hennah (1877), 13, Cox C.C., 547.
42. GOODHART, C.B. *J. Biosoc. Sci.*, **1**, 235, 1969.
43. *British Medical Journal*, **2**, 491, 1970.
44. *The Registrar General's Statistical Review of England and Wales* for the year 1968, Supplement on Abortion. H.M.S.O., 1970.
45. *British Medical Journal*, **3**, 362, 1970.
46. FINNIS, J.M. [1971] Crim. L.R. 9.
47. KARIM, S.M.M. *Conference on Prostaglandins.* New York Academy of Sciences, 1970.
48. KARIM, S.M.M. & FILSHIE, G.M. *Lancet*, **1**, 157, 1970.
49. KARIM, S.M.M. & FILSHIE, G.M. *Br. med. J.*, **3**, 198, 1970.
50. EMBREY, M.P. *Br. med. J.*, **2**, 258, 1970.
51. BEAZLEY, J.M. *Br. J. hosp. Med.*, **5**, 535, 1971.
52. KARIM, S.M.M. *Br. J. hosp. Med.*, **5**, 555, 1971.
53. COOK, R.G. *Br. med. J.*, **1**, 1045, 1938.

54. CAMERON, J.M. & DAYAN, A.D.   *Br. med. J.*, **1,** 1010, 1966.
55. *British Medical Journal*, **1,** 207, 1916.
56. GORDON.   *Clin. Proc.*, **4,** 135, 1945.
57. BROWN, R.L.   *Lancet*, **1,** 616, 1943.
58. SHAPIRO, H.A.   *J. forens. Med.*, **12,** 3, 1965.
59. DODDS, R.L. & MAYEUR, M.M.   *Br. med. J.*, **1,** 921, 1939.
60. FARNCOMBE, R.   *Lancet*, **2,** 825, 1935.

Chapter 14

INFANTICIDE OR CHILD MURDER

The killing of a newly born child is, in England, known as infanticide, and the crime may be committed either by acts of omission or by acts of commission.

Infanticide by an act of omission means neglect to do what is necessary for the continuance of the life of a newly born child, for example, neglecting to tie the umbilical cord after severance, since by omitting to do this the infant may bleed to death, neglecting to clothe it in a reasonable way so as to protect it from cold, or failing to remove such obstacles as would prevent it from breathing.

Infanticide by commission is the performance of any positive act which prevents a newly born child from living or which destroys its life.

In Scotland, the crime is known as child murder.

Law in England

Infanticide has been the subject of statutory enactments, the most recent being the Infanticide Act of 1938 by which, under certain circumstances, the killing of a newly born child by the mother is the crime of manslaughter. This Act provides that the offence of infanticide is committed when a woman by any wilful act or omission causes the death of her child, being under the age of twelve months, but at the time of the act or omission, the balance of her mind was disturbed by reason of her not having fully recovered from the effect of giving birth to the child or of lactation consequent upon the birth.

A jury may return a verdict of infanticide at the trial of a woman for the murder of her child, the child being under the age of one year, if they are of the opinion that she caused its death by an act or omission but that she was in the condition already described.

Nothing in the Act shall affect the power of the jury upon an indictment of murder of a child to return a verdict of manslaughter, or a verdict of guilty but insane, or a verdict of concealment of birth, in pursuance of section 60 of the Offences Against the Person Act, 1861, except that for the purposes of the proviso to that section a child shall be deemed to have recently been born if it had been born within twelve months before its death.

In every charge of infanticide the legal presumption is that the child is born dead, and the onus of proving that the child was born alive rests on the Crown.

As an alternative charge to infanticide the accused may be charged, under section 60 of the Offences Against the Person Act, 1861, with concealment of birth.   This section makes it an offence for every person who has endeavoured to conceal the birth of a child by any secret disposition of its dead body, whether the child died before, at, or after its birth.   If any person is tried for the murder of any child and is acquitted, the jury may find, if it so appears on evidence, that the child had been recently born, and that the accused did, by some secret disposition of the dead body of the child, endeavour to conceal the birth, in which case the court may pass such sentence as if the accused had been convicted upon an indictment for the concealment of the birth.

With the advent of the Infant Life (Preservation) Act in 1929, the law was amended with regard to the destruction of children at or before birth.   Child destruction is committed when any person, with intent to destroy the life of a child capable of being born alive, by any wilful act causes a child to die before it has an existence independent of its mother; provided that the prosecution must prove that the act was not done in good faith for the purpose only of preserving the mother's life. Thus this offence cannot be committed during the earlier stages of pregnancy.   For the purposes of the Act, evidence that a woman had at any material time been pregnant for a period of twenty-eight weeks or more shall be prima facie proof that she was at that time pregnant of a child capable of being born alive.

The Act, which applies to England only, also provides that in the trial of any person for murder or manslaughter of any child, or for infanticide, if the jury are of the opinion that the person charged is not guilty of any of these offences, but is shown by evidence to be guilty of child destruction, he may be so convicted and punished.

Law in Scotland

At common law in Scotland, there is no degree of difference between the murder of a child and the murder of an adult.   During the seventeenth century, however, the crime became one of such frequent occurrence and the difficulty of proving it so great, that an Act was passed in 1690 which provided that if certain indicia were proved, the jury were entitled to presume that the crime of child murder had been committed.   Owing to its severe nature, this enactment was repealed by the Concealment of Pregnancy Act, 1809, which reduced the crime to one of culpable homicide.

The Act of 1809 provides that if any woman conceals her being with child during the whole period of her pregnancy and does not call for and make use of help or assistance at the birth, and the child is found dead or amissing, she may be convicted and imprisoned.

Under this Act the onus is on the Crown to prove (1) that the woman was pregnant and that she concealed this fact during the whole period of pregnancy, (2) that she failed to call for or make use of help at the birth, and (3) that the child has been found dead or amissing.

It is a conclusive common law presumption that a woman who is pregnant and who does not reveal her condition or call for assistance at child-birth is recklessly indifferent to the life of the child.

It is advisable at this stage to give the legal definitions of certain terms. At common law, to constitute 'live-birth' the child must have been fully extruded from the parts of the mother, and have achieved an independent existence, but it is not necessary that the child should have breathed, or that the cord should have been cut, but the child must have given some active evidence of life.

The issue as to whether a child can have a separate existence before the umbilical cord is severed arose in a case of infanticide at Cambridge Assizes.[1] The ruling was that the entire child must actually have been born into the world in a living state, and the fact that it had breathed was not conclusive proof of separation, because it might have breathed during the act of separation. The fact that the child had breathed, although not conclusive, went some way toward the proof of independent existence. Before a child can be considered alive, it must have had an independent circulation and no longer derived its power of living by or through any connection with the mother. The fact that the child was still connected to the mother by the cord did not prevent the killing from being murder. The jury had to decide whether or not the child had shown a separate existence, if not, the mother must be acquitted of the charge of infanticide.

It will thus be seen that the legal definition of live-birth is divergent from the medical definition, as in the latter, evidence of respiratory action of the child whether initiated partly within or wholly without the maternal parts, is indicative of live-birth. Frequently, on account of the difficulty in determining by physical appearances of the body whether respiratory function was initiated while a portion of the child was within the maternal parts, or after complete extrusion, the alternative charge to infanticide or child murder, namely, a charge of concealment of birth, in England, or of pregnancy, in Scotland, is returned as the verdict of the jury.

When may a child be declared still-born?

The terms 'still-born' and 'still-birth' shall apply to any child which has issued forth from the mother after the twenty-eighth week of pregnancy, and did not at any time, after being completely expelled from its mother, breathe or show any other signs of life (pp. 141 and 148).

This question has arisen in a court of law in connection with a charge against a practitioner of alleged falsification of a birth certificate. During the evidence, a number of witnesses stated that the child was born alive about half an hour after the doctor had left the house of the mother, who was then in labour, that they heard it cry, or make a whining noise, and that it had died between three and six o'clock next morning.   The accused gave a certificate stating that the woman had been delivered of a still-born child.   He stated in his defence that the child was a six months' child, and that he inferred from this fact that it could not be born alive.   The jury gave the accused the benefit of the doubt, but stated that they believed he was guilty of gross carelessness in giving such a certificate.   It must be clearly understood that a child, irrespective of its intra-uterine development, which manifests signs of independent existence, as, for example, attempts at respiration, the act of crying, or the continuous action of the heart even for some minutes after birth, must be considered as born alive.

The following medico-legal questions arise in cases of infanticide or child murder:

Has the woman charged been recently delivered?
Is the body of the child found that of a viable child?
Is the body that of the child of the person accused?
Was the child born alive?
If the child was born alive, what caused its death?
How long has the child been dead?

Is the body of the child found that of a viable child?

The answer to the first question has already been discussed (p. 374). With regard to the second question, it should be explained that unless the child born has reached a stage of development which is consistent with the possibility of a living birth, a charge of infanticide or child murder will not usually be preferred against the mother.   In law, a fetus which has not attained the completion of the seventh month of intra-uterine life is held to be incapable of maintaining a separate existence, and is therefore non-viable.   Viability means, therefore, the capability of a fetus to maintain a separate existence after birth by virtue of a certain degree of development.   The presumption of the law, concerning the body of a child found dead and which shows evidence of less than seven months' intra-uterine age, is that the child has failed to live by reason of its immaturity.   On the other hand, should there be evidence that the immature fetus has lived after birth, and that it has been deprived of life by the act of the mother, a charge of infanticide or child murder would lie.

Is the body that of the child of the person accused?

Proof on this point is most usually established from the evidence of persons with whom the suspected woman has been more or less intimately associated in work or in social life.   A careful examination by the police of the wrappings which envelop the body of a child may throw some light on the identity of the mother.

Was the child born alive?

The answer to this question opens up a wide field for consideration.

A monster is generally considered to be incapable of living a separate existence, but this will depend upon the character of the monstrosity. Siamese twins have lived for many years. Acephalous, anencephalous, hemicephalous, ectocardiac, and other teratological subjects usually die quickly after birth, although an anencephalous monster has survived birth for sixty-one hours.

The body of a child may show evidence of maceration. This is a destructive aseptic process due to surface changes which occur within the uterus after the death of the child, and prior to its birth. It appears between 12 and 24 hours after fetal death and first reveals itself by blistering and peeling of the fetal skin. In certain cases, however, one has to decide whether such appearances were produced before or after birth, since many bodies which are examined show some evidence of decomposition.

Evidence of immaturity should be carefully noted. Infants of less than seven months of intra-uterine development are as a rule incapable of maintaining a separate existence (p. 402). Hoffmann, Greenhill, and Lundeen[2] have reported the birth and survival of a premature infant which weighed 735 g at birth. By the eighth day the infant had lost 140 g in weight. Whether or not any of the foregoing conditions are present, it must still be determined, by detailed examination of the body, whether there is evidence of live-birth or still-birth, since this question will arise in every case which is the subject of medico-legal inquiry.

The post mortem examination in all cases of infanticide or child murder must include a detailed investigation of:

> The condition of the lungs.
> The changes in the umbilicus.
> The changes in the digestive tract.
> The changes in the circulatory system.

Condition of the lungs

A detailed examination of the lungs will usually afford valid proof of the condition of the child with regard to respiration. Prior to independent life, the lungs are functionless, and it is only when the living child is born that they become organs of function. Before birth the lungs receive only a limited supply of blood necessary for their vitality and growth, but following birth the pulmonary circulation in the body of the child becomes established. In order that the process of aeration may be accomplished, respiration becomes operative. The establishment of these two vital functions, which occurs at the birth of a living child, produces physical changes in the lungs, in relation to volume, colour and weight.

Changes in volume of the lungs. Before birth the lungs do not fill the thoracic cavity, and the left lung does not even partially overlap the pericardium. In texture they resemble the consistence of liver tissue, are uniformly coloured, the lobes being indistinctly marked and the sharp edges lying in close contact. After the complete establishment of respiration they more or less fill the thoracic cavity, the degree of completeness depending upon the extent of the respiratory action. When complete aeration of the lungs has been in operation, the left lung more or less covers the pericardium. In the apex of the right lung, the appearances of inflation are usually most marked, since the air entry to this part of the lung meets with the least obstruction. Between the condition of non-inflation and complete inflation there are intermediate stages of incomplete inflation and, to determine the extent of the air entry, further examination is necessary.

Aeration of the lungs increases their weight as the vessels fill with blood once the pulmonary circulation is established. An increase from about 30 g or $\frac{1}{70}$ of the total body weight to 60 g is usual. This static test may interfere with histological examination and this can be omitted without altering the final opinion.

Colour of the lungs. Prior to respiration, the lungs are of a uniform dark bluish-red colour, but at the margins, where the tissue is thinner and therefore more translucent, they may appear lighter in colour. Unrespired fetal lungs do not present patches of different colour, but after respiration they become marbled in appearance; a dark bluish-red background with many red irregular patches may be seen, or the background may be of reddish colour, and the circumscribed patchy areas of dark bluish-red tint. The edges assume a more rounded contour. The marbling in appearance and colour is characteristic of natural inflation, and cannot be simulated by any artificial method. Fully respired lungs feel crepitant to the touch, whereas unrespired lungs feel solid and liver-like in consistence.

Hydrostatic test. This was the main test in the past and involved the determination of the buoyancy of the lungs. The test depends upon the ratio of the specific gravity of the lungs to that of water, as a lung containing air is lighter than water and will therefore float. Flotation of the lungs, however, may occur for a reason other than that of contained atmospheric air, while the lungs may sink as a result of disease or atelectasis, although the child may have breathed following birth. The test has been recognised as suspect for some time, and has no value when used alone.

Briefly it entails removing the larynx, trachea, and chest structures and placing the lungs in a sufficient amount of water, to observe the degree of buoyancy of each. Should they float, each is separated into its respective lobes and the procedure repeated after keeping two lobes for histology. If flotation again occurs, the lobes are chopped up into pieces and if they float they are wrapped in a cloth and stood upon to express putrefactive gases. If the lung has been aerated during life, it is almost impossible to squeeze out the contained air so that the pieces will sink.

Microscopy of the lungs. This is the most reliable means of deciding aeration or its lack in the lungs. The thoracic contents should be removed intact without touching the lungs themselves and fixed for 48 hours. Many samples for histology may be taken from the whole lung cut in cross-section.

In the typical still-birth, sections will show the alveoli and the bronchi collapsed, while in the aerated lung the alveoli, as well as the bronchi, are more or less expanded. The degree of dilatation of the vessels in their walls can also be ascertained and the existence of pathological processes in the lungs may be detected.

Sections may be stained specifically to demonstrate fat. The alveolar ducts may be lined by a fatty membrane, the origin of which has not yet been defined. Its formation probably indicates that the infant has breathed and was live-born. It is thought that limited distribution of this membrane is common[3] and can be found when the infant has survived its birth by at least one hour. It causes neonatal atelectasis.

In premature babies, by definition live-born and considered to have a birth weight of 2·5 kg or less, who survive at least one hour, there may be evidence of an eosinophilic hyaline membrane within dilated alveolar ducts. This membrane appears to be composed largely of fibrin, although it does not give the usual histochemical reactions of fibrin.[4] However, the membrane is not invariably present with other stigmata of idiopathic respiratory distress syndrome, viz. pulmonary resorption atelectasis, intense congestion, and sometimes intrapulmonary haemorrhages of widely variable extent. The membrane is accepted as a feature of neonatal death and is not seen in the still-birth fetus.[5, 6]

Other histological points of note are desquamation of bronchial epithelium and phagocytosis of meconium. Desquamation may give presumption of still-birth, provided the specimen was removed from the body by the correct technique and fixed for long enough. Phagocytosis of meconium by the cells lining the air sacs, provided artifact is excluded, indicates inhalation of liquor amnii and thus still-birth.

It is important to keep in mind the different possibilities which may occur during birth and to consider what effect they may have on the lungs of the newborn baby. This refers particularly to asphyxial deaths, for example strangulation of the umbilical cord, suffocation in extruded membranes or in blood between the mother's thighs or accidental overlaying (p. 411).

A consideration is now given to circumstances which complicate the investigation of lung aeration in the dead infant.

Breathing may occur while the child's head still remains in the vagina. Crying of the child while in the female genital tract is called 'vagitus uterinus'. Clouston[7] gives details of one of his cases. The patient was in labour with her third child and had been so for ten and a half hours. It was a brow presentation and the os was almost fully dilated. The head was firmly engaged and as he was withdrawing his hand, after the vaginal examination, the child began to cry. It was the normal crying of a newly born child and was heard by the mother, the nurse, and himself. A woman, in a cottage situated directly below the bedroom, also heard the crying. The loud crying persisted at frequent intervals for at least one minute. Four hours later the child was delivered by forceps. It was alive and normal. Vagitus uterinus is thought to be due to air present in the uterus and may result from suction of air along the examining hand during relaxation of the uterus. Air may also be sucked into the uterus during a uterine relaxation. It has been suggested that once there is air within the uterus it may suddenly be forced past a fold of membrane or the vagina by a contraction of the uterus and, as a result, there may be a sound which simulates a fetal cry. This seems an unsatisfactory explanation having regard to the description of the crying heard in several cases.

It is often said that artificial respiration applied to a child showing respiratory difficulty may cause sufficient lung expansion to obscure the issue. Manipulative procedures tend gradually to collapse the lungs, while mouth-to-mouth respiration does expand them. It is most unlikely that an untrained person could accomplish aeration, and thus the presence of air in the lungs from this cause can only be attributed to resuscitative treatment given by a skilled person, whose presence at the confinement would negative any criminal intent. Even then, inflation of fetal lungs by artificial means is difficult to accomplish.

Artificially inflated lungs do not exhibit the mottled or marbled coloration of naturally inflated lungs, only a portion being likely to be expanded by the process, and on cutting them, the exposed surfaces will present a dry appearance, whereas from the cut surfaces of naturally inflated lungs, blood-stained, frothy fluid will escape when pressure is applied. This is due to the fact that when respiration is established the pulmonary circulation becomes operative.   Without the normal function of breathing, there will be no more blood in the lungs than that which existed during the fetal condition, in which state the lungs still remain, except for the presence of air which has been introduced by artificial means.   Apart from these points of differentiation, there is no hard-and-fast method of distinguishing between lungs which have been partially inflated by respiration and those which have been partially distended by artificial means.

The gaseous products of decomposition in the lungs may assist in causing them to float, but there must be substantial evidence of putre-faction generally, together with a non-inflated state of the lungs, before flotation can be attributed solely to this cause.   Fetal lungs are resistant to the process of putrefaction and, therefore, marked evidence of putre-faction of the body is usually present in cases where these gaseous products prove an important factor in the flotation of the lungs.   When the lungs and the body generally are far advanced in decomposition, it becomes impossible for the examiner to determine whether flotation, if it takes place, is due to the presence of atmospheric air, or of putre-factive gases, or of a combination of both factors.   He should, therefore, frankly admit his inability to affirm that the child had breathed.   In cases where the degree of putrefaction is not far advanced, pressure on the portions of lung tissue, as already described, will expel these extran-eous gases without total destruction of the tissue, and their resultant behaviour in water will indicate the presence or absence of contained atmospheric air.

Occasionally a child may have breathed and yet the lungs sink.   In certain cases, breathing may be so shallow that the air in the alveoli is absorbed by the blood without appreciable expansion of the alveolar walls.   It has been shown experimentally that air which has entered the lungs may be entirely absorbed, after respiration has ceased, by the blood circulating through them.

Pulmonary collapse, resulting from atelectasis, and pulmonary consolidation, due to acute oedema, may cause respired lungs to sink in water.   If disease is present to this extent it will provide a sound reason for death quite apart from a homicidal act.

Much has been written in recent times about the microscopic appear-ances of the lungs in the fetus and the newly born, live-born child, and it has been pointed out that in some instances there is difficulty in distinguishing microscopically between these two conditions.

The minute differences in the microscopical appearances between the lungs of the child who dies immediately before birth, and those of the child who dies immediately after birth are, of course, of interest to physiologists and they are of some academic interest to medico-legal experts.   They are not, however, of assistance to the medico-legal practitioner or to the legal authorities in deciding whether or not there is sufficient evidence of live-birth on which to found a charge of infanticide.

As some confusion has been caused by the discussion of these matters in medico-legal journals and textbooks, the authors consider it might be of help to those engaged in medico-legal practice to detail the practical considerations involved.

If a case occurs which necessitates an investigation as to whether there has been a live-birth or not, the following procedure should be followed.

1. If the body is extensively putrefied, then this should be reported along with a statement that because of the extent of putrefaction it was impossible to give an opinion on the question of live-birth.

2. In the absence of extensive putrefaction, the hydrostatic test should be performed. If none of the lobes floats then it should be reported that there is no evidence that respiration has taken place.

3. If one or more lobes float then parts of the lung should be compressed as previously described. If these areas continue to float and the general appearances of the lungs are consistent with respiration, then it should be reported that there is evidence that respiration has taken place, and histological sections of expanded portions of the lungs should be retained for reference purposes.

Stomach-bowel test

A confirmatory indication of establishment of respiration, when associated with definite aeration of the lungs, is the presence of swallowed air in the stomach and upper small intestine. The infant gulps in air during its attempt at breathing. Double ligatures are applied to both the cardiac and pyloric ends of the stomach prior to removal. The intestine is similarly ligatured at different points. The various parts are tested by flotation, and if a positive result is shown they are punctured under water, when the contained air may be seen to escape to the surface. The important fallacy of the test lies in the presence of gases of putrefaction. When the test is negative, it cannot be inferred that breathing has not occurred.

Miron Hajkis[8] stated that the radiological demonstration of air in the upper alimentary tract was a corroborative sign of respiration. If air had reached the duodenum he considered this strong evidence of live-birth. Air was not shown in the stomach and intestine of the still-born even after 48 hours of insufflation. He was unable to inflate the lungs artificially in these still-births.

Changes in the umbilicus

The changes which occur in the stump of the umbilical cord are of value in determining the period a child has survived its birth. The first sign of separation of the stump from the abdominal wall may be apparent in from thirty-six to forty-eight hours after birth, and consists of an inflammatory line at their junction. The line of separation becomes deeper daily until separation is completed. Probably in the largest number of cases the separation is accomplished on the sixth day, in the next largest on the fifth, while in graded smaller proportions of cases, on the seventh, eighth, and ninth days, respectively. The scar at the site of the cord remains active for up to about 12 days.

It is important to note the mode of severance of the cord (p. 418).

Changes in the digestive tract

The important sign to be looked for in the stomach and intestines is the presence or absence of food, and if present, its character. The presence or absence of meconium in the large intestine should also be noted. The presence of food, such as partly digested milk, would point to the fact that the child had survived its birth, although its absence would not point to the opposite conclusion. With regard to meconium in the bowel, its absence does 'not necessarily indicate that the child has survived its birth, since, for example, in breech presentations, which, in the absence of skilled assistance, are perilous to the life of the child, the meconium may be voided, partly as the result of abdominal compression, and partly from asphyxial manifestations induced by pressure on the cord.

Changes in the circulatory system

The changes in the heart and circulatory system should receive attention, although not much practical benefit may accrue from the examination because of the comparative variations in time when the fetal structures close. The foramen ovale, ductus arteriosus, ductus venosus, and umbilical vessels are all patent in a newly born child, but they become closed at variable periods following birth. The foramen ovale, for example, does not become permanently closed till the second or third month. The ductus arteriosus and ductus venosus, however, begin to shrink within three or four days. The umbilical vessels are the first to become obliterated. They begin to contract some hours after birth, and are occluded within a few weeks.

Summary of factors indicative of live-birth

The following conditions, when found would warrant an examiner in affirming that a child had been born alive:

When the child is sufficiently mature to be able to live an independent existence.

When the lungs more or less completely fill the thoracic cavity.

When the colour of the lungs is marbled, or mottled.

When the lungs, or portions of them, after being duly tested, float in water.

When a blood-stained, frothy fluid exudes from the cut surfaces of the lungs on the application of pressure, and when fine bubbles of air are seen to escape when pressure is made on the cut surfaces of the lungs submerged in water.

When microscopical examination shows expansion of the alveoli, and patency of the vessels, and when alveolar duct membrane is present with widespread distribution in the lungs and consequent atelectasis.

A child has survived its birth for some appreciable time when there is evidence of:

Changes in the umbilical cord.

Presence of food in the stomach or intestinal tract.

If the child was born alive, what caused its death?

A child may be born alive in a weakly condition and may only survive its birth for a few minutes or hours. This may result from various causes, such as congenital debility, difficult parturition causing injuries of the brain or skull, and imperfect establishment of respiration.

The principal causes of perinatal deaths, which embrace all still-births and neonatal deaths within the first week of extra-uterine life, are asphyxia, the commonest, congenital abnormalities, low birth weight and its pulmonary complications, infections, cerebral birth trauma, and erythroblastosis.

Cerebral haemorrhage of the newly born used to be a relatively common occurrence, and infants who died within a few days of birth quite frequently showed lesions of the brain attributable to trauma sustained during delivery. The commonest site of intracranial injury with haemorrhage is the triangular area at the junction of the falx and tentorium. However, cerebral birth trauma has contributed less to perinatal deaths in recent years. Fractures of the skull are rare in normal labours, or even in difficult labours, unless the aid of forceps has been required. Mace[9] records the case of a woman of twenty-five, a multipara, who awoke in the middle of the night without pains. During the act of micturition the fetal head appeared at the vulva and was soon born. One of the parietal bones was fractured, although there had been no interference. The cord was unruptured, and the child did not fall to the ground.

In the case of an Rh-positive fetus, and a mother whose blood lacks Rh agglutinogen, anti-Rh agglutinins are formed in her plasma, due to the passage of the Rh agglutinogen from the fetus across the placenta, and these pass back across the placenta into the fetal circulation.   This results in the haemolysis of the fetal blood cells, which is the chief feature of the group of conditions known as erythroblastosis fetalis. Previous therapeutic abortion may be the cause of passage of Rh agglutinogen into the maternal circulation.   This may unwittingly put a future Rh-positive fetus at risk in the Rh-negative mother.

In the examination of the body of a newly born child, it is necessary to consider not only the cause of death but the manner in which death has been produced.   Where, for example, the cause of death is asphyxia, it might have arisen from accident attending the birth or from a criminal act.

A child may die at the moment of delivery from suffocation in the clothing of the mother, by bedclothes, or by discharges which accompany delivery, or by precipitate delivery into a vessel containing water, such as a water-closet.   The last-named event may be caused by the

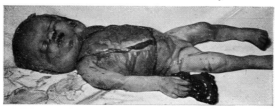

FIG. 209

Note that umbilical cord encircles the neck and is attached to placenta, beside right hand.   Commencing putrefaction of abdominal wall is seen, also lividity of face and upper part of chest

fact that, just before birth, the pressure of the head on the rectum and bladder frequently creates a strong desire on the part of the mother for evacuation, which, if acted upon, may, by the concurrence of a strong labour pain, cause the child to be projected into the lavatory-pan, and its death by drowning.   We have examined two cases of this kind.   In one of these, a young woman, in labour with her first child, delivered her child into a chamber-pot which contained a quantity of urine.   We found the child, a small one, head downwards in the position described. In the other, a married woman, in labour with her third child, went to the lavatory on a tenement stair-landing, and while there was seized with violent pains, and delivered the child into the closet-pan.   She shouted for help, and the child was removed and resuscitated.

In an isolated case, when a mark is found upon the child's neck, it may become necessary to decide between strangulation by natural causes and by applied violence.   Coiling of the umbilical cord round the neck of the child is by no means uncommon, and it is not difficult, therefore, to conceive a case in which a woman might be suspected of the murder of her child, when in point of fact, it has been strangled by the cord during birth. We have examined at least two cases in which this was the apparent cause. The mark produced by the umbilical cord on the neck is never well shown, and the death is not so much due to the constriction exercised as to asphyxia induced by interference with the placental circulation through the cord (Fig. 209).

Is the child viable or non-viable?

As has already been mentioned, a fetus under the age of seven months will not live under ordinary circumstances. According to law, a fetus which has not attained the completion of the seventh month of intra-uterine life is held to be incapable of maintaining a separate existence, and is therefore non-viable. In the examination of the body of a fetus, the determination of its stage of development is of great importance in cases of suspected infanticide or child murder (p. 76). The stage of development of the child can be ascertained by a careful examination of the ossification centres of certain bones, the calcaneum, the talus, the cuboid, the femur, and the tibia. The centres in the femur and tibia are situated at the lower and upper ends respectively. To examine the lower end of the femur, the leg should be flexed against the thigh, and an incision made across, and into the knee-joint, when the end of the femur is pushed forward through the wound. Thin slices of cartilage are then cut, in transverse plane, until the centre is exposed. The head of the tibia is next pushed forward through the wound, and examined in a similar manner. To expose the bones of the foot, an incision should be made through the interspace between the third and fourth toes and carried backwards through the sole of the foot and heel. The centres in the os calcis, talus and cuboid can then readily be examined.

The following is the order of appearance of these ossification centres:

Calcaneum . .	At fifth to sixth month of intra-uterine development.
Talus . . .	About seventh month of intra-uterine development
Lower end of femur .	About eighth month of intra-uterine development
Cuboid . . .	Usually at full-term
Upper end of tibia .	At full-term, or shortly after full-term

The centre of ossification in the lower end of the femur at birth usually measures from 5 to 7 mm in diameter.

In odd instances, even in an apparently mature child, the femoral ossification centres may not be visible. We have noted this in two cases.

It has been stated that the centre in the upper end of the tibia is present in about 80 per cent of full-term infants.

The absence of an ossification centre in the upper end of the tibia and in the cuboid bone does not necessarily imply immaturity, but their presence indicates maturity.

Death due to criminal violence

The bodies of illegitimate children are often concealed in strange places, and sometimes may so remain for long periods before discovery. We have examined bodies found in boxes, in trunks, and in other receptacles, the mothers being at the time of delivery in domestic service, and the births unknown to their employers. In some instances, the bodies of dead newly born infants are disposed of in the most casual fashion to avoid the expense of burial. The body may be thrown on to a waste-heap, into a receptacle for refuse, or into a river or canal. It should be appreciated that the character of the place in which the body may be found does not provide definite indication either that the child has been born alive or that it has met with a violent death. The examiner should therefore approach the case with an entirely open mind.

Frequently the bodies of newly born children are found bearing marks of violence. In such cases, careful deliberation is often necessary to differentiate between accident and homicide.

In the Glasgow district recently there has been a spate of disposing, or attempting to dispose of the bodies of newly born children in dust-bins. In the middle of winter a man walking past an ash-pit heard a cry and found a carrier bag containing a female child still attached to the placenta. The child was removed to hospital where she was found to be hypothermic. She weighed 2·15 kg and may have been slightly premature. With appropriate treatment she made sufficient progress to be discharged two weeks later. Despite wide publicity and extensive inquiry, the mother was never traced.

The staff of a cleansing department depot were able to stop the mechanism just before the body of a male child passed from hopper to destructor. The body weighed 3 kg. Its crown/heel length was 20 inches (51 cm) due to distraction of the cervical spine with sundering of the spinal cord. There was extravasation of blood throughout the tissues of the neck and signs of asphyxia in the organs of the chest. The child had been still-born. There is further interest in this case. The mother, aged 15, delivered herself at home. Her family, aware that she had put on weight, did not know that she was pregnant. She returned to work as a typist three days later, having thrown the body of the child into a dustbin. The placenta was flushed down the lavatory-pan.

In some instances there may be evidence of extensive injury, the result of brutal violence. In one of our cases the infant had been

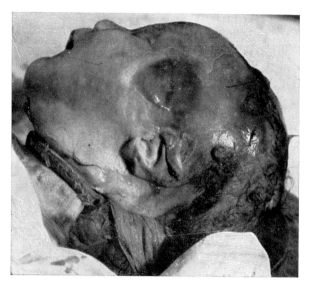

FIG. 210

Body of newly born child with silk stocking tied tightly
round neck.   Note signs of putrefaction

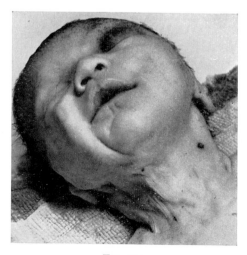

FIG. 211

A case of infanticide showing contusion of left
eye, associated with fracture of skull, and abrasions on neck due to compression

thrown from a window on the third floor of a building. It is obvious, however, that any method may be employed, as in cases of murder in which adults are the victims. In cases of infanticide or child murder there is a high incidence of asphyxial deaths, which result from suffocation, strangulation, throttling, drowning, or by the impaction of foreign bodies which have been deliberately inserted into the mouth or air-passages.

In some cases it is impossible to determine the cause of asphyxia, although this form of death is clearly demonstrated by the internal appearances, or whether it has been produced accidentally or homicidally. When a ligature is found tightly encircling the neck and internal signs of asphyxia are present, it is not difficult to arrive at an opinion (Fig. 209). In such cases the nature of the ligature should be noted, the ligature preserved, and the mark upon the neck carefully dissected for evidence of extravasation. The appearance of the lungs, froth in the air-passages, and blood-stained, frothy exudation on lung-section would point to drowning. The presence of foreign bodies in the mouth or air-passages when accompanied by internal signs of asphyxia points to homicidal suffocation.

In one case, a woman was convicted for having suffocated her newly born child by forcing pieces of paper into its mouth, presumably with the object of stifling its cries. In another case, where the body of a male child, contained in a box loaded with pieces of iron, was found in a river, post-mortem examination showed that it had been strangled.

Often children are throttled, and in such cases the plea of attempting self-delivery may be advanced.

If death is due to asphyxia and there is no clear evidence of criminal interference, weight is given to natural disease as the cause.

Precipitate labour is sometimes a defence in a case of infanticide or child murder, where fracture of the skull is present. The value of the relevancy of this plea may be established by the medical evidence obtained by an examination of both mother and child. The questions to be considered in the examination of the former are:

Whether the woman is a primipara or multipara.
Whether the pelvic parts are roomy.
Whether or not there is laceration of the perineum.

And in the examination of the latter:

Whether or not the umbilical cord is ruptured.
Whether or not the placenta and fetus are still united by the cord.
The character of the cranial lesions.
The presence or absence of a caput succedaneum.
The size and development of the fetus relative to the pelvis of the mother.

The condition of ossification of the fetal cranium.

The presence or absence of other marks of violence upon the body.

Careful consideration and review of all the circumstances will enable the examiner to test the plea offered, by the logic of the facts.

In precipitate labour, a child may be projected to the ground from the mother's body, while she is in the erect position, and thus sustain fatal injury to the skull.   To test this possibility, experiments have been made.   The dead bodies of twenty-five newly born children were dropped, head downwards, from a height of 30 inches (0·8 m) from the

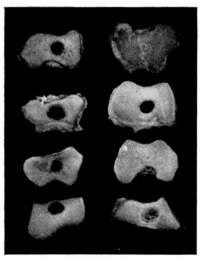

FIG. 212

The appearances of the centres of ossification in the lower end of the femur at different stages of development

ground, the average height of the female genitals from the ground in the standing posture.   Cranial fractures were produced in twenty-four of the bodies, and of these, twenty-two sustained fractures of either one or both temporal bones.

Another cause of death may arise from the deliberate omission to ligate the umbilical cord after cutting.   Such a case provides a typical instance of infanticide or child murder by omission.   The appearance of severance of the cord with a sharp instrument, the absence of ligature, and the comparatively bloodless condition of the body, are indications which would point in this direction.

It rarely happens that a child's death is caused exclusively by neglect and exposure after its birth, but such cases are not unknown.   In one case a young farm servant gave birth to a living male child in a cowshed and left it lying on the floor, in consequence of which the child died from pneumonia. She was found guilty.

Newly born children may be killed by poisoning. Such cases are rare, since a woman who desires to rid herself of a newly born child usually adopts the quickest and readiest means of preventing it from crying and thus announcing its birth.

When marks of violence are present, the effects of violence being the cause of death, and there is evidence of complete respiration, is there justification for expressing an opinion that the child was live-born, in the legal sense, at the time the injuries were inflicted?

If the violence on the body is so distributed, or is of such a character, that full delivery of the child is indicated, there would be adequate justification for stating that the child was live-born in the legal sense. If the child had survived its birth long enough to have been suckled, the presence of milk in the stomach would place the matter beyond dispute.

It would appear that by the law of Scotland, the destruction of a child during the parturient process does not constitute the crime of homicide. With the advent of the Infant Life (Preservation) Act, the law, as applicable to England, was amended with regard to the destruction of children before they have attained an independent existence (p. 400).

How long has the child been dead?

The answer depends upon the post-mortem changes present and the factors attendant on their production (see p. 114).

PROCEDURE AT AUTOPSY OF NEWLY BORN CHILD

External examination

The examination of the body of a newly born child is made in the same manner as the examination of the body of an adult, but the following points, after the wrappings of the body have been noted for identification purposes, demand special attention:

The general development of the body with respect to maturity or immaturity.

The appearance of the skin in relation to the absence or presence of vernix caseosa, indicative of whether the body has been washed or not. Vernix caseosa is a sebaceous secretion covering the fetus and protects its skin against maceration while in the liquor amnii.

The state of the natural orifices of the body, and in respect of the mouth and upper passages, the presence or absence of foreign bodies.

The presence or absence of marks of violence.

The condition of the cord; if the cord has been severed, the character of severance; length of the cord; if ligatured or not, and if tied, the character of the ligature.

Whether or not the placenta is still attached to the body by the cord.

The position and character of the caput succedaneum (the bruised swelling of the scalp due to the process of birth, particularly in a first labour).

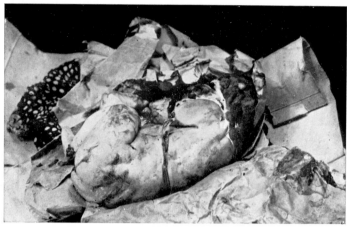

FIG. 213

Body of newly born child, the victim of infanticide, shown in wrappings as found. Early formation of adipocere affected the tissues of the neck. The umbilical cord can be seen encircling the trunk

Internal examination

Head. Examine as in adult cases, except that the brain may be exposed by cutting through the membranous connection of the skull bones. Should the brain substance be unduly soft, the skull may be divided with strong scissors and the brain cut across on a level with the bone incision, when it can be removed with the calvarium. The venous sinuses are examined for thrombus.

Neck. Examine carefully for marks of constriction.

Attention should be directed to the possibility of there being foreign bodies in the air-passages.

Chest cavity. Examine organs in natural position. Note the volume of the lungs and the space occupied by them; the position of the highest convex part of the diaphragm; the colour of the lungs, and their consistence by palpation; the presence or absence of petechiae or Tardieu's spots. The latter may be present in live- and still-births alike. It merely indicates the struggle to breathe. Remove lungs and apply the hydrostatic test.

Abdominal cavity. Avoid the umbilical site when making the primary incision through the skin and underlying tissues composing the abdominal wall. Note condition and appearance of organs in natural position; the condition of the umbilical vessels; the presence or absence of air and food in the stomach and intestines; the presence or absence of meconium in the large intestine, and if present, the amount and distribution.

Examination of the spine. Any injury or congenital defect, such as spina bifida, should be noted.

Examination of ossification centres in bones of foot, in lower end of femur, and in head of tibia. The following tabulated criteria will assist in the assessment of the development of a newly born child.

DIFFERENTIATION OF NEWLY BORN INFANTS AS TO AGE AT BIRTH

	Seven months	Eight months	Nine months (calendar)
Length . . .	32 to 37 cm	35 to 42 cm	45 to 60 cm
Weight . . .	1·3 to 1·8 kg	1·8 to 2·3 kg	2·9 to 3·2 and upwards
Ossification centres	Calcaneum, talus.	Calcaneum, talus. Centre in lower end of femur appears	Calcaneum, talus. Lower end of femur—size: 5 to 7 mm in diam. Cuboid—usually at full term. Head of tibia—frequently at full-term.

Infants at birth have occasionally been found to weigh as little as 1 lb (0·45 kg) or as much as 15 lb (7 kg). There is a reasonably close relationship between age and fetal weight, as well as for length from crown to heel. Length is a much better measure of maturity than weight but is more difficult to determine.

Up to 20 weeks' gestation fetal length represents the square of the age in months. After 5 months the length, in centimetres again, represents the age in months multiplied by 5.

At 28 weeks' gestation, the average weight of the fetus is about 1·3 kg, although when the weight is under 1·5 kg, estimates of age should be guarded.   At 32 weeks average weight should be 1·5 to 2 kg; at 36 weeks 2·5 kg; and at 40 weeks 3 to 3·5 kg.

ILLUSTRATIVE CASES

Application of violence

The body was that of a mature child.   Ossification centres were present in bones of foot, in lower end of femur, and in head of tibia. The placenta was attached to the cord which had not been severed from body.   A moderate-sized caput was present over right parietal bone. The undernoted injuries were present:

> Extensive bruising over anterior half of scalp, entire left side of scalp, left side of forehead, and left eyelid.   These areas contained a considerable quantity of extravasated blood.
> Two linear abrasions and three small punctured incised wounds were present on front of neck (Fig. 211).

Skull and brain.   There were extensive extradural and subdural haemorrhages, and the vault of skull on left side of frontal bone showed a stellate fracture, a limb of which involved roof of left orbit where it terminated in a curved fracture.   There was also a stellate fracture of left parietal bone which divided the bone into four portions with result-ant depression.   The right parietal bone was also the seat of a stellate fracture which divided the bone into three pieces and caused depression. There was a small laceration of right occipital lobe of cerebrum.

Neck.   Dissection of the tissues showed four small areas of bruising over sides and on the floor of the mouth.

Lungs.   These showed complete expansion and several punctate haemorrhages, or Tardieu spots, were present over the pleurae.   On section, copious, frothy, blood-stained exudate was expressed.

Heart.   Some Tardieu spots were present on the surface and the right ventricle was slightly dilated.

Stomach.   This organ was almost completely filled with liquid and clotted blood, together with some mucus.   The blood had resulted from an injury present on right side of pharynx.

Opinion.   The body was that of a mature child who had respired freely.   Death had resulted from the effects of asphyxia due to pressure applied to the neck, and multiple fractures of the skull with resultant cerebral haemorrhage.   From the character of the cerebral haemorrhage, the head injuries had been produced during life, and from the microscopical examination of tissue removed from the various sites of injury, these had also been produced ante-mortem. The body of the child was found in a suitcase together with blood-stained clothing and bed linen.

Cot deaths

The finding of a definite cause of sudden deaths in children under two years has always been a problem for pathologists. Frequently, the best that investigators can do is to eliminate the possibility of foul play and on occasion there may even be difficulty in this.

The unsatisfactory situation has worried all those who are concerned in the investigation of these deaths and there has been increasing research into the problem, especially in the United Kingdom and the United States.[10, 11, 12, 13] Sudden infant deaths number about 3,000 in Britain and about 25,000 in the U.S.A. per year. The incidence varies from about 1 to 3 per 1,000 live-births.[14] The infants are usually between one and six months old, with the majority aged between two and three months. In 1963, the first international conference on the subject of sudden infant death was held, and the second in 1970.[15, 16]

Professor Sir Samuel Bedson and Professor F. E. Camps were responsible for drawing the attention of the Ministry of Health to the importance of further study of sudden deaths in infancy. As a result of their efforts, a committee was formed and an inquiry started during 1954. This was continued for ten years and a report detailing the steps of the investigation and the conclusions of the committee was published during 1965.[17] The report considered that in these deaths there were three main factors: infection, suffocation, and hypersensitivity reaction.

The role of mechanical suffocation in causing sudden infant death, whether by choking on baby food, suffocation, or overlaying, is now considered to be very rare in a healthy infant, especially since the causes such as soft pillows have been reduced by education of the general public. The two main theories propounded now are infective, involving viruses, and allergic, where anaphylaxis due to inhaled cow's milk is the trigger mechanism. Attempts to isolate bacteria and viruses have often failed but where viruses have been isolated from respiratory and intestinal sites, no viraemia has been found.[18] Little evidence of circulating interferon, which might be taken as an indicator of recent infection, was obtained in those deaths investigated as having a viral cause.[18, 19]

That sudden unexpected death in infancy is less common in breast-fed babies at first sight supports the incrimination of cow's milk, but breast feeding tends to be associated with a higher general standard of mother care. The immunoglobulin IgA and other components in human milk are known to have positive antiviral and antibacterial activity in the baby while human milk is also believed to be non-allergenic to man.   If breast feeding is continued over the danger period for sudden infant death, some protection may be given to the child, though not guaranteeing safety.   There is no irrefutable evidence for either hypothesis.

As research proceeds, more and more possible causes have been suggested without substantiation, for example cortisol insufficiency, hypoparathyroid disease, laryngo-spasm, and cardiac arrhythmia. Interest is also now being shown in the reflexes affecting respiration in infants and the effect of their inhibition or failure.

Epidemiological study[20] has been attempted and although difficult, some patterns have appeared.   The children do tend to come from the age range stated above and to belong to social class 3 (skilled occupations).   Such deaths are more common in male infants.   Low birth-weight infants appear more susceptible and the highest incidence is in winter.   Most of the affected infants die in sleep without a sound, and a large number have a history of blocked nose.   Often the infant has been perfectly healthy previously, and this makes the death all the more tragic.

We have investigated a considerable number of sudden deaths in infants and most of our cases have shown a definite pattern.   They have come from poor homes; they have shown a napkin rash varying from moderate to severe; there have been multiple haemorrhages in the thymus gland, the heart and the lungs, and the lungs have been poorly expanded.

We would like to add one note of caution.   We have seen a number of sudden deaths in infants where a history was given which would have suggested a probable death from respiratory infection but subsequent investigation revealed that the children had been killed by one of the parents.

Attempt to dispose of body by burning

The child weighed 5¾ lb (2·6 kg) and its length was 20½ inches (51 cm).   The umbilical cord, attached to the body, measured 10 inches (25 cm) and appeared to have been evenly severed, but was not ligatured.   The finger- and toe-nails were well developed.   Putrefactive changes were present, and the right side and back of head, face, neck, right arm and hand, back and sides of body, and entire legs and feet showed effects of burning.   The scanty hair upon the scalp was singed and soot deposit was present in most of the areas affected by burning. On the right side of the skull was a gap, due to injury of the parietal and occipital bones, through which liquid brain tissue had escaped.   The edges of bone, over posterior part of gap, showed charring and powdering.   In the left lumbar region, the tissues were split for a distance of 5 inches (12·5 cm) and bowel protruded. The tissues over both groins and over right side of abdomen were similarly affected. In the last-named situation, the aperture communicated with the interior of abdominal cavity. The burns on body varied from third to sixth degree. Vesicles were absent. Microscopical examination of tissue from the areas of burning showed that these lesions had been produced after death, and similar examination of tissue from the edges of the apertures gave the same indication. The lungs did not show any evidence of establishment of respiration. The circumstances made it clear that an attempt had been made to dispose of the dead body of this illegitimate child by placing it in an open fireplace.

An unique case

The case of R. v. Lloyd and Hampson, Liverpool Assizes, June 1944, is exceptional. The accused were charged with the attempted suffocation of a newly born male child. The evidence was that a full-term child, weighing $8\frac{1}{4}$ lb (3·7 kg) had been buried in a garden, in the bank of an air-raid shelter, and that three hours later it was dug up alive. The after-birth was first unearthed, and when further digging was in progress a short sigh was heard. The remainder of the earth was then removed manually and the child was found. It lay on its right side, was naked, and the body was covered with wet soil. Seven inches of umbilical cord, which had been ruptured, but had not been tied, remained attached to the abdominal wall. The child showed signs of life and following clearance of the air-passages, a warm bath, and treatment for shock, recovery gradually ensued. There were a few superficial scratches and a small bruise on the body. The infant had been buried 18 inches to 2 feet below the soil which was wet due to falling rain.

References

1. *British Medical Journal*, **2**, 652 and 726, 1940.
2. HOFFMAN, S.J., GREENHILL, J.P., & LUNDEEN, E.C. *J. Am. med. Ass.*, **110**, 283, 1938.
3. OSBORN, G.R. In *Modern Trends in Forensic Medicine*, p. 53, ed. Simpson, K. Butterworth, 1953.
4. GITLIN, D. & CRAIG, J.M. *Pediatrics*, **17**, 64, 1956.
5. BARTER, R.A. *Lancet*, **2**, 945, 1958.
6. *Lancet*, **2**, 160, 1959.
7. CLOUSTON, E.C.T. *Br. med. J.*, **1**, 200, 1933.
8. HAJKIS, M. *Lancet*, **2**, 134, 1934.
9. MACE. *L'Obstét.*, **6**, 54, 1901.
10. CAMPS, F.E. *Br. J. hosp. Med.*, **4**, 779, 1970.
11. RAVEN, C. *J. forens. Med.*, **16**, 120, 1969.
12. COOKE, R.T. & WELCH, R.G. *Br. med. J.*, **2**, 1549, 1964.

13. FROGGATT, P., LYNAS, M.A., & MACKENZIE, G.   *Br. J. prev. soc. Med.*, **25,** 119, 1971.
14. *Lancet,* **2,** 1021, 1970.
15. BERGMAN, A.B., BECKWITH, J.B., & RAY, C.G. (eds.).   *Sudden Infant Death Syndrome.*   University of Washington Press, 1970.
16. *Proceedings of the Second International Conference on Causes of Sudden Death in Infants.*   University of Washington Press, 1970.
17. *Enquiry into Sudden Death in Infancy.*   Ministry of Health Report on Public Health and Medical Subjects, No. 113.
18. *British Medical Journal,* **4,** 250, 1971.
19. RAY, C.G. & HEBESTREIT, N.M.   *Pediatrics,* **48,** 79, 1971.
20. *Lancet,* **2,** 1021, 1970.

Chapter 15

RAPE AND OTHER SEXUAL CRIMES

SEXUAL crimes in England and Scotland are governed by different legislation, and in the following sections the differences in the enactments and their application are set out.

England

The Sexual Offences Act, 1956, a consolidating Act, defines two degrees of sexual assault—rape and indecent assault. Rape consists of having sexual intercourse with a woman or girl without her consent. Under section 24, proof of penetration is all that is required to constitute completion of the act of sexual intercourse, and not ejaculation. As to the degree of penetration necessary to constitute rape, it has been ruled that the slightest penetration of the penis within the vulva is sufficient, even to such a slight degree that the usual signs of virginity (p. 433) are not interfered with. Indecent assault is something that stops short of intercourse.

It is an offence for a man to have unlawful sexual intercourse with a female, although there may be some appearance of consent on her part, in the following circumstances:

   (i) coercing her into submission by fear of intimidation;
   (ii) impersonating her husband;
   (iii) inducing her by fraudulent practices to make a fundamental mistake, for example, where a singing master induced a girl to have intercourse with him by pretending to her that the act was part of the normal breathing exercises;[1]
   (iv) administering or causing to be taken substances producing in her a state of insensibility;
   (v) while she is asleep;
   (vi) while she is insensible through drink;
   (vii) where she is too young to give true consent;
   (viii) where she is too defective mentally to give true consent.

It is an offence for a man to have unlawful sexual intercourse with

   (i) a girl under the age of thirteen, whether by force or not, under section 5 of the Act;
   (ii) a female whom he knows to be an idiot or imbecile.

An offence is committed where a man has unlawful sexual intercourse with a female who is mentally defective, even if she has given consent.

Her consent, even if a true one, is no defence to this charge, but it is a defence that the accused did not know and had no reason to suspect that she was defective. Similarly, an offence is committed where the female is in an institution 'within the meaning of the Mental Health Act, 1959, or placed out on licence therefrom or under guardianship under the Act'. The degree of idiocy must be such as to render the female incapable of expressing assent or dissent. Consent produced by mere animal instinct would be sufficient to prevent the act from constituting rape, but it would still be an offence.

Under section 6 of the 1956 Act, it is an offence to have intercourse with a girl above the age of thirteen but below the age of sixteen except:

(a) where a marriage is invalid under the provisions of the Marriage Act, 1949, or the Age of Marriage Act, 1929 (the wife being under sixteen at the celebration of the marriage);

(b) where the man is under twenty-four and has not previously been charged with a similar offence and believes the girl to be sixteen or over, with reasonable cause for this belief.

Thus any male who has or attempts to have intercourse with a girl above the age of thirteen and under sixteen commits the offence of having or attempting to have unlawful sexual intercourse. It must be realised that unlawful carnal knowledge does not constitute rape, since the act is committed with the consent of the female, who being under sixteen, cannot give valid consent. Carnal knowledge of a female of any age without her consent is rape.

Consent after the age of sixteen eliminates the legal offence, but under the age of consent even solicitation on the part of the female would not avoid the criminality of the sexual act committed by the man.

To constitute the crime of rape, where the female involved is over thirteen, three features are necessary:

(a) the use of force to overcome the female's will to resist;
(b) resistance to the utmost by the female;
(c) penetration.

The necessary force is the overcoming of such resistance, and it is immaterial what means are used to this end. Actual violence is unnecessary so long as the woman's will to resist is overpowered. In the case of an adult woman in possession of all her faculties there must be resistance to the utmost by her for the commission of the crime. It would not amount to rape if the female, after half-hearted resistance, gave consent. Resistance must be maintained to the last and until the woman is overcome by unconsciousness, complete exhaustion, brute force, or fear of death. Rape may be committed against any female whatever her character, except when the relationship of husband and wife exists.   The use of force on the part of the husband does not constitute rape.   It should be noted however that it is the crime of rape for a husband to have intercourse with his wife against her will, while a separation order is in force.[2]   A husband may, however, be guilty as an accessory to the rape of his wife by aiding another person in its perpetration.   Where the assaulted female is physically incapable of resistance, force does not require to be proved and to a lesser degree this is the case when the victim suffers from weakness of mind not amounting to idiocy.   It is unnecessary to prove force in the cases of females under thirteen or of idiots.   They are regarded incapable of consent and the mere fact of penetration is enough.

In England, a boy under fourteen is presumed incapable of committing rape.   This is a presumption which is not rebuttable by evidence of precocious development (p. 358).   It would seem however that a boy under fourteen can be convicted of attempt to commit rape or of an indecent assault.

Sections 14 and 15 of the 1956 Act make it an offence to commit an indecent assault on a woman or man.   Children under the age of sixteen cannot in law give consent which would prevent an act being an assault for this purpose; but where a marriage is invalid because it was celebrated when the wife was under sixteen, the invalidity does not make the husband gulity of an indecent assault upon her if he believes her to be his wife and with reasonable grounds.   In other circumstances it is not a defence that the accused believed the girl had attained the age of sixteen and the special defence given to a man under twenty-four on a charge of unlawful sexual intercourse with a girl under sixteen has no application to a charge of indecent assault.

Indecent assault is an assault accompanied by circumstances of indecency on the part of the accused towards the allegedly assaulted person.   There must be a hostile gesture attending the indecent act.   Any touching of the body, such as the breasts, genitalia, or the thigh above the skirt may constitute indecent assault.   When it became clearly established that an invitation, unaccompanied by any hostile gesture, could not amount to an indecent assault, the Indecency with Children Act, 1960, was passed.   This makes it an offence for a person to commit an act of gross indecency with or towards a child under fourteen, or to incite a child under that age to such an act with him or another.

Scotland

Rape, under common law in Scotland, is the carnal knowledge of a woman forcibly and against her will, or, whether by force or not, of a female under *twelve* years of age, or of an idiot.   An idiot in Scotland is deemed incapable of giving consent whereas in England the state of idiocy must be such as to render the female incapable of expressing assent or dissent.

To constitute the crime in females above twelve three points must be proved in evidence:

(i) the use of force to overcome the woman's will to resist;
(ii) resistance to the utmost by the female;
(iii) penetration.

Carnal knowledge of a woman obtained by impersonating her husband is deemed to be rape under the Criminal Law Amendment Act, 1885. As in England, it is an offence to overpower a woman by drugging her into a state of insensibility for the purpose of having unlawful carnal knowledge, but in Scotland sexual connection with a woman found in a state of insensibility from intoxication does not constitute the crime of rape. Taking sexual advantage of a female while she is asleep is an indictable offence termed Clandestine Injury to a Woman.

The case of H.M. Advocate v. Grainger[3] is one of interest on the latter point. Two men were indicted on a charge that they did ravish a woman while she was in a state of insensibility or unconsciousness from the effects of intoxicating liquor. Their counsel maintained that the indictment was irrelevant in respect that it did not disclose the crime of rape according to the law of Scotland. The presiding judge sustained this objection.

In stating the objection counsel argued that, as rape (save in the exceptional cases of pupils and idiots) is the carnal knowledge of a woman forcibly and against her will, the crime could not be committed unless the woman is in a condition, physically and mentally, to exercise her will-power and offer resistance, and as the libel set forth that the woman was in a condition when she was incapacitated by reason of intoxication from offering any resistance or from exercising her will-power in the way of giving or refusing consent, the offence charged did not amount to rape.

In giving his decision the judge stated that it was not alleged that the accused supplied the liquor with which the woman became intoxicated. Had this allegation been made, the charge of rape might have been sustained, as it has been decided that it is rape to have connection with a woman whose resistance has been overcome by drugging her. It might be suggested, he continued, that the present case fell to be assimilated to that of a female idiot; but that did not seem to be a true analogy. The idiot had, in law and in fact, no will; in the present case the woman assaulted had a will, the activity of which had been but temporarily suspended by her intoxication. The true analogy seemed to him to be the case of the woman who was taken advantage of while asleep, and such an offence was not rape. Just as a sleeping woman was temporarily in a state of unconsciousness wherein she was incapable of exercising her will-power, so here it seemed that the woman was in the same temporary condition of unconsciousness by reason of intoxication. What was said to have been done by the accused, although not rape, was a criminal offence, the crime of inflicting clandestine injury on a woman, and must be indicted as such, and not as rape.

In the case of H.M. Advocate v. Logan,[4] the Lord Justice-Clerk in charging the jury directed that if the drink were administered by the accused with the object of overcoming the resistance of the victim, the crime might be rape; but that if the drink had been taken by the victim of her own free will and not been given with a view to overcoming her resistance, the crime, so far as it was possible to define it, came within the category of indecent assault.

Under section 4 of the Criminal Law Amendment Act, 1885, any person who unlawfully and carnally knows any girl under the age of thirteen years shall be guilty of felony, and any person who attempts the foregoing shall be guilty of a misdemeanour.

Section 5 enacts that any person who unlawfully and carnally knows or attempts to have unlawful carnal knowledge of any girl being of or above thirteen and under sixteen years of age, or of any female idiot or imbecile woman or girl, shall be guilty of a misdemeanour, provided that it shall be a sufficient defence to the first part of the section if it shall be made to appear to the court or jury that the prisoner had reasonable cause to believe that the girl was of or above the age of sixteen years.

By the Age of Marriage Act, 1929, which makes marriages under sixteen void, it is a defence for a man charged under section 5 of the Act of 1885, or charged with indecent assault, to prove that at the time of the alleged offence he had reasonable cause to believe that the woman in question was his wife.

The Criminal Law Amendment Act, 1922, amended the Act of 1885 with respect to offences against persons under the age of sixteen.

Under section 1 it is no defence to a charge or indictment for an indecent assault on a child or young person under the age of sixteen to prove that he or she consented to the act of indecency.

Section 2 provides that it is not a defence to a charge under section 5 of the Act of 1885, that there was reasonable cause to believe the girl was at least sixteen, except where a man is aged twenty-three or under. This defence is valid only on the first occasion a person is charged with an offence under this section.

Section 4 provides that any person who uses towards a girl of or above the age of twelve years and under the age of sixteen years any lewd, indecent, or libidinous practice or behaviour which, if used towards a girl under the age of twelve years would have constituted an offence at common law, shall, whether the girl consented to such practice or behaviour or not, be guilty of an offence against this Act.

As we have already seen, the law, under certain circumstances, permits a prisoner charged with having carnal knowledge of a girl between the ages of thirteen and sixteen, to show that he had reasonable cause to believe that she was over the age of sixteen years. A defence cannot be founded upon impressions formed from the appearance of the girl, for, if such a defence could be entertained, it would nullify the statute altogether, because the accused would only have to say that while the girl's age might be fourteen, he believed, and had grounds for believing from her appearance, that she was over sixteen. It must not be mere supposition on the part of the accused. It must be that he formed the opinion upon information, or other intelligible and reasonable grounds of belief. Credible information obtained perhaps from the girl herself, or from other sources, by a man twenty-three years of age or younger, is alone a valid defence. It is a matter of constant observation in daily life, and it is well known by medical men, that the evidences of physical maturity in girls between the ages of thirteen and sixteen are as variable as is their stature or their weight, and that there are many girls of such ages who might well be mistaken for a more advanced age than that of sixteen.

Where girls are under twelve, actions are usually taken at common law. Indecent practices between males are a crime at any age. In Scotland, there is no age fixed by law before which a male person is held incapable of committing rape. Probably the earliest age at which conviction has followed was that of a boy aged thirteen years and ten months.

Considerations in the Medico–legal Investigation of Rape

It is easy for a female to allege that she has been raped and frequently the story of the circumstances is fabricated by a 'victim' to account for facts which would otherwise be awkward to explain. Because of this and the severity of the charge, it is most important in cases of rape to obtain evidence that will corroborate the woman's statement and help establish the responsibility, if any, of the man she may be accusing of the crime.

The two main considerations in the examination are:

(i) signs of physical resistance;
(ii) local evidence of rape.

Signs of physical resistance

From what has been said respecting the legal interpretation of the kind of force and amount of penetration necessary to constitute rape, it will be obvious that from the medico-legal point of view the physical signs will vary in different cases, or may even be absent, although the crime has been committed.

It is easy to conceive the possibility of legal commission of the crime without any physical evidence whatever being found on the body of the female to justify a medical examiner in doing more than reporting the negative facts. Since the slightest degree of penetration, without emission, constitutes the crime, no physical signs of defloration may be produced; indeed, there may be no local evidence whatever of the juxtaposition of the male and female parts. Therefore, the medical examiner is not justified in affirming, because no such physical evidence is forthcoming, that rape has not been committed. If evidence exists, the range of physical signs will vary according to the capacity for physical resistance. In the case of young children, females who have been drugged, or those who are in a state of unconsciousness from any other cause, the evidence of resistance will probably be absent, while the local signs of accomplishment of the act are likely to be well marked, but even then the signs will depend upon whether or not the female has been accustomed to sexual intercourse. In cases of rape, we must therefore distinguish between the general signs of physical resistance and the local evidence.

Assuming that a healthy, vigorous young woman alleges that she has been ravished, the first thing the medical examiner must look for is evidence of the signs. If the woman has resisted to her uttermost, she will probably bear marks upon the body, face, neck, and limbs of her violent resistance, and probably, also, she will have inflicted injuries upon the body of her assailant. In such a case, therefore, the examiner should look for evidence of the signs of violence upon her body, such as wounds, bruises, or scratches. In the absence of these, he should exercise at first a healthy scepticism as to the truth of her statements, unless she avers that she had fainted, been overcome by fear, or had been drugged, and her sexual parts bear evidence of interference. At the same time, our experience has led us to the belief that this scepticism may be carried too far. There are, unquestionably, girls who become panic-stricken when an attack of this kind is made upon them, and are rendered incapable of offering serious resistance, with the consequence that their bodies do not bear evidence of injuries such as might be expected from a severe struggle, while locally there may be all the expected signs of the accomplished act of penetration. In such a case, the acts and demeanour of the girl immediately after the alleged commission of the crime should be subjected to very critical investigation, as these may provide valuable evidence, corroborative or otherwise, regarding the alleged ravishing. In the case of children, the examiner must not always expect evidence of physical resistance, since frequently children are incapable of exercising sufficient resistance to provoke injury.

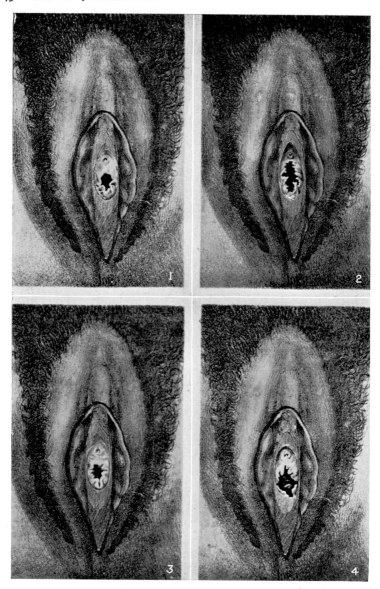

FIG. 214

Types of hymen. (Photographs of prepared models)
1. Intact—Annular, with natural notches
2. Intact—Fimbriated
3. Ruptured, following coitus
4. Ruptured extensively, following delivery

The breasts and nipples may be severely injured. In particular, they may be bitten, leaving a dental impression sufficiently clear for identification of the assailant (see p. 66).

Before considering the appearances of the sexual parts associated with recent loss of virginity, it is advisable to discuss the physical signs of virginity.

Signs of virginity

The following are the principal signs:

An intact hymen.
A normal condition of the fourchette and posterior commissure.
A narrow vagina with rugose walls.

These signs, taken together, may be regarded as evidence of virginity but taken singly they cannot be so reckoned.

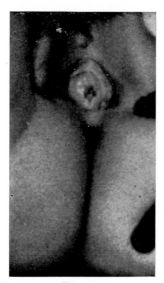

FIG. 215
Intact annular hymen with natural notches

The hymen, which varies greatly in shape and consistence, is found as a normal structure in most virgin females, except in certain cases in which from varied causes it has been more or less destroyed by factors other than sexual intercourse, principally masturbational acts, the insertion of foreign bodies, disease, scratching due to irritation of the parts from lack of cleanliness, gynaecological examination, operation, or accident. In cases of habitual masturbation, which is quite a prevalent habit in females, some hypertrophy of the labia and clitoris may be present (see Fig. 222). Mason[5] reports the case of a girl, aged seventeen, who was a confirmed clitoris masturbator from the age of eight, in whom the erected clitoris measured 5 centimetres in length and $1\frac{3}{4}$ centimetres at the base, and showed a similar measurement of the glans. The form of the intact hymen is variable in character and may show merely as a slight annular ring fringing the opening of the vagina, it may be tight and rigid or, very rarely, may exist in such pronounced form as to constitute an imperforate curtain which entirely shuts off the vagina from the external genitals (Fig. 202). Between these two extremes there are varying forms. The following types of intact hymen may be met with:

The infantile hymen with a small, slit-like opening near the centre.

The annular hymen.

The annular hymen with natural notches which may give a lobulated appearance.

The fimbriated, or irregularly notched hymen.

The hymen showing a septum and unequal openings, or with two openings, one serrated, and the other lobed.

The hymen showing a posterior rudimentary septum.

The hymen showing an irregular, puckered opening and undistended.

The crescentic hymen.

From a want of knowledge of these forms, mistakes may be made by examiners, since natural notches and fimbriations could be mistaken for rupture in sexual cases (see p. 432). While recent rupture of the hymen would signify the forcible introduction of an instrument of some kind, and while loss of the hymen does not necessarily indicate loss of virginity, its persistence does not unequivocally point to the existence of virginity. In odd cases, the hymen has remained unruptured after coitus and during resultant pregnancy, and has remained intact until ruptured by the birth of the child, or until incised to permit the passage of the child. In these rare cases, the hymen has been of annular and distensile type which has permitted the entry of the male organ without rupture. It should not be forgotten that pregnancy can occur even when penetration is impossible, since only the entry of spermatozoa is essential to achieve this.

In the virgin female the vagina is narrow and its walls are slightly rugose. The absence of these characteristics does not, however, necessarily indicate habituation to sexual intercourse, since masturbation, or repeated mechanical dilatation, may affect the virgin condition.

From a review of the foregoing signs, it will be apparent that they must be found conjointly to afford satisfactory evidence of the virgin state.

Local evidence of rape

We turn now to consider the signs in the sexual parts of a virgin female which when found would support the examiner in concluding that rape had been committed.

These are:

Recent rupture of the hymen.
Presence of blood, fresh or dried, about the vulva.
Marks of bruising, abrasions, or inflammation of the parts.
Presence of semen in the vagina.

Additional signs such as discomfort in walking or frequency of micturition may be present in certain cases, especially in young girls.

When there has been forcible attempted penetration or complete penetration of the vagina, evidence of rupture of the hymen will be present, as a rule, but both the character and extent of the injury will vary in different cases depending upon the nature of the hymen, the disproportion between the male and female parts, the extent of the penetration, and the amount of force used. The site of rupture presents a tear, or a series of stellate tears, in the membrane marked in recent cases by a blood-stained or inflamed line or lines. Such tears are usually in the posterior part of the hymen; anterior tears support the possibility of injury inflicted by a finger.

Rupture of the hymen is almost invariably accompanied by some degree of bleeding. The severed edges do not unite, but become rounded off in the process of healing which, in the case of slight tears, occurs in from two to three days; more extensive tears take a longer period to heal, usually about seven to ten days or even slightly longer, depending upon circumstances. It is not possible to date an injury of the hymen after it has completely healed. In women who are habituated to intercourse, and in those who have borne children, the remains of the hymen constitute what are known as carunculae myrtiformes which are situated round and close to the vaginal orifice and present the appearance of different-sized small, round, fleshy projections or tags.

Where an infant or young child is involved there may be a tear from the fourchette posteriorly to the rectum if any real attempt has been made at penetration. Usually no attempt at this is made and the attack is one of indecent assault involving fingering, or some other indecent practice.

Attention should be paid to the presence of blood about the vulva, thighs, and pubic area of the body, and on the clothing. Whether blood is present or not, and, if present, the amount will depend upon the extent of the injury and the vascularity of the hymen. It sometimes happens that, from the unusual quantity of effused blood, the examiner may be led to suspect that the assailant has also received injury to his genitals.   In three cases which we examined, the quantity of blood found on the girls' underclothing, and at the place where the crime was committed, was greater than would reasonably have been expected from an injury to the hymen.   On examination of the suspected males who had been apprehended, a recent rupture of the fraenum of the penis was found in each case.   Apart from such injury to the male, coitus may cause considerable bleeding where, in the hymen a small vessel has been incompletely torn.   We have not seen this in rape, but we have seen it in the case of the first coitus of marriage.   The examiner should be on the alert, however, that he is not deceived by a false charge of rape, and that the presence of blood is not merely menstrual.   There will be corroborative evidence of rape should bruising

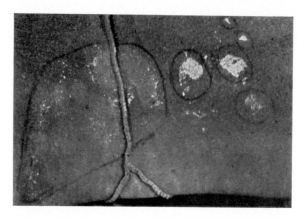

FIG. 216

Seminal stains, close to crutch of undergarment, photographed in filtered ultra-violet light

or abrasions of the genitals be found, since either of these conditions is indicative of violence.

Accompanying the foregoing signs, evidence of their cause is afforded when semen is found in the vagina.   In all cases of alleged rape, smears of vaginal fluid taken by swab or aspirated by pipette should be examined microscopically for spermatozoa.   The smears should be made at the time of examination.   Several microscope slides are lightly and evenly smeared with the vaginal fluid.   The smears should be thin. To some of the slides a drop or two of 0·3 per cent acetic acid or normal saline are added.   Cover-slips are applied and the preparations examined microscopically.   The remaining slides should be dried or fixed and a staining process employed (p. 442).   The pubic hair and the hair around the external genitals, together with any suspicious staining on the skin or clothing, should also be examined for evidence of seminal fluid.   Dried stains on the thighs should be moistened with saline and smears made on a glass slide using a throat swab.   The absence of semen, however, must not be interpreted as an indication that rape has not been committed since an emission is not a requisite of the crime.

The use of filtered ultra-violet light will prove helpful in the detection of seminal staining, whether upon hair, the body surface, or clothing. The ultra-violet lamps of Hanovia pattern have proved most useful in this respect.

A vaginal examination should be carried out with estimation of the degree of vaginal dilatation.   The opening in the hymen up to the age of about thirteen normally just admits the tip of the little finger. In most virginal adults, two fingers may just be inserted into the vagina through the hymen.   Undue dilatation of the vagina may point to intercourse in a child, but it can follow the insertion of foreign bodies like tampons.   In cases of violence, a rectal examination should include examination of the anus and the recto-vaginal septum, and a rectal swab should be taken.

In some cases, the victim of rape or unlawful carnal knowledge may become infected with gonorrhoea or syphilis.   Owing to the existence of a belief among persons of the lower classes that coitus with a young virgin will cure them of gonorrhoea, children are sometimes infected. In one of our cases two young children were affected with gonorrhoea, the result of sexual contacts with a male lodger who was suffering from the disease.   Many years ago, in Glasgow, a woman was tried and convicted on a charge of lewd, indecent, and libidinous practices and behaviour towards a boy, aged seven years, from which he contracted gonorrhoea.

A far more common cause of purulent discharge, however, is vulvo-vaginitis.   The differentiation between a simple vulvo-vaginal inflammation and gonorrhoeal infection should be determined by bacteriological examination.

Our case records show a wide variance in the extent and character of local injury in sexual cases.   In one instance, a child of seven years, violence had been extreme, and the perineum was so torn that the injury communicated with the rectum.   In the case of a girl aged sixteen, of muscular build, who alleged that forcible and complete intercourse had been performed upon her by five men on ten occasions within four hours, the hymen had not been recently torn, and there was only a small amount of dried blood on the labia.   There was no evidence of local injury or of inflammation.   In a series of thirty-six cases involving young females, there was evidence of a ruptured hymen, but only in sixteen of these was the rupture recent.   The ages of the girls varied from thirteen to seventeen years.   In eleven of these instances there was definite evidence of sexual trafficking.   The findings confirm the view that sexual offences with girls under sixteen are more common than the number reported to the authorities would indicate.

ILLUSTRATIVE CASES

A post-mortem examination of the body of a girl, aged seven, made by us, showed that the cause of death was asphyxia due to compression of the air-passages.   There were some bruising and abrasions of both legs.

Examination of the genital region showed that the private parts, fork of the legs, region of anus and lower parts of buttocks, were more or less covered with a thin layer of blood mixed with faeces.   Detailed examination showed that the tissues between the vagina and rectum had been completely torn for a distance of fully an inch.   In our opinion the injuries described in these parts had been produced either by the fingers of an assailant or by the forcible intromission of a male organ.

A man was indicted and tried at the High Court at Glasgow on a charge of rape and murder.   The post-mortem examination of the woman's body showed the following features: (1) vertical lacerated wound $1\frac{1}{2}$ inches long from bridge of nose upwards in the middle line, extending down to bone; (2) similar wound on eyebrow, $\frac{1}{2}$ inch long, and close to right of (1); (3) similar wound about 1 inch to left of (1), $\frac{1}{2}$ inch long; (4) oblique lacerated wound, $\frac{1}{2}$ inch above and outward from (3), 1 inch long and reaching bone; (5) severe bruising of right upper eyelid and neighbouring parts, and a lesser degree of bruising of left upper eyelid; (6) incised wound on front of nose extending into right nostril and separating right side of nose from underlying bone which was exposed; (7) perforating lacerated wound of lower lip, V-shaped, opening into mouth; (8) bruising of upper lip and extensive bruising of both sides of neck with abrasion of skin; and (9) severe and extensive bruising of upper and inner sides of both thighs, and a recent rupture of hymen with extensive blood-staining around vaginal orifice.

Examination of the scene of the crime showed a patch of blood-stained turf with a sharp stone projecting slightly from it.

Blood-stains were found upon nearly all the garments of the accused, including the trousers, and on these, seminal stains were found on the inside of the front opening.   Blood-stains were also found on all the garments of the deceased.   The piece of turf showed a blood-stained area 24 inches by 19 inches.   On the pubic hair of the dead woman, complete spermatozoa were found.

Hairs found on the trousers of the accused had been pulled out by the roots and corresponded, in microscopical characters, to the pubic hairs of the deceased.   At the trial a plea of not guilty was tendered, but a special defence was lodged that if the accused committed the crime, he was at the time either insane, or in such a condition mentally, as not to be responsible for his actions. After lengthy evidence for the Crown, including medical evidence as to the sanity of the accused, the defence called medical evidence as to his mental abnormality, which indicated in the opinion of these medical witnesses that accused was affected by sadism. The jury, however, found the accused guilty of rape and culpable homicide, and he was sentenced to fifteen years' penal servitude.

The next case illustrates a story of sexual assault fabricated by an imaginative girl of fourteen.

She lived with her widowed mother, a woman who prided herself on knowing each intimate detail of her daughter's life. The girl alleged that, while walking through a public park adjacent to her school playing fields, she had been accosted by a man aged about 48, whom she described in considerable detail. Being intelligent, she realised the futility of resistance, and allowed him to remove one leg of her pants and tights before submitting to intercourse. Only some days later did she tell this story to her mother, who promptly called the police.

Although confident of the truth of the tale, the mother was initially reluctant to permit examination. She insisted on being present.

There was no injury to the private parts, the hymen being intact. The introitus just admitted two fingers, but these were firmly clasped. The opinion had to be given that this girl was *virgo intacta*, there being no evidence of any sexual interference.

Another case is rather unusual. A man was charged with rape. His defence was that intercourse had taken place with consent. Examination of the woman did not show any extensive injury of the body. Local examination revealed oozing of blood from the vulva a few hours after the alleged assault. The hymen showed two recent tears, the first, situated on the left side, close to junction of upper and lower quadrants and associated with bruising, the second, on the right side in approximately a corresponding position. The latter tear also showed some bruising. A tear, $\frac{1}{4}$ inch long, was present close to midline of fourchette. Spermatozoa were found on the vaginal swabs. Examination of the accused did not show any evidence of injury affecting the genitals. In flaccid condition, the penis measured $4\frac{1}{4}$ inches from base to tip, circumferential measurement around mid-part was $3\frac{3}{4}$ inches, and similar measurement around coronal part was 4 inches. The size of the penis was thus in considerable excess of the average in European subjects. The defence raised the question of penile dimensions as an explanation of the infliction of injury during the act of coitus with consent. The jury unanimously found the accused not guilty of rape.

Examination of the accused

As the examination of an accused person may disclose evidence which would tend to connect him with the charge preferred against him, it can only be made with his full consent.   Such consent should be obtained in the presence of a third person, after cautioning the accused of the possible results of the proposed examination and informing him of his right to withhold consent (see p. 56).   Scratches upon the face or hands of the accused, bites on his body or limbs, or bruises on his legs from kicks, are strong corroboratory evidence of the averment of the complainant that she resisted vigorously.   Rupture of the fraenum of the penis, in rare cases, may be found, and affords evidence of forcible intromission of the organ into an incommensurately smaller passage.   This was found in one case where a man was charged with the rape of a girl, whose underclothing was saturated with blood.   The floor of the vestibule where the crime was committed was also heavily stained with blood.   The man denied any knowledge of the crime, but the finding of blood in the seams of the front part of his trousers, which showed evidence of recent washing, and on the nails and soles of his boots, heightened the suspicion of his guilt.   He pleaded guilty at his trial.

Apart from general or local injury, the penis may show evidence suggestive of recent turgescence, the effects of friction, or of moisture at the meatus due to seminal fluid.

Examination of seminal stains

It is usually necessary, as corroborative evidence of sexual offences, to examine the clothing of the person assaulted, and that of the person accused, for the presence or absence of seminal stains and blood-stains. Such work is nowadays more commonly performed by specialist forensic scientists, but the medical examiner must have a knowledge of the principles involved and the limitations of many of the techniques used.

The underclothing in such cases is frequently not characterised by its cleanliness, and consequently the examiner may expect to find a variety of stains ranging in colour from red, brown, or yellow to a faint, almost imperceptible, greyish colour.   Those of a reddish colour are commonly composed of blood; of a yellowish colour, from vaginal discharge, or urine; of a brownish colour, from faeces; while those of a greyish appearance may be due to semen.   To narrow the line of investigation, a preliminary examination of the garments under filtered ultra-violet light should be made, when stains, such as those composed of urine, leucorrhoeal discharge and seminal fluid, will show a bright fluorescence. The fluorescence of seminal stains is of a bluish-white colour, and stains reacting in this manner should first be selected for examination (Fig. 217). Whenever a photograph is taken by filtered ultra-violet light with the view to producing it in court, an ordinary photograph should also be taken. Courts are inclined to distrust photographs which may not record what is normally seen but show only what is normally not seen. This also applies to infra-red photography (pp. 73, 291).

Seminal stains, when dry, assume a greyish-white appearance, impart a stiffened feeling to the fabric, and show an irregular, map-like contour. Many leucorrhoeal stains exhibit similar characters and microscopical examination will have to be employed to determine the difference. The stains when they are presented for examination are usually in a dried condition, and before their constituents can be examined

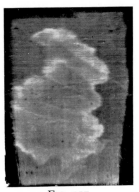

FIG. 217

Photograph of a seminal stain during exposure to filtered ultra-violet light

microscopically they must be moistened in order to obtain an extract. Excellent results are obtained by microscopical examination of scrapings, taken from the surface of a stain, following the addition of a drop or two of a 0·3 per cent solution of glacial acetic acid in distilled water to the scrapings on a slide. In the majority of cases, particularly when the stains are fairly thick and not of recent origin, this method has been found preferable to the soakage method, and is recommended. The cutting edge of a scalpel is a suitable instrument to employ when making the scraping, but care should be taken to avoid the use of an excess of the material and to exclude, so far as possible, fibres from the fabric. The procedure for the soakage method is as follows:

Excise a portion from the stains, keeping each in a separate watch-glass.

Add sufficient 0·3 per cent solution of glacial acetic acid in water (preferably distilled) to moisten the stained material.

Place the specimens in an air-tight container until there is complete saturation of the fabric.

Prepare a series of six clean glass slides, and with a pair of flat-bladed forceps smear each with the moistened stain.

On three of them place cover-slips. These are now ready for examination. Dry the other three slides, and stain with haemalum, gentian violet, or methylene blue, with eosin as a counter-stain, or with any other suitable dye.

We strongly recommend the following staining methods:

(*a*) haemalum and eosin.

The smears must be thin and spread uniformly on the slide.

Dry by fanning.

Fix with methyl alcohol.

Refix, for five minutes, first with 95 per cent and then with 70 per cent ethyl alcohol.

Rinse quickly in water.

Stain for twenty minutes with haemalum. (A 2 per cent solution of crystalline haematin in 90 per cent alcohol is added to a 5 per cent solution of potassium alum.)

Steep in running water for thirty minutes or longer.

Restain with haemalum for five minutes.

Rinse in water for ten minutes.

Stain, for contrast, with 3 per cent alcoholic eosin solution for three minutes.

Differentiate in sequence of 70 per cent, 90 per cent, and absolute alcohol.

Clear in carbol-xylol.

Mount in canada balsam.

Apply cover-slip.

(*b*) Papanicolaou

The solutions required, which may be purchased commercially, are Harris's haematoxylin, OG 6 and EA 50. After fixing in a mixture of equal parts ether and alcohol for thirty minutes, the smears are rinsed in 70 per cent alcohol, then water, before staining for four minutes with haematoxylin. Next, the smear is differentiated in 0·5 per cent hydrochloric acid, then rinsed in tap water before dehydrating in alcohol. The smear is then stained for three minutes in OG 6 and EA 50, with rinses in alcohol between each. Before mounting, it is dried in absolute alcohol and cleared in xylol.

The preparations are thus examined in the unstained and stained conditions. The $\frac{1}{6}$ inch objective should be employed.

The characters of seminal fluid

The normal quantity of seminal fluid in a single ejaculate is from 2 to 5 ml, and on the average about 4 ml, although the volume varies widely even in the same person.   Volumes of 6 ml and over may be regarded as excessive, but a case has been reported of an ejaculate amounting to 13·5 ml.   The total number of spermatozoa in an ejaculate from a healthy young man is about 400 to 500 millions, but it must not be forgotten that seminal stains may not disclose the presence of spermatozoa if the subject from whom the seminal fluid came suffers from aspermia or oligospermia.   Such states may be either temporary or permanent.   In these instances, since the finding of spermatozoa is necessary to prove that stains are seminal, there is a considerable chance of guilty persons evading conviction.   The fresh ejaculate is of a

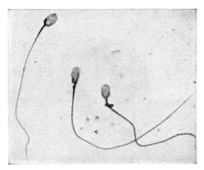

FIG. 218

Spermatozoa.   Stained   preparation—
methylene blue.   × 850

gelatinous, sticky character, but after it has been exposed to the air for about a quarter to half an hour, it tends to become more liquid, probably due to enzymic action.   Semen consists of two unities, seminal fluid and certain formed cellular elements including spermatozoa, and epithelial cells and crystals, composed of choline and lecithin. It is slightly alkaline in reaction.

It is not difficult to recognise a spermatozoon when it is seen entire because of its large and obvious head, which is about 4·5 μ in length, and its neck and filamentous tail, which are about 50 μ long.   The seminal fluid of young male subjects frequently contains spermatozoa, and we have found them plentifully in stains produced by the ejaculate of boys of thirteen.

Although stains are proved to be of seminal origin when spermatozoa are present, their absence does not prove that the stains have not been produced by human semen.   For medico-legal purposes, we hold the view that if spermatozoa, or at least one complete spermatozoon, are not found in the stain, we cannot positively affirm that such stains are seminal, and that the apparent absence of these bodies does not permit of an opinion that the stain has not been produced by human seminal fluid.   In the latter instance, an examiner should merely state that, as the result of his examination, he was unable to detect the presence of spermatozoa.   The discovery of spermatozoa in stains is not always an easy matter, for the obstructive elements are many.   The important responsible factors are the character of the fabric, the age of the stain, and the conditions to which it has been exposed before reaching the laboratory for examination.   Spermatozoa have been discovered in stains long after their emission.   We have found many complete sperms in a stain upon a garment after the elapse of five months following the sexual offence, the garment having been in police custody during that period.   The undergarment in question, apart from the seminal staining, was clean and relatively new.   On the other hand, we have frequently examined seminal stains which, when moist and fresh, were found to contain spermatozoa, but which did not reveal them after they had become dried from exposure to the air of a warm room, even after comparatively short intervals of time.   Desiccation would seem, therefore, in some cases, to lead quickly to disintegration of spermatozoa.   We have been able, however, in unequivocal stains kept in stoppered bottles, to detect spermatozoa after the lapse of six months.   Our view is that it is not so much the continuous desiccation which militates against their discovery on fabrics, as the occurrence of decomposition in the early stage before the stains become dried, due to their admixture with urine or other discharges which undergo rapid decomposition.   Readily identifiable spermatozoa may be found in the vagina for a considerable period after death.   The writer has had no difficulty in detecting complete and well-preserved spermatozoa in a vaginal swab after some eighty-five hours, the estimated interval between death and the taking of the swab.   A number of circumstances play an important part in the preservation or early destruction of sperms within the vagina of the cadaver.   (For their survival period within the vagina of the living subject see p. 372.)

The acid phosphatase test.   The fact that the prostatic secretion element of seminal fluid contains a very much higher percentage of acid phosphatase than any other body fluid has been used as a test for seminal fluid.

The test is a quantitative one and is usually carried out by measuring fixed quantities, e.g., 1 square centimetre, of stained material and estimating the amount of acid phosphatase present.   The estimation is made by calorimetry.   When it is found that there is a considerably higher quantity of acid phosphatase present than could have been caused by contamination from any other source, then it is presumed that the stain is composed of seminal fluid.[6] We have found this a useful sorting test but are of the opinion that it should not, by itself, be relied upon as definite evidence of the presence of a seminal stain for court purposes.

Florence test. This is merely a preliminary chemical test, and is not regarded for medico-legal purposes as a positive test for seminal fluid. The reagent employed consists of a solution of 1·65 g of potassium iodide and 2·54 g of iodine in 30 ml of distilled water. The reaction is shown by the formation of dark brown crystals, rhombic or needle-shaped, when the reagent is mixed with an aqueous extract of seminal fluid. The test is employed as follows: The seminal extract is prepared by warming the stains in a little water on a water-bath, acidifying with dilute hydrochloric acid, cooling and adding some dry ammonium sulphate. The extract so treated is filtered, the reagent is added, and the mixed fluid examined microscopically. In most instances, the reaction is obtained simply by adding a drop of the reagent to a wet film of seminal solution, placing a cover-slip on the slide and examining microscopically. The reaction is due to choline. The crystals are composed of periodide of choline, which may also be produced by tissue extracts. Forbes[7] states that if the result is negative, the spermatic fluid may not have reacted due to a very low choline content, the stain may have been over-diluted, or it may not have been composed of seminal fluid. When positive, one need not necessarily find spermatozoa since it may be a case of aspermia. In his opinion, a fallacy might be due to tissue extracts in the stain.

The attention of the examiner must not be confined solely to seminal stains. It is important, especially in cases where there has been recent rupture of the hymen, that blood-stains also should be examined for spermatozoa, since they may be present in the blood which flows from the breach in the hymen.

Leucorrhoeal stains are characterised by an abundance of squamous epithelial cells, and if the discharge has been mucopurulent, by pus cells also, the compound nuclei of which can be rendered apparent by treatment with weak potassium hydrate.

In conclusion, it should be stressed that the presence of at least one spermatozoon must be established to identify positively the stain as semen, and that no one should undertake this examination without adequate experience.

Precipitin or serological test with seminal fluid. The spermato-precipitins are of value in the identification of seminal fluid in certain cases, admittedly few in number, for example, in bestiality cases, where it may be desirable to differentiate between the seminal fluid of man as opposed to animal, by having a corroborative serological test to substantiate an opinion based on the microscopical differences in character of the spermatozoa. To apply the test, an immune serum must be prepared by injecting a rabbit with human seminal fluid or the seminal fluid of a particular animal, in the same manner as for the production of anti-blood serum. Anti-human semen serum is available commercially. With a properly prepared serum, 1 ml of seminal fluid extract to which 0·1 ml of immune serum has been added will give a reaction in one hour at room temperature (for technique see p. 349).

Determination of the group of seminal fluid. Serum from Group A and serum from Group B are mixed with saline to form dilutions of 1 : 2, 1 : 4, 1 : 8, 1 : 16, etc. 0·1 ml of each dilution of each serum is added to the same amount of seminal fluid in a small test tube. The tubes are allowed to stand for two hours at laboratory temperature when they are centrifuged, the supernatant fluid tested with cells of Group A and Group B, respectively, and the effects of the previous absorption carefully noted. In this manner the group of the seminal fluid is determined. By this means, it is therefore possible in certain cases to show that the group of seminal fluid found on stained articles differs from that of the seminal fluid of a suspect who may be charged with a sexual offence.

Examination for venereal disease

The examination for the presence of venereal infection in an accused or assaulted person must include both clinical and laboratory procedures and should be conducted only by those specialised in the appropriate fields.

Can a healthy adult female be raped by one man?

There is no doubt that rape can be perpetrated in the instance of a woman who has become exhausted by the resistance which she has offered, or when, on account of fear or injury, she has lost consciousness. One should refrain, however, from expressing an opinion on this important point until careful consideration has been given to all the facts of the particular case. There have been many undoubted cases in which a woman has been raped by an unaided man, despite the fact that so long as a woman retains complete possession of her senses it does not require great physical strength to deny sexual entry by apt disposition of her limbs. When the act has been accomplished, one is almost forced to the conclusion that the victim must have become physically exhausted and incapable of further resistance, or that from fear or injury there had been temporary loss of consciousness, or that there was marked disproportion in strength between the woman and her assailant, or that she finally became acquiescent to the sexual act. On the other hand, it must not be forgotten that an assailant might have overcome her resistance by an appropriate disposition of her clothing.

When marked disproportion of age, size, and apparent strength in favour of the female are present, a charge of rape is often unsuccessful, because consent is likely to have been given. In most cases of this kind, however, such questions will probably not be asked of a medical witness, because the judge and jury are able to form their own opinions. The duty of the medical witness is to decide from the appearances of the body of the female, whether carnal knowledge of the woman has been effected forcibly, and the court will form its own opinions on the other points.

It is obvious that rape might be perpetrated quite easily when there is more than one assailant.

Is it possible for a woman to be violated during ordinary sleep without her knowledge?

The answer to this question is that it is highly improbable in the case of a virgin. We should say that it is impossible, because of the pain attendant upon a first coitus. In the case of women who are accustomed to sexual intercourse, it is unlikely, although not impossible.

By the law of Scotland this offence is not rape but clandestine injury to a woman (p. 428). In our experience we have only known one attempt of this kind. The prisoner tried to impersonate the husband of a young woman and entered her bed, but the woman, awaking when he tried to have coitus, raised the alarm, whereupon the man fled. On examination we found her to be six months pregnant but not to have sustained any injury.

Carnal knowledge during unconsciousness

Cases of violation of females during a state of unconsciousness occasioned by fits, faints, hysteria, and anaesthetics have occurred. That the act may be accomplished under such circumstances is obvious. It is unfortunately true that medical men and dentists, by reason of their professional work, are liable occasionally to have baseless charges of this kind preferred against them by women following the administration of an anaesthetic. A chaperon obviates such an accusation.

Procedure in examination of females in cases of alleged rape

In proceeding to the examination of persons in connection with a charge of rape or unlawful carnal knowledge, there are certain points which should prove useful to the inexperienced.

When such a charge is laid with the police, the practice is that a doctor is requested to examine the complainer, who, by laying the charge, is presumed to be willing to afford all the evidence, even to the examination of her person. Expressed consent to make the examination must, nevertheless, be obtained (p. 56). It may be necessary to explain the need for examination, making the point that without the evidence thereby obtainable, proceedings against the accused become difficult, if not impossible. Another female should always be present during the examination. In cases of unlawful carnal knowledge and other sexual offences with girls under the age of sixteen, the consent of the girl is insufficient, since she is held incapable of giving or withholding consent until she has attained the age of sixteen. The consent of her parent or

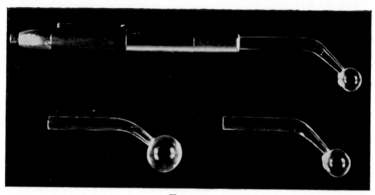

FIG. 219

Graduated plastic rods for deployment of hymeneal edges during examination with pen-torch also fitted. (By courtesy of City of Glasgow Police).

guardian is, therefore, first required. A detailed history, patiently taken and in the complainer's own words, is of immense value and should be recorded; quiet discussion with the girl often helps her to relax and become more co-operative. The subsequent examination may elucidate discrepancies in the story.

When making a local examination of the genitals, modesty must not be allowed to obstruct a detailed investigation. Either the lithotomy or knee-chest position may be utilised for the purpose, adequate illumination must be available, and the subject under examination should be treated with consideration.

In cases which present an annular notched hymen or a hymen which shows an irregular purse-like opening, it may be, and frequently is, a difficult matter to differentiate between the natural notches and the results of old and small lacerations. Practice has shown that this matter is greatly simplified by the use of a glass rod with a small, spherical head.   This is gently passed through the hymeneal aperture and then eased forwards, when the edges of the hymen become slightly everted. By slowly rotating the sphere, around which the edges are deployed, natural notches are readily differentiated from tears, recent or old. This method does not cause either pain or injury, and its use by us over a long period has amply demonstrated its value.   These rods, originally made for the late Professor Glaister in Pyrex glass, are now available in plastic.   The cylindrical part fits into a pen-torch (Fig. 219).   The rod should be at body temperature before insertion.

The following examination should be made in such cases:

The general physical appearance, her demeanour, and her emotional state.

The presence or absence of marks of violence upon her body; their character, and position, when present.

The presence or absence of marks upon the clothing when the assault is alleged to have taken place in the open.

The condition of the genitals, with respect to: (1) the presence or absence of blood; (2) the signs of bruising, or other injury; (3) the condition of the hymen with regard to old or recent injury, together with the character, extent, and situation of the injury; (4) whether, from the character of the vagina, the female has been habituated to coitus.

Some vaginal secretion for microscopical examination should be obtained as already described (p. 436).

If a muco-purulent or purulent discharge is present, a specimen should be taken for bacteriological examination (see p. 437).

The examination of stains on garments for spermatozoa should be made subsequently.

In cases where the woman alleges that she was raped under the influence of alcohol or drugs, samples of blood, urine, and faeces should be collected and put into a sealed container for analysis (p. 609).

INDECENT AND LEWD PRACTICES

The provisions of the Criminal Law Amendment Act, 1885, as applicable to Scotland, in relation to these offences, have already been described (p. 429).   Such practices have assumed a varied form and have covered a wide range of indecent conduct towards girls and boys in the many cases which we have investigated.   Among the most prevalent, are handling of the private parts, including the introduction of the finger into the vagina, masturbatory acts performed upon the girl, inducing her to handle the male organ, mutual masturbatory acts, intercrural connection, and lingual contact with the private parts.

When the subjects of such offences are under the age of puberty, girls of twelve years and boys of fourteen years, the crimes are generally under common law, but where the girls are above the age of twelve and under the age of sixteen the charge is brought under the Criminal Law Amendment Act, 1922, section 4.

The age of the girl, if under sixteen, must be set out in the indictment and must be proved at the trial.   In the case of gross indecency between males, whether in public or in private, puberty, for obvious reasons, is not made the limit of a charge.   Further, in the case of boys, consent cannot legitimise the offence, and where a boy old enough to consent, has consented, instead of the act not constituting an offence as in the case of females over the age of sixteen, the act becomes a crime in both parties.   In cases of indecent assault between females, if the assaulted person is over sixteen the defence of consent could be employed, since an adult and consenting woman may behave indecently in private, but this is not permitted by law between males.   Conversely, it is an offence for a female to commit an indecent assault upon a boy.

In the case of R. v. Hare,[8] a woman was convicted of indecent assault on a boy of twelve.   On appeal it was argued that the offence of indecent assault on a male referred to in section 62, Offences Against the Person Act, 1861, could not be committed by a woman, since offences in that section were limited to sodomitical offences.   Mr Justice Avory in dismissing the appeal, pointed out that 'unnatural offences' did not govern the words 'any indecent assault upon a male person' and said there was no ground for limiting these words in the manner suggested.

In all cases of indecent practices, it is held to be an aggravation of the offence when the offender is in a relation of trust to the person offended, as for instance, a teacher or a nurse.   It is also an aggravation if venereal disease is communicated, or if previous convictions for indecent, lewd, and libidinous practices have been recorded against an accused person.

The examination of the subjects resolves itself into an examination of the private parts of the offended girls or boys, and we have not infrequently found that such practices have been made by one offending male against a series of girls or boys of tender age.   In some cases, injury to the hymen may be found due to the insertion of the finger of the offender.   The only evidence of any value as to whether the male organ has been used and emission of semen has taken place, is obtained by an examination of the underclothing, bedding, or other material. On a number of occasions, we have had to examine the male offender where there was a charge of communicating venereal disease to the offended girl or girls.   Reviewing the records of several hundred cases of indecent practices with girls, we find that in the majority of them more than one girl was molested by the accused man, and in several instances the accused was responsible for indecent practices with no fewer than four, five, six, and seven young girls. Drink played an important role. One of the men charged was an epileptic. Venereal disease was occasionally communicated to the young victims. Many of the offenders were married and the father of children. The ages of the male accused varied from sixteen to sixty-four, while the age range of those molested was four to fifteen years, the commonest ages being between seven and twelve.

With regard to cases of unlawful carnal knowledge, venereal disease was not infrequently transmitted, and pregnancy resulted in many cases between the ages of thirteen and sixteen.

UNNATURAL SEXUAL CRIMES

Allen[9] states that 'the law of the land discourages any public manifestation of sex, no matter how normal it may be'. Any transgression of this tends to be regarded as an act of indecency and may be punished accordingly. Apart from 'natural' manifestation, there are six so-called 'unnatural offences' which are punishable. These are:

1. Incest.
2. Buggery.
3. Bestiality.
4. Masturbation, if publicly performed.
5. Indecent exposure.
6. Tribadism, if publicly performed.

Incest

The crime of incest is statutory in Scotland (the Act of 1567), while it is an offence against the canon law, and also against statute law in England (Sexual Offences Act, 1956). Incest is the crime of carnal connection between persons held to be within the forbidden degrees of relationship. The forbidden relationships mentioned in Leviticus, chapter 18, verses 6 to 18, have been grouped as follows:[10]

(i) Direct ascendants and descendants (for example, son and mother, grandfather and granddaughter).
(ii) Siblings, whether of full or half blood.
(iii) Aunt and nephew, uncle and niece.

In England, it is unnecessary that the relationship should be traced through lawful wedlock. There must have been actual sexual connection to constitute the crime. An attempt to commit incest is rarely if ever charged; it is accepted that where incest is charged, the jury may convict of an attempt only.[11] The parties must know that they were related within the prohibited degrees, but if coitus is established the onus of disproving presumed relationship is thrown on the persons

accused.   The Criminal Procedure (Scotland) Act, 1938, has enacted
that carnal knowledge between a man and a woman whose marriage to
each other is authorised by the Marriage (Prohibited Degrees of
Relationship) Acts, or would be authorised on the death of any person,
is not incest.

Medical evidence in such cases resolves itself into affirmation of non-
virginity of the female, or the existence of pregnancy.   We have examined many girls for evidence of this crime, and in all of them there were
definite signs of trafficking in the sexual parts, and in some, pregnancy
resulted, while in others seminal stains on the undergarments were
found.

In one of the many cases in which we have made examinations, the
incestuous intercourse was between brother and sister, both under the
age of majority.   The girl at the time of our examination was seven
months pregnant.   In many other instances, the intercourse was between father and daughter.

In one case, two sisters were involved in incestuous intercourse with
their father.   The elder, aged sixteen and ten months, explained that
the acts of intercourse had occurred twice weekly over a period of eight
years; the younger, aged fourteen stated that her father had had
connection with her on at least ten occasions, over a period of two years.

In reviewing many cases of incest, we found that the father of the
victim was involved in numerous instances, and the relationship of
stepfather, uncle, or brother was frequently encountered.   The ages
of the females ranged from six to twenty-three years, the most frequent
age incidence being fifteen years.   Pregnancy resulted in some cases.
In one of these, the girl was twelve and a half years old.   In two cases
where the sexual relationship took place between brother and sister,
the age of the girls was fifteen and that of the brothers seventeen and
eighteen respectively.   Another case involving three adults was most
unusual, since the woman, already married and with one child, committed incest on many occasions not only with her adult brother but
with her aged father.

Buggery

The offence of buggery consists of sexual intercourse per anum by
man with man; or by man with woman; or sexual intercourse by man
or woman in any manner with an animal.   Buggery is made an offence
under section 12 of the Sexual Offences Act, 1956, in England.   Nevertheless, section 1 of the Sexual Offences Act, 1967, provides that an act
of buggery, or gross indecency between two men shall not be an offence,
provided it is in private, the parties consent, and they have both attained
the age of twenty-one.

In Scotland, the crime of sodomy, defined as unnatural carnal connection between males, is prosecuted at common law or under section 11 of the Criminal Law Amendment Act, 1885. There is no provision for consenting males over any age even in private. Prosecution under section 11 of the Criminal Law Amendment Act, 1885, in such cases, is as an alternative charge to that of sodomy where the facts, which can be proved, fall short of what is necessary to sustain a charge of sodomy, or a definite attempt to commit sodomy, but where the act committed is one of gross indecency between males. This section has therefore widened the scope of the law, with respect to the commission of indecent offences by two or more male persons, whether in public or private, but does not of itself necessarily deal with the crime of sodomy. It includes such offences as penile friction on the gluteal folds, handling of the male parts, mutual masturbation, or intercrural connection. Persons involved in homosexual activities may be active or passive participants or they may alternate.

Proof of penetration, but not emission, is necessary to constitute the act of sodomy. In R. v. Wiseman,[12] a man was indicted for having committed this offence with a woman, and in R. v. Jellyman[13] for committing the offence on his wife. Anal intercourse with women is probably not a crime in Scotland. Paederasty is the form of sodomy in which the passive agent is a boy. This unnatural crime is, perhaps, more common than is supposed, but charges frequently break down at, or before, trial for want of adequate evidence.

The disproportion between the penis and the anal orifice, together with the absence or use of violence, and the use or otherwise of a lubricant, in the course of penetration, are important factors in determining whether injury to the anus will result.

Medical evidence is restricted, in the main, to an examination of the passive agent, but, in either, there may be evidence of trauma to the penis or of recent seminal staining, traces of lubricant, faeces, or anal secretion. Clothing may be contaminated by faeces or semen.

Consent for examination must be obtained.

The lesions which the examiner should look for, in the passive agent, are:

Recent lacerations, bruising, or inflammation of the anal mucous membrane.

Dilatation of the anus, absence of puckering of the anal orifice, and diminished sphincter grip, in varying degree, in habitual cases.

An infundibuliform shape of the anus in confirmed passive sodomists.

The presence of old lacerations, as indicated by scarring, and of external piles.

Incriminating stains.

The buttocks should be pulled apart, because in habitual homosexuals the anus gapes and mucous membrane is exposed due to the lack of sphincter tone. This differs from the normal reflex contraction on separating the buttocks. A rectal examination with the passive agent in the knee-elbow position should be performed to judge the tone of the anal sphincter. Swabs should be taken from the anus and surrounding area for examination for spermatozoa, venereal infection, and presence of lubricant.

It must be remembered that dilatation of the anus may exist from changes due to natural disease, and, in the dead, from putrefaction.

This unnatural crime may be committed in ways which leave no lesions behind them, and consequently, in many cases, the crime either goes undetected, or fails to be proved through lack of evidence.

Sodomy most frequently results from the condition of male sexual inversion or homosexuality. A review of a number of cases of sodomy

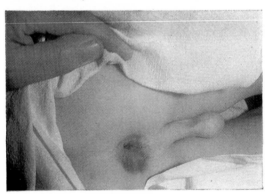

FIG. 220
Case of sodomy—passive agent—a boy
(By courtesy of Dr James Imrie)

shows that the age of the active agent varied from twenty-five to sixty-four years, whereas that of the passive agent was from six to forty-three years. In some instances, the active partner had previously been convicted of sodomy, and in others, with the offence of gross indecency with another male. A case (reported to us by the late Dr Mearns) is of special interest, since it shows precocity of the active agent. He was a boy of fourteen, who suffered from urethral gonorrhoea and had experienced sodomitic relations with several men whom he had importuned for the purpose of gratifying his perverted sexual urge.

So far as boys are concerned, in Scotland charges at common law are usually preferred when the boy is below the age of puberty. Such cases can still be brought at common law when the youth is above that age but usually such charges are brought under section 11 of the Criminal Law Amendment Act, 1885, in Scotland and section 13 of the Sexual Offences Act, 1956, in England.

With regard to gross indecency between males, points which emerge from our records are:

The ages of the accused varied from twenty-five to forty five;
The assaulted males varied in age from six to twenty-six;
One of the accused had four previous convictions for sodomy and indecent practices, one had five convictions for lewd practices and was found to be insane, another had a conviction for sodomy and gross indecency with a male, and several had previous convictions for gross indecency.

Taylor's[14] monograph on homosexual offences and their relation to psychotherapy contains some very interesting information, and allusions to it are freely made. He states that in 1946, ninety-six persons were received into Brixton Prison charged with homosexual offences. Of these, thirty-nine were charged with indecent assault on boys, twenty-four with importuning, seventeen with gross indecency, and sixteen with the crime of sodomy. Of the ninety-six cases, fifty-seven involved offences against boys, including all the indecent assaults. He classified all the cases into four groups:

1. those with heterosexual tendencies in whom the homosexual offence was in the nature of a substitution for the normal heterosexual act and who were classified as 'pseudo-homosexuals';
2. 'bisexuals', individuals in whom strong heterosexual, as well as homoseuxal, tendencies were obvious;
3. prostitutes, individuals who would have fallen into the 'pseudo-homosexual' group, but were characterised by the fact that the homosexual acts were carried out for gain; and
4. 'true inverts', which numbered only thirteen in the total of ninety-six cases. Of the 'true inverts', eight were charged with importuning, three for gross indecency, and two for sodomy. Of the thirteen, only one was interested in boys, but twelve were attracted to men. Five were always passive, two were always active, three were either active or passive, and in three the act was in the form of mutual masturbation.

Androgynous physique was present in six cases. Of the two active men, one was quite effeminate in appearance. Of the five preferring the passive role, three were of feminine, and two were of masculine build. Perversions were much more evident in those preferring the passive role. Fellatio was admitted by four men. Of the true inverts, thirteen cases in all, seven had had treatment with improvement, three refused treatment, and only one of the remainder was considered likely to benefit by treatment.

ILLUSTRATIVE CASES

Two young men assaulted a boy, and while one held him the other committed the act. On examination, we found four recent linear lacerations of the anal mucous membrane with evidence of bleeding.

A man was charged with repeated acts of sodomy with a boy aged eight over a period of seven months. Examination of the anal parts showed irritation around the entrance, and a healing fissure on the mucous membrane, together with an infundibuliform shape of the rectal orifice. The boy suffered from incontinence of faeces.

In a case of sodomy, involving two adults, smears from the glans penis and urinary meatus of one of the men and from the rectum of the

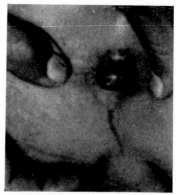

FIG. 221

Case of sodomy. Passive agent was a boy of ten. Some dilatation of anus, together with bruising and inflammation, were present

other showed numerous spermatozoa. Stains from the jacket, rain-coat, and trousers of the former man, and from the overcoat and trousers of the latter, also disclosed the presence of many spermatozoa.

In a case of attempted sodomy by a man with a boy, examination under filtered ultra-violet light of the pyjamas worn by the boy showed a fluorescence of certain oleaginous stains which was identical to the fluorescence given by the contents of a jar of vaseline said, by the boy, to have been used by the accused.

Bestiality

Bestiality is the term applied to sexual intercourse between a person and an animal, whether by the anus or by the vagina. In England, it is indicted under the Sexual Offences Act, 1956. In Scotland, bestiality is an offence at common law. There is no reported case in Scotland of bestiality by a woman, but in England a woman may be guilty of the crime. Any evidence of a medical character must either be supplementary to that of eye-witnesses, or purely circumstantial. When in the latter form, it usually consists in finding upon the person of the accused evidences of contact with the animal as, for example, hairs which correspond with those of the animal in question, or the presence of human seminal fluid in, or around, the parts of the animal.

ILLUSTRATIVE CASES

A man was tried for bestiality with a mare. A pair of trousers which the accused was wearing at the time of apprehension, and hair from the hinder parts of the mare, were examined. Stains consisting of blood were present in the fork of the trousers, and also a hair, similar to the hairs from the mare, was found. Certain other whitish stains on the trousers were examined and some were found to contain squamous epithelium. When fluid from the neighbourhood of the genitals of the mare was examined, immediately following the offence, spermatozoa were found. The accused pleaded guilty, and, having been previously convicted of a similar crime, was sentenced to a long period of imprisonment.

At the Circuit Court, Glasgow, a man was tried for bestiality with a cow.

At the High Court, Dumfries, a man was convicted of bestiality with domestic fowls.

A man was apprehended near Renfrew after having been seen attempting to have unnatural intercourse with a duck. On examination as to his mental condition, he was found to be of unsound mind and unfit to plead.

At Fort William, a man was charged with committing this offence with a female goat, and was convicted.

OTHER SEXUAL PERVERSIONS

Sadism

The term is applied to the association of sexual desire and the inflicting of cruelty or violence. The condition is frequently associated with 'lust' murder (Fig. 191, p. 332).

Masochism

This is the opposite of sadism, since the condition is the association of sexual desire with the desire for submission to cruelty and violence or mutilation.

Fetichism

Fetichism is sexual gratification produced by contact with, or the sight of, an object that normally does not exercise a sexual influence on the mind.   An infinite variety of sexual references may thus be developed among different individuals.

Indecent exposure or exhibitionism[15]

These terms apply to the acts of men whose sexual desire consists principally of the exhibition of the genitals with or without performances of masturbatory acts in the presence of woman or young girls.   Occasionally women may expose themselves in public.

Female sexual inversion, tribadism, or lesbianism

These terms are applied to sexual relationships between females (see Fig. 223).

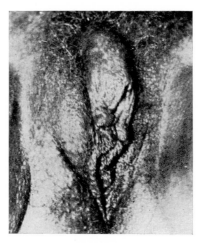

FIG. 222
Abnormal enlargement of clitoris in a
woman long habituated to lesbianism

Male sexual inversion or homosexuality

These terms are applied to sexual relationships between males (p. 452). The strictly sexual aspects have already beeen considered.   Rupp[16] has pointed out that sudden unexpected and violent death is commoner in the homosexual because of the clandestine nature and promiscuity of his sex life.

Transvestism or eonism

Transvestism is the name given to the perversion in which males find sexual pleasure in wearing female apparel. This condition is sometimes found in females who dress themselves in male attire.

Necrophilia

The term is applied to the act of defiling the dead by sexual intercourse. The case of John Christie in 1953, about which several books have been written, is instructive.

References

1. R. v. Williams [1923] 1 K.B., 340.
2. R. v. Clarke [1949] 2 All E.R., 448.
3. H.M. Advocate v. Grainger 1932, S.L.T. 28.
4. H.M. Advocate v. Logan 1937, S.L.T. 104.
5. MASON, L.W.   *Am. J. Obstet. Gynec.*, **25,** 144, 1933.
6. WALTHER, G.   *J. forens. Med.*, **18,** 15, 1971.
7. FORBES, G.   *Police J.*, **13,** 162, 1940.
8. R. v. Hare [1934] 1 K.B., 354; 24 Cr. App. R. 108.
9. ALLEN, C.   *The Sexual Perversions and Abnormalities.*   Oxford University Press, 1940.
10. H.M. Advocate v. Aikman & Martin, 1917, J.C.8.
11. GORDON, G.H.   *The Criminal Law of Scotland.*   Edinburgh: Green, 1967.
12. R. v. Wiseman (1718), Footes Rep., 91
13. R. v. Jellyman (1838), 8 C. & P., 604.
14. TAYLOR, F.H.   *Br. med. J.*, **2,** 525, 1947.
15. ROOTH, F.G.   *Br. J. hosp. Med.*, **5,** 521, 1971.
16. RUPP, J.C.   *Medicine Sci. Law,* **10,** 189, 1970.

Chapter 16

MENTAL DISORDER IN ITS MEDICO-LEGAL ASPECTS

ALTHOUGH the statutory enactments dealing with mental illness are mainly administrative in character, it is necessary for his intelligent and legal conduct that the practitioner of medicine should be familiar at least with those provisions by which his relations to the person of unsound mind are regulated. His relationships with the public will doubtless bring him sooner or later into contact with such cases. He may be required: (1) to certify mental unsoundness; (2) to pronounce an opinion on the mental capacity of a prisoner to instruct counsel for his defence, or to plead to a given charge; (3) to pronounce an opinion regarding testamentary capacity; or (4) to certify in other contingencies, such as in the appointment of a curator to a person who, owing to mental unsoundness, is unable to manage his own affairs.

The legislation dealing with the care, treatment, protection, and safeguarding of the property and affairs of mentally disordered persons is contained in the Mental Health Act, 1959, and the Mental Health (Scotland) Act, 1960. These Acts also contain provisions concerning mentally disordered persons involved in criminal proceedings.

A principal purpose of both these acts is to ensure that, wherever possible, the mentally disordered patient can have the same ready access, without formality, to care and treatment as the patient suffering from some physical disorder.

THE MENTAL HEALTH ACT, 1959

The Act begins by dissolving the Board of Control and makes provision for the establishment of Mental Health Review Tribunals in the Regional Hospital Board areas. It gives a number of definitions of the terms which are used in the Act.

Mental disorder means mental illness, arrested or incomplete development of mind, psychopathic disorder, and any other disorder or disability of mind.

Severe subnormality (including the idiots and imbeciles of pre-1959 legislation) means that the patient is incapable of living an independent life or guarding himself against serious exploitation because of arrested or incomplete development of the mind.

Subnormality is a lesser degree ('feeble-minded') which requires or is susceptible to medical treatment or special care.

Psychopathic disorder means a persistent disorder or disability of mind (whether or not including subnormality of intelligence) which results in abnormally aggressive or seriously irresponsible conduct on the part of the patient, and requires or is susceptible to medical treatment. Before 1959, there was a category of 'moral defectives' who were considered to suffer from mental disorder by reason only of promiscuity or other immoral conduct; such are excluded by the Act.

COMPULSORY ADMISSION TO HOSPITAL

Admission for observation

This must be based on the written recommendations of two medical practitioners in the prescribed form, stating that the patient is suffering from mental disorder of a nature or degree which warrants the detention of the patient in a hospital under observation for at least a limited period, and that he ought to be so detained in the interests of his own health or safety or with a view to the protection of other persons.

A patient admitted to hospital under an application for observation may be detained for a period not exceeding twenty-eight days, unless he has become liable to be detained by virtue of a subsequent application for further detention.

Admission for treatment

A patient may be detained in hospital for treatment on an application accompanied by the written recommendations of two medical practitioners.

The application. The regulations concerning this apply both to applications for observation and treatment. The application must be made either by the nearest relative of the patient or by a mental welfare officer and must specify the qualifications of the applicant: it must be addressed to the managers of the hospital to which admission is sought. The applicant must have seen the patient within the fourteen days ending with the date of the petition.

The medical recommendations. These must state that the patient is suffering from, in the case of a patient of any age, mental illness or severe subnormality, and in the case of a patient under the age of twenty-one years, psychopathic disorder or subnormality, and that it is necessary in the interests of the patient's health or safety, or for the protection of other persons, that the patient should be detained. The reasons for the opinions expressed must be given and a statement that other methods of dealing with the patient are not appropriate. The patient must be described in each of the recommendations as suffering from the same form of mental disorder. The recommendations must be signed on or before the date of the application and the doctors must have examined the patient either together or at an interval of not more than seven days.   One of the medical recommendations must be given by a practitioner who has been approved for this purpose by a Local Health Authority.   One of the recommendations must also, if practicable, be given by a practitioner who has previous knowledge of the patient.   One of the recommendations may be given by a practitioner in the hospital in which the patient is to be detained.   This is not permissible in the case of mental nursing homes and private patients.

The medical recommendations cannot be given by any of the following:

(*a*) the applicant;

(*b*) a partner or assistant of the applicant or of the doctor making the other recommendation;

(*c*) a person who receives or has an interest in the receipt of any payments made on account of the patient or, except as previously mentioned, a practitioner on the staff of the hospital to which the patient is admitted;

(*d*) various relatives of the patient and of the doctor giving the other recommendation.

The effect of the application.   The properly completed application, if presented within fourteen days of the date of the most recent medical examination, is sufficient authority for removal and detention of the patient in hospital.

There are provisions for the rectification of errors in the application and medical recommendations.

The authority to detain lapses at the end of a year, but it may then be renewed for a year and, on subsequent expiry, for periods of two years if the responsible medical officer, after examining the patient, considers that it is necessary in the interests of the patient's health or safety, or for the protection of other persons, that he should continue to be detained. The responsible medical officer must report this to the managers of the hospital, and this is the authority for renewal of the detention.   The managers of the hospital must notify the patient, who has a right to apply to a Mental Health Review Tribunal.

A patient who is detained for treatment as a psychopathic or subnormal patient cannot be detained beyond the age of twenty-five years, unless the authority for his detention is renewed under the special provisions of the Act.

Emergency admission

In cases of urgent necessity an application can be made by a Mental Welfare Officer or by a relative.   This must be accompanied by a statement that it is of urgent necessity for the patient to be detained, and compliance with the procedure required for admission for observation would involve undesirable delay, and a medical recommendation from one doctor who must examine the patient within a period of three days ending with the date of the application, verify the urgency and if practicable, have previous acquaintance with the patient.

This emergency application ceases to have effect on the expiration of a period of seventy-two hours from the time the patient is admitted, unless a properly completed second medical recommendation is received by the managers of the hospital.

Leave of absence from hospital and absence without leave

The responsible medical officer may grant to any patient who has been detained, leave of absence either indefinitely or for a specified period.

A patient cannot be taken into custody and returned to the hospital after he has absented himself without leave for the following periods:

(a) in the case of patients over twenty-one years who are detained as psychopathic or subnormal patients, six months;
(b) in any other case, twenty-eight days.

Discharge of patients

An order for discharge of a patient detained for observation or treatment may be made by the responsible medical officer or by the managers of the hospital.

An order for discharge can also be made by the nearest relative of the patient, after giving at least seventy-two hours' notice in writing to the managers of the hospital, but this order will be of no effect if during the period of notice the responsible medical officer furnishes a report to the managers certifying that the patient, if discharged, would be likely to act in a manner dangerous to other persons or to himself.   Under these circumstances no further order for the discharge of the patient can be made by the relative during a period of six months following the report.

When the responsible medical officer furnishes the above report, the managers must notify the nearest relative, who can within a period of twenty-eight days appeal to a Mental Health Review Tribunal.

Detention of patients concerned in criminal proceedings

This procedure is described in Part V of the Act and its provisions should be read along with those of the Criminal Procedure (Insanity) Act, 1964.

When a Court is satisfied after hearing evidence from two doctors, one of whom must be approved as having special experience in the diagnosis and treatment of mental disorder, that the delinquent is suffering from mental illness and that this is the most suitable method of disposing of the case, it can make an order for admission to hospital. The Supreme Court (Appeal Court, High Court, Crown Court) is empowered to make orders restricting discharge. These may be for a period specified in the order or unlimited. An order restricting discharge can only be made if one of the doctors has given oral evidence in Court. Magistrates' Courts can commit the delinquent to the Supreme Court for the purpose of obtaining a restricting order.

The patient can be released only by order of the Home Secretary.

If the Home Secretary is satisfied, by reports from at least two medical practitioners, one of whom must be approved for the purpose, that a person serving a sentence of imprisonment is suffering from mental illness, psychopathic disorder, subnormality or severe subnormality, and this is of a nature or degree which warrants detention in a hospital for medical treatment, then he can direct that the person be removed from prison and detained in hospital.

THE MENTAL HEALTH (SCOTLAND) ACT, 1960

The Act establishes the Mental Welfare Commission, which consists of not fewer than seven and not more than nine Commissioners, including at least one woman. At least three of these must be medical practitioners and one must be a solicitor or member of the Faculty of Advocates of five years standing.

The duty of the Commission is to exercise a general protective function in respect of persons who by reason of mental disorder are incapable of adequately protecting themselves or their interests. Throughout the Act the general term 'Mental Disorder' is used to cover both mental illness and mental deficiency.

COMPULSORY DETENTION IN HOSPITAL

So far as possible, people suffering from mental disorder will go into hospitals on the advice of their own doctors and this does not require any legal formality. Some patients, however, still require compulsory detention and, as this is a serious interference with liberty, appropriate legal procedure is detailed in the Act. The three essentials are:

1. An application;
2. Recommendations by two medical practitioners;
3. Approval by the Sheriff.

The application

This must be made in the prescribed form to the board of management of the hospital to which admission is sought by the nearest relative, or by a mental health officer.   If the application is made by a mental health officer, he must take such steps as are reasonably practicable to inform the nearest relative of the patient of the proposed application and of his right to object to the Sheriff.

The application for admission is not valid unless the person making the application has seen the patient within the period of fourteen days ending with the date on which the proposed application is submitted to the Sheriff.

The medical recommendations

These recommendations must be signed on or before the date of the application by two medical practitioners, neither of whom is the applicant, who have personally examined the patient separately at an interval of not more than seven days, or where no objection has been made by the patient or his nearest relative, together.   The certificates explain why it is necessary for the patient to be detained.

One of the recommendations must be given by a practitioner who has been approved for this purpose by a Regional Hospital Board as having special experience in the diagnosis or treatment of mental disorder, and the other recommendation should, if practicable, be given by the patient's general medical practitioner or another medical practitioner who has previous acquaintance with the patient.

One only of the recommendations can be given by a practitioner on the staff of the hospital named in the application.   In the cases of private patients and admissions to private hospitals, neither recommendation may be given by a practitioner on the staff of the hospital named in the application.

Not more than one of the recommendations can be given by a medical officer in the service of a local authority.

The recommendations must contain a statement as to whether the person signing the recommendation is related to the patient and declare any pecuniary interest which he may have in the admission of the patient to hospital.

This differs basically from the situation in England, where the Mental Health Act, 1959, allows the detention of a person after the provision of two medical certificates; there no quasi-judicial procedure is necessary.

The approval by the Sheriff

The application for admission must be submitted to the Sheriff for his approval within seven days of the last date on which the patient was examined for the purposes of the medical recommendation.

The Sheriff may make such inquiries and hear such persons, including the patient, as he thinks fit.   When there is an objection to the application by the nearest relative, he must hear the relative and any witness whom he may call.

The effect of the application

Approval by the Sheriff of an application for admission is the authority for removal of the patient to the hospital named in the application, and when the application has been forwarded to the board of management, for the admission of the patient to that hospital at any time within a period of seven days from the date on which the Sheriff approved the application.

The authority to detain lapses at the end of a year, but it may then be renewed for a year and, on subsequent expiry, for periods of two years if the responsible medical officer, a doctor authorised for the purpose by the board of management or local health authority, obtains from another medical practitioner a report on the condition of the patient and reports that a further period of detention is necessary in the interests of the patient's health or safety, or for the protection of other persons. The patient must be informed of the renewal of his detention, and may appeal to the Sheriff to order his discharge.

When a patient has been admitted to a hospital as a result of an application approved by a Sheriff, the board of management must, within seven days, notify the Mental Welfare Commission of the admission and send them a copy of the application and medical recommendations.

There are two classes of patient who are not liable to admission to hospital under compulsion if they are over the age of twenty-one years. These are persons who, though mentally defective, are not so defective as to be unable to lead an independent life or to guard themselves against serious exploitation, and mentally ill persons with a persistent disorder manifested only by abnormally aggressive or seriously irresponsible conduct.   Persons in these categories who have been detained, or subjected to guardianship, must be discharged on reaching the age of twenty-five years, unless likely to act dangerously.

Emergency admission

In cases of urgent necessity, an emergency recommendation may be made by one medical practitioner.   This must state that by reason of mental disorder it is urgently necessary for the patient to be admitted and detained in a hospital, but that compliance with the formal procedure for admission would involve undesirable delay.

An emergency recommendation provides authority for the removal of the patient to hospital at any time within a period of three days from the date on which it was made and for his detention for a period not exceeding seven days.   The emergency recommendation must be made by the medical practitioner on the day on which he examined the patient. Where practicable the consent of a relative or mental health officer must be obtained, and a statement that this has been done must accompany the recommendation.   If it has not been practicable to obtain such consent, a statement of the reasons for this must accompany the recommendation.

Leave of absence

The responsible medical officer in a hospital may grant leave of absence to any patient.   Where periods of leave of more than twenty-eight days are granted, the Mental Welfare Commission must be informed about this and also about the patient's return.

A patient cannot be taken into custody and returned to the hospital after he has absented himself without leave for the following periods:

(*a*) in the case of patients detained by reason of suffering from mental deficiency, three months;

(*b*) in the case of patients detained in pursuance of an emergency recommendation, seven days;

(*c*) in any other case, twenty-eight days.

Discharge of patients

Orders for discharge of a patient can be made by the responsible medical officer, and the Mental Welfare Commission, if they are satisfied that the patient is not suffering from mental disorder, or that it is not necessary in the interests of his health or safety, or for the protection of other persons, that he should continue to be detained.

An order for discharge can also be made by the nearest relative of the patient after giving not less than seven days' notice in writing to the board of management of the hospital, but this order will be of no effect if during the period of notice the responsible medical officer furnishes a report certifying that the patient, if discharged, would be likely to act in a manner dangerous to other persons or to himself.   If such a report is made the board of management must report this to the nearest relative, who can within twenty-eight days appeal to the Sheriff to order the discharge of the patient.

An order for discharge of a patient can also be made by the board of management of the hospital: this order becomes effective only after a period of seven days and with the consent of the responsible medical officer.   If he refuses consent he must provide the board with a report certifying that in his opinion the patient cannot be discharged without being a danger to himself or others.

Detention of patients concerned in criminal proceedings

The procedure is described in Part V of the Act.   The Act consolidates the old law and adds a number of new provisions.

Section 54 empowers a Court, where it appears that a person charged before the Court is suffering from mental disorder, to remand him to an available mental hospital, rather than in custody. Written or oral evidence of one doctor is sufficient to support the request for such a remand, the purpose of which is psychiatric assessment by the responsible medical officer who reports back to the Court.

Under section 63, where persons are found insane in bar of trial (that is, unfit to plead) or acquitted of a charge on indictment on grounds of insanity, it is the duty of the Court to record this finding. Where a person is charged on indictment and evidence is brought that he was insane at the time of doing the act and he is acquitted, the Court must direct the jury to find whether the person was insane at the time of doing the act, and declare whether the person was acquitted by them because of his insanity.   In both cases the Court makes an order for detention in a State Hospital, or such other hospital as the Court may for special reasons specify.   Such an order carries an automatic restriction on discharge, which continues in force until the Secretary of State is satisfied that the patient may be released without danger to the public (formerly, these patients were detained 'at her Majesty's pleasure'). The law with regard to insanity in bar of trial also applies to summary procedure in the Sheriff Court.

The Secretary of State, if he is satisfied on the reports of two doctors that a person detained in prison is suffering from a mental disorder, can direct that he should be transferred to hospital, under sections 65 and 66.   The Secretary of State can issue directions restricting the discharge.   Section 65 deals with persons awaiting trial or sentence, while section 66 deals with those already serving a term of imprisonment.

If it appears to the prosecutor of any Court that a person charged may be suffering from mental disorder, it is the duty of the prosecutor to provide the Court with such evidence of mental disorder as may be available.

In the *Glasgow Herald* of 22nd January 1971, a case is reported of a judge sentencing a man to imprisonment rather than sending him to the State Hospital, because one of three psychiatrists felt detention in the State Hospital to be unwarranted.   The judge's fear was that the State Hospital staff might take the same view and 'instead of serving a substantial sentence he will go scot-free'.   A recommendation that the prison authorities would arrange psychiatric treatment was made.

The case was linked editorially with that of a man who had been released from the State Hospital after less than five months, whereas his co-accused was serving a five-year sentence.

TESTAMENTARY CAPACITY

The duty of giving evidence as to the testamentary capacity of a testator usually falls upon medical witnesses, although it is not confined to them.

In the case of a disputed will in which the ground of action is the incapacity of the testator to make such will, doubtless the evidence of the medical attendants of the testator would, as a general rule, prove of the greatest value.   It is therefore advisable for practitioners, in order to maintain an attitude free from the semblance of bias or partiality, to avoid being witnesses to documents of a testamentary nature.

In probate suits, the ultimate burden of proving testamentary incapacity rests on the party contesting the will.

For a will to be valid, from the medico-legal point of view, the testator must be in possession of a 'sound and disposing mind'.   This state of mind, however, may be quite consistent with certain departures from sanity, and it may be inconsistent with an absence of insanity in the ordinary sense, where, for example, by reason of degenerative changes in the brain of an old person, the mind has become weakened and facile. If the legal definitions of what constitutes a sound and disposing mind are reviewed, it will be found that probably one of the best definitions is that given by Lord Cockburn in the case of Banks v. Goodfellow.[1] He stated that if the human instincts and affections, or the moral sense, became perverted by disease, if insane suspicion or aversion took the place of rational affection, if reason and judgment were lost and the mind became a prey to insane delusions, calculated to interfere with and destroy its functions, and to lead to a testamentary disposition due only to their baneful influence, then the will was bad.   If, however, the testator had an insane delusion, but it did not affect the general faculties of the mind and had no effect on the will, the mere fact that he had it did not take away his testamentary capacity.

The law admits that there may be sufficient intelligence remaining, although reduced from an average standard, for the legal exercise of the disposition of an estate.   This is well exemplified in many legal decisions in cases in which the testators were the acknowledged subjects of delusions, sometimes of a most definite character.   Further, the reasonable nature of the document is an important element.   It is therefore apparent that the law allows considerable latitude in the interpretation of the mental state with reference to testamentary capacity.

A lucid interval is not necessarily a complete restoration to mental vigour previously enjoyed nor is it merely the cessation or suppression of the symptoms of insanity.   The burden of proof of a lucid interval rests on the party asserting its existence.

The testator should have a sound and disposing mind either at the time of giving instructions for the preparation of the will or at the actual moment of its execution. The law does not demand that this state of mind should exist on both these occasions, but in the case of a holograph will it must exist at the time when the will is made and signed by the testator. The testator must fully comprehend:

the nature of a will and that he is disposing of his property to the person or persons named;
the extent of his possessions of which he is disposing;
the nature and effect of his act in its bearings on the moral claims of others, which should have had his consideration.

It is also necessary that:

the instructions for the preparation of the will have been given, and its subsequent execution made voluntarily and without any undue influence by any other person.

Thus the question which the medical practitioner has to answer is whether the testator is, or was, in a mental condition, by reason of natural incapacity, old age, illness, or insanity, such as to render him incapable of understanding that he is, or was, disposing of his property to a certain person or persons, or of knowing the extent of his estate, and of understanding the nature and effect of his act with relation to the natural claims of those excluded from the will. The only means available to the practitioner for answering the question are afforded by the behaviour and statements of the testator, either in connection with the act of testamentary disposition, or with reference to the acts of his daily life and his contacts with those around him. Even with evidence of mental impairment in one direction, it still remains to be considered whether the degree and character of the impairment prejudices the ability of the testator to dispose of his estate in a proper fashion. The testamentary capacity of an aphasic person can only be measured by the character and extent of the brain lesion and its effects upon the receptivity of the mind.

Care must be taken by the medical practitioner in prescribing drugs, particularly hypnotics and sedatives, to a person about to test a will.

MANAGEMENT OF PROPERTY OF PERSON MENTALLY INCAPACITATED

When a person, by reason of mental incapacity, is precluded from managing his affairs efficiently, a legal application to the Court may be made by relatives or friends of that person for the appointment of someone to administer his affairs.

Procedure in England[2]

Part VIII of the Mental Health Act, 1959, makes provision for the management of the property and affairs of mental patients. The person responsible for this is a Judge of the Court of Protection, an office of the Supreme Court, and he is appointed by the Lord Chancellor. He is given wide powers of administration when, after consideration of medical evidence, he is satisfied that a person is incapable, by reason of mental disorder, of managing and administering his property and affairs. The Court of Protection has thus been able to authorise the execution of a settlement of the property of a person suffering from mental disorder by the receiver on the patient's behalf. Additional power has now been granted to this office under Part III of the Administration of Justice Act, 1969, which amends section 103 of the Mental Health Act, 1959. Hereby the Court has the power to authorise the execution of a will on the patient's behalf. Medical evidence supporting the lack of testamentary capacity again must be presented to the Court before the Court can practise this jurisdiction.

In England, the age of majority must be reached before the will can be validly executed. By the Family Law Reform Act, 1969, this age is now eighteen.

Procedure in Scotland

In Scotland, the affairs of an insane person are administered exclusively by a curator bonis or judicial factor who is appointed on petition to the Court of Session (or Sheriff if the estate is small). The person whose estate is thus administered may still make a will the validity of which is upheld by the Court unless absence of testamentary capacity can be proved.

With the petition for appointment of a curator bonis go certificates signed by two practitioners, 'on soul and conscience', to the effect that the person is incapable of managing his affairs and stating specifically the cause and its duration, copies of which are appended to the petition. One of the certificates at least should be given by a doctor unconnected with the hospital should the person be detained. The certificates should include the date and place of interviewing such person, and should be dated within the period of one month prior to the presentation of the application. The petitioner usually nominates a curator bonis, but if the nomination is objected to on the ground of adverse interest or for other reason, and such objection is upheld, the Court may appoint some other suitable party.

Under the Mental Health (Scotland) Act, 1960, section 91, Local Health Authorities have a duty to petition the Court for the appointment of a curator bonis when this is required in connection with a person in their area, and no other arrangements have been made on his behalf.

In Scotland, persons reaching the age of minority have full legal capacity to make a will. This age is twelve in respect to girls and fourteen to boys. The law also allows for the signing of a will for a person who is unable physically to sign it.

CRIMINAL RESPONSIBILITY

The law presumes that every person is sane and accountable for his actions until the contrary is proved. The burden of proving otherwise rests upon the person setting up the defence of insanity. There are many people tainted with insanity who are, nevertheless, influenced by the same motives as ordinary persons and to whom the fear of punishment has a sufficiently strong deterrent effect. For such individuals the defence of insanity would be unsuccessful.

The present law on the defence of insanity is based upon the answers given by fourteen judges to certain questions put to them on abstract issues by the House of Lords in 1843. The principal decisions which were then taken are embodied in what are called the M'Naghten Rules, drawn up following the trial of a man named M'Naghten.[3] He was tried for the murder of Mr Drummond, whom he shot in the belief that he was Sir Robert Peel, for whom he had lain in wait. His acquittal followed on the ground of insanity. Medical evidence was led to the effect that a person of otherwise sound mind might be affected with morbid delusions and that the prisoner was in that condition. The evidence also indicated that a person labouring under a morbid delusion might have a moral perception of right and wrong, but that in the case of the prisoner it was a delusion which carried him beyond the power of his own control, leaving him no such perception, and that he was not capable of exercising any control over acts which had a connection with his delusion. The answers which the jury gave to the questions put to them were to the effect that at the time the act was committed the prisoner did not have the use of his understanding so as to know that he was doing a wrong and wicked act, and that the prisoner was not sensible at the time he committed the act that he was violating both the laws of God and man.

Put briefly, the M'Naghten Rules are that, to establish a defence on the ground of insanity, it must be clearly proved that at the time of committing the act the accused was labouring under such a defect of reason from disease of the mind that he did not know the nature and quality of his act, or if he did, that he was not aware that he was doing wrong.

Legislation has not yet disturbed the criteria of insanity laid down by the judges in the M'Naghten case. Those falling within the M'Naghten Rules must be held to be without a criminal mind or mens rea. Nevertheless, an act may be a crime although the mind of the person who commits it is affected by disease, if such disease does not in fact produce upon his mind one or other of the effects above mentioned. With respect to the legal interpretation, in this connection, of the term 'wrong', the criterion is not legal right and wrong, but moral right and wrong. It must be a knowledge which is not merely general and abstract, but a knowledge which must exist with regard to the particular act under consideration.

The interpretation of the law differs, however, in the rulings of different judges. Some adhere to its literal terms, and hold that the medical evidence must be confined to a description of the state of mind of the accused at the time the act was committed, which, in many cases, may be absolutely impossible, although an opinion might be hazarded on the point from a consideration of his mental condition at the time of the examination. Other judges leave the jury to say from the evidence led whether the accused was prevented by any disease affecting his mind from controlling his own conduct.

This certainly enlarges the purview, and it permits of medical evidence being led regarding the mental condition of the accused at the time of examination, and, based upon that, as to whether any disease then present was likely to have existed at the time of the commission of the act, thus preventing him from controlling his conduct. Other judges put the question to the jury, whether the accused knew the nature and quality of the act, and whether he was of sound mind. This is still a more liberal interpretation of the law, since, by implication, a person may be insane who at the time he committed the act knew the nature and quality of the act, and, consequently, any relevant medical evidence would be admitted which had relation to the mental condition of the accused. It will be obvious that the interpretation which different judges may place on the law will affect the range and character of the medical evidence which is permissible.

Assuming, however, that the witness is permitted to offer such relevant evidence as will throw light upon the mental condition of the accused at the time of the examination, and, by implication, of his mental state at the time of the commission of the crime; what kind of evidence would justify the witness in offering an opinion of the insanity and irresponsibility of an accused person? Generally, the existence of delusions, especially delusions bearing upon the particular crime which has been committed, would be strong evidence, because their existence betokens dissociated cerebral action. A delusion may cause abnormality either of the whole mental outlook or only of certain actions.

A man may be the subject of a delusion which, although it affects his actions, does not offer any causal connection with the crime he has committed.

It must not be forgotten, however, that the intellect may have been so abnormal at the time when the crime was committed that, in the ordinary process of reasoning on the part of the examiner, the connection between the delusion and the crime cannot be traced. If delusions are found to exist in a person who has committed a criminal act, it would be the duty of the examiner to discover, if possible, how far the processes of ideation and volition are affected thereby, and to demonstrate the path by which he has arrived at the conclusion that the person is sane or insane.

A delusion is a persistent and incorrigible belief that things are real which exist only in the imagination of the patient and which no rational person can conceive that the patient, when sane, could have believed. It is usually associated with the personality of the individual, and consists of a belief in some beneficial or prejudicial influence. When the delusion is believed to be prejudicial to the affected individual, acts of violence either towards himself or others frequently result. A delusion differs from an hallucination in that the latter is expressive of a disordered sense, and is a perception by one or other of the senses without external causation, for example, a person labouring under an hallucination may state that he hears voices speaking to him, when in point of fact no one is speaking.

The medical witness must rely solely upon his examination of the accused to arrive at an opinion as to sanity or insanity, and the evidence obtained will depend upon the range and method of that examination.

The examiner must take into account such factors as the mental history of the progenitors, the physical condition of the accused, together with his personal mental condition, in relation to the character of the crime committed. Frequently, the crime is purposeless or motiveless in character, is committed upon persons usually held dear by the culprit, or upon those who are strangers to him, and its perpetration is accompanied by complete unawareness on the part of the perpetrator. The mental history of the accused, together with his present condition, must be exhaustively inquired into, so that from the complete examination, the examiner may be able, in giving evidence, to place all the facts before the Court in such a way that they may be appreciated by laymen.

The case of John Thomas Straffen is of interest in the consideration of mental disorder and its relation to criminal responsibility. Straffen was born on 27th February 1930. He was placed on probation during 1939, after having been convicted of a number of petty offences. Shortly after this he was certified as a mental defective.

During July 1951, a child, Brenda Goddard, was throttled, and although Straffen was suspected by the Bath police, there was no evidence against him. In August 1951, another child, Cicely Batstone, was found throttled in the same region and Straffen was identified as having been seen at the site of the crime in the company of the victim. He was charged with murder and was found insane and unfit to plead and committed to Broadmoor.

On 29th April 1952, Straffen escaped and four hours elapsed before he was recaptured. During this period a little girl, Linda Bowyer, was found to have been throttled.

On 21st July 1952, Straffen's trial for the murder of Linda Bowyer started at Winchester Assizes. He pleaded not guilty. This was surprising, as less than a year earlier he had been found unfit to plead to a similar charge. The only possibility left to the defence was to bring Straffen within the M'Naghten Rules. A number of psychiatrists gave evidence about his mental condition, but none of them could satisfy the court that Straffen did not know that he had killed Linda Bowyer, and that he did not know that it was wrong to kill her. He was found guilty and sentenced to death. During the time he was awaiting execution, an inquiry was held into his mental state by order of the Home Secretary in accordance with the provisions of the Criminal Lunatics Act, 1884. On 29th August 1952, Straffen was reprieved and committed to Wandsworth Prison.

The Straffen case demonstrates well the various levels at which the mental state of a criminal may come within the consideration of the legal authorities.

For the descriptions of the various types of insanity and states of aberration of the mind, the reader is referred to treatises which deal with the clinical aspects of this subject. Neither from a statutory nor a legal point of view is a definite diagnosis of the specific form of insanity required, although a record of all the facts indicative of insanity is essential.

The M'Naghten Rules do not form part of Scots law,[4] although they influence a judge's charge to the jury.

The Criminal Procedure (Insanity) Act, 1964

This Act applies to England and is concerned with the methods of dealing with those who are found insane at the various stages of criminal proceedings. It is to a considerable extent the result of the passing of the Mental Health Act, 1959.

Its principal provisions are:

The alteration of the form of verdict. The English Law now recognises that where there is insanity there is no guilt.

The 'special verdict' is therefore changed to that of not guilty by reason of insanity.

There is a right of appeal to the Court of Criminal Appeal against 'special verdicts'.

When the question of unfitness to plead may be under consideration the Court is given the power to postpone consideration of this question until the opening of the case for the defence and if, before this, the jury return a verdict of acquittal, the question of fitness to plead shall not be determined.

Uncontrollable or irresistible impulse

In 1923, Lord Justice Atkin's Committee, which was appointed to review the criteria of insanity as incorporated in the M'Naghten Rules, reported that they reaffirmed these criteria, but made a recommendation that it should be recognised that a person charged criminally with an offence is irresponsible for his act when the act is committed under an impulse which the person was, by mental disease, deprived of any power to resist.   This is the criterion of uncontrollable or irresistible impulse.   The only attempt to add this to the M'Naghten Rules was made in the House of Lords in 1924, by Lord Justice Darling in moving the second reading of the Criminal Responsibility (Trials) Bill which he had introduced.   This was opposed so strongly that the Bill was withdrawn.   It has been suggested, from time to time, that allowance, which reduced full criminal responsibility, should be made for persons who suffer from an abnormal mental condition which renders them liable to commit crimes under the influence of an irresistible impulse. It has been felt, however, that if such a defence was recognised, the resulting exemption would be more than a potential risk that violent tempered persons would make less effort to control their tempers and then avail themselves of such an excuse.

At the hearing of the appeal of Kopsch[5] in 1925, the Lord Chief Justice said that the fantastic theory of uncontrollable impulse was not yet part of the criminal law, and it was to be hoped that the time was very far distant when it would be made so.

In Sodeman v. R.,[6] before the Judicial Committee of the Privy Council, the defence was that the accused had a mind which could not resist doing meaningless acts.   It was suggested that the M'Naghten Rules were no longer to be treated as an exhaustive statement of the law relating to insanity, and that there must be grafted on to it a rule that where a man knew that he was doing wrong, none the less, he might be insane if he was caused to do the act by an irresistible impulse produced by disease.   This view was not accepted by the Court.

The Homicide Act, 1957, introduced the principles of diminished responsibility to English law.   Section 2 enacts that a person shall not be convicted of murder if he was suffering from such abnormality of mind as substantially to impair his mental responsibility; for this purpose the abnormality of mind may arise from arrested or retarded development, any inherent cause, or disease or injury.   The section provides that in such cases the conviction shall be for manslaughter.

In contrast to Kopsch (supra) consider R. v. Byrne,[7] where, in reviewing the terms of the Homicide Act 'mental responsibility for his acts' was held to require consideration of the extent to which the accused's mind is answerable for his physical acts.   Byrne's abnormality of mind was defined as a state of mind so different from that of the ordinary human being that the reasonable man would term it abnormal.

Diminished responsibility

Turning now to Scotland, it has long been part of the law that the established proof of diminished responsibility may reduce a charge of murder to that of culpable homicide. In the case of H.M. Advocate v. Savage,[8] Lord Alness stated that the law had come to recognise those who, while they may not merit the description of being insane, were nevertheless in a condition as to reduce the quality of their act from murder to culpable homicide. In such cases there must be proved aberration or weakness of mind, some form of mental unsoundness, a state of mind bordering on, though not amounting to, insanity, a mind so affected that responsibility is diminished from full responsibility to partial responsibility, and the prisoner must be only partially responsible for his action.

The case of H.M. Advocate v. Kirkwood[9] is also worthy of note in this connection. The accused was tried for murder before the Lord Justice-Clerk. A special defence was put forward that at the time of the crime charged the accused was insane and not responsible for his actions. At the close of the medical evidence, counsel for the defence tendered a plea of guilty of culpable homicide, and this plea was accepted by the Crown on the ground of diminished responsibility of the accused. In passing sentence, the presiding judge, Lord Aitcheson, said: 'It is quite impossible for me to assess what the precise degree of your responsibility is, but the only sentence I can pronounce upon you that can in any way be commensurate with the crime you have committed and adequate in the public interest, is that you be detained in penal servitude for life.' The accused appealed against the sentence, and it was argued for the appellant that it was the duty of the presiding judge to discriminate between what was due to responsibility and what to irresponsibility, and to assess to what extent the accused was responsible for the crime. It appeared that the accused had been subject to epileptic fits for several years and had been treated in hospital. These fits were frequent and sometimes prolonged, and were on occasions accompanied by violence. On one occasion there had been an attempt to commit suicide. A medical witness gave evidence to the effect that the appellant was sane at the time of his examination and also when the crime was committed, but that he was not, at the time of the crime, a fully responsible individual. Other medical witnesses went further, and stated that there were circumstances connected with the actual crime which would lead them to say that the appellant was quite insane in what he did and that he had no idea what he was doing.

In intimating the refusal of the appeal, which was heard before eleven Judges of Justiciary, the Lord Justice-General, Lord Normand, stated that the defence of impaired responsibility was somewhat inconsistent with the basic doctrine of Scots criminal law that a man, if sane, is responsible for his acts and, if not sane, is not responsible. It was a

modern variance of the doctrine, justified by medical testimony directed
to the special facts of some particular case.   Mental weakness, short of
insanity, was regarded by our law as an extenuating circumstance having
the effect of modifying the character of the crime or justifying a modification of sentence or both.   But it might be impossible to assess the
degree of responsibility and, further, the diminished responsibility of the
accused was not the only relevant circumstance.   The interests of
society included the reformation of the criminal, the prevention of the
repetition of the crime by him or by others, and the protection of other
members of the community.   Inquiry had satisfied him that Kirkwood's mental and physical condition would be carefully considered,
that, if necessary, ameliorative treatment would be given to him, and
that his condition would be reviewed from time to time by the authorities who had power to control his treatment and to order his eventual
release.   There was nothing which would justify the Court in interfering with the sentence.   It has been held[10] that if the mental condition
of an accused person did not bring him within the category of diminished
responsibility when sober, he could not place himself within that category by taking drink.

Amnesia in relation to crime

Hopwood and Snell[11] have thrown light on this subject as the result
of an investigation based on the examination and histories of a hundred
male inmates of what was then known as the State Criminal Asylum at
Broadmoor.   Their views are that the defence was not as successful as
its frequency of presentation would presuppose, that amnesia cannot be
diagnosed on the patient's word alone, but must be checked by known
facts, since independent evidence is essential, and that real recovery
does not occur until some weeks or months after the crime.   A history
of chronic alcoholism, indication of a psychopathic personality, or
neuropathic heredity was frequently elicited.   They consider that the
commencement and especially the end of the amnesic period are of
special importance and are frequently blurred.   In cases where there is
partial amnesia, the patients were found to have a confused recollection
of their acts, and the ideas which were accompanied by marked emotion
were remembered, but those less emotional in character were not.   They
hold the further opinions that statements made soon after the crime,
which are indicative of a knowledge of the crime, are not inconsistent
with a genuine amnesia due to a subsequent repression.   Touching
upon the nature of the crime, they add that it is frequently without
obvious motive, is unpremeditated, and that the perpetrator makes no
effort to escape the consequences.   A sudden return of memory almost
certainly indicates malingering.

Amnesia cannot be pled in bar of trial, as it does not of itself lessen the accused's understanding of the charges and the proceedings, nor does it interfere with communication between accused and counsel.[12, 13]

Inebriety

The abuse of alcohol by persons may, under certain circumstances, bring them within the category of insanity and irresponsibility. Although chronic alcoholism is one of the more indirect causes of insanity, nevertheless the direct effects of alcohol frequently induce insanity of a temporary nature, for example, delirium tremens. The common law rule is that mere drunkenness cannot be pleaded as an excuse for crime, but a state of mental unsoundness produced by alcohol can be so pleaded, and if established by proof, would be held to be so. The position, therefore, resolves itself into the question whether or not an accused person who has committed a crime while under the influence of alcohol was sane or insane.

In a trial on a charge of murder, counsel for the accused asked the presiding judge to direct the jury that, if they were of the opinion that the accused, while acting in self-defence, had exceeded what was reasonably necessary as retaliation because of a temporary loss of reason caused by an attack of the deceased while he, the accused, was under the influence of drink, they were bound to acquit him of culpable homicide. The presiding judge directed the jury to the contrary effect, namely, that if, although provoked, the accused exceeded in brutality what the ordinary man should have done, drink could not palliate the brutality of his acts. The accused was convicted of culpable homicide. The court, in an appeal on the ground of misdirection, held that drunkenness, short of proved incapacity to form the intent necessary to commit the crime, could not palliate retaliatory violence in excess of what was reasonably necessary, and refused the appeal.[14]

The position with regard to inebriety and criminal responsibility can be summed up shortly. Drunkenness is ordinarily neither a defence nor excuse for crime unless the intoxication is such as to prevent the individual from restraining himself from committing the act in question or to take away from him the power of forming any specific intention.[15] The reason why ordinary drunkenness is not an excuse for crime lies in the fact that the offender did wrong in getting drunk. If distinct disease of mind is caused by drinking, as opposed to drunkenness, and obliterates the knowledge between good and evil, the jury may bring in a verdict as in the case of insanity.

It will, therefore, be understood that in cases of delirium tremens the defence will be one of insanity, but that in certain cases of drunkenness the condition of drunkenness at the time when the crime was committed, although not an excuse for the crime, may be pleaded as a mitigation and, provided the degree of intoxication is proved to be such that it deprived the accused of the power of forming any specific intention, the charge of murder may be reduced to that of manslaughter in England, or to culpable homicide in Scotland.

The Homicide Act, 1957, does not change the foregoing principles. Mr Justice Donovan has stressed this, stating that the section in the Homicide Act dealing with diminished responsibility was not intended to be, nor was it, a charter for drunkards.[16]

Mutism

The legal procedure adopted at the trial of an accused person who is mute differs in England and Scotland.

English procedure

Any question whether the accused is mute of malice or by visitation of God is determined by a jury sworn to try the preliminary issue. If their verdict is 'mute by the visitation of God', a second issue must be determined, namely, whether the accused is able to plead and understand the proceedings at the trial. If he is not, he is treated as insane, unless the incapacity is temporary. In the case of R. v. Governor of Stafford Prison,[17] a prisoner who was totally deaf and could neither read nor write was arraigned for a felony. He stood mute, and a jury was impanelled and sworn to ascertain whether he was mute by the visitation of God. They found that he was, and were then sworn again to try whether he was capable of pleading to the indictment. They found that he was incapable of pleading to, and taking his trial upon, the indictment and of understanding and following the proceedings by reason of his inability to communicate with, or be communicated with, by others. Upon this verdict the judge, acting under section 2 of the Criminal Lunatics Act, 1800, ordered him to be kept in custody until His Majesty's pleasure should be known. It was held that this judgment amounted to a finding that the prisoner was insane within the meaning of the Act, and that the order was properly made.

Scottish procedure

In 1817, for the first time in Scotland, the question as to whether a person deaf and dumb is an object for trial and punishment, came to be tried. The case concerned a woman, Jean Campbell, alias Bruce, who was indicted at Glasgow for the murder of her child.[18] The question was a new one and the Lords on the Circuit certified the case for the consideration of the High Court. The Court was satisfied that she had the power of communicating her thoughts, and showed intelligence of right and wrong. She was committed for trial and the case was remitted to the judges at the next circuit at Glasgow, when she pleaded not guilty by communicating by a deaf and dumb show. Her evidence, given by signs and gestures, was that the child had fallen accidentally from a parapet into the River Clyde and had drowned. A verdict of not guilty was returned.

In February 1942, at the High Court in Glasgow,[19] a man was charged with murder, and after six doctors had stated that he was fit to instruct his defence, the presiding judge decided that he was insane within the meaning of the Lunacy Act, 1857. The accused man was deaf, unable to talk properly, could not read, was said to be feeble-minded, but was not certifiably insane. Five judges in the High Court decided that the prisoner should stand trial on the charge, and that the question of his sanity should be left to be determined by the jury. The accused was tried at a later date and acquitted.

If mutism or insanity be accepted as a plea in bar of trial, there is no way of the panel's establishing his innocence.[20]

Epilepsy

Many persons suffering from epilepsy experience changes of mood in relation to seizures. The most common forensic aspect of this disease is the severe psychic disturbance preceding or immediately following the motor fit. Acts of violence and grave criminal assaults may be committed without the perpetrator being properly aware of the facts. Confusion following a seizure may precipitate automatic acts of unlawful sexual behaviour, assault, and murder.[21] When applied as a defence, it may be regarded as such aberration or defect which partially removes responsibility, that is, diminished responsibility.[9]

References

1. Banks v. Goodfellow (1870), L.R. 5 Q.B., 549.
2. JENNINGS, R. *Br. med. J.*, **2**, 801, 1970.
3. M'Naghten's Case, (1843) 10 C. & Fin., 200.
4. Breen v. Breen, 1961, S.C., 158.
5. Kopsch v. R. [1925], 19 Cr. App. R., 50.
6. Sodeman v. R. [1936] 2 All E.R. 1138.
7. R. v. Byrne [1960] 2 Q.B. 396.
8. H.M.A. v. Savage, 1923, J.C. 49.
9. H.M.A. v. Kirkwood, 1939, J.C. 36; 1939, S.L.T. 209.
10. H.M.A. v. Macleod, 1956, J.C. 20; 1956, S.L.T. 24.
11. HOPWOOD & SNELL. *J. mental Sci.*, **79**, 27, 1933.
12. Russell v. H.M.A. 1946, J.C. 37.
13. R. v. Podola [1959] 3 All E.R. 418.
14. H.M.A. v. Reid, 1947, S.L.T. 150.
15. D.P.P. v. Beard [1920] A.C. 479.
16. R. v. Dowdall, *The Times*, Jan. 22, 1960.
17. R. v. Governor of Stafford Prison [1909], 2 K.B. 81.

18. H.M.A. v. Campbell (1817), Hume, i, 45.
19. H.M.A. v. Wilson, 1942, J.C. 75.
20. WHITEHEAD, J.A.   *Lancet*, **2**, 376, 1969.
21. FENTON, G.W.   *Br. J. hosp. Med.*, **7**, 57, 1972.

Chapter 17

LAWS RELATING TO POISONS

DRUGS and poisons cannot be separated into watertight compartments. The poisonous action of drugs at therapeutic dose is perhaps best seen in the anti-mitotic group, for example, cyclophosphamide, used in the treatment of malignant disease, but interference with cell metabolism is basic to the pharmacology of such widely used drugs as digoxin, penicillin, and the thiazide diuretics. Conversely, a substance familiar as a poison in one context, for example warfarin, is more correctly described as a drug in another.

Of all types of murder, poisoning must be the one most often undetected. At post-mortem no cause of death can be more perplexing.

Toxicology, which has been defined as the knowledge of the sources, characters, and properties of poisons, the symptoms which they produce, the nature of the fatal results, and the remedial measures which should be employed to combat their actions or effects, is the subject of the remaining portion of this volume. This chapter is concerned with the legal regulation of the manufacture, sale, and supply of drugs and poisons.

The law does not define poisons, leaving each substance to be considered in the context of the particular case. In England, the appropriate statute, the Offences Against the Person Act, 1861, speaks of 'any poison or other destructive or noxious thing'. The Criminal Law (Scotland) Act, 1829, mentions 'any deadly poison or other noxious and destructive substance or thing, with intent thereby, or by means thereof, to murder, or disable, or do other grievous bodily harm'.

STATUTES REGULATING THE SALE OF POISONS

The Acts of Parliament by which the sale of poisons and the practice of pharmacy in England and Scotland are regulated include:

Pharmacy and Poisons Act, 1933, and Statutory Rules and Orders made thereunder.
Pharmacy and Medicines Act, 1941.
Dangerous Drugs Act, 1965, and Statutory Regulations and Orders.
Dangerous Drugs Act, 1967.
Therapeutic Substances Act, 1956, and Regulations.
Drugs (Prevention of Misuse) Act, 1964.

The **Medicines Act, 1968,** and the **Misuse of Drugs Act, 1971,** will also be considered, although at the time of writing few of their important provisions have been activated. These two Acts, taken together, will go far to simplify our legislative approach to poisons and drugs.

Pharmacy and Poisons Act, 1933

The Poisons List[1] is divided into two parts:

> Part I of the List consists of those poisons which are not to be sold by retail except by a person who is an *authorised seller of poisons,* for example, a registered pharmacist whose business premises are registered with the Pharmaceutical Society of Great Britain.
>
> Part II of the List consists of those poisons which are not to be sold by retail except by a person who is an authorised seller of (Part I) poisons or whose name is entered in a list, kept by a local authority, of persons who are entitled to sell poisons in this part of the List (*listed seller*), or who carries on the business of an authorised seller of poisons at one or more chemist's shops to sell drugs, but not Part I poisons, or at other shops where no pharmacist is employed and which are registered by the Pharmaceutical Society and not by a local authority.

In determining the distribution of poisons as between Part I and Part II of the List, regard was given to the desirability of restricting Part II to substances in common use or likely to come into common use, for purposes other than the treatment of human ailments, and which it is reasonably necessary to include in Part II if the public are to have adequate facilities for obtaining them. The Secretary of State may from time to time, after consultation with, or on the recommendation of, the Poisons Board, by order, amend or vary the List as he thinks proper, and the List as in force is referred to as 'The Poisons List'.[1]   In this Act the expression 'poison' means a poison included in the Poisons List.

The division of the Poisons List into Parts I and II, together with the distribution of the various substances contained therein, is of subordinate interest to members of the medical profession.   The regulations regarding the sale of poisons contained in Parts I and II, however, demand consideration and are important.   Details affecting each poison may be found in *Poisons and T.S.A. Guide.*[2]

For example, many Part II poisons may be sold by a listed seller only in certain forms.   Schedule Five of the Poisons Rules[3] contains a large number of these, mostly in forms suitable for horticulture and agriculture, for example, sheep dips, rodent poisons, fungicides.   If the poison is in any other form, or wanted for any other purpose, even Part II poisons may only be sold by authorised sellers.

Further exemptions are contained in the Third Schedule. Such substances may be sold by unqualified persons from unregistered premises. No restriction is placed on the sale of, for example, adhesives, enamels, glue, lacquer solvents, matches, photographic paper, and varnishes. Exemption is given also to preparations of poisons otherwise controlled, for example, surgical spirit containing not more than 0·015 per cent brucine, nicotine in tobacco, anti-histamines for external use containing not more than 1 per cent of anti-histamine, paraquat in pellet form, quinine in soft drinks, fluoride in toothpaste.

Wholesalers are permitted to sell Part I poisons only to those they know to be authorised sellers or to those who tender a signed statement to the effect that the purchaser does not intend selling the poison on any premises connected with his retail business. Containers must be impervious to the poison. Bottles with vertical fluting are used (with some exceptions) for medicines for external use. The label must show the name and address of the seller, the name of the poison, its proportion in any mixture, and the word 'POISON' with other cautionary phrases appropriate to particular substances.

A Part I or Part II poison which is not otherwise controlled may be dispensed without a prescription given by a duly qualified medical practitioner, dentist, or veterinary surgeon. If such a poison be dispensed **not** on prescription, a record must be kept of the date of supply; the ingredients and quantity supplied; the name of the person to whom the poison was supplied. If the substance is dispensed on prescription, the prescriber's name is also recorded. None of the requirements applies to National Health Service prescriptions.

The label must show the name and address of the seller and the words' For external use only' when the substance is for example, a lotion.

It should be noted that if any medicine sold comes within the Dangerous Drugs Acts (see p. 505) the proper entry must be made in the Dangerous Drugs Register.

Under the **Poisons Rules,**[3] **1971,** made by the Secretary of State as empowered under the Act, certain substances are relegated to specific Schedules. The First and Fourth of these Schedules, to which special restrictions apply, are of high importance to members of the medical profession who should have a clear knowledge regarding the classes of poisons contained therein, and of the restrictions imposed on their sale.

FIRST SCHEDULE

Substances included in the Poisons List to which special restrictions apply unless exempted by Rule 11

Acetorphine; its salts; its esters and ethers; their salts.
Acetyldihydrocodeine; its salts.
Alcuronium chloride.

Alkaloids, the following; their quaternary compounds; any salt, simple or complex, of any substance falling within the following:

Aconite, alkaloids of, except substances containing less than 0.02 per cent of the alkaloids of aconite.

Atropine except substances containing less than 0·15 per cent of atropine or not more than one per cent of atropine methonitrate.

Belladonna, alkaloids of, except substances containing less than 0·15 per cent of the alkaloids of belladonna calculated as hyoscyamine.

Brucine except substances containing less than 0·2 per cent of brucine.

Calabar bean, alkaloids of.

Coca, alkaloids of, except substances containing less than 0·1 per cent of the alkaloids of coca.

Cocaine except substances containing less than 0·1 per cent of cocaine.

Codeine; its esters and ethers; except substances containing less than 1·5 per cent of codeine.

Coniine except substances containing less than 0·1 per cent of coniine.

Cotarnine except substances containing less than 0·2 per cent of cotarnine.

Curare, alkaloids of; curare bases.

Ecgonine; its esters and ethers; except substances containing less than the equivalent of 0·1 per cent of ecgonine.

Emetine except substances containing less than 1 per cent of emetine.

Ephedrine; its optical isomers; except when contained in liquid preparations or preparations not intended for the internal treatment of human ailments and except solid preparations containing less than 10 per cent of ephedrine or its optical isomers otherwise than in an inert diluent.

Gelsemium, alkaloids of, except substances containing less than 0·1 per cent of the alkaloids of gelsemium.

Homatropine except substances containing less than 0·15 per cent of homatropine.

Hyoscine except substances containing less than 0·15 per cent of hyoscine.

Hyoscyamine except substances containing less than 0·15 per cent of hyoscyamine.

Jaborandi, alkaloids of, except substances containing less than 0·5 per cent of the alkaloids of jaborandi.

Lobelia, alkaloids of, except substances containing less than 0·5 per cent of the alkaloids of lobelia.

Morphine; its esters and ethers; except substances containing less than 0·2 per cent of morphine calculated as anhydrous morphine.

Nicotine.

Papaverine except substances containing less than 1 per cent of papaverine.

Pomegranate, alkaloids of, except substances containing less than 0·5 per cent of the alkaloids of pomegranate.

Quebracho, alkaloids of.

Sabadilla, alkaloids of, except substances containing less than 1 per cent of the alkaloids of sabadilla.

Solanaceous alkaloids, not otherwise included in this Schedule, except substances containing less than 0·15 per cent of solanaceous alkaloids calculated as hyoscyamine.

Stavesacre, alkaloids of, except substances containing less than 0·2 per cent of the alkaloids of stavesacre.

Strychnine except substances containing less than 0·2 per cent of strychnine.

Thebaine except substances containing less than 1 per cent of thebaine.

Veratrum, alkaloids of, except substances containing less than 1 per cent of the alkaloids of veratrum.

Yohimba, alkaloids of.

Allylisopropylacetylurea.

Allyprodine; its salts

Alphameprodine; its salts.

Alphaprodine; its salts.

Amino-alcohols esterified with benzoic acid, phenylacetic acid, phenyl-propionic acid, cinnamic acid or the derivatives of these acids, except substances containing less than 10 per cent of esterified amino-alcohols and except procaine when in a preparation containing any substance to which Part II of the Therapeutic Substances Act 1956 for the time being applies; their salts.

Amphetamine; its salts.

Anileridine; its salts.

Antimonial poisons except substances containing less than the equivalent of 1 per cent of antimony trioxide.

Apomorphine; its salts; except substances containing less than 0·2 per cent of apomorphine.

Arsenical poisons except substances containing less than the equivalent of 0·01 per cent of arsenic trioxide and except dentrifices containing less than 0·5 per cent of acetarsol.

Barbituric acid; its salts; derivatives of barbituric acid; their salts; compounds of barbituric acid, its salts, its derivatives, their salts, with any other substance.

Barium, salts of.

Benzethidine; its salts.

Benzoylmorphine; its salts.

Benzphetamine; its salts.

Benzylmorphine; its salts.

Betameprodine; its salts.

Betaprodine; its salts.

Bezitramide; its salts.

Busulphan; its salts.

Cannabinol and its tetrahydro derivatives, prepared wholly or partly by synthesis; their 3-alkyl homologues; any ester or ether of any substance falling within this item.

Cannabis; the resin of cannabis; extracts of cannabis; tinctures of cannabis; cannabin tannate.

Cantharidin except substances containing less than 0·01 per cent of cantharidin.

Cantharidates except substances containing less than the equivalent of 0·01 per cent of cantharidin.

Carbachol.

Carperidine; its salts.

Chloroform, except substances containing not more than 5 per cent of chloroform or when in preparations not intended for the internal treatment of human ailments.

Chlorphentermine; its salts.

Clonitazene; its salts.

4-Cyano-2-dimethylamino-4,4-diphenylbutane; its salts.

4-Cyano-1-methyl-4-phenylpiperidine; its salts.

Dehydroemetine; its salts.

Demecarium bromide.

Desomorphine; its salts; its esters and ethers; their salts.

Dexamphetamine; its salts.

Dextromethorphan; its salts; except substances containing less than 1·5 per cent of dextromethorphan.

Dextromoramide; its salts.

Dextrorphan; its salts.

Diacetylmorphine; its salts.

Diacetylnalorphine; its salts.

Diampromide; its salts.

Digitalis, glycosides and other active principles of, except substances containing less than one unit of activity (as defined in the British Pharmacopoeia) in two grams of the substance.

Dihydrocodeine; its salts; its esters and ethers; their salts.

Dihydrocodeinone; its salts.

Dihydrocodeinone O-carboxymethyloxime; its salts; its esters; their salts.

Dihydromorphine; its salts; its esters and ethers; their salts.

Dimenoxadole; its salts.

Dimepheptanol; its salts; its esters and ethers; their salts.

Dinitrocresols (DNOC); their compounds with a metal or a base; except winter washes containing not more than the equivalent of 5 per cent of dinitrocresols.

Dinitronaphthols; dinitrophenols; dinitrothymols.

Dinosam; its compounds with a metal or a base.

Dinoseb; its compounds with a metal or a base.

Dioxaphetyl butyrate; its salts.

Diphenoxylate; its salts; except preparations containing, per dosage unit, not more than 2·5 milligrams of diphenoxylate calculated as base and not less than twenty-five micrograms of atropine sulphate.

Dipipanone; its salts.

Disulfiram.

Dithienylallylamines; dithienylalkylallylamines; their salts.

Drazoxolon; its salts.

Dyflos.

Ecothiopate iodine.

Embutramide.

Endosulfan.

Endothal; its salts.

Endrin.

Ethylmorphine; its salts; its esters and ethers; their salts; except substances containing less than 0·2 per cent of ethylmorphine.

Etonitazene; its salts.

Etorphine; its salts; its esters and ethers; their salts.

Etoxeridine; its salts.

Fencamfamin; its salts.

Fentanyl; its salts.

Fluanisone.

Fluoroacetamide; fluoroacetanilide.

Furethidine; its salts.

Gallamine; its salts; its quaternary compounds.

Guanidines, the following:
  polymethylene diguanidines; di-*p*-anisyl-*p*-phenetylguanidine.

Hydrocyanic acid except substances containing less than 0·15 per cent, weight in weight, of hydrocyanic acid (HCN); cyanides, other than ferrocyanides and ferricyanides, except substances containing less than the equivalent of 0·1 per cent, weight in weight, of hydrocyanic acid (HCN).

Hydromorphinol; its salts: its esters and ethers; their salts.

Hydromorphone; its salts; its esters and ethers; their salts.

Hydroxycinchoninic acids; derivatives of; their salts; their esters; except substances containing less than 3 per cent of a hydroxycinchoninic acid or a derivative thereof.

Hydroxypethidine; its salts; its esters and ethers; their salts.

Hydroxyurea.

Isomethadone (isoamidone); its salts.

Ketobemidone; its salts; its esters and ethers; their salts.

Laudexium; its salts.

Lead, compounds of, with acids from fixed oils.

Levamphetamine; its salts.

Levomethorphan; its salts.

Levomoramide; its salts.

Levophenacylmorphan; its salts; its esters and ethers; their salts.

Levorphanol; its salts; its esters and ethers; their salts.

Mannomustine; its salts.

Mebezonium iodide.

Mephentermine; its salts.

Mercaptopurine; its salts; derivatives of mercaptopurine; their salts.

Mercuric chloride except substances containing less than 1 per cent of mercuric chloride; mercuric iodide except substances containing less than 2 per cent of mercuric iodide; nitrates of mercury except substances containing less than the equivalent of 3 per cent, weight in weight, of mercury (Hg); potassiomercuric iodides except substances containing less than the equivalent of 1 per cent of mercuric iodide; organic compounds of mercury except substances, not being aerosols, containing less than the equivalent of 0·2 per cent, weight in weight, of mercury (Hg).

Mescaline, and other derivatives of phenethylamine formed by substitution in the aromatic ring; their salts.

Metazocine; its salts; its esters and ethers; their salts.

Methadone (amidone); its salts.

Methadyl acetate; its salts.

Methylamphetamine, its salts.

Methyldesorphine; its salts; its esters and ethers; their salts.

Methyldihydromorphine; its salts; its esters and ethers; their salts.

2-Methyl-3-morpholino-1,1-diphenylpropanecarboxylic acid; its salts; its esters; their salts.

Methylphenidate; its salts.

1-Methyl-4-phenylpiperidine-4-carboxylic acid; esters of; their salts.

Metopon; its salts; its esters and ethers; their salts.

Mitobronitol.

Monofluoroacetic acid; its salts.

Morpheridine; its salts.

Mustine and any other N-substituted derivative of di-(2-chloroethyl) amine; their salts.

Myrophine; its salts.

Nalorphine; its salts.

Niclofolan.

Nicocodine; its salts.

m-Nitrophenol; o-nitrophenol; p-nitrophenol.

Noracymethadol; its salts.

Norcodeine; its salts; its esters and ethers; their salts.

Norlevorphanol; its salts; its esters and ethers; their salts.

Normethadone; its salts.

Normorphine; its salts; its esters and ethers; their salts.

Norpipanone.

Nux Vomica except substances containing less than 0·2 per cent of strychnine.

Opium except substances containing less than 0·2 per cent of morphine calculated as anhydrous morphine.

Organo-tin compounds, the following:
 Compounds of fentin.

Ouabain.

Oxycodone; its salts; its esters and ethers; their salts.

Oxymorphone; its salts; its esters and ethers; their salts.

Pemoline; its salts.

Phenacemide.

Phenadoxone; its salts.

Phenampromide; its salts.

Phenazocine; its salts; its esters and ethers; their salts.

Phencyclidine; its salts

Phendimetrazine; its salts.

Phenomorphan; its salts; its esters and ethers; their salts.

Phenoperidine; its salts; its esters and ethers; their salts.

Phentermine; its salts.

2-Phenylcinchoninic acid; 2-salicylcinchoninic acid; their salts; their esters.

4-Phenylpiperidine-4-carboxylic acid ethyl ester; its salts.

Pholcodine; its salts; its esters and ethers; their salts; except substances containing less than 1·5 per cent of pholcodine.

Phosphorus compounds, the following:

  Amiton.

  Azinphos-ethyl.

  Azinphos-methyl.

  Chlorfenvinphos except sheep dips containing not more than 10 per cent, weight in weight, of chlorfenvinphos.

  Demeton-O.

  Demeton-S.

  Demeton-O-methyl.

  Demeton-S-methyl.

  Dichlorvos.

  Diethyl 4-methyl-7-coumarinyl phosphorothionate.

  Diethyl p-nitrophenyl phosphate.

  Dimefox.

  Disulfoton.

  Ethion.

  Ethyl-p-nitrophenyl phenylphosphonothionate.

  Mazidox.

  Mecarbam.

  Mevinphos.

  Mipafox.

  Oxydemeton-methyl.

  Parathion.

  Phenkapton.

  Phorate.

  Phosphamidon.

  Schradan.

  Sulfotep.

  TEPP (HETP)

  Thionazin.

  Triphosphoric pentadimethylamide.

  Vamidothion.

Picrotoxin.

Piminodine; its salts.

Pipradrol; its salts; its esters and ethers.

Piritramide; its salts.

Polymethylenebistrimethylammonium salts.

Proheptazine; its salts.

Propoxyphene; its salts.

Racemethorphan; its salts.

Racemoramide; its salts.

Racemorphan; its salts; its esters and ethers; their salts.

Savin, oil of.

Sodium 4-(dimethylamino)benzenediazosulphonate.

Strophanthus, glycosides of.

Thallium, salts of.

Thebacon; its salts.
Tretamine; its salts.
Triaziquone.
Trimeperidine; its salts.
Zinc phosphide.

This Schedule, which contains certain poisons from both Part I and Part II of the Poisons List, imposes the following restrictions:

1. The purchaser must be known to the seller or to one of his qualified assistants to be a person to whom the poison may properly be sold.

2. If this condition cannot be complied with, then the purchaser must show a written certificate signed by a householder, and this has to be endorsed by a police officer in charge of a police station, unless the householder is known to the chemist to be a responsible person of good character.

3. Following the sale of the poison, this certificate must be retained by the seller.

4. An entry of the sale must be made in a book kept for this purpose together with the date, the name and address of the purchaser, and the person granting the certificate, the name and quantity of the poison sold, and the stated purpose for which it was required.   The purchaser must sign the Poisons Register before the poison is delivered.

These restrictions do not apply to the following articles (Rule 11):

(*a*) machine-spread plasters;
(*b*) surgical dressings;
(*c*) articles containing barium carbonate or zinc phosphide, and prepared for the destruction of rats and mice; or
(*d*) corn paints in which the only poison is a poison included in the Poisons List under the heading of 'Cannabis'.

Doctors, dentists, and veterinary surgeons may obtain poisons contained in the First Schedule from any authorised seller by a written order or by personal attendance at the premises of the seller and by signing the Poisons Register.   If an order is sent, it must be signed, and contain the name and address of the purchaser together with the reason for the purchase of the poison.   In the case of emergency, a medical practitioner, dentist, or veterinary surgeon may obtain poisons contained in the First Schedule if they are required in the course of his profession, by giving an undertaking that he will furnish a written order within twenty-four hours.   Failure to furnish the order after the drug has been supplied is an offence.

The following provisions govern the supply of poisons by medical practitioners, dentists, and veterinary surgeons:

1. It is not necessary for a medical practitioner to keep a record of a medicine supplied unless it is a substance included in the First Schedule.
2. Dentists and veterinary surgeons must keep a record of all medicines which contain a poison and which have been dispensed or supplied by them.
3. The date on which the medicine was supplied, the ingredients, quantity, and the name of the person to whom the medicine was supplied must be entered in a book used for the purpose.
4. All medicines containing poisons supplied by medical practitioners, dentists, and veterinary surgeons must be labelled and bear the name and address of the practitioner.

Strychnine may not be sold or supplied unless as an ingredient in a medicine except:

(a) by wholesale;
(b) for export;
(c) to doctors, or veterinary surgeons, for use in their practices; or
(d) to a person or institution concerned with scientific education, research, or chemical analysis, for these purposes;
(e) under certain conditions for the purpose of killing moles, and not exceeding 4 ounces at one time; or
(f) to a person authorised by the Secretary of State to purchase strychnine for the purpose of killing seals.

It is unlawful to sell or supply Monofluoroacetic acid or any salt thereof, except by way of wholesale dealing or for export outside the United Kingdom, or to a person or institution concerned with scientific education or research or chemical analysis, for the purposes of that education or research or analysis, or by reason of certain additional exemptions, connected with its use as a rodenticide.

FOURTH SCHEDULE

The Fourth Schedule contains a list of the following substances subdivided into Parts A and B. All these substances can only be sold by retail upon a prescription given by a qualified medical practitioner, registered dentist, registered veterinary surgeon, or registered veterinary practitioner.

PART A

Alcuronium chloride.
Allylisopropylacetylurea.
Barbituric acid; its salts; derivatives of barbituric acid; their salts,

compounds of barbituric acid, its salts, its derivatives, their salts, with any other substance.

Busulphan; its salts.

Demecarium bromide.

Dinitrocresols (DNOC); their compounds with a metal or a base, except preparations for use in agriculture or horticulture.

Dinitronaphthols; dinitrophenols; dinitrothymols.

Disulfiram.

Dithienylallylamines; dithienylalkylallylamines; their salts; except diethylthiambutene, dimethylthiambutene and ethylmethylthiambutene.

Gallamine; its salts; its quaternary compounds.

Hydroxyurea.

Mannomustine; its salts.

Mercaptopurine; its salts; derivatives of mercaptopurine; their salts.

Mitobronitol.

Mustine and any other N-substituted derivatives of di-(2-chloroethyl) amine; their salts.

Phenacemide.

Phencyclidine; its salts.

2-Phenylcinchoninic acid; 2-salicylcinchoninic acid; their salts: their esters.

Polymethylenebistrimethylammonium salts.

Tretamine; its salts.

Triaziquone.

Part B

Acetanilide; alkyl acetanilides.

Acetohexamide.

Acetylcarbromal.

Amidopyrine; its salts; amidopyrine sulphonates; their salts.

p-Aminobenzenesulphonamide; its salts; derivatives of p-aminobenzenesulphonamide having any of the hydrogen atoms of the p-amino group or of the sulphonamide group substituted by another radical; their salts; except when contained in ointments or surgical dressings or in preparations for the prevention and treatment of diseases in poultry.

Aminorex; its salts.

Amitriptyline; its salts.

Androgenic, oestrogenic and progestational substances, the following:
Benzoestrol.
Derivatives of stilbene, dibenzyl or naphthalene with oestrogenic activity; their esters.
Steroid compounds with androgenic or oestrogenic or progestational activity; their esters.

Azacyclonol; its salts.

Benactyzine; its salts.

Benzhexol; its salts.

Benztropine and its homologues; their salts.

Bromvaletone.

Captodiame; its salts.

Caramiphen; its salts; except tablets containing not more than the equivalent of 7·5 milligrams of caramiphen base, and liquid preparations containing not more than the equivalent of 0·1 per cent of caramiphen base.

Carbromal.

Carisoprodol.

Chloral; its addition and its condensation products other than alphachloralose; their molecular compounds; except when contained, in the form of chloral hydrate, in preparations intended for external application only.

Chlordiazepoxide; its salts.

Chlormethiazole; its salts.

Chlorothiazide and other derivatives of benzo-1,2,4-thiadiazine-7-sulphonamide1,1-dioxide, whether hydrogenated or not.

Chlorphenoxamine; its salts.

Chlorphentermine; its salts.

Chlorpropamide; its salts.

Chlorprothixene and other derivatives of 9-methylenethiaxanthen; their salts.

Chlorthalidone and other derivatives of *o*-chlorobenzene sulphonamide.

Clomiphene; its salts.

Clorexolone.

Clorprenaline; its salts; when contained in aerosol dispensers.

Colchicum, alkaloids of; their salts.

Corticotrophins, natural and synthetic.

Cyclarbamate.

Cycrimine; its salts.

Desipramine; its salts.

Diazepam and other compounds containing the chemical structure of dihydro-1,4-benzodiazepine substituted to any degree; their salts.

3-(3,4-Dihydroxyphenyl)alanine; its salts.

Diphenoxylate and its salts in preparations containing, per dosage unit, not more than 2·5 milligrams of diphenoxylate calculated as base and not less than twenty-five micrograms of atropine sulphate.

Dothiepin; its salts.

Ectylurea.

Emylcamate.

Ephedrine; its optical isomers; their salts; when contained in aerosol dispensers.

Ergot, alkaloids of, whether hydrogenated or not; their homologues; any salt of any substance falling within this item.

Ethacrynic acid; its salts.

Ethchlorvynol.

Ethinamate.

Ethionamide.

Ethoheptazine; its salts.

Ethylnoradrenaline; its salts; when contained in aerosol dispensers.

Fenfluramine; its salts.
Flufenamic acid; its salts; its esters; their salts.
Glutethimide; its salts.
Glymidine.
Haloperidol and other 4-substituted derivatives of N-(3-p-fluorobenzoyl-propyl) piperidine.
Hexapropymate.
Hydrazines, benzyl phenethyl or phenoxyethyl; their α-methyl derivatives acyl derivatives of any of the foregoing substances comprised in this item; salts of any compounds comprised in this item.
Hydroxy-N,N-dimethyltryptamines; their esters or ethers; any salt of any substance falling within this item.
Hydroxyzine; its salts.
Imipramine; its salts.
Indomethacin; its salts.
Iprindole; its salts.
Isoaminile; its salts.
Isoetharine; its salts; when contained in aerosol dispensers.
Isoprenaline; its salts; when contained in aerosol dispensers.
Mebutamate.
Meclofenoxate; its salts.
Mefenamic acid; its salts; its esters; their salts.
Mephenesin; its esters.
Meprobamate.
Metaxalone.
Metformin; its salts.
Methaqualone; its salts.
Methixene; its salts.
Methocarbamol.
Methoxsalen.
Methoxyphenamine; its salts; when contained in aerosol dispensers.
Methylaminoheptane; its salts; when contained in aerosol dispensers.
Methylpentynol; its esters and other derivatives.
α-Methylphenethylamine, β-methylphenethylamine and α-ethylphen-ethylamine; any synthetic compound structurally derived from any of those substances by substitution in the aliphatic part or by ring closure therein (or by both such substitution and such closure) or by substitution in the aromatic ring (with or without substitution at the nitrogen atom), except ephedrine, its optical isomers and N-substituted deriva-tives, fenfluramine, hydroxyamphetamine, methoxyphenamine, phenyl-propanolamine, pholedrine and prenylamine; any salt of any sub-stance falling within this item.
Methyprylone.
Metoclopramide; its salts.
Mitopodozide; its salts.
Nortriptyline; its salts.
Orciprenaline; its salts; when contained in aerosol dispensers.
Orphenadrine; its salts.
Oxethazaine.

Oxyphenbutazone.
Oxytocins, natural and synthetic.
Paraldehyde.
Paramethadione.
Pargyline; its salts.
Pemoline; its salts.
Pentazocine; its salts.
Phenaglycodol.
Phenbutrazate.
Phenetidylphenacetin.
Phenformin; its salts.
Phenothiazine, derivatives of; their salts; except dimethoxanate, its salts and promethazine, its salts and molecular compounds.
Phenylbutazone; its salts.
5-Phenylhydantoin; its alkyl and aryl derivatives; their salts.
Pimozide; its salts.
Pituitary gland, the active principles of, other than corticotrophins, oxytocins and vasopressins; except when contained in inhalants or in preparations intended for external application only.
Procainamide; its salts.
Procarbazine; its salts.
Procyclidine; its salts.
Promoxolan.
Propylhexedrine; its salts; except when contained in inhalers.
Prothionamide.
Prothipendyl; its salts.
Quinethazone.
Quinine; its salts; except in preparations containing less than 10 per cent of quinine or its salts.
Rauwolfia, alkaloids of; their salts; derivatives of the alkaloids of rauwolfia; their salts.
Salbutamol; its salts.
Styramate.
Sulphinpyrazone.
Sulphonal; alkyl sulphonals.
Suprarenal gland medulla, the active principles of; their salts; except when contained in preparations intended for external application only or in inhalants (other than inhalants in aerosol dispensers containing adrenaline or its salts), rectal preparations or preparations intended for use in the eye.
Suxamethonium; its salts.
Syrosingopine.
Tetrabenazine; its salts.
Thalidomide; its salts.
Thiocarlide; its salts.
Thyroid gland, the active principles of; their salts.
Tofenacin; its salts.
Tolbutamide.
Tribromethyl alcohol.

2,2,2-Trichloroethyl alcohol, esters of; their salts.
Trimipramine; its salts.
Troxidone.
Tybamate.
Vasopressins, natural and synthetic.
Verapamil; its salts.
Zoxazolamine; its salts.

The following restrictions apply to Part A only. The prescription must be in writing and must be signed and dated by a duly qualified practitioner, registered dentist, or registered veterinary surgeon. Provided that where an authorised seller of poisons is reasonably satisfied that a person ordering any such poison and who is a duly qualified medical practitioner and who is by reason of some emergency unable to furnish such a prescription immediately, he may, notwithstanding that no such prescription has been given, if the said person undertakes to furnish him within the twenty-four hours next following with such a prescription, deliver the poison ordered in accordance with the directions of the said person, so, however, that notwithstanding anything in such directions, the supply shall not be repeated unless such a prescription has been given. If any person by whom any such undertaking has been given fails to deliver to the seller a prescription in accordance with the undertaking, or if any person for the purpose of obtaining delivery of any poison under the foregoing proviso, makes a statement which is to his knowledge false he shall be deemed to have contravened the provisions of this Rule. The prescription must specify the address of the person giving it, except in the case of a National Health Service prescription, and the name and address of the person for whose treatment it is given, or, if the prescription is given by a veterinary surgeon, of the person to whom the medicine is to be delivered. If the prescription is given by a dentist, it must bear the words 'For dental treatment only', or, if given by a veterinary surgeon, the words 'For animal treatment only.' The total amount of the medicine to be supplied, unless the preparation is contained in the British National Formulary, and the dose to be taken have to be added. The person who dispenses the prescription must comply with the following requirements:

1. The prescription must not be dispensed more than once unless the prescriber has stated thereon either that it may be dispensed a stated number of times or that it may be dispensed at stated intervals.

2. If the prescription contains a direction that it may be dispensed a stated number of times or at stated intervals, it must not be dispensed otherwise than in accordance with the direction. A prescription which contains a direction that it may be dispensed a

stated number of times but no direction as to the intervals at which it may be dispensed shall not be dispensed more often than once in three days, and a prescription which contains a direction that it is to be dispensed at stated intervals but no direction as to the number of times that it may be dispensed shall not be dispensed more often than three times.

3. At the time of dispensing or, where a poison has been delivered in an emergency, on the subsequent receipt of the prescription there must be noted on the prescription above the signature of the prescriber the name and address of the seller and the date on which the prescription was dispensed or, as the case may be, the poison was delivered.

4. Except in the case of a National Health Service prescription, or a prescription which may be dispensed again, the prescription must, for a period of two years, be retained on the premises on which it was dispensed in such manner as to be readily available for inspection.   When a repeat prescription is dispensed for the last time, it must be retained by the chemist.

The drugs in Part B are also obtainable only on prescription, but the prescription is by law only required to bear the usual signature of the doctor, and to be dated by him.

FIFTEENTH SCHEDULE

It is unlawful to sell any poison included in the Fifteenth Schedule to these Rules and intended for use as weed-killer or in the prevention or treatment of infestation by animals, plants, or other living organisms unless there has been added to the poison a dye or other substance which renders it a distinctive colour whether dry or wet or in solution.   This rule does not apply to poisons or sheep dips which are already of a distinctive colour.

Arsenical poisons.
Drazoxolon; its salts.
Fluoroacetamide; fluoroacetanilide.
Monofluoroacetic acid; its salts.
Organo-tin compounds, the following:
    Compounds of fentin.
Phosphorus compounds, the following:
    Azinphos-ethyl.
    Azinphos-methyl.
    Chlorfenvinphos.
    Dichlorvos.
    Disulfoton in solution.

Ethion.
Mecarbam.
Mevinphos.
Oxydemeton-methyl.
Phenkapton.
Phorate in solution.
Phosphamidon.
Thionazin.
Vamidothion.

DRUGS (PREVENTION OF MISUSE) ACT, 1964

This act is concerned with amphetamine compounds and substances having a similar action. To these were added lysergamide (LSD), mescalin and related substances in 1966; methaqualone was included in 1971. It makes it unlawful for a person to have possession of any of these compounds unless it is by virtue of the issue of a prescription by a duly qualified medical practitioner, registered dental practitioner or registered veterinary practitioner, or unless he is a registered manufacturer of, or dealer in bulk in, these substances. Those who have possession of these drugs in the legitimate course of their employment are also exempt, e.g. doctors, dentists, and veterinary practitioners. There are also restrictions on their importation.

A constable may arrest without warrant a person who is found committing, or is reasonably suspected of having committed an offence under the Act if he reasonably suspects that person will abscond unless arrested, or the person's name and address are unknown or cannot be verified (section 2).

Section 3 provides for the granting of search warrants by a justice of the peace (or in Scotland, a sheriff or magistrate) on sworn evidence that there are reasonable grounds for suspecting that one of the controlled substances is in any premises in contravention of section 1.

The Dangerous Drugs Act, 1967, section 6, materially increases police powers to detain and search persons and vehicles when the officer has reasonable grounds to suspect a contravention of the 1964 Act.

THE PROVISIONS OF THE DANGEROUS DRUGS ACTS AND STATUTORY RULES AND ORDERS

The medico-legal relations of the medical practitioner to these Acts and to the Statutory Rules and Orders are of importance.

The 1965 Act, a consolidating one, regulates the Importation,

Exportation, Manufacture, Sale, and Use of Opium and other Dangerous Drugs. Part III deals with prevention of the improper use of certain drugs of addiction and controls their manufacture, sale, possession, and distribution except on premises licensed for the purpose. It also regulates the issue, by medical practitioners, of prescriptions containing any of these drugs, and the dispensing of any such prescriptions, and requires persons engaged in their manufacture, sale, or distribution to keep such books and furnish such information in writing or otherwise as may be prescribed. The regulations under this part of the Act provide for authorising any person who lawfully carries on business in accordance with the provisions of the Pharmacy and Poisons Act, 1933, as an authorised seller of poisons, to manufacture at the shop, in the ordinary course of his retail business, any preparation, admixture, or extract of any drug to which this part of the Act applies, and to carry on at the shop the business of retailing, dispensing, or compounding any such drug, subject to the power of the Secretary of State to withdraw the authorisation in the case of a person who has been convicted of an offence against the Act.

By the Dangerous Drugs Act 1967, where the Home Secretary suspects that a medical or dental practitioner is supplying or prescribing dangerous drugs illegally, or is administering them to himself unlawfully, he may summon him to appear before a tribunal composed of a representative from the General Medical Council, the British Medical Association, the Royal Medical Corporations, and a legal assessor. If the charges are proved, on the recommendation of this tribunal, the Home Secretary may withdraw the practitioner's authority to issue such drugs.

Drugs to which the Dangerous Drugs Act, 1965, Orders and Regulations apply

1.

Acetorphine.
Acetyldihydrocodeine.
Allylprodine.
Alphacetylmethadol.
Alphameprodine.
Alphamethadol.
Alphaprodine.
Anileridine.
Benzethidine.
Benzylmorphine
   (3-benzylmorphine).
Betacetylmethadol.
Betameprodine.
Betamethadol.
Betaprodine.

Bezitramide.
Clonitazene.
Cocaine.
Codeine.
Desomorphine.
Dextromoramide.
Diamorphine.
Diampromide
   (N-[2-(N-methylphenethyl-
   amino)-propyl-]propionanilide).
Diethylthaimbutene.
Dihydrocodeine.
Dihydrocodeinone-O-carboxy-
   methyloxime.
Dihydromorphine.

Dimenoxadole.
Dimepheptanol.
Dimethylthiambutene.
Dioxaphetyl butyrate.
Diphenoxylate.
Dipipanone.
Ecgonine.
Ethylmethylthiambutene.
Ethylmorphine
   (3-ethylmorphine).
Etonitazene.
Etorphine.
Etoxeridine.
Fentanyl.
Furethidine.
Hydrocodone
   (dihydrocodeinone).
Hydromorphinol.
Hydromorphone.
Hydroxypethidine.
Isomethadone.
Ketobemidone.
Levomethorphan.
Levomoramide.
Levophenacylmorphan.
Levorphanol.
Metazocine.
Methadone.
Methadyl acetate.
Methyldesorphine.
Methyldihydromorphine
   (6-methyldihydromorphine).
Metopon.
Morpheridine.
Morphine.
Morphine methobromide,
   morphine-N-oxide and other
   pentavalent nitrogen morphine
   derivatives.
Myrophine.

Nicocodine.
Nicomorphine
   (3,6-dinicotinoylmorphine).
Noracymethadol.
Norcodeine.
Norlevorphanol.
Normethadone.
Normorphine.
Norpipanone.
Oxycodone.
Oxymorphone.
Pethidine.
Phenadoxone.
Phenampromide.
Phenazocine.
Phenomorphan.
Phenoperidine.
Pholcodine.
Piminodine.
Piritramide
Proheptazine.
Properidine (1-methyl-4-
   phenylpiperidine-4-carboxylic
   acid isopropyl ester).
Racemethorphan.
Racemoramide.
Racemorphan.
Thebacon.
Thebaine.
Trimeperidine.
4-Cyano-2-dimethylamino-4,4-
   diphenylbutane.
4-Cyano-1-methyl-4-phenyl-
   piperidine.
1-Methyl-4-phenylpiperidine-4-
   carboxylic acid.
2-Methyl-3-morpholino-1,1-
   diphenylpropanecarboxylic acid.
4-Phenylpiperidine-4-carboxylic
   acid ethyl ester.

2. Any ester (other than one expressly mentioned in paragraph 1 above) or ether (other than one so mentioned) of a substance for the time being specified in that paragraph.

3. Any salt of a substance for the time being specified in paragraph 1 or 2 above.

4. Any derivative of ecgonine which is convertible to ecgonine or to cocaine.

5. Concentrate of poppy-straw (that is to say, the material arising when

poppy-straw has entered into a process for the concentration of its alkaloids).

6. Medicinal opium.

7. Any extract or tincture of cannabis.

8. Any preparation, admixture, extract or other substance containing any proportion of a substance for the time being specified in paragraph 1 above or in any of paragraphs 2 to 7 above.

The principal restrictions imposed under the Regulations are:

1. A person duly authorised shall not manufacture, or carry on any process in the manufacture of a drug otherwise than in accordance with the terms and conditions of the authority issued to him and then only on the premises authorised.

2. A person shall not supply or procure, or offer to supply or procure, to or for any person, including himself, or advertise for sale, a drug or preparation unless he is duly authorised to do so and does so in accordance with the terms and conditions of his authority, and the person supplied is authorised to be in possession of the drug or preparation.

The administration of a drug or preparation by, or under the direct personal supervision *and in the presence of,* a duly qualified medical practitioner, or by, or under the direct personal supervision and in the presence of, a registered dentist, in the course of dental treatment, or a certified midwife, shall not be deemed to be the supplying of a drug or preparation.

A person to whom a drug or preparation is lawfully supplied on a prescription lawfully given by a duly qualified medical practitioner, a registered dentist, or a registered veterinary surgeon, or person registered in the Supplementary Veterinary Register in pursuance of the Veterinary Surgeons Act, 1966, or to whom a drug or preparation is lawfully supplied by a duly qualified medical practitioner or a registered veterinary surgeon or person registered in the Supplementary Veterinary Register in pursuance of the Veterinary Surgeons Act, 1966, who dispenses his own medicines, shall be deemed to be a person authorised to be in possession of the drug or preparation so supplied.

Persons who are members of the following classes:

(*a*) duly qualified medical practitioners;

(*b*) registered dentists;

(*c*) registered veterinary surgeons and registered veterinary practitioners;

(*d*) registered pharmacists who are employed or engaged in dispensing medicines at a public hospital or other public institution;

(*e*) sisters or acting sisters for the time being in charge of a ward, theatre, or other department in such a hospital or infirmary;

(*f*) persons in charge of a laboratory for purposes of research or instruction and attached to an institution approved for the purpose by the Secretary of State;

(*g*) public analysts for the purposes of the Food and Drugs Act, 1955, or the Food and Drugs (Scotland) Act, 1956;

(*h*) persons acting as sampling officers under these Acts;

(*i*) inspectors appointed by the Pharmaceutical Society of Great Britain;

are authorised, so far as may be necessary for the practice or exercise of their respective professions or employments, to be in possession of, and to supply, drugs or preparations, provided that a dentist shall not be authorised to supply drugs or preparations otherwise than by the personal administration to persons receiving treatment from him.

The term 'institution' means a university, university college, public hospital, or other like institution.

It should be noted that a certified practising midwife is authorised to purchase, to be in possession of, and to administer, medicinal opium, tincture of opium, and pethidine preparations, including Pethilorfan, so far as is necessary for the practice of her profession or employment as midwife. Notification to the local supervising authority of her intention to practise is prerequisite.

The preparations controlled by the Dangerous Drugs Acts are now relegated to one of three groups.[2]   Those in the first group (D.D.) are subject to full control. Less severe control is exercised over 'D.D. Reg.' and 'D.D. Inv.' preparations.

D.D. and D.D. Reg. drugs in the actual custody of an authorised person must be kept in a locked receptacle which can be opened only by the authorised person. A qualified employee may have access to such drugs. Storage of D.D. Inv. preparations is not regulated, unless the drug is also in the First Schedule to the Poisons List.

A prescription for the supply of any drug in the D.D. category must comply with the following requirements:

1. It must be in writing or typewriting, must be dated, signed by the medical practitioner, dentist, or veterinary surgeon, with his usual signature, and address, and must specify the name and address of the person for whose use the prescription is given. The prescription must specify the total amount of the drug to be supplied, or if the preparation is to be found in the B.P., B.P.C., B.N.F., or the Dental Practitioners' Formulary, or is a Drug Tariff Formulation, the total amount of that preparation. In the case of ampoules, the prescription may state either the total amount, including overage, to be supplied, or the amount intended to be

injected. In prescriptions issued under the National Health Service Acts, on the forms provided, the address of the practitioner need not be included.

2. A prescription shall only be given by a medical practitioner when required for purposes of medical treatment. When given by a dentist, it must be marked 'For local dental treatment only', and when by a veterinary surgeon, shall be marked 'For animal treatment only.'

3. The drugs shall not be supplied more than once on the same prescription, provided that if the prescription so directs, the drugs may be supplied on more than one but not exceeding three occasions, as directed in the prescription, at intervals to be specified therein. Repeats may not be ordered on a National Health Service prescription.

4. The prescription shall be marked with the date on which it is dispensed and shall be retained by the person, firm, or body corporate by whom the prescription is dispensed, and, unless for the purposes of the National Health Service Acts, shall be kept in the premises where it is dispensed and shall be available for inspection. In no case may the prescription be returned to the patient.

Every person authorised to supply dangerous drugs or preparations shall comply with the following provisions:

(a) He shall keep a register and enter therein, in the forms set out in Part I and Part II of the First Schedule in the Dangerous Drugs (No. 2) Regulations, 1964, true particulars with respect to every quantity of any drug or preparation obtained by him, and with respect to every quantity of any drug or preparation supplied by him.

A separate register or a separate part of the register shall be used with respect to each class of drug and its preparations.

(b) The required entry in ink or indelible pencil must be made on the day on which the drug or preparation is received or on which the transaction with respect to the supply thereof takes place, or, if that is not reasonably practicable, on the following day.

(c) So much of this Regulation as requires a person to enter in the register particulars with respect to drugs or preparations supplied to him shall not apply to:

(1) A duly qualified medical practitioner who enters in a day-book true particulars of every drug or preparation supplied by him to any person, together with the name and address of that person and the date of the supply, and enters in a separate book a proper reference to each entry in the day-book which relates to the supply of any drug or preparation.

Entry in the register or day-book will be deemed to have been complied with if there is entered as the amount obtained or supplied, true particulars as to either the total quantity of the drug or preparation, or the total quantity intended to be administered or injected.

(2) An authorised seller of poisons, who enters in a separate book a proper reference to each entry in a Pharmacy Act book which relates to the supply of any drug or preparation.

Every register, separate book, day-book, or Pharmacy Act book must be kept on the premises, and be available for inspection.

The Dangerous Drugs Act, 1967, and the Dangerous Drugs (Supply to Addicts) Regulations, 1968, forbid medical practitioners to administer or supply cocaine or heroin (or any preparation containing these drugs) to any person addicted to the drug, save for the relief of pain.   Addicts are defined as those who, as a result of repeated administration, have become so dependent upon the drug that they have an overpowering desire for its administration to be continued.   Certain practitioners are licensed by the Secretary of State to treat addicts by, if need be, the administration of the drugs to which the patient has become addicted.

The Dangerous Drugs (Notification of Addicts) Regulations, 1968, lay an obligation on any medical practitioner who attends a person whom he considers is addicted to any drug to write to the Chief Medical Officer at the Home Office giving particulars, if known, of the name, address, sex, date of birth, and National Health Service number of that person, the date of attendance and the name of the drug or drugs concerned.

Control of Dangerous Drugs and Poisons in Hospital

In hospitals with Pharmaceutical Departments, medicines containing a poison may be supplied only on a written order signed by a duly qualified medical practitioner, registered dentist, or sister in charge. The label must indicate that the medicine is to be stored in the poisons cupboard.   Such a cupboard is inspected at least four times a year by the pharmacist.

A Dangerous Drugs Register is kept by the pharmacy.   A sister is not legally obliged to keep one, but is required to keep copies of all orders for D.D. and D.D. Reg. preparations.   In practice, such a register is kept in all wards and departments.   Prescriptions must be in writing in the case sheet and be signed or initialled by the prescriber.

Therapeutic Substances Act, 1956, and Regulations

This Act controls the manufacture, sale, importation, purity, and standards of certain therapeutic substances used in the treatment of disease and capable of causing danger to the health of the community if used without proper safeguards. These include such substances as vaccines, antitoxins, corticosteroids, and antibiotics.

Pharmacy and Medicines Act, 1941

This Act amends the Pharmacy and Poisons Act, 1933. It restricts the publication of advertisements of: (1) Substances used for treatment of Bright's disease, cataract, diabetes, epilepsy or fits, glaucoma, locomotor ataxy, paralysis or tuberculosis, except in special cases where there is a professional interest. (2) Anything calculated to lead to its use for procuring the miscarriage of women (p. 385).

The Medicines Act, 1968

This compendious statute makes new provisions with respect to medicinal products and related matters, together with consolidation of large parts of the legislation already discussed. Part I of the Act requires the Health Ministers to appoint a Medicines Commission of at least eight members drawn from the medical and pharmaceutical professions. The Commission is empowered to tender advice to the Ministers on all matters relating to medicinal products. Committees are to be established to consider safety, quality, efficacy, and so on.

The Ministers will grant licences authorising importation, manufacture, wholesale dealing, and sale, with appropriate exceptions for pharmacists, midwives, and other professional classes.

Part III provides for 'general sale lists' of products which can with reasonable safety be sold otherwise than by, or under the supervision of, a pharmacist, for example by means of automatic machines. This part also regulates the introduction of new remedies and the maintenance of standards contained in the British Pharmacopoeia or other similar publications.

Parts IV, V, and VI regulate pharmacies, labelling, advertising, and storage.

Part VII concerns the British Pharmacopoeia and other publications. The Pharmacopoeia is no longer under the direction of the General Medical Council, but is to be published by the new British Pharmacopoeia Commission (p. 9).

A start has been made in implementing parts of the Act by establishing the Medicines Commission, the Committee on Safety of Medicines, and committees under the respective chairmanship of Lord Rosenheim and Sir Derrick Dunlop concerned in drawing up a General Sales List and a list of products to be supplied on prescription only.

The Misuse of Drugs Act, 1971

This Act, which has not yet come into force, repeals the Drugs (Prevention of Misuse) Act, 1964, and the Dangerous Drugs Acts, 1965 and 1967, without invalidating regulations made under these Acts.

The Act strikes at overprescribing by doctors (sections 10 to 13); at trafficking more than mere possession of controlled drugs (Schedule 4). It is designed to be much more flexible in approach to an ever-changing drug 'scene'. To this end, section 1 constitutes an Advisory Council on the Misuse of Drugs, which body is charged with the duty of keeping under review the situation in the United Kingdom and advising the Minister on measures which ought to be taken:

(a) for restricting the availability of such drugs or supervising the arrangements for their supply;

(b) for enabling persons affected by the misuse of such drugs to obtain proper advice, and for securing the provision of proper facilities and services for the treatment, rehabilitation, and after-care of such persons;

(c) for promoting co-operation between the various professional and community services which in the opinion of the Council have a part to play in dealing with social problems connected with the misuse of such drugs;

(d) for educating the public (and in particular the young) in the dangers of misusing such drugs and for giving publicity to those dangers; and

(e) for promoting research into, or otherwise obtaining information about, any matter which in the opinion of the Council is of relevance for the purpose of preventing the misuse of such drugs or dealing with any social problem connected with their misuse.

Schedule 2 classifies controlled drugs according to relative harmfulness. Class A, the most dangerous, includes cocaine, heroin, morphine, LSD, and opium. Amphetamines, cannabis, and codeine are in Class B. Drugs such as methaqualone are included in Class C.

Strangely enough, the barbiturates appear in none of the Classes (nor do alcohol and tobacco!).

It is to be hoped that this useful Act will come into force with less delay than has attended the bringing to life of the Medicines Act. Central to both Acts are bodies of professional people charged with advising the appropriate Minister. Perhaps part of the delay may be attributed to the reluctance of persons of sufficient calibre to staff yet another committee.

References

1. *The Poisons List Order*, 1970, S.I. 1970/797
2. *Poisons and T.S.A. Guide*, 10th ed. The Pharmaceutical Press, 1971.
3. *The Poisons Rules*, 1971, S.I. 1971/726

Chapter 18

GENERAL ACTION OF POISONS, EVIDENCE AND TREATMENT OF POISONING

General action of poisons

THE action of poisons may be local, remote, or both. They may kill either by direct interaction with the tissues or by being transferred to some remote situation where more specific interactions may disrupt essential life processes. Although corrosive substances cause lesions in the parts with which they are brought into contact, the proximate cause of death may well be due to indirectly related phenomena such as shock. With regard to the remote action of poisons, some of them act on certain organs more than others, for example opium, morphia, the barbiturates, and alcohol affect the brain, digitalis and oxalic acid involve the heart, strychnine, the spinal cord, and chlorine, gaseous in form, the lungs. Certain other poisons, notably arsenic trihydride, carbon monoxide, potassium chlorate, pyrogallic acid and many of the nitro- and amino-derivatives of benzene and its homologues act upon the blood. Poisons which are frequently swallowed and cause death are phenol and phenol derivatives, prussic acid and cyanides, corrosive acids and alkalis, oxalic acid and oxalates, opium derivatives, barbiturates and aspirin, strychnine and nux vomica, arsenic and mercury salts, phosphorus, atropine and belladonna. The dosage of potent drugs can be divided, in arbitrary manner, into two groups, namely, those in which the lethal dose lies far in excess of the active dose and those in which it lies close to the active dose. Of the drugs which may be relegated to the former group, atropine may be mentioned, while of those belonging to the latter group, strychnine is an example. There is a very definite distinction between the terms 'toxic dose' and 'fatal dose', since the former merely causes symptoms of poisoning while the latter induces poisoning to such a degree that death results.

Circumstances modifying the action of poisons

Quantity. The question of dosage has already been touched upon. The larger the quantity and the greater the severity of the symptoms, the more rapid usually is the fatal result. It must not be forgotten, however, that the actual excess, in respect of some poisons, may prove beneficial by inducing both rapid and effective emesis. The question of quantity, which separates the medicinal action of a poisonous drug from its toxic action, has prompted the law to differentiate between a poison and a noxious thing.

Condition of administration.

Condition of administration. A poison acts most rapidly when inhaled in gaseous or vaporous form, or when injected intravenously; next, when injected intra-muscularly or subcutaneously; and least rapidly when swallowed. Further slowing down of absorption occurs when the substance which is ingested is only partly soluble. With decreasing rapidity, absorption takes place from the mucous surfaces and the unbroken skin.

Chemical combination and mechanical mixture.

Chemical combination and mechanical mixture. When two substances, both of which may be dangerous poisons, combine chemically the product has unique properties. The toxicity is not related to the original materials. Small modifications in the structural skeletons of organic materials can cause small differences in properties when the new material is compared with the old but often the new material is quite different. If the metabolic processes can reverse any chemical change the properties of the original material become apparent again.

Mechanical mixing does not change the properties. All the components exhibit their own actions. It is possible that one substance may make another in the mixture appear more active. For example death occurs from barbiturate poisoning at considerably lower levels when alcohol is present. It should be noted that mixtures occurring in the body are as potent as those formed outside and then ingested.

When a powdery poisonous substance is administered with fluids of much lighter specific gravity, the substance is liable to sediment in the vessel, and thus the quantity actually swallowed is less than when the vehicle of administration has been a fluid of specific gravity more nearly approaching that of the powder. It is by adopting the latter principle that the poisoner who uses arsenic administers it in a fluid which by its colour will mask the presence of the poison, and which is heavy and viscid. When a poison is administered by the mouth, the stomach being empty, its action will be much more rapid than when swallowed after a meal.

Habit.

Habit. Habit diminishes the effects of certain poisons, since a tolerance towards them is gradually developed. It is a matter of common observation, for example, that continuous indulgence in alcohol and tobacco confers a comparative immunity from danger from poisonous doses. Similarly, the morphine habit may be contracted to such an extent that immense doses may be taken with impunity. From continued use, strychnine and arsenic may be taken in doses which otherwise would be liable to act poisonously.

Condition of bodily health. A relatively small dose, from which a stronger person would probably recover, may kill a weakly person. In certain diseases, some drugs can be given, with impunity, in doses which, in other circumstances, would be likely to prove harmful. In some diseases, on the other hand, certain drugs cannot be administered even in small doses without toxic effects. This is seen in cases of renal disease, when mercury and morphia should only be administered with the greatest caution.

Age. Adults are more tolerant to certain drugs, such as narcotics, than children and old persons.

Idiosyncrasy. Among persons, there is a varying degree of susceptibility. From time to time this is seen when such drugs as morphia, cocaine, quinine, iodine, and bromide are administered.

Cumulative action. Certain poisons tend to accumulate within the body as the result of slow excretion, and therefore the continued administration of relatively small doses may occasion symptoms of poisoning, for example, lead, mercury, digitalis, and carbon monoxide.

Evidence of poisoning in the living body

The evidence of poisoning will depend upon whether the poisoning is acute or chronic.

In acute poisoning the symptoms appear suddenly while the individual is in good health. The person is affected with a group of symptoms of a definite character out of consonance with his previous state of health. This feature of the attacks stands out prominently in all recorded cases of poisoning. Not all or even most of the common symptoms may be seen in any given case. At the same time, certain manifestations of disease which simulate poisoning may have a sudden onset, and such a possiblity should receive due consideration.

In chronic poisoning, the onset of the symptoms is more gradual and insidious, on account of the small quantity of poison which has been administered on each occasion, since it is often the intention of the poisoner to kill his victim gradually by persistent administration of small doses in the hope of averting suspicion. In such cases, the possibility of detection lies in the absence of causal relationship between the condition of the patient and the symptoms from which he suffers, in the fitful coming and going of the symptoms, in their appearance, usually after food or liquid has been taken, and in their complete disappearance on the patient's removal from his usual surroundings.

In acute poisoning especially, and in chronic poisoning generally, the symptoms frequently appear soon after food, medicine, or fluid has been taken.   It must be borne in mind, however, that it is precisely under such circumstances that symptoms of disease, for example gastro-intestinal conditions, may arise.

When more than one person has eaten similar food, and when they are similarly affected, there is strong presumptive evidence of poisoning.

The strongest proof of criminal or suicidal administration of poison, however, is established by the discovery of poison in the food taken, in the vomited matter, or in body excretions, provided it can be shown that such could not have occurred from accidental contamination.

Duty of a medical practitioner in cases of suspected poisoning

Should a doctor be called to a patient who he suspects is suffering from chronic poisoning, what points should he attend to, apart from the treatment of the patient?

These may be summarised broadly as follows:

The time of the occurrence of the symptoms, and their character, should be carefully noted.

Their relation, in point of time, to the taking of food, fluid, or medicine, and the order in which they appear, should be fully investigated.

It should be observed whether the symptoms intermit, or increase steadily in severity.

The previous condition of health of the person affected should be ascertained.

If there has been vomiting, the vomited matter should be inspected and, if possible, a sample taken for analysis.

A sample of the suspected peccant food, fluid, or medicine, and a sample of urine and faeces should be obtained for analysis.   These should be placed in suitable containers, sealed, and labelled.

If food is suspected, inquiry should be made as to whether similar food has been eaten previously without ill-effect, and whether or not any person other than the one affected has eaten it without resultant illness, or has been affected more or less simultaneously.

Explanations offered or remarks made, regarding the onset of symptoms, should be noted.

When the symptoms do not conform to ordinary illness, and when, in spite of appropriate treatment, they continue, the environment of the patient and the conduct of those looking after him, should be carefully observed, and the services of both a nurse and a consultant obtained.

Should there be suspicious circumstances, the patient should be removed to hospital or to a nursing home where he can be under close observation and supervision remote from his usual environment.

General lines of treatment in acute poisoning

Matthew[1] says that the management of poisoned patients is often described by experts in associated fields such as pharmacologists or forensic pathologists and that as a result the literature contains much inaccurate information. He suggests the practising clinical toxicologist as a better source of knowledge and goes on to outline a number of points where there is error or controversy.

Bearing this in mind the general lines of treatment may be summed up in a few sentences, but the mode and extent of their application must be left to the judgment of the practitioner according to the needs of individual cases.

First. The poison should be removed from the stomach expeditiously even if the delay suggests that the stomach may be empty.

Second. Antidotes should be administered if available.

Third. The poison should be eliminated from the body by the natural channels.

Fourth. Symptomatic treatment should be administered and stimulation of the respiratory and circulatory systems should be resorted to immediately indications present themselves.

The best and most expeditious method for the removal of poisons from the stomach is by the use of the stomach tube, which is easily introduced, and, when intelligently used, can do no injury. The tube, which is composed of flexible rubber, should be about 12 mm, or slightly less, in diameter, and about 1·5 m in length. It should be marked at a point about 50 cm above the lower end, which should be perforated by more than one opening. The actual termination of the lower end should be rounded off in order to avoid friction when the tube is passed. A filter-funnel should be inserted into the upper end of the tube. The average distance between the lips and the cardiac end of the stomach in the adult subject is approximately 45 cm, and it is for this reason that the tube is marked in the manner described, so that the operator may have some indication when the end of the tube has reached the interior of the stomach. In the case of young children, a tube of narrower calibre and of shorter length should be employed. In using the stomach tube, it is advisable that the head of the patient, face downwards, should be placed over the end of the bed. In this position, the mouth and pharynx will be at a lower level than the larynx and trachea, and thus regurgitated fluid, around the tube, will not enter the airpassages. After the tube has been warmed and smeared with a lubricant, such as glycerine or vaseline, it is passed into the stomach by depressing the tongue with the finger, sliding the tube along the finger into the pharynx, directing the tip to the back of the pharynx, and thus into and down the oesophagus. Water, of body temperature, first tested against the cheek or lip of the administrator, is then poured in by the funnel. The water may contain a suitable dissolved antidote. While pouring in the fluid, the funnel should be held above the patient's head. As the last portion of water is being poured in, and the tube and a portion of the funnel are full of water, the tube at its junction with the funnel is pinched between the finger and thumb, and the tube is then lowered below the level of the stomach. The stomach contents will then syphon out and a sample may be retained for analysis. The process may be repeated as often as required. To perform complete gastric lavage, about 2 gallons of water in all should be used. About 1 pint of fluid should be employed for each separate lavage. When the poison which has been swallowed is known, a suitable chemical antidote may be dissolved in the solution used for lavage, and when the process is nearing completion, a quantity of the fluid should be allowed to remain in the stomach.

In cases of strychnine poisoning, it is imperative that before attempting to introduce the tube, the patient should first be anaesthetised, otherwise the attempt will induce spasm and frustrate the effort. When a patient is conscious and a stomach tube is not available, simple emetics, such as mustard and water, or salt and water, should be freely used. If the patient refuses or is unable to swallow, an emetic, such as apomorphine, should be given hypodermically.

The stomach tube should not be employed in poisoning by strong corrosives on account of the danger of perforation of the stomach by the tube, following the effects of the corrosive lesions. In such cases it is preferable, when possible, to counteract their effects by causing the patient to drink neutralising demulcent fluids. In poisoning by certain substances, which by irritant action cause nephritis, it is necessary to assist excretion. Perspiration may be induced by hot baths and warm packs.

To dilute the poison which has been absorbed into the bloodstream and aid its elimination from the body, intravenous infusion of normal saline solution or glucose saline will be found most beneficial in certain cases. Blood transfusion will be found useful in poisoning due to toxic substances causing blood changes. When asphyxial manifestations threaten, and in certain stages of gaseous poisoning, oxygen is valuable. To clear the airway, the patient should be placed face downward to allow fluid to drain from the mouth and upper passages. When there is a tendency for the tongue to fall back, its position should be carefully controlled. When breathing ceases, artificial respiration must be employed without delay. Oedema glottidis may call for intubation.

In cases of prolonged unconsciousness the bladder should be catheterised. The treatment of symptoms should be applied as indications arise, and such stimulatory measures as are necessary must also be utilised. The detailed lines of treatment in cases of specific poisoning are described later under the appropriate headings.

Antidotes

The effects of a limited number of poisons can be counteracted by antidotes, which may be divided into three groups, in accordance with their mode of operation, namely: (a) physical, (b) chemical, and (c) physiological.

Physical antidotes. These are few in number. Some of them have also a chemical action to a limited extent. For example, egg albumen or flour and water are mechanical antidotes in poisoning by corrosive sublimate. At the same time, by the formation of albuminate of mercury, which is practically insoluble in the stomach, egg albumen acts partly as a chemical antidote. Charcoal may be reckoned as a physical antidote in alkaloidal poisoning, as by strychnine. Physical antidotes also exercise a beneficial effect in other cases, since they dilute the poison and thus may limit its effects. Demulcent fluids act in this manner both in corrosive and irritant poisoning.

Chemical antidotes. These neutralise poisons by forming new compounds which are either insoluble or less active; thus alkalis in acid, and dilute acids in alkali, poisoning may be taken as the simplest type. Magnesium sulphate may be used in poisoning by carbolic acid, and sulphates of the alkalis in poisoning by lead or barium. Freshly precipitated oxide of iron, made by treating tincture of perchloride of iron with excess of ammonia, filtering the precipitate, and adding water, may be used in arsenical poisoning as a chemical antidote since it forms the comparatively insoluble ferric arsenite. Tannin and its preparations produce an insoluble tannate in poisoning by antimony. Potassium permanganate is a powerful antidote in morphine poisoning.

Physiological antidotes. The mode of action of these is widely divergent. Chloroform may be said to exercise an antagonistic effect in strychnine poisoning by inducing general anaesthesia, thus overcoming the tetanic contractions and giving an opportunity for the elimination of the poison from the stomach and from the body generally. Atropine, within limits, is a physiological antidote to morphia and to the organic phosphorus compounds. Physiological antidotes are not reliable in their action.

Intravenous injections of normal saline or glucose saline, also blood transfusions, in certain cases of poisoning, yield very beneficial results.

Evidence of poisoning in the dead

Evidence from post-mortem appearances. The post-mortem appearances found will be described in detail when specific poisons are considered. In conducting a post-mortem examination where poisoning is suspected, evidence of disease must be differentiated from lesions due to the effects of a poison. Should any doubt exist in the mind of the examiner, histological examination should be made. Adequate and appropriate material for analysis must be secured, and in this respect the nature and characters of the lesions present, if any, together with the history of the case should provide the necessary indications. When such indications are not available, all the organs, together with a specimen of blood and urine, should be retained.

Evidence from chemical analysis. The most important proof of poisoning is the detection of the poison within the body. This evidence may not be available due to the destruction of the poison itself or the introduction of massive amounts of foreign material as may happen in embalming. Special difficulties may occur when the products of putrefaction obscure materials of closely similar character.

In the toxicological section which follows, descriptions of the methods of analysis have been omitted. Toxicological analysis is a highly specialised branch of science which has fallen appropriately within the sphere of the skilled chemist and those who wish to examine this subject in depth should consult such works as Stewart and Stolman,[2] *Methods of Forensic Science*,[3] Curry,[4] Clarke,[5] or one of many others.

Those who want more general information may find some help in the appendices to this book. These include the following sections:

Simplified explanations with examples of some of the more used techniques including spectrometry and chromatography.

Interpretation of results and sources of error.

A selection of data obtained using ultra-violet spectrometry, gas chromatography, thin layer chromatography, and colour reactions.

References

1. MATTHEW, H. *Br. med. J.*, **1**, 519, 1971.
2. STEWART, C.P. & STOLMAN, A. *Toxicology*. London: Academic Press, 1960.
3. *Methods of Forensic Science*, vols 1 and 2, ed. Lundquist, F.; vols 3 and 4, ed. Curry, A.S. London: Interscience.
4. CURRY, A.S. *Poison Detection in Human Organs*, 2nd ed. Springfield: Thomas, 1969.
5. *Isolation and Identification of Drugs*, ed. Clarke, E.G.C. The Pharmaceutical Press, 1969.

Chapter 19

TOXIC MATERIALS

ACETIC ACID (*Vinegar*)

Properties and Uses

PURE acetic acid is an ice-like solid below about 16°C, hence it is often described as glacial acetic acid. Above that temperature it is a colourless liquid with a characteristic odour. The specific gravity is 1·05 at 20°C. The dilute acid is found in most homes in the form of vinegar. It has a number of medical uses, e.g. neutralisation of caustic alkalis in poisoning.

Symptoms

Dilute acetic acid acts simply as an irritant but the glacial acid is corrosive. The parts with which the acid comes into contact are softened, and assume a whitish or pale yellowish colour. Laryngeal complications, because of the volatility of the acid, are commonly found in such cases. Vomiting is usual. The action, locally, is therefore that of a corrosive, and such effects are apparent in the mouth.

The Annual Report of the Chief Medical Officer of the Ministry of Health for the year 1937, refers to cases of acetic acid poisoning. In one case a man who in a restaurant took a quantity of vinegar which was labelled 'Highly Concentrated Vinegar', died soon afterwards. The contents of the bottle consisted of approximately 60 per cent acetic acid. If the directions on the label had been followed, the contents should have been diluted to about one part in thirteen, prior to use.

Treatment

The stomach should be washed out, and an alkali, such as lime-water or magnesia, administered. A stomach tube, if strong acid or if severe tissue damage is evident, should not be used. Avoid alkaline carbonate. Milk or olive oil may be used as demulcents. Special symptoms should be treated as they arise.

Post-mortem findings

The mucous membrane of the oesophagus and stomach will be affected in varying degree, and there may be evidence of corrosive action. The upper air-passages will show marked congestion.

Analytical findings

The acid is generally detected and measured in the stomach.   As it is present in most biological materials a significant quantity must be found.

Fatal dose and time of death

The fatal dose is variable but is probably about 50 g, though 4 g of the glacial acid has killed a child.   An adult has recovered after taking as much as 180 g.

Note.   Vinegar which is about a 4 or 5 per cent solution does not appear to cause much harm.   Polson and Tattersall[1] quote the case of a woman drinking over 2 litres and recovering after only a mild illness.

ACETYLSALICYLIC ACID (Aspirin)

Aspirin is a colourless crystalline powder (m. pt 136°C) which is moderately soluble in water (0·25 g/100 ml).   It is well known to the public and is used for a variety of conditions, including headache, influenza, and rheumatism.   This drug has a mild soporific action. It has also antipyretic and antirheumatic properties.   In very excessive doses, or as the result of idiosyncrasy, toxic effects may ensue.

A significant number of deaths are due to aspirin each year.

Symptoms

The symptoms of poisoning include vomiting, giddiness, buzzing in the ears, oedema of the face and eyelids, skin rash, cyanosis, acidosis and dehydration.   In acute poisoning the patient is seldom unconscious and if drowsy this is of serious significance.   It is more common for children to be drowsy or even in coma.

Hyperpnoea is an important indication of this form of poisoning and is caused by stimulation of the respiratory centre.   This leads to hyperventilation, which in turn produces a respiratory alkalosis.   The subsequent disturbance of the acid–base balance is of complex nature. Occasionally these cases may be mistaken for diabetic coma.   Hyperpyrexia and profuse perspiration occur.   Delirium is present in certain cases.   Severe and even fatal haemorrhages due to hypo-thrombinaemia may supervene.

Treatment

If the patient is conscious and is seen shortly after ingestion of the poison, gastric lavage should be carried out.   The subsequent treatment should be dictated by the requirements of the individual case as the reactions to the poison are frequently variable. For this reason, sustained attention should be directed to the electrolytic balance and specially to the possibility of potassium loss. Respiratory depression may be treated by administering artificial respiration with oxygen. If there is abnormal bleeding vitamin K may be given.

Post-mortem findings

A typical finding in aspirin poisoning is congestion of the gastro-intestinal tract perhaps with areas of erosion. The lungs, liver, and kidneys may show degenerative changes.

Analytical findings

Materials submitted for examination are analysed for 'salicylate' content, as aspirin is rapidly de-acetylated in the blood. Very often low values are found due to the subject having survived in hospital for some time. In such cases values found in post-mortem blood ranged from 15 to 26 mg salicylate/100 ml. The values recorded for subjects found dead from aspirin poisoning ranged from 52 to 126 mg salicylate/100 ml blood.

Fatal dose and time of death

Death has followed ingestion of 2·5 g aspirin by a two-year-old child and 30 g in an adult but recovery has followed doses of 90 g and 85 g. The fatal dose is, therefore, very variable; a lower limit in the region of 5 g is probable. Death may be rapid but survival for a day or two is common.

Illustrative case

The following case, for the details of which we are indebted to Drs Glen, Millar, and Shanks, Victoria Infirmary, Glasgow, is illustrative of most of the findings in aspirin poisoning: The patient swallowed 45 g of aspirin, in addition to two sleeping powders of unknown composition. She was admitted to hospital, about seven hours afterwards, when she was mentally clear and rational. Prior to admission, she had suffered from violent vomiting and diarrhoea, also buzzing in the ears. The pulse-rate was fast, the extremities were moist and cold, but there was no cyanosis although breathing was rapid. Shortly after admission, she had a convulsion, of short duration, at first tonic and later clonic. Following this, she became rather confused and perspired freely. Her condition deteriorated and she gradually sank into coma. Breath-ing became progressively more acidotic and ultimately there was extreme 'air-hunger'.   She showed cyanosis and died within twenty-six hours of admission.

The treatment employed consisted of gastric lavage, which yielded a dirty green result, but no tablets were seen.   Shortly after this, the patient was able to retain four-hourly doses of alkali.   She was also given four-hourly rectal saline with glucose.

Post-mortem examination showed moderate cyanosis of the face and finger-tips.   The right heart was dilated.   The myocardium was soft. The lungs were intensely congested.   The liver, pancreas, and kidneys were also deeply congested.

Note.   Other salicylates such as methyl salicylate (oil of wintergreen) have similar effects.

Methyl salicylate is a colourless liquid, with a characteristic odour, which boils at 223°C and is only slightly soluble in water (0·074 g/100 ml at 30°C).   This fluid may be swallowed accidentally or suicidally. The symptoms are those of gastro-enteritis.   Post-mortem findings include evidence of gastro-enteritis, submucous haemorrhages in the pelves of the kidneys, petechial haemorrhages in the renal cortex, and visceral congestion.

Townsend[2] reports a fatal case of poisoning of a man who drank about four ounces of methyl salicylate liniment in a gulp mistaking it for alcohol.   He vomited and then collapsed.   Two and a half hours later he was fully conscious although much distressed with vomiting. Gastric lavage and copious fluids, including sodium bicarbonate, milk, and water were the principal lines of treatment used.   Next morning his condition had deteriorated and fine crepitations were present at the base of the lungs.   He became delirious and death supervened twenty-four hours after drinking the liniment.

Derobert and Gascoin[3] describe a fatal case.   A three-year-old child died in about three hours after swallowing methyl salicylate.   The autopsy findings included intense congestion of all viscera, especially the lungs and kidneys.   Subpleural petechiae were present.

ACONITINE

Aconitine is obtained from the dried root of the plant *Aconitum napellus*, or Monkshood.   The root has caused poisoning, having been eaten in error for horse-radish.

Aconite root when tasted produces tingling and numbness of the tongue, mouth, and lips, and when cut slowly reddens.   Horse-radish root when tasted is hot and pungent, but does not cause tingling, and when cut remains white.

From the fresh leaves and flowering tops of the aconite plant an extract is made, and from the root, a tincture and a liniment.

Aconitine is usually a white amorphous powder. Other alkaloid derivatives have been obtained from the aconite class.

Symptoms

The signs and symptoms may be described as follows: Their onset develops from a few minutes to an hour after taking the poison: numbness, burning, and tingling of the mouth and throat; a feeling of constriction and burning in the throat; severe pain and tenderness in the stomach; nausea and vomiting; numbness, loss of power, and pain in the limbs; giddiness, singing in the ears, deafness, and impairment of vision; indistinct articulation, and ultimate loss of the power of speech; unconsciousness, convulsive gasps, or convulsions; contraction and later dilatation of the pupils. The cause of death is either cardiac or respiratory failure due to paralysis of the centres in the brain.

Treatment

Delay absorption by giving milk or activated charcoal and then remove by gastric lavage or emesis. Digitalis may be used to counter-act cardiac depression. Atropine is used to prevent vagal slowing of the heart. Respiratory embarrassment may necessitate the use of artificial respiration and oxygen inhalations.

Post-mortem findings

These may be as follows: Pallor of the mucous membrane of the mouth; congestion or engorgement of the brain and lungs; inflammation of the mucous membrane of the stomach; congestion of the liver and kidneys.

Fatal dose and time of death

The fatal dose is about 250 mg of plant extract. The fatal amount of pure substances is probably about 2 mg; 4 mg has certainly caused death. Death usually occurs somewhere between 45 minutes and a day.

AMITRIPTYLINE, IMIPRAMINE, and NORTRIPTYLINE

These and the related drugs are used as antidepressants. These materials block parasympathetic responses and may be potentiated by amine oxidase inhibitors or alcohol.

Symptoms

The symptoms include drowsiness, blurred vision, constipation, urine retention, hypotension, tachycardia, tremors, confusion, and abdominal pain.   Acute overdose may result in convulsions, cyanosis, coma, fall in blood-pressure, respiratory depression, and cardiac disturbances.   Ventricular fibrillation may precede death.

Treatment

Treatment involves gastric lavage or emesis.   Artificial respiration may be used as necessary.   Maintain blood-pressure by giving fluids and treat other symptoms as they arise.

Post-mortem findings

Liver damage may be present but the findings are non-specific.

Analytical findings

These drugs may be detected and measured in tissues and fluids but the levels are rather low and care is required if the measurement is to be successful.   In fatal poisoning the blood levels may be much less than 1 mg/100 ml.   The liver levels are usually greater than 1·0 mg/100 g and the urine levels may well be of the order of ten's of mg/1co ml.

Fatal dose

The fatal dose of these drugs varies but is somewhere in the region of 1 to 2 g, though recoveries after ingestion of quantities of this order are reported.

Note.   Other antidepressant drugs such as phenelzine (Nardil) have a monoamine oxidase-inhibiting action and when taken with some foods such as cheese or sliced broad bean pods result in severe reactions.   These combined effects include headache, rise in blood pressure with possible intracranial haemorrhage, and acute cardiac failure.

AMMONIUM HYDROXIDE ('Ammonia')

Properties and uses

The concentrated solution is a colourless liquid with a characteristic pungent odour and is less dense than water (sp. gr. 0·88).   This material is used widely in industry in various strengths and purities.   It is commonly met with in the home in the form of more or less dilute solutions used for cleaning purposes.   In medicine, it is used as smelling salts or as a restorative.

Symptoms

In two of our cases, suicide had been attempted by drinking ammonia sold for domestic purposes.   In both cases, which recovered, the symptoms of dyspnoea and dysphagia were very marked, and the former were accompanied by some degree of cyanosis.   In one of the cases, the mouth and throat showed patchy corrosion, and the tongue and pharynx were congested and oedematous.   Following recovery from the initial symptoms, stricture of the lower third of the oesophagus developed, which, however, was overcome by the use of graduated bougies.   In neither of the cases was the amount of fluid swallowed ascertained.   The strength of the ammonia, which had been taken, was 9·8 per cent.   Liquor ammoniae fortis contains 35 per cent by weight of ammonia.   Serious symptoms of poisoning have followed the swallowing of ammonium carbonate.   When ammonia is swallowed, there are more or less immediate symptoms of acute irritation involving the mouth, upper air-passages, oesophagus, and stomach.

The urgent symptoms in poisoning by ammonia are due to the ammoniacal fumes which are liberated.

Treatment

The treatment is as described under potassium hydroxide.

Post-mortem findings

These consist of a raw, inflamed condition of the lips, mouth, tongue, pharynx, and larynx, with patchy erosion of the mucous membrane. The oesophagus is also involved and the lining membrane is usually of whitish-yellow colour and sodden in appearance.   Frequently there is irregular desquamation with exposure of underlying tissue.   Oedema of the glottis is sometimes present.   The gastric mucosa may show a similar picture to that of the oesophagus, although the colour is usually darker.   Patchy submucosal extravasations of blood may be seen. As a rule, there is intense congestion.   When a quantity of the fumes has been inhaled, the bronchi are covered with a fibrinous membrane which is easily stripped and leaves a raw surface beneath.   The lungs are congested and oedematous, or evidence of bronchopneumonia may be present.

Analytical findings

Usually restricted to detection and estimation in the stomach. If any decomposition is present, special care is required because ammonia-like substances are produced.

Fatal dose and time of death

About 30 ml of strong ammonia is probably a fatal dose. The shortest survival period known is four minutes: however, periods beyond a day are common.

Note. *Ammonia.* Ammonia is a colourless gas, with a characteristic odour, which condenses to a liquid at $-33.4°C$. The chemical formula for this gas is NH_3. The term 'ammonia' is often used in the home and industry for the solution of the gas in water. This material has the formula NH_4OH. The chemical combination is loose so that the gas (NH_3) may be expelled easily from solution, e.g. by a rise in temperature.

Poisoning from ammonia fumes occurs industrially in the course of the manufacture of ammonia, the handling of containers, and among other sources, in working with refrigeration plant. This gas affects the tissues with which it is brought into contact and is not absorbed into the system. A concentration which is dangerous for an exposure of half an hour is 2,500 to 4,500 parts of the gas per million parts of air. The excellent report on forty-seven cases of ammonia gas poisoning, published by Caplin,[4] has covered the salient points in this connection, and we take the liberty of quoting freely from this authoritative contribution.

The cases in question occurred during a heavy air raid in London, as the result of a connecting pipe of an ammonia condenser in a cellar having been damaged by a piece of flying metal. Caplin divides the case into three groups, according to the nature of the symptoms shown by the poisoned persons, namely, mild, moderate, and severe. The mild group comprised nine cases. These persons showed irritation of the conjunctivae and upper respiratory passages. They also suffered from inflammation of the lips, buccal mucosa, and swelling of the fauces. The moderate group, which included twenty-seven cases, in addition to the above symptoms, suffered from hoarseness, dysphagia, and bronchitis. Eleven cases, relegated to the severe group, showed evidence of shock, cyanosis, intense dyspnoea, persistent cough, with frothy sputum, and suffered from bronchitis and pulmonary oedema. All cases, classified as mild, recovered. Three cases in the moderate group died after thirty-six hours from pulmonary oedema; nine others developed bronchopneumonia, and three of these cases also died within two days. Of the cases relegated to the severe group, four died within forty-eight hours following admission to hospital, and three other cases died later. The cause of death in all instances was broncho-pneumonia.

The treatment was directed to shock. Electric cradles and morphia (10 to 15 mg in severe cases) were used. The dose of morphia was reduced when dyspnoea and cyanosis were present. Oxygen inhalation by intratracheal catheter was administered to relieve cyanosis. When moist sounds in the lungs were pronounced, 0·6 mg of atropine was given and repeated at two-hourly intervals. To neutralise the ammonia on the buccal mucous membrane, diluted vinegar was first used as a gargle and mouth-wash, and later liquid paraffin was applied. For pain and oedema of the mouth and throat, a cocaine and adrenalin spray was employed. The condition of the eyes was relieved by irrigation with boracic solution and the instillation of a few drops of castor oil.

AMPHETAMINE (*Benzedrine*)

Amphetamine is a colourless liquid (b. pt 200°C) which is soluble in water. Amphetamine sulphate is a white powder which melts with decomposition at 300°C and is easily soluble in water. It has a marked stimulating effect on the central nervous system, manifested by a diminution in the sensation of fatigue, an increase in mental activity, and euphoria, and thus its clinical use is wide and varied.

Symptoms

In toxic doses the symptoms include restlessness, irritability, dry mouth, and perhaps abdominal cramps. Collapse and even syncope may follow.

There appears to be the possibility of addiction and the victims may exhibit symptoms which may lead to a faulty diagnosis of schizophrenia.

Treatment

Gastric lavage is recommended and activated charcoal to hinder absorption. Barbiturates may be used but caution is required. (Barbiturates are often formulated with amphetamine and may be present and contributing to the toxicity.) The patient should be kept in a warm, darkened room.

Post-mortem findings

These include reddish blotches on the skin, generalised oedema of the lungs, and pulmonary petechial haemorrhages. The adrenals may show haemorrhagic discoloration.

Analytical findings

Amphetamine may be found unchanged in the fluids and tissues.

Fatal dose and time of death

The fatal dose is probably somewhat under 200 mg. Death has followed five days after ingestion of 140 mg.

Note. Other central nervous system stimulants such as dexamphetamine (the dextrorotary isomer of amphetamine), diethylpropion hydrochloride, methyl phenidate hydrochloride, methylamphetamine, phenmetrazine hydrochloride, and phentermine all have toxic effects similar to amphetamine.

AMYL NITRITE

This is a pale yellow liquid which is less dense than water (0·85 g/ml at 20°C) and only slightly soluble in it. It has a fragrant odour but inhalation of large amounts results in toxic effects. It is used in medicine as a very rapid vasodilator for the relief of angina.

Symptoms

Toxic doses produce vomiting, cyanosis, dyspnoea, Cheyne–Stokes breathing, coma, and death due to cardio-vascular collapse. Methaemoglobin may be formed.

Treatment

This consists of gastric lavage, injections of adrenalin or ephedrine, to counteract the vasodilating effect, artificial respiration, and oxygen inhalations. To counteract the formation of methaemoglobin, small amounts of methylene blue should be administered. When doses are small they bring about the conversion of methaemoglobin to haemoglobin, thus exercising the opposite effect of methylene blue in high concentrations. In severe cases, an immediate exchange transfusion may be life saving.

Post-mortem findings

The post-mortem findings are usually oedema of the lungs and brain, lividity of slate-grey colour, and a brownish colour of the blood due to methaemoglobin. The kidneys may show degenerative changes.

Analytical findings

Amyl nitrite may be difficult to find due to its rapid destruction in the body, but amyl alcohol may be found.

Fatal dose and time of death

These are not known, though recovery following the ingestion of 10 g is reported.

ANAESTHETICS

Chloroform and ether are described in the text. A selection of others are given below with a few notes on each.

Ethyl chloride like chloroform enters into chemical union with the blood. It acts as a stimulant on the central vasomotor system. In 10 per cent concentration and upwards it produces paralysis of the myocardium comparable with that produced by chloroform in one-twentieth of this concentration.

It is used as a general anaesthetic for minor operations of short duration.

Nitrous oxide is the commonest anaesthetic for dental work, and is perhaps the safest anaesthetic for any short-period anaesthesia. The mortality arising from its use has been reckoned to be about one per million. The use of continuous nitrous oxide and oxygen, with or without ether, is also a prevalent form of anaesthesia for certain operations.

One of the dangers which arises is the production of anoxia. We have investigated cases in which, following the completion of anaesthesia, unconsciousness has persisted for long periods and has resulted in death from this cause.

Divinyl ether vapour, which is highly inflammable, is capable of producing a rapid anaesthesia with good muscular relaxation. Post-anaesthetic complications are rare following its use, but it should be noted that prolonged anaesthesia may bring about liver damage, and thus patients with liver insufficiency should be regarded as unsuitable subjects.

Cyclopropane is supplied as a liquid in cylinders. It becomes a vapour at atmospheric temperature and pressure, and is inflammable. Cyclopropane is used in a closed circuit apparatus and is a powerful anaesthetic which in low concentration does not irritate the respiratory passage, but has a tendency to depress respiration. It is much less toxic than chloroform, and anaesthetists hold the opinion that respiratory failure precedes failure of circulation.

Tribromethyl alcohol is a basal narcotic, used for the purpose of anaesthesia, and is administered by the rectum. 70 to 90 mg per kg of body-weight is the amount given. Toxic dosage causes death by respiratory paralysis. A number of deaths have been recorded.

Curare injection (combined) with light general narcosis for surgical operative purposes has been in use for some time, and the view that such procedure gives the advantages of a high spinal block with practically none of the disadvantages is held by many. A small dose of curare is recommended since this can be added to subsequently if there is indication. Prostigmine is the physiological antidote for overdosage. The following preparations of curare, among others, are available: intocostrin, curarine chloride, and tubarine. Myanesin has been recommended as a synthetic curare substitute. The use of curare is not without danger and its use should be restricted to those who are fully experienced in the administration of anaesthetics.

Spinal anaesthetics comprise synthetic drugs having a similar composition to cocaine, for example stovaine and novocaine, also nupercaine, a drug allied to quinoline. Of these, nupercaine is regarded as probably the least toxic. Death has resulted from the use of these drugs as spinal anaesthetics. Death from spinal anaesthesia usually occurs as the result of a fall in blood-pressure following vasomotor paralysis, or from diminished respiration due to abdominal or intercostal paralysis rather than medullary ischaemia.

Local anaesthesia is induced by means of nerve blocking or by local infiltration. Cocaine on account of its toxicity is never injected and its use is confined to surgery of the eye, nose, mouth, and throat where it may be applied to the surfaces in a diluted solution. Local anaesthetics are cocaine derivatives such as procaine or novocaine and amethocaine, or quinine derivatives such as quinine and urea hydrochloride or quinine hydrochloride and urethane.

Death under anaesthesia

The expectation of death under an anaesthetic has been estimated at about 1 in 1,000. It is the duty of the authorities who are charged with the investigation of the causes of sudden deaths to make inquiry regarding every death which occurs during the administration of an anaesthetic, or following the administration of an anaesthetic, or under circumstances in which the anaesthetic may be regarded as a contributory cause of death. For the purpose of inquiry the term anaesthetic includes all general, spinal, and local anaesthetics. It is most desirable that the public should be assured from such inquiries that due care has been exercised prior to, and during, the administration of the anaesthetic, and that appropriate measures have been taken to resuscitate the patient. In Scotland, deaths under anaesthesia must be reported to the Procurator-Fiscal, and those in England to the Coroner.   An inquiry in accordance with the rights and duties of his office is held by each official.   With the announcement of the death to the Fiscal in Scotland a report by the patient's doctor is furnished on a form, supplied from the office of the Fiscal, in which are specified the circumstances of the death, including the following details: (1) Full name of patient; (2) Age; (3) Address; (4) When admitted to Hospital or Nursing Home; (5) Nature of disease or ailment; (6) Date of operation and hour of death; (7) When, and by whom, patient was informed that anaesthetic was necessary; (8) What precautions were used in preparing patient for its administration; (9) When, and by whom, patient was examined as to condition of the heart, lungs, and urine, and what was their condition; (10) Anaesthetist, anaesthetic, method of administration; time during which patient was under influence of anaesthetic; (11) What physicians were present at operation; (12) Who was the operator.   This report is sent by the Procurator-Fiscal to a medico-legal examiner, who, from the facts found on inquiry into the circumstances attending the death, and from the post-mortem examination, gives his opinion on the following points in his report: (1) The cause of death; (2) Whether the patient was medically examined before it was decided that an anaesthetic should be administered; (3) Whether all due precautions were observed during the actual administration of the anaesthetic; (4) Whether there were any symptoms about the patient which might and should have been discovered by examination indicating that the administration of an anaesthetic would be attended by special risk to life; and (5) whether prompt and adequate resuscitative measures were employed.

It is difficult, if not, indeed, impossible, to lay down a rule regarding the question of apportionment of responsibility between the surgeon who operates and the anaesthetist who administers the anaesthetic, because there are several conceivable sets of relationships between these persons.   The general position would appear to be that the decision to operate rests with the surgeon, that the control of the operation is in his hands, but that with a skilled anaesthetist, the assessment of the fitness, or otherwise, of the patient to take the anaesthetic must rest with the anaesthetist.   The circumstances of each individual case must determine this issue.

Responsibilities of an anaesthetist

An anaesthetist is only bound to show a reasonable degree of skill and care.   He is not responsible for an error in judgment.   The skilled anaesthetist is an independent expert.   The duties of an anaesthetist include the satisfactory working of the anaesthetic assembly as well as the administration of the anaesthetic, and thus he is responsible for ensuring that the cylinders are in their correct positions and that the gas passing through each flowmeter is actually the one which the flow-meter indicates. With so many and varied anaesthetics used singly and in combination, it is inevitable that the apparatus for their administration has become complicated in design. Special precautions are therefore necessary to avoid the risk of accidents, including explosion arising from defective circuits or static sparks. Burning of a patient by contact with liquid ether or chloroform is yet another hazard to be avoided. The responsibility of the anaesthetist extends to the question of a patient's safety prior to removal from the operating theatre at the conclusion of an operation, and such points as the prevention of partial or complete obstruction to breathing due to vomiting, falling back of the tongue, and dropping of the jaw. Respiratory depression, shock, and collapse are matters for close attention.

Causes of death under anaesthesia

Most anaesthetic deaths fall into one of four groups:
1. Deaths primarily due to the condition of the patient.
2. Deaths incidental to the anaesthetic, such as vomiting.
3. Deaths primarily due to the anaesthetic.
4. Deaths resulting directly or indirectly from defects in the anaesthetic apparatus or errors in the exhibition of drugs.[5]

The principal accidents which occur under general anaesthesia include asphyxia caused by vomiting, failure of respiration, and failure of circulation. Of the many cases which we have investigated, a large percentage of the patients were in a critical condition prior to anaesthesia.

Before it can be established that the anaesthetic was the principal factor in the cause of death, it must be established that the general health of the patient was good before the operation, that the operative shock could not be regarded as the major factor in the death, and that post-mortem examination did not disclose any condition which might have proved a contributory factor. In most cases, the anaesthetic may be regarded merely as a contributory factor.

Primary cardiac failure is most frequently due to the advent of ventricular fibrillation, while primary respiratory failure may be brought about by depression of the respiratory centre, deficient oxygen intake, or obstruction of the airway as a result of a variety of causes.

Cardiac failure may result from overaction of the sympathetic nerves, or vagus nerve, or from primary depression of the cardiac musculature.

Treatment

In primary respiratory failure, having ensured a clear airway, artificial respiration with oxygen administration should be promptly initiated and maintained for a prolonged period. Tongue traction should be undertaken. Hypodermic medication, to stimulate the respiratory centre, may usefully be adopted.

When cardiac failure ensues artificial respiration and direct cardiac massage are the two most important measures to be employed. To be successful, cardiac massage must be undertaken within five minutes of cardiac arrest. When the circulation has ceased for a longer period, anoxaemia of the brain cells is thought to bring about irreversible changes in the central nervous system.

Post-mortem findings

The findings are similar in both respiratory and cardiac failure. In cases of primary respiratory failure, lividity of the exterior of the body and visceral congestion are usually more marked than in cases of primary cardiac arrest.

ANILINE (*Phenylamine*)

Aniline is a colourless oily liquid which is slightly more dense than water and soluble in it to a limited extent (3·4 g/100 ml at 20°C). This material which has a characteristic aromatic odour may develop a brown shade on standing. Dangerous concentrations of vapour may occur in such trade processes as dye manufacturing, dye-using works, leather polish works, rubber works, textile-dyeing works, and in chemical manufacture. Toxic results may follow absorption through the skin, inhalation, or ingestion. Industrial aniline poisoning is notifiable and must be reported to the Home Office.

Symptoms

The symptoms in acute poisoning consist of bluish-ashen coloured cyanosis of the lips, ears, fingers, face, and mucous membranes, headache, giddiness, nausea, vomiting, palpitation, tachycardia, shortness of breath, mental confusion, excitement, delirium, and convulsions. The action of the heart becomes enfeebled and the temperature is subnormal. An odour of aniline may be perceived in the breath and from perspiration and urine. Aniline haemolyses blood cells and methaemoglobin is formed in the blood. The urine becomes dark in colour. Chronic poisoning presents such symptoms as anorexia, headache, digestive disturbances, anaemia, and neurasthenia. The so-called 'aniline' tumours of the bladder have been shown to be produced by β-napthylamine.[7]

Treatment

Free gastric lavage should be employed and cardiac treatment may have to be administered without delay. Use artificial respiration and oxygen inhalations if necessary. In certain cases, benefit may be obtained from the use of intravenous saline or blood transfusions. If severe methaemoglobinemia is present methylene blue should be injected.

Post-mortem findings

The post-mortem signs are not characteristic. The blood is dark and the peculiar colour of post-mortem lividity will attract attention. The heart, liver, and kidneys will show a varying degree of fatty degenerative change.

Analytical findings

Aniline may be found in the tissues and fluids. The concentration of methaemoglobin is used as an indication of the intensity of exposure.

Fatal dose and time of death

The fatal dose is very variable. Death has been reported following ingestion of 1 and 25 g of aniline but recovery has followed 30 and 70 g. If the subject survives for twenty-four hours recovery is usual. Serious disturbances follow exposure to concentrations of 100 to 160 part per million for more than an hour.

Notes. 1. Phenylenediamine and toluenediamine, used as dye intermediates in dyeing hair and furs, are toxic. As a hair dye, a 2 per cent solution, with a 1·5 per cent solution of sodium hydroxide, is applied, followed by an oxidising agent such as a 5 per cent solution of ferric chloride, if a brown shade is desired, or a 3 per cent solution of hydrogen peroxide when a black colour is required. The use of phenylenediamine in dyes may cause local dermatitis and serious toxic manifestations. Israels and Susman[8] point out that an attempt to remove the dye with hydrogen peroxide, or sodium thiosulphate, should never be made, since by the production of aniline the symptoms are intensified. The general symptoms of poisoning are giddiness, weakness, insomnia, epileptiform convulsions, coma, and death. Toluenediamine produces destruction of the red blood cells, methaemoglobin, and toxic jaundice with accompanying degenerative changes. The amino compounds are also absorbed by inhalation, but the toxic effects are less serious than those of the phenyl compounds. The risk of poisoning industrially is present in the manufacture of colours and in the process of dyeing furs.

2. Pyridine when pure is a colourless liquid which is slightly less dense than water and miscible with it in all proportions. When impure it may have the appearance of a yellow oily liquid. It has a characteristic odour which resembles that of the purple-coloured solution sold as 'methylated spirits' of which it is a minor constituent.

When swallowed, pyridine acts as a gastro-intestinal irritant and frequently causes evidences of asphyxia. Cerebral symptoms are common. In fatal cases the cause of death is asphyxia.

If the fumes are inhaled the symptoms chiefly affect the respiratory system. The upper air-passages and lungs become congested, an irritating and persistent cough is a frequent accompaniment, and the eyes become suffused.

ANTIHISTAMINES

The antihistamines include such materials as antazoline, chlorpheniramine, cyclizine, diphenhydramine, meclozine, pheniramine, promethazine, thonzylamine, tripelennamine, and others, usually in the form of the hydrochloride. These substances are used to counteract the action of histamine but many have other actions such as anticholinergic, anti-adrenaline, and anti-serotonin effects. Cases of poisoning, particularly among children and juveniles, have occurred.

Symptoms

The general picture is one of sedation and ranges through drowsiness, muscular weakness, dizziness, incoordination and loss of the ability to concentrate, to deep sleep. There may be coma or convulsions with intervening periods of unconsciousness and death may result from respiratory failure.

Treatment

Gastric lavage should be used and at the conclusion a small amount of sodium bicarbonate solution should be left in the stomach. Paraldehyde should be used to control convulsions as barbiturates are not so effective. Oxygen inhalations and artificial respiration may be required. Respiratory infection may be controlled with antibiotics.

Post-mortem findings

There may be signs of cerebral and kidney damage but in general the findings are non-specific.

Analytical findings

Levels reported for promethazine in poisoning are under 1 mg/100 g of liver and ten times less in the blood.   Fatalities involving drugs in this group have been reported as having only 'trace' quantities of drug present.

Fatal dose

The fatal dose is not known and is variously estimated anywhere between 0·1 g and 10 g but is probably somewhat under 1 g.

Note. The antihistamine phenindamine has stimulant side effects rather than the sedative effects exhibited by the others of this group.

ANTIMONY AND ITS COMPOUNDS

Antimony is used widely as an alloy and its compounds are used in the textile and pottery industries.   Inorganic and organic compounds of antimony are used extensively in the treatment and control of infestations such as bilharziasis.   As with arsenic, antimony is available in many types of compounds and the variation in toxicity is similar.

The principal salt of antimony with which cases of poisoning have been associated is antimony-potassium tartrate, or tartar emetic, which has a diaphoretic and emetic action.   Tartar emetic occurs in the form of a whitish or whitish-yellow powder, which contains 36·5 per cent of antimony.   It is soluble in boiling water, one in three, is about six times less soluble in cold water, and is insoluble in alcohol.

Symptoms

Acute.   The following signs and symptoms are common: An astringent metallic taste in the mouth; a sensation of heat and constriction in the throat; dysphagia, to some extent; gastric pain followed by vomiting of an incessant character and accompanied or succeeded by diarrhoea; faintness and profound prostration: there may, or may not, be intense thirst; the pulse is small, rapid, and weak; the skin is covered with a cold, clammy perspiration; there may be cramps in the abdomen and limbs, which before death may assume almost a tetanic character; partial or complete coma usually precedes death.

Chronic.   The symptoms consist of marked nausea followed by vomiting, and sooner or later the stomach contents show the presence of bile-stained mucus; watery diarrhoea, or diarrhoea alternating with constipation; the pulse gradually becomes weak; there is progressive weakness and loss of weight; the patient develops a loathing for food, since vomiting is sometimes associated even with the sight of it; cachexia accompanied by prostration generally precedes death.

Treatment

The first line of treatment is to empty the stomach with a stomach tube. If vomiting is not frequent, and when the tube is not available, emesis should be induced by simple emetics, and strong tea or tannic acid given to form the insoluble tannate. When the tube is used, warm water alone is sufficient for lavage. Stimulants should be administered in the event of threatened collapse, and the patient should be kept warm. Sedatives should be used when improvement in the pulse and general condition indicate that the patient is out of immediate danger. Careful dieting is necessary for some time following recovery from the immediate effects of poisoning.

Treatment with B.A.L.—dimercaptopropanol—has been recommended. The initial dose by intramuscular injection is $2 \cdot 5$ mg/kg. This should be repeated at four-hourly intervals for a total of four to six injections on each of the first two days. Then two injections should be given daily for a period of ten days, or until complete recovery. Liberal administration of glucose and high protein diet with calcium salts, methionine and B complex vitamins are necessary.[9]

Post-mortem findings

The mucous membranes of the pharynx, larynx, oesophagus, and stomach are congested. The gastric mucosa is frequently covered with tenacious mucus, and scattered, irregular areas of submucous petechial haemorrhages may be seen. These are prevalent on the greater curvature and at the cardiac orifice, although they may be distributed generally. The mucous lining of the duodenum shares the same appearances. The contents of the stomach are usually scanty in amount, dark in appearance, and sometimes blood-stained.

In chronic poisoning the findings may not be well marked. The tongue is usually dirty and the buccal mucous membrane may show aphthous patches. The gastro-intestinal tract will show evidence of irritation, and patches of ulceration may be found either in the stomach or intestines, or in both. There is considerable emaciation of the body.

Fatty degenerative changes involving the liver, kidneys, and myocardium are frequently found.

Analytical findings

Antimony is normally present in the body in small amounts (Appendix III). When tissue levels are being interpreted this should be borne in mind, together with the possibility of medical or industrial exposure.

Fatal dose and time of death

The amount is indefinite, and depends both upon the constitution of the individual and upon the fact that the emetic action of the drug readily induces vomiting.   600 mg have killed a boy of five, and a similar quantity a girl of three.   However, recovery has followed doses of 4, 11 and 25 g.

4 g produced death in an adult in ten hours.   In the boy and girl above mentioned, 600 mg proved fatal in eight and twelve hours, respectively.

Notes.   Untoward results may follow an intravenous injection either as the result of susceptibility or of anaphylaxis.   Asphyxial signs developed in the case of a woman following an intravenous injection of 60 mg in a 6 per cent solution, although recovery took place following an intracardiac injection of adrenalin.   A number of deaths have been recorded after intravenous injection of normal amounts of antimony compounds in the treatment of bilharziasis.

2. The effects of antimony trihydride (stibine) are similar to those of arsine but it is considered to be less toxic.   Production of the antimony trihydride is more difficult and it is, therefore, less hazardous.

ANTIMONY TRICHLORIDE (Butter of Antimony)

Properties and uses

The pure substance is a colourless, crystalline solid which absorbs moisture from the air.   It is very soluble in water acidified with hydrochloric acid.   If the water is not acidified a white precipitate is formed. The commercial material is usually a yellow to red liquid which gives a buttery-looking precipitate with water.   Antimony trichloride has limited use in industry and in veterinary medicine.   It is not normally found in the home.

Symptoms

The symptoms produced are more markedly those of a corrosive than of an irritant.   In the cases recorded, the prominent signs and symptoms were persistent vomiting, severe burning pain in the mouth, throat, oesophagus, and stomach, and general signs of collapse.

Treatment

Treat as for a typical acid corrosive but bear in mind the possibility of antimony poisoning coming to the fore.   A large volume of water would change any of the remaining chloride to the much less soluble and, therefore, much less toxic antimony oxychloride.

Post-mortem findings

Evidence of corrosion of the parts with which the poison has come into contact, with denudation of the mucous membranes, may be found post-mortem.

Analytical findings

The amount of antimony in the stomach may be found and if antimony poisoning as opposed to corrosion enters the picture the concentration in other tissues is of value. See under antimony.

Fatal dose and time of death

The amount which constitutes a fatal dose has not been established with precision. Taylor records a case in which an army surgeon took, suicidally, from 60 to 90 ml and died. A boy of ten years, however, has recovered after taking about 15 ml.

ARSENIC AND ITS COMPOUNDS

Arsenic and its compounds have many uses in industry such as dyeing, glass making, the manufacture of sheep dips and agricultural sprays. Also there is some use in medicine for the treatment of skin disease and as an antisyphilitic drug. Tonics containing arsenic are still available. The following Table gives a brief list of the types of compounds.

Table 1. Examples of Compounds of Arsenic

Class	Example
Element	Arsenic (As_4)
Arsenious compounds .	. Arsenious oxide (As_2O_3)
Arsenic compounds .	. Arsenic pentoxide (As_2O_5)
Arsenites . . .	. Sodium arsenite ($NaAsO_2$)
Arsenates . . .	. Sodium hydrogen arsenate (Na_2HAsO_4)
Organic compounds .	. Sodium cacodylate ($C_2H_6O_2AsNa,3H_2O$)
	Arsphenamine ($C_{12}H_{12}O_2N_2As_2,2HCl,2H_2O$)

All arsenic compounds are toxic but not to the same extent. Trivalent compounds are more toxic than pentavalent ones and these in turn are more toxic than the organic arsenicals. Superimposed on this picture is the fact that the low-solubility compounds are less toxic than the more easily soluble compounds.

Arsenic trioxide, arsenious oxide or white arsenic is the substance most commonly employed in homicidal arsenical poisoning. As met with in commerce, it is either in the form of cakes, broken lumps, or a white, gritty powder. It is not very soluble in cold water, which will only dissolve 1 g per 100 ml at 2°C. When, however, it is mixed with boiling water and is boiled for some time, about 11·5 g per 100 ml will be held in solution so long as the water remains hot, but when the water cools again the excess comes out of solution to form a deposit in the vessel. By reason of this insolubility, when the fine powder is placed in water or other liquid, some of it forms a whitish film on the surface of the fluid, and the heavier particles fall to the bottom of the vessel. Experiments have shown that 6 g of arsenious acid mixed with two teaspoonfuls of cocoa, milk, and boiling water in a teacup, could not be detected either by appearance, taste, or smell, but that on stand-ing, the milk curdled and the arsenic sedimented. With arrowroot and gruel similar results were observed.

Organic compounds of arsenic are less poisonous than the inorganic ones. Cacodylic acid, although containing 54·3 per cent of arsenic, is relatively non-toxic, as are also its salts or cacodylates.

There are numerous organic arsenical preparations available for therapeutic treatment, which consist of arsenic either in trivalent or pentavalent compounds. As the result of exhibition of these drugs, there is a liability to occurrence of jaundice, especially in sensitive subjects. The jaundice is rarely severe, but acute yellow atrophy of the liver may occur and cause death. Arsenic is to some extent stored in body tissues from where it is gradually excreted without toxic symptoms.

Symptoms

Acute. The intensity of the symptoms is regulated to some extent by the physical form in which the arsenic is taken, whether in solid form, in suspension, or in solution, and by the quantity ingested. When the amount taken is a large one it is suggestive of suicide or accident rather than homicide. The onset of symptoms is also regulated by these and other factors, including whether or not a meal has been recently taken. Usually, however, the symptoms appear within about an hour, although in some cases, where even large doses have been given, they may be late in appearance. In one case, 2 g of powdered arsenious acid was taken when the stomach was empty and symptoms did not appear until after two hours. In a second case, where the quantity was similar, the symptoms did not develop for seven hours, while in a third case, ten hours intervened before symptoms appeared. When the poison is introduced into the rectum or vagina, days may elapse before the symp-toms manifest themselves.

The symptoms of poisoning are often initiated by nausea, faintness, and a burning pain in the stomach and epigastrium, which is increased by pressure. These are followed by retching and vomiting, which become severe, continuous, and persistent. The vomited material varies in appearance during the course of a case. At first, it consists of stomach contents, but later becomes blackish or greenish in colour, due to the presence of bile, and latterly consists of mucus mixed with altered blood in varying quantity. Insistent and painful diarrhoea, accompanied by tenesmus, is common, the stools being streaked or tinged with blood. The patient may complain of a sense of oppression, coldness, and collapse. There is usually an intense thirst, the gratification of which, however, only increases the vomiting. Painful cramps may be present in the muscles of the lower limbs. The pulse becomes small, rapid, feeble, irregular, and almost imperceptible, the face appears anxious and pinched, the skin becomes cold and clammy, and death is usually preceded by restlessness, convulsions, or coma, although it may supervene suddenly from cardiac failure. When successive sublethal doses of arsenic have been taken, the clinical picture of the patient may be one of subacute or chronic poisoning.

In subacute poisoning the symptoms are less intense and many may be absent.

Chronic. When small repeated toxic doses of arsenic have been taken over a period, or when several sublethal doses, with short intervals between them, have been given, symptoms of chronic poisoning are likely to appear. Such doses are highly suggestive of homicidal administration. The general symptoms are remarkably constant in their character. Probably one of the earliest signs is gradual loss of weight due to malnutrition, and accompanying this there may be falling out of the hair and pigmentation of the skin. The eyes are suffused and watery, the conjunctivae being congested, and there are symptoms of coryza. The tongue is either reddened or is covered with a thick white coating. Eczematous eruptions may be present on the body, usually accompanied by increased pigmentation of the skin which may assume the form of dark brown or blackish patches, thought to be due to a melanin derivative, or the skin may assume an earthy or jaundiced appearance. The patient will probably complain of general malaise, nausea, disinclination for food, and diarrhoea or diarrhoea alternating with constipation. There may be intermittent vomiting. There is frequent complaint of numbness of the hands and feet, and the patient may walk with an unsteady and uncertain gait, if able to walk at all. These symptoms are due to peripheral neuritis. The palmar surfaces of the hands and the plantar surfaces of the feet are frequently the sites of hyperkeratosis. There may also be mental hebetude, or delusions. Though this appears to be a formidable and unmistakable list of symptoms they are not all present at one time, arsenic poisoning is easily mistaken for a whole series of ailments. Usually it is not until after many treatments that arsenic is suspected, if indeed it ever is.

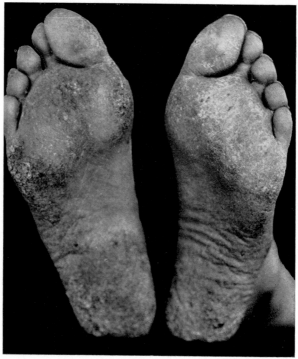

FIG. 223

Chronic arsenical poisoning showing hyperkeratosis

The phenomenon of improvement in hospital, deterioration at home, is a significant indicator.

Treatment

The stomach should be emptied without delay, either by the use of an emetic or preferably by a stomach tube. Gastric lavage must be thorough. Treat other symptoms such as dehydration, anuria or liver damage as they arise. Dimercaprol is used as a chelating agent for the removal of arsenic. The maximum recommended treatment is 4 mg/kg every 4 hours for 48 hours and then every 12 hours for a total of 10 days.

Post-mortem findings

The character of these appearances depends very largely upon the quantity taken and the period which has elapsed before death. The stomach is primarily the seat of post-mortem appearances, although the poison may have entered the body by means other than the mouth. When the poison has been swallowed the mucous membrane will show a varying degree of inflammation, with injection of the vessels, which is patchy in distribution and corresponds to the deposits of arsenic, round which the inflammatory changes centre. Arsenious oxide is converted into the yellow sulphide in the stomach and particles may be observed either with or without the aid of a magnifying glass. When seen, certain of the particles should be collected for subsequent chemical examination. The surface of the membrane may be thinly coated with mucus and streaked with blood. Submucous petechial haemorrhages are very often seen. The contents of the stomach are frequently of a darkish-brown colour. The cardiac and pyloric ends of the stomach are often congested. Congestion of the wall of the intestinal tract is frequently found, and the tract as a whole may contain a considerable quantity of dark fluid. Congestion of the vessels of the lining membrane of the pharynx and larynx is also common. Sub-endocardial ventricular haemorrhages are not infrequent. The liver is very often enlarged and pale in colour, due to fatty degenerative changes. The kidneys and myocardium are similarly affected in many cases.

The above appearances persist for variable intervals after death, and arsenic may be recovered from the stomach after relatively long periods, despite vomiting, due to its tenacious association with the gastric mucosa.

While the foregoing may be taken as descriptive of the appearances in the average fatal case when the poison has been ingested, their incidence is but little changed no matter by what other channel the arsenic enters the body. They are found, for example, in cases of respiratory poisoning by arsenic trihydride, and even when the arsenic has been introduced by the vagina.

The preservative influence of arsenic upon the tissues of those poisoned by this substances has been repeatedly observed and noted following exhumation, despite assertions to the contrary.

Analytical findings

Arsenic, quickly absorbed, is stored in the liver, and from there passes into the general circulation. It is slowly excreted by the urine, faeces, and sweat. Although the intestinal tract eliminates some of the arsenic from the body, the kidneys are the principal excretory organs. After a single dose, arsenic may be found in the urine in less than an hour and may continue to be present in small amounts for about ten to fourteen days or even longer. After a series of doses, excretion of arsenic may persist for about one month. Absorbed arsenic is found in greatest quantity in the liver, and in the course of a few days produces fatty changes. In two to three weeks following recovery from a single dose, all traces of the poison may have left the body with the exception of the hair, nails, skin, and bones. Arsenic will not be found in the hair above the skin level until a few days after ingestion though it is measurable in the roots after as little as thirty minutes. The amount of the poison found in different parts of the intestinal tract is highly important in fatal cases in relation to the interval of time which has elapsed between ingestion and death. When it is present in the upper part of the small intestine, the interval would be about three to six hours approximately. About ten hours would be necessary for it to reach the lower part of the small intestine and about twelve hours to reach the caecum. It must not be forgotten that arsenic, by its irritant action, hastens peristalsis.

The hair and nails irreversibly fix arsenic from the blood stream. Since these keratin tissues are slow in growth, the portions that are formed during the time the arsenic is being excreted will retain arsenic. Hair grows at the rate of about 13 mm a month and it has been stated that the weekly growth is from 1 to 3 mm. The rate of growth of the nails is about 3 mm a month. Thus the trapping of arsenic in these keratin structures enables the analysis of successive short lengths of hair, from the base to the tip, and of portions of the nails, from the base to the tip, to give an approximate indication of arsenic dosage or the intermittent periods of such administration. It is necessary to ensure that these structures have not been contaminated by arsenical fluids from the body from which they have been removed or, when exhumation has taken place, by contamination of the soil. Both hair and nails should be cleaned prior to analysis.

Hair when soaked in an arsenical solution is capable of absorbing arsenic, but such absorption will show a more or less even distribution as opposed to natural excretion into growing hair, when, if the administration has been intermittent, the deposit of arsenic will be irregular in distribution. Experiments have shown that arsenic which has been excreted into the hair cannot be removed by prolonged steeping in normal cleaning fluids.

Arsenic is always present in human tissues. It is a normal environmental contaminant and from this source small amounts enter the body. In order, therefore, to establish that death resulted from arsenical poisoning, the history of the symptomatology prior to death must receive careful consideration, and there must be a sensible amount of arsenic isolated.

The average amounts of arsenic normally present in human tissues are given in appendix III. When these values are exceeded by four to six times a source of abnormal exposure should be suspected. The resultant interpretation must take into account such factors as industrial exposure, unusual soil concentrations, and other sources, including therapeutic administration.

Fatal dose and time of death

The smallest recorded fatal dose is 125 mg. Recovery has, however, occurred after large doses. A woman, intent on suicide, took about 14 g of arsenious acid, was violently ill three hours later with vomiting, and seven hours after swallowing the poison, with watery diarrhoea. Despite these symptoms, her general condition remained fairly good. On the third day she developed haematemesis and melaena, but on the fourth day improvement commenced, and her recovery was complete within a fortnight.

Death has occurred in individual cases at the end of twenty minutes and ten hours, respectively, but the fatal period is very variable and may range from several hours to several days. In one case, for example, when 13 g were swallowed, death did not ensue until the seventh day. Twelve to thirty-six hours, however, may be taken as an average period.

Illustrative case

The post-mortem examination showed that the mucous membrane of the pharynx, epiglottis, and larynx were congested and the vessels injected. Both chambers of the right side of the heart were considerably dilated. The left auricle was also dilated. A number of small sub-endocardial haemorrhages were present in the left ventricle over an area situated immediately below the posterior cusp of the mitral valve. The liver was pale in colour and enlarged. The stomach contained about 1 pint of darkish, yellowish-brown fluid. There were numerous patchy groups of petechial haemorrhages in the submucosa. These were most marked nearer the pyloric end of the stomach. The intestinal tract, as a whole, was more or less filled with darkish-brown fluid. The lining of the small intestine showed slight, generalised congestion. That of the large intestine showed more marked congestion which was patchy in distribution although generalised in extent. Microscopical examination of the liver and kidney tissue showed the presence of fatty degenerative changes.

A number of tissues were analysed and the results are shown in Table 2.

The stomach and intestinal contents were equivalent to approximately 700 mg of arsenious oxide.

Forty-seven days after death the body was exhumed and the following specimens were submitted for analysis: Earth adjacent to the coffin, portions of the shroud and coffin lining, head hair, portions of the left femur, muscle and skin overlying the left femur, skin from the soles of the feet, and the nails from the hands and feet. No abnormal amounts of arsenic were found in any of the burial material. The arsenic levels found in the other tissues are given in Table 3.

The large amounts of arsenic present in the entirely fluid contents of

Table 2.   Case of Arsenic Poisoning

Wet tissue	Arsenic (µg/g)
Brain	0·7
Stomach	19·0
Stomach contents . .	654·0
Intestine	41·0
Intestine contents . .	369·0
Liver	61·0
Spleen	4·4
Kidney	21·0
Pancreas	0·9
Heart	1·5
Adrenals	7·3
Lungs	2·4
Urine	11·0
Bile	4·3

Table 3   Arsenic in other tissues

Material	Arsenic (µg/g)
Hair (scalp end to 25 mm.)	7·6
,, (remaining 65 mm.)	2·9
Femur (marrow)	0·6
,, (bone)	0·9
Thigh (muscle)	2·5
,, (skin)	2·1
Foot (epidermis)	4·1
,, (dermis)	4·1
Finger-nail (root end)	43·0
,, (tip end)	35·0
Toe-nail (root end)	48·0
,, (tip end)	35·0

the stomach was consistent with a lethal dose of arsenic having been ingested shortly before death, certainly within a day.

The presence of arsenic in the proximal and distal portions of nails and proximal and distal portions of hair was consistent with it having been taken throughout the minimum period of six months before death. The relative amounts of arsenic present in the various portions of nails and hair were consistent with larger amounts having been taken towards the end of life.

Note. *Non-fatal poisoning.* The materials available for examination are limited to those exterior to the body. These are exposed to the environment and may be heavily contaminated. Workers in the manufacture of glass and tin smelters who were investigated showed hair and nail levels as high as hundreds of parts per million. Details of the interpretation of arsenic in hair are given in a publication by Smith.[10]

ARSENIC TRIHYDRIDE (*Arsine*)

This is a colourless, inflammable gas with a garlic-like odour. It burns in air with a blue-white flame. The gas is formed when metals react with acids or alkalis in the presence of arsenic impurities or by the action of water on calcium, magnesium, or sodium arsenide, or by the action of dilute acid on other metallic arsenides.

Poisoning by this gas has arisen in a variety of industrial and scientific pursuits.

Arsine exerts its poisonous action after absorption into the blood stream through the lungs.

When arsine is absorbed into the blood stream, gradual and progressive haemolysis of the red cells follows, with liberation of haemoglobin and methaemoglobin. The conversion of these substances by the liver into bile pigments, excessive in amount, produces jaundice. Haemoglobin and methaemoglobin are also excreted by the kidneys with resultant tubular degeneration of the kidneys. The continued haemolysis of the corpuscles leads to progressive anaemia.

Symptoms

Malaise, shivering, headache, and great weakness, giddiness, faintness, pains in the head, epigastrium, and loins, sense of oppression in breathing, with, perhaps, some cyanosis, nausea, sickness, and vomiting. These manifestations are followed by continuous vomiting, with bile or blood in the vomit, jaundice, with enlargement of the liver, varying in tint from golden-yellow to mahogany, thirst and dryness of the throat, haemorrhages from one or more parts of the body, and haemoglobinuria or haematuria, oliguria, or complete anuria. The urine varies in colour from red to reddish-brown depending on the amount of unaltered haemoglobin, methaemoglobin, or bile pigments. It contains albumin and casts. The patient who is on occasion delirious gradually becomes comatose, and there is progressive deterioration of the pulse until death.

Treatment

Blood transfusion, about 500 ml on each occasion, is most beneficial, but should be given slowly. Diuresis must be encouraged by the administration of fluids by the mouth or rectum to avoid blockage of the renal tubules by cellular debris. A close estimate of the intake and output of fluid must be made to exclude the possibility of oedema. Glucose, with or without insulin, should be used, and this line of treatment is of special importance when there is necrosis of the liver. Oxygen inhalations are necessary in the condition of excessive anaemia. Other treatment must follow lines indicated by individual cases. Dimercaprol is used to remove arsenic. The treatment is described under arsenic.

Post-mortem findings

Jaundice is usually present. The lungs are congested. In the pericardium and pleurae, reddish or reddish-brown coloured serum may be found. The myocardium very frequently shows fatty degenerative changes, and subendocardial haemorrhages may be present. The liver is enlarged, and the gall-bladder distended with bile. The colour of the liver is often abnormal, ranging from yellow to deep indigo. The kidneys are also changed in colour, from dark red to indigo, and are enlarged. The spleen also is very frequently enlarged and altered in colour. In the stomach there are congestion of the mucous membrane, submucous petechial haemorrhages, and, occasionally, patches of erosion, in which changes the intestines often share. Fatty degenerative changes are also found in the liver and kidneys. The urine contains haemoglobin, methaemoglobin, red blood cells, casts, bile pigments, and albumin. Microscopical examination of the blood shows a considerable reduction in the number of red cells, an alteration in the shape and colour of the red cells, and the presence of 'shadow cells'. The blood-spectrum is frequently that of methaemoglobin.

Analytical findings

The arsenic levels of any tissue may be found and interpreted against the usual levels given in Appendix III.

Fatal dose and time of death

Exposure to a concentration of over 30 p.p.m. for an hour or more is dangerous. The fatal period is in the region of five to seven days.

ATROPINE

The following notes apply equally to atropine, hyocyamine, hyoscine, and synthetic substitutes, e.g. benzhexal, caramiphen, dicyclomine, homatropine, probanthine. Poisoning is almost exclusively accidental and is due either to excessive amounts of medicines or to ingestion of toxic plant materials. It is believed that hyoscine (scopolamine) was the poison used in the Crippen case.

Symptoms

These are giddiness, drowsiness, mental confusion, great thirst, due to parching of the mouth and throat, the result of diminished secretion, indistinct articulation and difficulty in swallowing. In the earlier stages, the patient is talkative, chattering, active and in a state of delirium which is often turbulent or violent. The face is flushed, the pupils are widely dilated and immobile, and the temperature is elevated. In cases which end fatally, the drowsiness lapses into deep sleep, then coma, during which the face usually assumes a livid colour. Finally, there are convulsions, and death.

Treatment

Delay absorption with milk or activated charcoal and then remove by gastric lavage or emesis. Excitement may be controlled by the use of sedatives or mild hypnotics. Artificial respiration, or the use of oxygen, may become necessary. Treat other symptoms as they arise.

When the berries of *Atropa belladonna* have been eaten and have remained for some time in the stomach, they tend to resemble raisins, with which they should not be confused, since the seeds of the former are smaller and darker than raisin seeds. In such cases it is expedient to use an emetic rather than a stomach-tube since the berries may readily block the tube.

Post-mortem findings

In the case of children, the stomach contents should be carefully examined for portions of berries or seeds. The post-mortem signs are generally those of comato-asphyxia, and oedema of the lungs may be present.

Analytical findings

Atropine and related drugs may be found in the urine after ingestion of the drug or vegetable material containing it.

G M J—NN

Fatal dose and time of death

The fatal dose of atropine is about 10 mg for children and 125 mg for adults. A number of adults have recovered following doses of 230, 250 and 330 mg of atropine. Doses of 125 mg hyoscyamine and 30 mg of hyoscine have caused death. About 30 berries of *Atropa belladonna* (deadly nightshade) cause serious poisoning in children.

There may be some delay in the onset of symptoms after ingestion of atropine-containing materials, thereafter death occurs within a day.

BARBITURATES

Generally these are white crystalline solids which are slightly soluble in water as the free acid but easily soluble in the form of the sodium salts. A list of barbiturates with common names is given in Appendix IV. These drugs may be roughly divided into three groups depending on the rate of action of the drugs. The first is the slow-acting group of which phenobarbitone is almost the only one used. The second is the intermediate acting group of which pentobarbitone, butobarbitone, amylobarbitone, and quinalbarbitone are the commonly encountered examples. This group is often subdivided to give slow- and fast-acting subgroups. The third group is the fast-acting group of which thiopentone is an example. These drugs are used widely as sedatives, hypnotics for pre-anaesthetic medication, and for the treatment of psychiatric conditions. They have a depressant effect upon the central nervous system and affect the cardiac and respiratory centres. Respiration becomes shallow and rapid or slow and laboured. When narcosis is of long duration, pulmonary oedema or broncho-pneumonia is prone to develop. In some cases there is idiosyncrasy, and in all cases, if the administration is continued, the risk of addiction is ever present. In cases of fatal poisoning, death is usually caused by respiratory failure. Barbiturates are contra-indicated when there is impairment of the liver or kidneys, since excretion is normally slow and these drugs are cumulative.

Barbiturates cause many more deaths by suicide or accident than any other drug or poison and the frequency increases each year.

Symptoms

The following signs and symptoms are indicative of poisoning: Giddiness, indistinct articulation, occasional nausea, diplopia, stupor, coma, shallow and rapid or slow and laboured respiration, slowing of the pulse-rate, and subnormal temperature. The reaction of the pupils varies. As poisoning advances, the face tends to become progressively cyanotic. Oliguria may be present. Bullous changes may affect the skin over the distal parts of the legs. Coma usually continues for one or two days, but the period of survival may be much shorter. When oedema of the lungs, or broncho-pneumonia, complicates the condition, death may result from cardiac failure.

Treatment

The stomach should be washed out thoroughly by means of the stomach tube. In a few cases in which blood barbiturate levels were monitored frequently during treatment it was found that the levels continued to rise for up to one day. At post-mortem examination in other cases where treatment had been attempted for a significant time large masses of barbiturate were recovered from the stomach. The airway must be kept clear, by aspiration if necessary, and oxygen should be administered continuously. Artificial respiration should be employed when there is indication. The patient should be kept warm and roused and not submitted to muscular exertion. Penicillin or other antibiotics may be given in cases in which respiratory function is depressed or in which coma has supervened. If the coma is prolonged, intravenous fluids should be given until improvement becomes manifest. The bladder will require catheterisation.

As an adjunct to this conservative treatment bemegride and other materials have been used. There is considerable opposition to these now on the grounds that they are not likely to be effective when severe respiratory depression is present. It is probable that the initial stimulation of the medullary centres may be followed by greater depression. The following procedure may be adopted in the administration of bemegride and amiphenazole if their use is decided on. Firstly, a 5 per cent glucose intravenous infusion is set up. Every five minutes, 1 ml of a 1·5 per cent solution of amphenazole in saline should be added to the drip. This should be followed immediately by 10 ml of a 0·5 per cent solution of bemegride in saline. These injections are continued until the pharyngeal and laryngeal reflexes return and the patient reaches a state of light anaesthesia from which spontaneous recovery should take place in about eight hours.[11, 12, 13]

Clemmesen[14] describes seventy cases of barbituric-acid poisoning, which included seven with respiratory paralysis. In each of these seven cases brief treatment with megimide and amiphenazole restored respiration.

Forced diuresis and alkalinisation of the urine have recently been used to treat successfully severe cases of barbiturate intoxication. Urea was used as the diuretic and sodium lactate as the alkalinising agent. This treatment resulted in a considerable increase in the elimination rate of barbiturate.[15]

Post-mortem findings

The post-mortem signs are not in any way characteristic. The general picture is that of comato-asphyxia. There may be evidence of commencing, or established, broncho-pneumonia, or of oedema of the lungs.

Analytical findings

Barbiturates may be measured and identified in any of the tissues. Commonly blood only is submitted for analysis and is all that is necessary in most investigations. However, in a small number of cases little or no barbiturates are discovered in the blood when massive amounts have been found in the stomach. Investigation of liver barbiturate levels in these cases resulted in the finding of barbiturate, but in levels under 1 mg/100 g. Table 4 gives a summary of some levels of barbiturates found in a survey of fatal poisonings.[16]   See also the note on barbiturates and alcohol.

Table 4.   Barbiturate Levels in Fatal Poisonings

Tissue	Intermediate-acting group		Phenobarbitone	
	Range	Average	Range	Average
Blood (mg/100 ml) .	0·7– 9·6	3·3	3·3–9·3	6·5
Brain (mg/100 g) .	1·1– 7·9	3·5	—	—
Liver (mg/100 g) .	1·5–33·0	9·6	—	—

Fatal dose and time of death

The minimum dose of the intermediate barbiturates is not known for certain but is probably somewhat over 1 g, and for the long-acting barbiturates the value is probably about twice this. Recovery has followed doses in the order of ten times these amounts of phenobarbitone and butobarbitone. Death may not occur for some time and is then due to pulmonary complications.

Note.   1. Barbiturates and alcohol are a lethal combination and account for over 50 per cent of the cases investigated. The taking of barbiturates with alcohol to get the enhanced effect is not widespread but common enough to cause concern and a significant number of genuine accidents do occur. In a typical case, an adult male in a public house was discussing the advantages of whisky and barbiturates (pentobarbitone). He elected to demonstrate this by ingesting a 'handful' of capsules which he 'washed down' with a 'reasonable' amount of whisky. Within a 'few minutes' he became intensely cyanosed and was found to be dead on admission to hospital. The blood alcohol was 126 mg/100 ml and the pentobarbitone was 9·6 mg/ 100 ml. In another case, an adult female was out for an evening during the course of which she took an unknown quantity of pentobarbitone and alcohol. She died within four hours and post-mortem analyses gave values of 160 mg alcohol/100 ml of blood and 1·9 mg pentobarbitone /100 ml of blood.

Table 5 gives a brief summary of the levels of barbiturate found, when alcohol was present, in a survey of fatal poisonings.[16] The values are significantly lower than those found when no alcohol was present.

Table 5. Blood Barbiturate Levels in Fatal Poisonings when Alcohol was also Present

Barbiturate	Range (mg/100 ml)	Mean (mg/100 ml)
Intermediate	0·4–6·9	2·0
Phenobarbitone	0·9–5·1	2·6

Note. 2. Primidone is metabolised to phenobarbitone in the body and as a result this source should be considered when phenobarbitone is found. To produce equivalent blood phenobarbitone levels five times as much primidone as phenobarbitone is required. In a typical primidone poisoning case in which about 30 g was ingested thirty-two hours before death, the following values were found: 6·7 mg phenobarbitone /100 ml of urine, 9·3 mg phenobarbitone/100 ml of blood, 7·5 mg phenobarbitone/100 g of brain and 27·5 mg phenobarbitone/100 g of liver. These values are typical of those found in phenobarbitone poisoning.

BARIUM AND ITS COMPOUNDS

Barium and its salts have wide specialised uses in industry. The sulphate is common in medicine as a radio-opaque material for x-ray diagnosis. Due to its very low solubility, barium sulphate is non-toxic. In the home, barium sulphide may be found as a depilatory preparation and the chloride or carbonate may be present in some pesticides. The soluble salts of barium are toxic and the metal is dangerous due to its property of reacting with any water with which it comes in contact. This causes extensive tissue damage aggravated by the caustic hydroxide formed in the reaction.

Symptoms

Nausea and vomiting of a watery mucus; convulsive movements of hands and feet; general convulsions. To these symptoms must be added diarrhoea with tenesmus, grave signs of shock, loss of motor power and sensation. The heart is embarrassed in its action, and the breathing laboured and slow.

Treatment

Wash out the stomach with a solution of magnesium sulphate (6 g /l). Give 30 g dose of sodium sulphate, well diluted, and repeat if necessary. Treat general condition along usual lines. Cardiac or respiratory stimulants may be necessary.

Post-mortem findings

Inflammation of the stomach and intestines. The kidneys may show necrosis and there may be some liver damage.

Analytical findings

A list of normal barium levels is given in Appendix III.

Fatal dose and time of death

The fatal dose is variable but is probably in the region of 1 g of an absorbable salt, though recovery, after treatment, followed ingestion of 6 g of the chloride. The time of death varies from a few hours to days.

Illustrative cases

Morton[17] describes severe poisoning of eighty-five British soldiers in Persia by barium carbonate, intended for use as rat poison, which was accidentally mixed with flour and made into pastry. Sauer[18] records the case of a woman who was given about 7 g of barium chloride in error. Recovery followed treatment. When seen three hours after taking the dose she was collapsed and her pulse, which was thready, was 120 per minute. Four teaspoonfuls of crystalline magnesium sulphate were given in water followed by a hypodermic injection of 0·6 mg of atropine sulphate and 15 mg of morphine sulphate. The pain was relieved almost at once, and on the following day the patient felt perfectly well.

BENZENE, TOLUENE, XYLENE

These materials are the simplest of the aromatic hydrocarbons. They are all colourless liquids at room temperature with pleasant odours. All these substances are used widely in industry as solvents and, as a result, are easily available. They may cause poisoning by ingestion or inhalation. Industrial benzene poisoning is notifiable and must be reported to the Home Office.

Symptoms

When benzene is taken by mouth, there is gastro-intestinal irritation with vomiting. Cerebral symptoms quickly supervene.

Acute poisoning follows the inhalation of a large quantity of the vapour, and the symptoms are giddiness, nausea, vomiting, muscular prostration, dyspnoea, delirium, convulsions, coma, and death, due to severe haemorrhage or toxaemia.

Chronic poisoning is characterised by general malaise, headaches, giddiness, impairment of vision, nervousness, gastro-intestinal disturbances, anaemia, loss of weight, insomnia, loss of memory, and neuritis. The blood picture shows a leucopenia and poikilocytosis of red cells. Benzene is a bone-marrow poison.

Treatment

Poisoning by inhalation is treated by the use of oxygen together with intravenous saline and dextrose. Symptoms are treated generally. If the material is ingested, gastric lavage is recommended. Blood transfusion may be necessary.

Post-mortem findings

Acute poisoning is indicated by purpuric spots on the mucosa of the nose, mouth, and throat, and sometimes on the uterus. The blood may not be coagulated and there may be general congestion of the organs. Chronic poisoning may result in degenerative changes of the heart and liver and the bone marrow may be damaged.

Analytical findings

The hydrocarbon may be found in the tissues and organs. Fatty tissues may tend to store rather more than other tissues. Patty[19] quotes a value of 0·2 mg benzene/100 ml of blood when the subject is exposed to air containing 100 p.p.m. and proportionally greater with respect to the air concentration. Exposure to benzene is often assessed by the urinary sulphate ratio, i.e. inorganic sulphate to total sulphate. With no exposure the value is 86 per cent. An eight-hour exposure to a concentration of 200 p.p.m. gives a value of 38 per cent. Phenol excretion in urine has also been used as a measure of exposure. Hippuric acid in urine has been used as a measure of toluene exposure.

Fatal dose and time of death

A volume of 15 to 20 ml of benzene will cause serious, if not fatal, illness. The maximum allowable concentration in air is about 200 p.p.m. for toluene and xylene and nearly an order of magnitude less for benzene. Exposure to about 20,000 p.p.m. of benzene is almost immediately fatal, to about 2,000 p.p.m. for an hour produces marked depression. Death may occur rapidly or at any period up to about three days.

Note. The aromatic hydrocarbons are extensively discussed in a monograph by H. W. Gerarde[20]

BERYLLIUM

Beryllium is used in the preparation of many alloys. Its compounds are met with in the form of ores and as chemicals used for the coating of discharge tubes. Exposure may occur during the handling of the ores or the purified materials or during the handling of the metal itself, e.g. in turning or machining; Browning[21] and Tepper and others[22] describe such exposures and the subsequent treatment and implications.

Symptoms

The toxic reactions include dermatitis, chronic skin ulcers, and inflammatory changes in the respiratory system. Severe exposure may result in a chemical pneumonitis typically shown by dyspnoea, substernal pain, cyanosis, and cough with blood-stained sputum. X-ray examination of the lungs some two or three weeks after the onset of symptoms showed diffuse haziness of both lungs, soft, irregular intervals of infiltration with perbronchial markings, and the appearance of large or conglomerate nodules in the lung fields. The lung fields cleared after one to four months.

Treatment

Remove from exposure and treat symptoms as they arise. Cortisone has been used to control symptoms but they may recur when the treatment ends.

Post-mortem findings

The usual finding is atypical pneumonitis. There may also be some liver damage.

Analytical findings

Beryllium may be demonstrated in the tissues in greater than normal concentrations. A list of normal levels is given in the appendix. Beryllium is said to be stored in tissue for a considerable period. Post-mortem levels after chronic poisoning were found to be in the region of 7 to 10 p.p.m. in liver and lungs. Very high values (2,000 p.p.m.) have been quoted for the lungs in acute poisoning.

Fatal dose

Acute toxic reactions may occur at 25 μg/m^3 of air and it is suggested that this is the highest level allowable for short exposure. If exposure is repeated, a maximum value of 2 μg/m^3 is recommended. A monthly average concentration of not greater than 0·01 μg/m^3 has been proposed.

BISMUTH AND ITS COMPOUNDS

Bismuth and its compounds are used in metallurgy and the pharmaceutical industry. Injected bismuth salts are used for the treatment of syphilis and yaws. Orally administered bismuth salts are used to relieve the symptoms of gastric and duodenal ulcers and dyspepsia. Some preparations are used as radio-opaque materials for x-ray diagnosis. Poisoning is caused by the soluble salts and is mainly the result of injection.

Symptoms

The toxic effects include stomatitis, colitis, and nephritis. Bismuth compounds are contra-indicated in cardiac disease, since bismuth is liable to induce weakness and irregularity of the action of the heart. In chronic cases a 'bismuth line' may appear in the gums.

Treatment

Sodium thiosulphate, 0·5 g in a 10 per cent solution given intravenously. Gastric lavage. Symptomatic and general treatment should be employed.

Intramuscular injections of B.A.L. have been recommended. A dose of 2·5 mg/kg should be given initially and thereafter repeated at four-hourly intervals up to a total of four to six injections on each of the first two days.   The treatment should then be reduced to two daily injections for about three weeks or until recovery.[9]

Post-mortem findings

Added to the above symptoms liver damage may be found and the blood may contain methaemoglobin.

Analytical findings

A list of normal values is given in Appendix III.

Illustrative cases

Roe[23] reports the case of a child one month old who, suffering from diarrhoea, had become dehydrated.   600 mg of bismuth subnitrate were given every two hours, and death occurred two days later.   Methaemoglobin was found in the blood, and there were small haemorrhage in the cortex of the brain.   Dowds[24] describes three deaths due to subcutaneous injections of sodium bismuth tartrate.   In two of these there was intense stomatitis, and the urine was loaded with albumin and contained bismuth.

BORON COMPOUNDS

Compounds of boron have wide but fairly specialised uses in industry. The commonest compounds are boric acids and the salts formed with them.   Orthoboric acid (boracic acid) and sodium tetraborate (borax) are commonly present in medicine chests as the pure compounds for use in solution as mild antiseptics or in mixtures, as for example talc with borax.   Although these compounds appear harmless they are responsible for a large number of accidental poisonings, many fatal.

Goldbloom and Goldbloom[25] have traced 105 cases of boric acid poisoning in adults and children.   Thirty-eight of these were under one year and showed a mortality of 70 per cent.   Valdes-Dapena and Arey[26] report 172 cases of poisoning, 83 of which were fatal.

Symptoms

Borates act as depressants on the central nervous system.   Other symptoms include malaise, nausea, hiccough, vomiting, diarrhoea, an erythematous skin eruption, fall of temperature, convulsions, coma, and collapse.   The erythematous rash may be accompanied by papules, vesicles developing between the fingers and on the backs of the hands. In one of our cases, in which 300 mg doses were administered internally for a chronic bladder condition, the patient developed symptoms of weakness out of all proportion to the ailment, and a papular rash over certain parts of the body. Nephritis occasionally develops and there may be a few submucosal haemorrhages. Sanders recounts the facts of his personal experiences of toxic effects of boric acid. Suffering from dysentery, a solution of the acid in warm water was used as a rectal douche daily for some time. He developed a rash, resembling bromide rash, over the entire body, became delirious, had a feeble pulse, and was unable to sleep. After a fortnight, during which his condition was serious, he commenced to recover.

Treatment

Empty the stomach with a stomach tube, or by means of an emetic, and thereafter give a purgative dose of magnesium sulphate. Plasma transfusions if necessary.

Post-mortem findings

These include necrosis of the gastro-intestinal tract and of the renal tubular epithelium. Gonzales[27] reports that in three cases there was a cystitis characterised by a severe haemorrhagic oedema of the submucous layer of the bladder.

Analytical findings

Fifty per cent of the acid is excreted in the urine within twelve hours, the rest remains in the body up to three to four days, and thus may accumulate as the result of repeated dosage. Analysis is usually restricted to detection in the stomach or urine. Normally tissue contains somewhat under 1 μg/g. The highest boron levels after poisoning are found in the brain, liver, and fat. Pfeiffer and others[28] investigated boric acid poisoning and quote values of above 1 μg/g.

Fatal dose and time of death

The fatal dose is probably somewhere in the region of 20 g. Death occurs in two days to a week.

Note. Compounds of boron bonded to hydrogen called boranes are being used in the rubber industry and as fuels. These materials are much more toxic than the borates, being irritant to the lungs and kidneys. Death is probably due to pulmonary oedema.

BROMIDES

The commonest salts are the sodium and potassium bromides.   Both are soluble, colourless crystalline solids.   They may occur in the home as photographic chemicals or sedatives.   As sedatives, their use is widespread in a variety of conditions and occasionally toxic manifestations appear.   These may be mild, but severe and even fatal cases sometimes occur.   The rate of excretion is dependent chiefly on the efficiency of the kidneys and the daily fluid and sodium chloride intake. Bromides replace the chlorides in the body.   The symptoms show a wide variation and may be acute or chronic.   There is also personal idiosyncrasy. The symptomatology is not peculiar to bromide intoxication, and diagnosis with certitude can only be established by ascertaining whether the blood bromide is raised and by the gradual disappearance of the symptoms when the bromide administration is withheld.

Symptoms

Furred tongue, anorexia, constipation, slurring speech, listlessness, giddiness, gingivitis, lachrymation, coryza, tachycardia, irregular pulse, occasional diarrhoea, alteration in the tendon reflexes, rash, tremors, and toxic-delirium states with confusion and hallucinations.

Treatment

Stop bromide.   Give large quantities of bland fluid and 2 g sodium chloride capsules, four hourly.   If it is not possible to give sodium chloride orally then normal saline may be given intravenously at the rate of 1 l every four hours to a maximum of 4 l daily.   In cases of delirium sedatives are dangerous but, if imperative, paraldehyde is recommended.

It may take several weeks for the symptoms to disappear.

Analytical findings

Bromide may be estimated in any of the fluids or tissues but the interpretation of the results should be careful to take into account the levels normally found.   In cases of intoxication the levels are above 150 mg/100 ml of serum.   More serious toxicity is found when the level exceeds 250 mg/100 ml.   Shaw[29] quotes a value of 288 mg/100 ml of blood in a case of driving while intoxicated with bromide.

BROMINE

This is a dense, dark-brown liquid with an acrid odour.   The vapour has a deep yellow/brown colour.   Solutions in water are yellow to brown.

Symptoms

The symptoms are those of an irritant poison. When the gas is inhaled, its action involves the entire respiratory tract.

Treatment

The treatment is that applied in the case of chlorine.

Post-mortem findings

The mucous membranes show a brownish-yellow discoloration. Oedema of the glottis sometimes results and oedema of the lungs is common.

Analytical findings

Quantitative analyses for bromine or the estimation of bromide may give significant results.

Fatal dose

The fatal dose of bromine is estimated at about 1 g. The maximum permissible level of vapour in the air is 0·1 p.p.m.

CADMIUM AND ITS COMPOUNDS

Cadmium and its compounds have many specialised uses in industry but no medical applications and are not normally found in the home. There is a definite hazard of poisoning in industry and almost all cases arise from this source.

Symptoms

The signs and symptoms of poisoning by inhalation consist of headache, irritating cough, metallic taste in the mouth, nausea, vomiting, sometimes accompanied by diarrhoea, and tachycardia. After some twenty-four to thirty-six hours, breathlessness, pain in the chest, and more marked gastro-intestinal symptoms make their appearance. The urine may assume a brownish colour. When cadmium is swallowed, its emetic action usually obviates fatality, but vomiting, with or without diarrhoea, is marked.[30]

Treatment

There is no specific treatment for cadmium poisoning. Calcium gluconate may be given as a prophylactic measure.

Post-mortem findings

When death occurs, post-mortem examination usually shows congestion of the gastro-intestinal and respiratory tracts. Bronchitis, nephritis, and fatty changes in the heart and liver may be found.

Analytical findings

Tissues and fluids may be analysed for the cadmium level. A list of normal levels is given in Appendix III.

CANNABIS INDICA (*Indian hemp, hashish*)

Hashish is produced by compressing the resinous exudate and dried flowering tops of *Cannabis sativa* into hard masses or slabs. The active principle, tetrahydrocannabinol, which is not an alkaloid but a lipoid-soluble, non-nitrogenous substance, is contained in the resin. The drug is extensively used in the Near and Far East on account of its aphrodisiac, hypnotic, and analgesic actions. It is sold in native bazaars under different names and in different forms; for example, it may be smoked mixed with tobacco, taken as an adulterant in confections, coffee, or swallowed in capsules. Little tolerance is acquired and although a drug of addiction, it does not frequently lead to physical deterioration or to withdrawal symptoms.

Symptoms

Taken in very large doses, acute poisoning with fatal results may ensue. In small doses, it produces symptoms similar to the early stages of inebriation, namely, a sense of elevation and superiority. With increased doses, drowsiness is likely to supervene, and addicts relate that during this stage erotic and other visual impressions are usually experienced. After large doses, the stage of drowsiness is accompanied by numbness and a sense of loss of power of the limbs, feeble but quiet respiration, weak and irregular pulse and faint heart action, dilatation of pupils and deep unconsciousness. Fatal cases are unusual. Acute mental disorders are much more frequent than chronic ones. People with excitable temperaments may become violent if interfered with while under the influence of the drug.

Treatment

Stimulants may be given by rectum, or by mouth if the patient is able to swallow, and artificial respiration should be employed, if indicated.

Analytical findings

Analysis of biological material for cannabis usually results in negative findings. Vegetable materials and perhaps stains on fingers caused by cannabis smoking may be successfully analysed for cannabis.

CANTHARIDIN

This is a colourless crystalline solid which sublimes at 84°C and melts at 218°C and is almost insoluble in water (3·3 mg/100 ml). It is the active principle of the dried *Cantharis vesicatoria* or 'Spanish Fly' (Fig. 224) found in Southern Europe. Cantharides powder contains

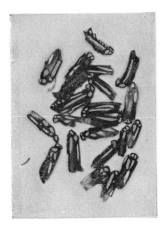

FIG. 224

Cantharis (Lytta) vesicatoria, or
'Spanish Fly'

not less than 0·6 per cent of cantharidin, which, when absorbed, is chiefly eliminated by the kidneys and intestinal tract. Popularly it is believed to have a marked aphrodisiac action in both sexes, and it is also believed to have an abortifacient action. It has been used criminally for both purposes. Among the medicinal preparations are: acetum cantharidini and tinctura cantharidis, and liquor epispasticus. Besides these, there are several proprietary blistering preparations.

It is usually administered for abortifacient purposes in the form of powder, but other preparations have been given.

A case of poisoning by cantharides with fatal result is reported by Nickolls and Teare.[31] Two young women died after eating coconut ice containing cantharidin. A man was charged with manslaughter and pleaded guilty. It was stated that the contaminated sweet was given to one of the girls to stimulate sex desire, while the other ate a portion by accident.

Symptoms

When cantharides is applied to the skin an inflammatory reaction results in a few hours and later vesicles form.   When swallowed, there is burning pain in the throat and stomach, subsequently difficulty in swallowing, nausea, abdominal pain, and vomiting, the vomited matter containing blood.   Intense thirst, and possibly diarrhoea, with perhaps blood and mucus also occur.   Pain on micturition, with great tenesmus and the passage of blood-stained urine, is a prominent symptom.   In the male, priapism may occur, and in the female there may be engorgement of the vulva.   In fatal cases, coma with convulsions usually precedes death.

Treatment

Free gastric lavage with tepid water.   After vomiting has ceased, the excretion of urine should be aided by the use of warm demulcent drinks, and other measures, and magnesium sulphate, but not castor oil, should be given.   Morphia may be used to control pain.

Post-mortem findings

Gastro-intestinal inflammation, due to the vesicating action of the cantharidin.   This is chiefly marked on the mucous membrane of the mouth, throat, stomach, and small intestine.   The kidneys, ureters, bladder, and urethra show signs of congestion and inflammation, macroscopically and microscopically, and blood-stained urine may be found in the bladder.   The pelvic viscera are usually engorged.

Analytical findings

In view of the fact that the poison may be in the form of the ground fly (cantharides) the stomach and intestinal tract should be examined closely for the remains of the shining elytra or wing cases of the insect. Analyses may then be made for the poison in the tissues and fluids.

Fatal dose and time of death

The lethal dose is probably under 60 mg.   Severe symptoms have been experienced after an estimated 1·5 mg.   About 1·5 g of powdered fly have produced death but recovery following larger doses is recorded. Death usually occurs within twelve to twenty-four hours after ingestion.

CARBON DIOXIDE

This is a colourless, odourless gas and is occasionally associated with carbon monoxide, as in choke-damp, lime-burning, and brick-burning. Because carbon dioxide is more dense than air it tends to collect in low-lying places when the ventilation is poor, and as a result forms a dangerous invisible hazard. It is the cause of fatalities in workmen associated with well-sinking, well-cleaning, breweries, fermentation vats, and aerated water factories.

Symptoms

When small percentages are present in the atmosphere the symptoms include somnolence, lassitude, and breathlessness. Constant exposure to air of ill-ventilated apartments produces anaemia, malnutrition, and other manifestations. High concentrations rapidly produce powerlessness, insensibility, and death.

Treatment

Fresh air, artificial respiration, and oxygen are all used. The body temperature should be maintained.

Post-mortem findings

The findings are typical of asphyxia.

Fatal dose

Concentrations over 30 per cent rapidly cause death.

CARBON DISULPHIDE

The pure compound is a colourless liquid which boils at 46°C. This material has an aromatic odour but the commercial product has a characteristic rancid odour. The vapour from this substance, when inhaled, rarely causes fatal acute poisoning, but it is held that a concentration of 1 in 300 to 1 in 500 will produce serious illness and a danger of mania and coma in about half an hour. Chronic poisoning is by no means infrequent among those employed in occupations in which it is used as, for example, in rubber works, especially in the 'curing-rooms', or in the manufacture of artificial silk by the viscose process. Acute poisoning is usually due to swallowing the liquid.

Symptoms

Acute.   The signs and symptoms in the acute form are: Unconsciousness, dilated and fixed pupils, embarrassment of breathing, with cyanosis, general symptoms of shock, due to the absorption of liquid, and an odour of carbon disulphide in the breath.   Acute mental disturbances, including mania, may occur.

Chronic.   The symptoms of chronic poisoning are many and varied. Any part of the central or peripheral nervous system may become affected.

Nausea, vertigo, headache, fatigue, insomnia, irritability, anaemia, and a perceptible odour in the breath are commonly found.   If the exposure is continued, there may be impairment of vision and memory, tremors, evidence of optic neuritis with amblyopia, polyneuritis, impotence, emaciation, depression, and mental disturbances including acute hallucinatory psychoses.   Pylorospasm may develop.   As a rule the prognosis is good and mental disturbances subside rapidly with restoration approaching normal in about three to four weeks.

Treatment

When the poison has been swallowed, gastric lavage should be used until the returned fluid is non-odorous.   Stimulants may be given. When inhaled, oxygen should be administered.

Post-mortem findings

When the poison has been swallowed, the manifestations include an odour of carbon disulphide in the cavities of the body, especially in the stomach and abdomen generally.   The lungs and other organs are congested and there may be gastric submucosal haemorrhages.   When fumes have been inhaled, the respiratory system shows evidence of congestion and there is often oedema of the lungs.

In chronic poisoning there may be changes in the ganglion cells of the cerebral cortex, and parenchymatous degeneration of the peripheral nerves.

Analytical findings

Sulphate in the urine is not reliable due to the many other possible sources.   Carbon disulphide may be estimated in the blood or urine.

Fatal dose and time of death

The fatal dose is somewhat below 15 g.   Atmospheric concentrations above 50 p.p.m. may be dangerous if inhaled for several hours.   Death may supervene at any time up to a few days.   Recovery from serious poisoning is usually not complete.

Carbon Monoxide

This is a colourless, odourless, non-irritant gas.   Among the principal sources are gases from ignition of explosives, from blast furnaces, the slow combustion of blaes or iron-waste heaps, coal-gas itself, and coal-gas admixed artificially with variable proportions of water-gas, the fumes from geysers in bathrooms, paraffin heaters, lime-kiln burning, the air of mines, and exhaust gas from internal combustion engines. Explosions in confined spaces, such as in mines, produce poisonous quantities of carbon monoxide.

Most deaths from carbon monoxide are suicidal, some are accidental and only a few are homicidal.   Illuminant gas is very commonly employed for the purpose of committing suicide.   In the investigation of cases of death due to carbon monoxide, it must not be forgotten that this gas may be used for the purpose of homicide as well as of suicide, and, for this reason, great care should be exercised.   In one case, for example, the dead body of a man was found lying on a bench in his workroom, and the gas jet above his head was turned on.   A piece of gas-tubing with an attachment for fixing to the jet lay beside the body. Examination of the blood showed that it was almost completely saturated with carbon monoxide.   The skin on various large areas of the body was of cherry-red colour.   Post-mortem examination revealed a fracture on each side of the lower jaw.   Two men were apprehended and charged with murder.   A watch, chain, and money, belonging to deceased, were acknowledged by one of the accused to have been stolen by him. Owing to insufficient evidence connecting the accused with the assault and with the gas incident, one was found guilty of robbery and the other was discharged.

'Town's gas' contains a very considerable percentage of carbon monoxide, varying according to the method of production.   In the vertical retort, steaming is introduced and the percentage is high, often reaching 22 per cent.   Carbon monoxide is an odourless gas, but when mixed with ethylene gas the odour of the latter is always perceptible. A considerable number of deaths has been caused by the use of gas geysers in bathrooms, since, occasionally, they may generate carbon monoxide.   The fractured gas main is a further source of poisoning.

Exhaust gas from internal combustion engines contains from 1 to 7 per cent of carbon monoxide depending on the richness of the mixture. A twenty horse-power motor-car engine will produce sufficient carbon monoxide, within five minutes, to render the atmosphere of a single-car garage deadly, provided the engine has been run with the garage doors closed.   It is therefore evident that fatalities may readily occur in this way.   Defects in the exhaust pipe of a motor car may permit the entry of carbon monoxide into the car and, depending upon the amount, may produce symptoms.

Choke-damp, which is a mixture of carbon monoxide and carbon dioxide, is liable to form in all collieries at 'dead-ends', where the ventilation is imperfect.   Blasting in mines and pit explosions are relatively common causes of fatal poisoning by carbon monoxide.   In burning buildings the carbon monoxide in smoke is the cause of a considerable number of deaths.   Occasionally cases occur under unusual circumstances.   We made a post-mortem examination of the body of a man found dead in a boiler which he had been repairing, and his blood showed evidence of death by carbon monoxide.

Dangerous effects may also result from coke-stoves, and the use of flueless braziers.   Owing to the use of gas in industry, chronic poisoning by carbon monoxide also occurs.   Signs of chronic poisoning may become manifest in persons who have been exposed to regular small, yet toxic, amounts of this gas over a considerable period, but these are very variable in character and degree.

There is a definite susceptibility to carbon monoxide under certain conditions.   This is seen at extremes of age, in anaemic subjects, and those who suffer from cardiac and respiratory conditions.   Chronic alcoholics are also susceptible.

Symptoms

Acute.   The symptoms of poisoning by carbon monoxide vary, depending upon the degree of saturation of the blood.   Haldane has found that when the blood has absorbed carbon monoxide to the extent of 20 per cent, the symptoms only manifest themselves on exertion, when there is a slight degree of shortness of breath and giddiness.   Thirty per cent saturation of the blood gives rise to symptoms when the individual is at rest.   When 50 per cent saturation is reached, the afflicted person shows inco-ordination, and staggers; loss of consciousness may be induced by exertion.   Death occurs when the saturation of the blood reaches from 60 to 80 per cent.   The action of carbon monoxide is cumulative, and even although there is only a small percentage of the gas present in the atmosphere, it is progressively linked up with the haemoglobin, with displacement of oxygen, until a condition of oxygen starvation is established by the formation of carboxyhaemoglobin. When a person is at rest, 0·1 per cent of carbon monoxide in the atmosphere inhaled may produce a blood saturation of 50 per cent in two and a quarter hours, but with exercise, an hour would suffice.   Carbon-monoxide poisoning in mines is usually a gradual process induced by small percentages of this gas.   When the amount of oxygen is 300 times greater than carbon monoxide, half of the haemoglobin can combine with the carbon monoxide and half with the oxygen, and this has been estimated as about the degree of blood saturation at which unconsciousness occurs. As the concentration of carbon monoxide in the air rises, the saturation of the haemoglobin increases and the oxygen-carrying capacity of the blood progressively diminishes until symptoms of anoxaemia occur. Only in this respect can carbon monoxide be regarded as cumulative in action. The onset of symptoms of poisoning may be insidious; a feeling of lassitude may merge into a state of drowsiness with a dulling of the senses which is succeeded by unconsciousness. On the other hand, the prodromal symptoms may be giddiness, palpitation, breathlessness, weakness of limbs, which may preclude escape, and, finally, unconsciousness.

The affinity of carbon monoxide for haemoglobin has been estimated as 300 times greater than that of oxygen.

In cases of acute carbon-monoxide poisoning the signs and symptoms are: deep coma; frequently the presence of a rosy tint affecting the lips and cheeks, but sometimes the face is pale and bedewed with perspiration or it may show, especially in deep coma, a leaden tint; the eyes are staring and glassy, the pupils are dilated and fixed; a small quantity of frothy fluid is usually present at the mouth; the breathing is shallow and quiet; the pulse is weak and almost imperceptible; the temperature is usually subnormal; coldness of the body. The patient suffers from anoxaemia and his state of oxygen lack may be as severe as that of blue-black victims of obstructive asphyxia. The rosy colour of the victim, which is due to the presence of carboxyhaemoglobin, is very misleading, especially since the action of respiration is apparently unembarrassed due to anoxic depression of the respiratory centre. Should the patient recover from the severe symptoms, it may take months before he is restored to his former health. Pneumonia is by no means an uncommon complication in severe cases and may cause death within a few days following exposure to the gas. In the various stages of acute poisoning, the symptoms might be confused with those due to drunkenness or acute alcoholic poisoning.

Shillito, Drinker, and Shaughnessey[32] have recorded data based on an investigation of nervous and mental sequelae in carbon-monoxide poisoning. The New York Metropolitan area was chosen for this study, since at least 21,142 acute exposures occurred there in a ten-year period. For the same period, a survey of the state mental institutions serving this area showed thirty-nine certain cases of sequelae of carbon-monoxide poisoning. When nervous or mental damage occurred, the intoxication had been extreme. None of the cases followed chronic poisoning from exposure over a long period. In two-thirds of these cases, the symptoms started immediately following exposure, and in the remaining third, within one to three weeks. The mental sequelae consisted of confusional psychosis, with disorientation, lack of judgment, and amnesia. Nervous sequelae ranged from altered reflexes to advanced Parkinsonism. Out of a total of forty-three cases, twenty-three patients made a complete recovery, nine suffered permanent nervous or mental sequelae, and eleven died.

Martland[33] states that in cases showing post-asphyxial encephalitic syndromes, due to prolonged anoxaemia, there is bilateral degeneration in the globus pallidus of the lenticular nuclei consisting of elongated, brownish areas, strongly resembling thrombotic softening and measuring 1 to 2 cm in diameter.

Chronic. When there has been exposure to repeated small yet toxic doses of carbon monoxide, the following comprise the commoner symptoms: headache, giddiness, gastro-intestinal disturbances, anaemia, tachycardia, palpitation, praecordial pain, faintness, breathlessness on exertion, muscular cramps, depression, irritability, and general nervousness. In women the menstrual periods may be irregular.

Gettler and Mattice[34] have shown that the average carbon-monoxide content of the blood of eighteen persons, living in New York City under conditions of minimal exposure, was from 1 to 1·5 per cent saturation. The average content of the blood of twelve persons, confined to a state institution in an ideal rural surrounding, was less than 1 per cent. The blood of twelve New York street cleaners was about 3 per cent, and the blood of two taxi-cab drivers was between 8 and 19 per cent on several occasions. Hanson and Hastings[35] report that, in a short series of normal individuals who did not smoke, the haemoglobin was saturated with carbon monoxide to the extent of 1·5 per cent. In subjects who were smokers, the saturation varied from 3 to 5 per cent.

It would appear that such factors must receive consideration in the interpretation of the results of blood estimations.

Treatment

In a case of carbon monoxide gas poisoning, it should be remembered that the linkage with haemoglobin is reversible in the presence of oxygen. The patient must be removed from the vitiated atmosphere at once. Often this is followed by collapse, more especially if he is taken into the open air. The reason for this lies in the fact that the atmospheric carbon dioxide is much less than in the vitiated atmosphere, and since carbon dioxide plays an important part in carbon monoxide dissociation, the effects of deprivation are shown clinically. The body should be well wrapped up after hot-water bottles, suitably covered, have been applied. This is important since carbon monoxide disturbs the heat-regulating centre with reduction in the processes of oxidation. To commence with, artificial respiration should be applied if breathing is only slightly embarrassed or irregular. If respiration is poor, oxygen should be given with a mask, and this treatment should be continued until normal respiration has been restored, and thereafter careful observation of the patient is necessary to detect an early indication of relapse.   Before applying this treatment the airway should always be clear.   Blood transfusion is of little benefit unless performed within an hour of the patient's removal from the poisoned atmosphere.   The position of the patient should be changed from time to time to prevent accumulation of fluid in the bronchi and dependent parts of the lungs.

Haggard and Greenberg[36] state that intravenous injection of methylene blue is contra-indicated, that it is not an antidote, that its use probably exerts deleterious effects, and that it may produce fatalities which would not otherwise occur.

Prolonged rest is essential.

Post-mortem findings

There is usually a pink coloration of the face and a similar, but patchy, colour of various surfaces of the body.   Post-mortem staining is of pinkish hue.   The blood is of a bright red colour.   The lungs are congested, often oedematous, and some frothy fluid is usually present in

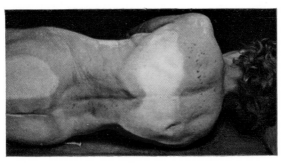

FIG. 225

Accentuated colouring of hypostasis, or post-mortem staining, in carbon monoxide poisoning.   Note areas of contact
flattening

the upper air-passages.   The muscles and organs also show the bright red colour.   The rosy-coloured markings on the body may not always be found.   Petechial haemorrhages may be seen on the meninges or surface of the brain, or both, and similar haemorrhages may be present in the cortical substance and in the corpus striatum.   The ventricles may contain blood-stained fluid.   The brain may be oedematous. Microscopical examination of sections may show lenticular degeneration.

Analytical findings

The carboxyhaemoglobin concentration of the blood is measured and values of 60 per cent or greater imply death from carbon monoxide poisoning. In many deaths, the level may be below this figure but in these cases death is usually from some other cause; the carbon monoxide making the victim unable to help himself out of a dangerous situation or contributing to the effects of drugs or alcohol. Carbon monoxide is quite rapidly eliminated from the blood of those who survive exposure, and therefore a sample of blood for examination should be secured as quickly as possible. In fresh air, and more especially when respiration has been stimulated, about half the total quantity of carbon monoxide will be eliminated probably during the first hour, the remainder in greater degree in the next six to ten hours, and all traces of it will probably have disappeared within twenty-four hours.

Fatal dose

The fatal dose depends on time of exposure and concentration and Henderson and Haggard[37] give the following guide. If the time of exposure (hours) multiplied by the concentration (part per million) is below 300 there is no perceptible effect. If the value is 600, the effect is just appreciable. At 900 there is headache and nausea and at 1500 there is danger to life.

CARBON TETRACHLORIDE (*Tetrachloromethane*)

Carbon tetrachloride is a dense, colourless, volatile liquid (boiling-point 76°C) with a characteristic odour. This material is used as an industrial solvent and as a dry-cleaning fluid. It is found in the home as a stain-remover or in some forms of fire-extinguisher. It has some use in medicine in the treatment of ankylostamiasis. Poisoning may result from drinking the fluid or by inhalation of the vapour. When the fluid is sprayed on burning material or hot metal, the chief decomposition product is phosgene. Thus, when carbon tetrachloride is used as an extinguisher, poisoning may result from its fumes or those of the decomposition products. When swallowed or inhaled, it exerts a soporific action, depressing both cardiac and respiratory centres.

Symptoms

The chief symptoms of poisoning are nausea, vomiting, pain in the epigastrium, faintness, loss of consciousness, and convulsions. Clinical manifestations of impaired renal function are common and vary in degree. The urine may be dark-coloured and this manifestation is frequently followed by jaundice. The urine may be loaded with casts and albumin, and death may result from uraemia. The liver may also be damaged, with accompanying symptoms of jaundice, bradycardia, haematemesis and melaena.

Treatment

Respiratory failure should be treated by artificial respiration in the open. If the poison has been swallowed, stomach lavage must be employed without delay. The patient should be kept warm and symptoms, which may include renal or hepatic failure, treated along usual lines. McGuire[38] states that serious cases should be treated with adrenalin, caffeine sodium benzoate, and digitalis, together with calcium lactate. He holds the view that calcium deficiency and the use of alcohol render the individual more susceptible, and that calcium therapy is particularly indicated in treatment. A beneficial line of treatment is the administration of 10 ml of 10 per cent solution of calcium gluconate intravenously two or three times daily with 12 g calcium gluconate, or 8 g of calcium lactose by mouth.

Post-mortem findings

These vary with the mode of administration. A characteristic odour is usually perceived, and there may be fatty degeneration of heart, liver, and kidneys. The larynx, bronchi, and lungs will be congested, in varying degree, and evidence of broncho-pneumonia may be present if the fumes have been inhaled, while the gastric mucosa and the lining of the oesophagus will probably show evidence of inflammatory irritation with or without areas of haemorrhage, when the drug has been swallowed. Jaundice, following liver involvement, and acute nephritis are frequently present.

Analytical findings

Carbon tetrachloride may be sought for in any of the tissues or fluids. If the subject survived for any length of time the amount found, if any, may be small. Tompsett[39] quotes a value of $2 \cdot 0$ mg/100 ml blood in a non-fatal poisoning when the subject consumed about 30 ml.

Fatal dose

The fatal dose is probably in the region of 10 g and the maximum permitted level in the atmosphere is 10 p.p.m.

Note. 1. The other chlorinated hydrocarbons such as trichloroethane and ethylene dichloride have similar properties.

2. Tetrachloroethane is a dense ($1 \cdot 6$ g/ml), colourless, volatile

liquid. The vapour is heavier than air, consequently it is apt to fall to lower levels of working places and does not readily mix with the atmosphere. It is used widely in industry as a solvent. It is exceedingly toxic to workers, probably being the most toxic of all the chlorinated derivatives, and a large number of cases of poisoning have occurred from its use. Poisoning may be acute or chronic. Several cases of suicide have been caused by drinking 'silk cleaning fluid'.

The symptoms, which are many and varied in character, are most frequently produced by inhalation of the fumes. They consist of malaise, anorexia, drowsiness, headache, mental confusion, nausea, and sometimes vomiting. When the toxic effects are severe, the symptoms shown are stupor, delirium, convulsive twitchings, nephritis, and coma, preceded or accompanied by a haemo-hepatogenous jaundice. Cholangitis affects the finer bile-ducts and produces bile-flow obstruction, with fatty degeneration and necrosis of the liver cells in some instances. Prognosis is always grave in severe cases. Dermatitis and visual disturbances may be present.

Treatment consists in the administration of oxygen, intravenous saline, sodium carbonate or calcium gluconate, blood transfusion, and catharsis.

On post-mortem examination, the liver is usually the chief organ affected. When the poison has been swallowed, the gastric mucosa will show congestion, with or without small erosions, and there will also be congestion of the lungs, kidneys, and intestinal tract. When death has been rapid the liver may be only congested, but when death has been delayed, necrosis or fatty degenerative changes will probably be present.

3. Trichloroethylene (trilene) is a dense (1.46 g/ml) colourless liquid. It is a volatile substance with a characteristic odour used in commerce as a solvent for tar, rubber, and in dry-cleaning. It is also employed for the extraction of oils and fats, degreasing metals, enamelling, cleaning photographic plates, and textile manufacture. Cases of trigeminal neuralgia have been treated by the inhalation of 0.5 to 1.0 ml. Trilene is used as an anaesthetic.

The fumes, if containing disintegration products, when inhaled may affect the central nervous system and give rise to such symptoms as headache, vertigo, fainting, drowsiness, cardialgia, paraesthesia of the limbs, coma, and death.

Post-mortem findings may consist of encephalitis, subpleural petechial haemorrhages, and desquamation of the renal tubular epithelium with fatty degenerative changes.

CHLORAL HYDRATE

Chloral hydrate is a colourless crystalline solid (m. pt $52\,°C$) which is very soluble in water. It has a pungent odour and has a burning bitter taste. The drug is used as a hypnotic, but due to irritant action on the stomach, it should be given in a dilute form. It is of special value in the treatment of nervous and mental conditions, is sometimes used for suicidal purposes, and has been employed criminally by mixing it with alcoholic beverages.

Symptoms

The principal manifestations are drowsiness, merging into unconsciousness, slow, shallow respiration, with cyanosis of lips, and gradual weakening of the pulse. Chloral hydrate is a central nervous system depressant which, in toxic doses, paralyses the respiratory and cardiac centres.

Treatment

Free gastric lavage should be employed and the body heat maintained. Forced diuresis or dialysis may be used in severe poisoning. Artificial respiration and oxygen inhalations may be necessary.

Post-mortem findings

There are no typical findings.

Analytical findings

Any of the post-mortem materials may be examined, but as metabolism to trichloroethanol is rapid this latter is more likely to be found. Jain and others[40] report a value of 0·9 mg trichloroethanol per 100 ml of blood in a fatal chloral hydrate poisoning. They found no chloral hydrate. Bonnichsen and Maehly[41] report chloral hydrate levels of 5·8 and 3·4 mg/100 ml blood in two fatal chloral hydrate poisonings.

Fatal dose and time of death

The fatal dose is uncertain. Death of an adult followed ingestion of 13 g while a sixteen-year-old boy recovered from the effects of 28 g. Death usually occurs in ten to fifteen hours but may be delayed for two or three days.

CHLORATES

The commonest salts are sodium and potassium chlorates, both of which look very like sugar in the crystalline form. They dissolve in water to give colourless solutions. Sodium chlorate is used extensively in gardening and path-laying as a total weed killer, and as a result is common in the home where it may be ingested accidentally. Potassium chlorate is often found in solutions used as gargles. The chlorates are commonly present in fireworks.

Symptoms

In large doses, these salts act as acute haemolytic poisons and produce signs and symptoms which may be summarised as follows: severe vomiting, pain in the epigastrium and abdomen generally, profuse diarrhoea, dyspnoea and deep cyanosis, lowered blood-pressure and cardiac weakness, also headache, giddiness, muscular weakness, restlessness, coma, and death. Oliguria or anuria are manifestations and any urine passed is first dark in colour, then reddish-brown, and contains haemoglobin, methaemoglobin, haematin, blood cells, casts, and albumin. The urine on standing shows a considerable quantity of chlorates. The blood corpuscles are destroyed and spectroscopic examination of the blood, which frequently is of chocolate colour, shows the spectrum of methaemoglobin. The sclera are sometimes icteric. Asphyxia occurs when the methaemoglobin prevents the blood from carrying the available oxygen. In subacute cases, death usually results from renal changes following obstruction of the renal tubules with fragmented red cells. The body, after death, may vary in colour from white to bluish-green or chocolate, due to methaemoglobin.

Treatment

Evacuate the contents of the stomach by free lavage. Transfusion of blood may be necessary to replace the destroyed blood cells. Intravenous sodium bicarbonate or methylene blue has been recommended. Diuresis should be encouraged by the administration of alkaline drinks. Administer oxygen, also cardiac and respiratory stimulants, if necessary. Oliguria should be treated by a high caloric protein-free diet.

Post-mortem findings

The blood may be chocolate-coloured due to the presence of methaemoglobin. The heart may be soft and flabby with extensive fatty degeneration. The kidneys may be large, the tubules being filled to distension with disintegrated corpuscles and blood pigment. This gives a peculiar striped appearance of the pyramids. Fatty degeneration of the liver and gastro-enteritis may also be present.

Analytical findings

Chlorate is most likely to be found in the stomach contents and urine. It rapidly disappears from other tissues due to chemical action. In a case where a large quantity of sodium chlorate was ingested the post-mortem urine chlorate level was 600 mg/100 ml. In another case where 15 g of sodium chlorate was found in the stomach the kidney chlorate level was 19·4 mg/100 g.

Fatal dose and time of death

The fatal dose is probably over 20 g but death has occurred after 12 g. Death usually occurs in a day or two, but Timperman and Maes[42] report one case where death occurred after 1 hour and 40 minutes.

Illustrative case

A woman took, by mistake for Rochelle salts, two tablespoonfuls of chlorate. Within twenty-four hours she was profoundly prostrated. Her temperature was 37·2°C, and the pulse and respiration rates were 136 and 32, respectively. The body surface was cyanotic, the breathing rapid but not laboured, and the pulse rapid but not feeble. She had vomited freely, and was still vomiting after admission to hospital. Two hours later, the temperature rose to 40·0°C. Three dark brown motions had been passed, and dark-coloured urine was voided involuntarily. The urine contained blood cells, methaemoglobin, and copious albumin. Next day, the skin, conjunctivae, and lips were of chocolate tint. She died thirty-seven hours after the poison had been taken. Coma preceded death.

Note. Hypochlorite solutions recommended for use as a sterilising agent for baby feed bottles may decompose to form appreciable amounts of chlorate. This may cause chlorate poisoning as the solutions are not rinsed from the bottles before use. Harris[43] reports such a poisoning incident involving a number of babies.

CHLORDIAZEPOXIDE, NITRAZEPAM, AND DIAZEPAM

These are the related tranquillisers Librium, Mogadon, and Valium. They are used as mild tranquillising agents in the treatment of neurotic conditions where there is anxiety and tension. There is also some muscle-relaxant activity. Nitrazepam is often described as a non-barbiturate hypnotic with an action similar to the intermediate-acting barbiturates.

Symptoms

These include drowsiness, weakness, and inco-ordination, which may be followed by cyanosis, coma, and respiratory depression. Other effects such as hypotension, blurred vision, impaired memory, and slurred speech may also be present.

Treatment

The absorption should be delayed by the use of activated charcoal or milk and then gastric lavage or emesis should be employed. Treat coma or respiratory depression as they arise and maintain blood-pressure.

Post-mortem findings

The findings on post-mortem examination are non-specific.

Analytical findings

These drugs may be separated and measured in tissue and fluids but careful analysis is required to eliminate interfering materials. The levels found after fatal poisoning are usually somewhat over 1 mg/100 ml of blood but recovery has followed levels of 1·8 mg/100 ml of blood.

Fatal dose

The fatal dose is not known but is estimated to be of the order of 10 g.

CHLORINE

Chlorine is a greenish-yellow gas, two and a half times heavier than air, with a smell resembling bleaching powder. When inhaled, it exercises both an irritant and suffocative effect. Industrial poisoning is caused by accidents in the course of its manufacture and from its use in the chemical industry. Chlorine inhalation is not an uncommon occurrence in workers engaged in the manufacture of hydrochloric acid and bleaching powder, but fatal results in such occupations are rare, and when they occur are more often due to pulmonary complication than to general constitutional effect.

Symptoms

The symptoms of acute poisoning are intense irritation of the eyes and mucous membrane of the respiratory passages, with extreme dyspnoea, nausea and vomiting, and spasm of the glottis. Death is caused by cardiac failure following inflammatory oedema of the lungs and pulmonary congestion. Should the patient survive for forty-eight hours, septic broncho-pneumonia may be a later and fatal complication. Chlorine inhalation in repeated small amounts may give rise to a chronic condition resulting in anaemia, cachexia, dental caries, and phthisis. Bronchitis and emphysema are common.

Treatment

Rest and maintenance of body warmth are imperative; the chief danger is acute pulmonary oedema; oxygen from an inhaler should be administered promptly and continuously while oedema is present and until there is no return of cyanosis after withdrawal; venesection is necessary when there is deep cyanosis and venous engorgement; 300 to 400 ml of blood should be withdrawn up to a total quantity of 700 ml if necessary; contra-indications are leaden grey colour with circulatory failure, low blood-pressure, and a small, rapid, or impalpable pulse; transfusions and infusions are contra-indicated in pulmonary oedema, but intravenous injections of saline may otherwise be given to reduce the high viscosity of the blood; expectoration should be encouraged by posture and not by expectorant mixtures; atropine, digitalis, and alcohol are contra-indicated; morphia should be restricted to 10 mg doses; when infective bronchitis or broncho-pneumonia develops, antibiotics should be given.

Post-mortem findings

These are principally asphyxial due to acute pulmonary oedema. The lungs are heavy and water-logged. On section, considerable congestion, occasional thrombosis of the network of pulmonary vessels, an abundant outpouring of fluid, and disruptive emphysema of weakened lung tissue, due to coughing, may be observed. Petechial haemorrhages may be visible on the pleural surfaces, and the pleural cavities will probably contain a variable quantity of serous or blood-stained fluid. Infective bronchitis, broncho-pneumonia, or pleurisy may be present. The chambers on the right side of the heart will be dilated and contain a considerable quantity of blood, as will the associated large vessels.

Analytical findings

Chlorine is not likely to be found as such, due to the rapid conversion to chlorides and other compounds.

Fatal dose and time of death

The maximum permissible level is 1 p.p.m. Exposure for even short periods to concentrations in the region of 1,000 p.p.m. may be fatal.

Death may occur immediately or after some days due to pulmonary oedema.

CHLOROFORM

Chloroform is a dense ($1 \cdot 5$ g/ml), colourless, volatile liquid with a characteristic odour. It is used industrially as a solvent and in medicine as an anaesthetic. Poisoning may follow ingestion or inhalation.

Symptoms

When inhaled chloroform has a paralysing effect upon respiration and causes a fall in blood-pressure. Chronic exposure to chloroform may result in liver damage. Gaddum[44] writing on the subject of ketosis

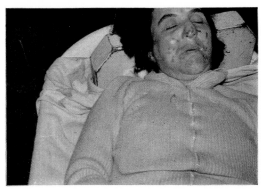

FIG. 226

Facial lesions caused by pressure on chloroform-soaked cloth

following chloroform anaesthesia states that the toxic action affects the liver, heart, and kidneys, which undergo fatty changes, and the patient develops ketosis and vomits. Ketosis is due to the incomplete oxidation of fats which leads to the accumulation of acid ketone bodies, such as aceto-acetic acid and hydroxybutyric acid. The occurrence of this condition following anaesthesia is possibly a consequence of the fact that anaesthetics have a specific inhibitory action on carbohydrate metabolism, which leads to a compensating increase of fat metabolism. Ingestion of chloroform results in a similar overall picture. Liquid chloroform may irritate the skin and cause 'burns'.

Treatment

The patient should be kept warm and given artificial respiration and oxygen. After ingestion liquid paraffin should be given followed by gastric lavage.

Post-mortem findings

There may be some congestion of the stomach and intestines with a few scattered extravasations of blood. Necrosis of the liver may be present.

Analytical findings

Tissues and fluids may be analysed for chloroform. During anaesthesia levels below 25 mg chloroform per 100 ml blood may be found. In a fatal case of chloroform inhalation a level of 12·5 mg per 100 g of liver was recorded. In general the dangerous level is thought to be somewhat over 40 mg/100 ml of blood.

Fatal dose and time of death

Deaths have been recorded after ingestion of 30, 45, 60 and 90 ml of chloroform but recovery had followed 120 and 150 ml doses. Death may supervene rapidly or may be after some days due to liver damage. A small quantity of chloroform may kill when inhaled in a concentrated mixture, while a comparatively large amount may be safe in a concentration below 2 per cent.

Illustrative cases

Hayward records a fatal case of a woman who drank 60 ml of chloroform. Her face was blanched, the lips and fingers were livid, the body and extremities were cold, the pulse was imperceptible, the heart sounds very feeble, the breathing shallow but regular, the corneae insensitive, and the pupils were equal, semi-dilated, and feebly responsive to light. She had vomited. Under treatment her condition at first improved, but when she recovered consciousness, a sudden and fatal collapse ensued.

Post-mortem examination showed that the right side of the heart contained dark, uncoagulated blood. The stomach contained about 30 ml of dark, chocolate-coloured fluid which emitted an odour of chloroform, the walls were slightly congested, and a few scattered extravasations of blood were present. The small intestines were intensely congested throughout, the mucous membrane being swollen, velvety, and of dark cherry-red colour with numerous extravasations, and contained a quantity of dark red fluid smelling strongly of chloroform.

A few cases of homicidal administration have been recorded (see Fig. 226). When a saturated pad has been applied with some degree of pressure to the region of the mouth and nostrils it tends to produce small, irregular areas of abrasion and excoriation. We have seen these appearances in two such cases.

An interesting suicidal case was that of a man who fatally chloro-formed himself by means of a service respirator, the inlet of which he closed with cellophane. Both the inlet to the face-piece and the outlet had been stuffed with cotton-wool impregnated with chloroform.

COCAINE

This is a colourless crystalline solid (m. pt 98°C) which is slightly soluble in water. The hydrochloride is very soluble in water. It has a bitter taste and imparts a numbness to the tongue and mucous membrane of the mouth. Cocaine has the property of desensitising the terminal nerves of the part into which it is injected or absorbed, and in a large dose produces paralysing effects upon the central nervous system. When injected for minor operations, such as the extraction of teeth, it has produced toxic effects and death. Many synthetic drugs have been substituted for cocaine and are employed as local and spinal anaesthetics. These include novocaine, nupercaine, stovaine, neocaine, and planocaine. In some persons, hypodermic injection, or snuffing, of cocaine has become an addiction and fatal poisoning has resulted.

Symptoms

Pallor of the face, dilatation and immobility of the pupils, dyspnoea, headache, giddiness, cramps, vomiting, fainting, unconsciousness, convulsions, and rapidity of pulse, quickly slowing down and becoming intermittent and feeble. In fatal cases, asphyxial manifestations supervene, and death results from depression of the respiratory and cardiac centres.

Addicts usually have an initial psychopathic tendency, or an unstable nervous system. The stimulating effect of the drug is responsible for the acquired habit. When the effects wear off, however, there are irritability and restlessness. In addition to the signs of physical degeneration which are apparent, addicts frequently suffer from psychical degeneration, which commonly assumes the form of insanity. Anorexia is a frequent symptom. In such persons, complaint is often made of a sensation in the skin as if grains of sand or insects or other small bodies were lying in, or under, it. Further, they become tolerant to the drug, the dosage of which is gradually increased. The cause of addiction may be attributed to the fact that cocaine quickly banishes fatigue and mental exhaustion, which are replaced by a feeling of mental and physical vigour. The effects of cocaine lead to increased erotic tension in women with the removal of normal inhibitions, which may ultimately lead to a state of nymphomania. In men the physical component decreases while the mental component is increased, this condition leading to many sexual perversions. Hallucinations may also be present. Cocaine may be taken either by the nose, in the form of snuff, or by hypodermic injection.

Treatment

The stomach should be washed out with a dilute solution of potassium permanganate or tannic acid. Medicinal charcoal may also be employed. If the drug has been administered hypodermically these remedies will be ineffective. To control convulsions, sodium amytal, 3 to 10 ml of a 10 per cent solution given intravenously, at the rate of 1 ml per minute, has been recommended. Artificial respiration and oxygen should be resorted to in the event of threatened asphyxia. If poisoning has resulted from the contact of cocaine with the mucous membrane, an endeavour should be made to remove as much of the substance as possible by washing the affected surface.

Post-mortem findings

In cases of acute poisoning, these are valueless as indicative of the character of the poison. Death being due to asphyxia, or cardiac failure, the signs of these forms of death are likely to be found.

Analytical findings

About 15 per cent of a dose of cocaine appears in the urine and may be detected there. Metabolism occurs in the liver.

Fatal dose and time of death

The fatal dose is about 1 g, though death has followed much smaller amounts. Generally death occurs within a very short period and survival beyond an hour is usually followed by recovery.

Illustrative case

A fatal case is recorded in which, for temporary relief of a urethral stricture to enable a catheter to be passed, 2 ml of a 10 per cent solution of cocaine hydrochloride was injected into the urethra, the meatus of the penis being held to prevent regurgitation of the fluid. In a few minutes the patient, a man of fifty-six, was in a state of clonic convulsion. His jaws were moving spasmodically, and he had bitten his tongue. The face was somewhat cyanosed, the breathing very spasmodic and slightly stertorous, the eyeballs fixed, and eyelids half closed.

A pulse could not be felt at the wrist, but the heart was beating.   About a minute later, respiration ceased, the cyanosis increasing.   Artificial respiration was at once commenced, and other measures employed, but the patient was dead in about three minutes.

Note.   The cocaine substitutes such as procaine are not habit-forming.   The toxicity of these materials is of the same order as cocaine and the symptoms are similar.

COPPER AND ITS COMPOUNDS

Copper salts when taken in large doses produce toxic effects.   Probably the most poisonous are the sulphate or blue vitriol, and the subacetate or verdigris.   They are seldom used for criminal purposes because of their striking blue or green colour.   The sulphate, however, has been taken with the hope of inducing abortion.   Workers in copper are said to suffer occasionally from toxic effects produced by inhalation of copper dust.   An outbreak of eighteen cases of gastro-enteritis occurred in a Liverpool factory canteen owing to the contamination of tea by copper from a corroded geyser.[45]

Symptoms

If 15 g of sulphate or subacetate has been taken, the following are signs and symptoms which may be looked for: pain in the mouth, oesophagus, and stomach; bluish or greenish coloration of the mucous membrane of the mouth; sickness, which produces a bluish or greenish vomit; there may be diarrhoea accompanied by colicky abdominal pains; convulsions and cramps of the limbs may sometimes occur.   If the case terminates fatally, death is preceded by convulsions, paralysis, or coma.   In chronic poisoning, which is but rarely observed even among workers in the metal or its salts, the main indications are on a parallel with salts of lead.   There are evidences of progressive emaciation, gastro-intestinal irritation, vomiting, loss of appetite, diarrhoea or constipation, a coloured line on the gums, and perhaps a coloration of the teeth, the colour being bluish, greenish, or purplish, may be found. The evidences of implication of the nervous system are also very similar to those from lead poisoning, namely, peripheral neuritis, and atrophy of the muscles of the shoulder, arm, and forearm, with wrist-drop in some cases.

Treatment

Empty stomach by emetic or tube. Potassium ferrocyanide, 600 mg in water, is recommended for its antidotal properties.   Treat symptoms along ordinary lines.

Post-mortem findings

Perhaps the most striking appearance is the bluish or greenish coloration imparted to the gastric mucosa. The mucous membrane is congested and injected, and occasionally shows eroded patches. The intestinal mucous membrane may share the same appearances. The coloration by bile may be mistaken for that of copper, but on touching copper staining with ammonia the blue colour becomes intensified or the green is changed to blue.

Analytical findings

Copper is an essential element in human metabolism and, therefore, any copper levels must be interpreted against the normal background present in all tissues. These levels are given in Appendix III. Values above four times the average should always be suspect though some may be caused by disease.

Fatal dose and time of death

14 g of subacetate, and 28 g of the sulphate, have caused death. The minimum dose has not been ascertained with precision but is probably of the order of 10 g. A child who swallowed an unknown quantity of copper sulphate died in four hours. A man who took 28 g died in twelve hours.

Illustrative case

A fatal poisoning[46] followed the injection of 9 ml of a 10 per cent solution of copper sulphate into a tuberculous fistula in a boy of six. There was severe parenchymatous injury of the heart, liver, and kidneys. Chemical analysis showed the bulk of the copper to be in the liver.

COPPER SULPHATE (*blue vitriol, blue stone*)

Properties and uses

The pure substance is a blue crystalline substance which is easily soluble in water (31·6 g/100 ml at 0°C). Copper sulphate is used in industry and to a limited extent in medicine where it appears as an astringent, a fungicide, or an emetic. Its use in the home is limited mainly to garden fungicides.

Symptoms

The solid form or very concentrated solutions act as a corrosive to a limited extent, otherwise the action is typical of an irritant (see under Copper).

Treatment

Usually emesis is spontaneous but if not, this should be provoked or the stomach may be washed out after giving milk or albumen. Potassium ferrocyanide is a useful precipitant.

Post-mortem findings

These are typical of a corrosive poison.

Analytical findings

The copper in the stomach may be estimated. The copper levels in other tissues may be measured but interpretation must be careful in view of the significant normal levels of copper in the body (see under Copper).

Time of death

Simpson[47] reports the death of a sixteen-month-old child, four hours after ingestion, and of a farm labourer twenty-four hours after exposure for $1\frac{1}{2}$ working days when he was spraying copper sulphate solution.

CORROSIVE POISONS

General action

There is more or less destruction of the parts with which the corrosive substance comes in contact, due to coagulation and destruction of protein and the extraction of water from the tissue. As a rule there is no remote systemic action, with the exception of shock. The signs and symptoms after swallowing a corrosive consist of burning, acute pain in the mouth, pharynx, oesophagus, and stomach, continuous retching and vomiting of shreddy blood-stained material, intense thirst, and probably some involvement of the air-passages. There will be signs of corrosion of the mouth or lips or both. Certain of the acids, being volatile, may readily act as irritant vapours. Consciousness is usually retained and death may result from shock, due to the extensive destruction of tissue, suffocation from implication of the larynx, or perforation of the stomach. Cicatricial contraction of the oesophagus is an occasional sequela.

Post-mortem findings

These may be expressed generally as signs of corrosion and partial destruction of the parts with which the fluid has been in contact and vary in extent from localised patches to extensive areas, particularly in the stomach.

MINERAL ACID CORROSIVES

Signs and Symptoms

The symptoms come on immediately. There is pain, which extends from the mouth to the stomach, gaseous frothy eructations, and brownish- or blackish-coloured vomit, sometimes mixed with portions of discoloured mucous membrane. There is intense thirst, the efforts to swallow in appeasing it causing difficulty and pain, and there may be considerable dyspnoea from swelling of the epiglottis and larynx. The mouth and lips are excoriated, their mucous membranes being sodden and discoloured, the colour depending upon the nature of the acid which has been swallowed. Articulation is often indistinct. If the acid has been taken from a spoon, or bottle, the lips may escape injury. The vomiting and retching being more or less continuous, the patient becomes prostrated, but the mental faculties usually remain clear until the terminal phase of the illness is approached. Death may result from convulsions, suffocation, exhaustion, shock, and from perforation of the stomach. Recovery may follow prompt attention but death may supervene subsequently from the effects of stricture of the oesophagus. When the ingested acid is weaker the intensity of the symptoms may be much less and some may well be absent.

General treatment

It is generally regarded as inadvisable to perform lavage in corrosive acid poisoning on account of the danger of resultant perforation. This is not a fixed rule but should be borne in mind. The specific circumstances of each case should decide the matter. For example, in a case seen very shortly after a strong acid has been swallowed, the potential benefit which might accrue from immediate lavage should probably be allowed to outweigh the possible danger of perforation. Alkalis, such as lime water, calcined magnesia, and milk of magnesia, may be employed, but alkaline carbonates which liberate carbon dioxide should not be used, on account of gaseous distension of the stomach. Later, diluent, demulcent drinks, such as barley-water, milk, or thin gruel, should be given freely. To combat respiratory failure, artificial respiration may be employed and oxygen used. When there is oedema of the glottis, tracheotomy may have to be performed. When there is circulatory shock, due to fluid loss and blood concentration, the patient should be given a continuous intravenous infusion of normal saline or saline with glucose. This should be maintained until the feeling of thirst has passed, the mouth is moist and urine is being secreted.   To alleviate pain, morphia should be administered with caution and other symptoms should be treated as they arise, including the administration of antibiotics, if necessary.

Post-mortem findings

The lips may be stained a yellow, whitish, or brownish colour. The mucous membrane of the mouth is corroded, the tissues being softened and discoloured, and the oesophagus is similarly affected. There may also be irregular patches of extravasated blood.   The gastric mucosa is frequently discoloured, and the colour variation will depend upon the nature of the ingested corrosive.   Extravasations of blood are common, and the mucous membrane is corrugated.   The stomach may be perforated.

OTHER CORROSIVE MATERIALS

The more common corrosive materials are described in the general text.   Table 6 gives a few facts about some of the less common ones.

Table 6.   Corrosive Materials

Compound	Description	Estimated fatal dose*	Comment
Acetic anhydride	Colourless liquid	ii	Irritant odour
Aluminium chloride	White solid	i	Deliquescent
Chromic acid	Red solid	i	Deliquescent
Formic acid	Colourless liquid	ii	Characteristic odour
Hydriodic acid	Colourless liquid		Often brown due to iodine
Hydrobromic acid	Colourless liquid	i	Often yellow due to bromine
Hydrofluoric acid	Colourless liquid	i	
Mercuric chloride	White solid	i	Not very soluble
Osmic acid	Yellowish solid	i	
Perchloric acid	Colourless liquid	i	
Phosphoric acid	Colourless liquid	i	Syrupy appearance
Potassium dichromate	Orange solid	i	
Stannic chloride	White solid	i	
Trichloroacetic acid	Colourless liquid	i	
Zinc chloride	White solid	i	
Calcium oxide	White solid	iii	
Calcium hydroxide	White solid	iii	
Cement, Portland	Grey-white solid	iii	
Ethanolamine	Colourless liquid	iii	
Sodium carbonate	White solid	iii	
Sodium phosphate	White solid	iii	

* i, under 5 g   ii, 5 to 20 g   iii, 20 to 60 g.

They have corrosive properties but also may have toxic reactions secondary to the corrosive effect and possibly much more important.

DI-ETHYL ETHER (*Ether*)

Ether is a colourless volatile liquid with a characteristic odour. It is less dense than water (0·7 g/ml) and slightly soluble (7·5 g/100 ml at 20°C) in it. The boiling-point is about 35°C and the vapour is very inflammable. Ether is widely used as a general anaesthetic. The use of ether as an intoxicant is not uncommon, and, like alcohol, a tolerance to quantity may be established by repeated use. It is much less toxic and much more rapidly stimulant in action than chloroform. Those who begin the habit take, at first, doses of about 10 to 15 ml, but when the habit is confirmed the amount may be several times this figure.

Symptoms

Death while under the influence of ether, employed as a general anaesthetic, is less frequent than in the case of chloroform and is brought about by paralysis of the respiratory centre. Only occasionally does death result from syncope as a direct result of ether administration.

Pulmonary complications, including bronchitis, bronchopneumonia, and, rarely, pulmonary oedema, sometimes follow ether administrations.

Treatment

The subject should be kept warm and given artificial respiration and oxygen. If convulsions occur, these may be controlled with barbiturates given intravenously.

Post-mortem findings

The viscera may show signs of congestion and smell of ether, but otherwise the findings are not characteristic.

Analytical findings

Ether may be found in the tissues or fluids. The lungs, as the main excretion route, are recommended.

Fatal dose and time of death

The fatal dose is not established but is probably somewhat over 30 ml. Anaesthesia is normally produced with a 6 to 7 per cent ether mixture and the dangerous level is somewhat above 10 per cent. Death may occur rapidly or be delayed and due to pneumonia, but death from liver damage is rare.

Note.   Dioxan (diethylene dioxide) is a colourless liquid miscible with water in all proportions. It is used as an intermediate in the synthesis of certain other compounds, as a solvent for waxes, resins, fats, oils, greases, celluloid, cellulose acetate or nitrocellulose, as a lacquer diluent, and sometimes as a fumigant. The fumes are irritating and have narcotic properties. The irritation affects the eyes and respiratory tract. Poisoning occurs when there is exposure to air in close proximity to the liquid contained in tanks and vats since high concentrations accumulate there.

Barber[48] reports five cases in workers who died from the effects of haemorrhagic nephritis and necrosis of the liver following Dioxan poisoning, after an acute illness lasting five to eight days.

DIGITOXIN

The glycosides from *Digitalis purpurea* (foxglove), a number of glycosides from other species, and some derived materials have similar reactions to digitoxin. Examples of the other species include *Digitalis lanata*, *Adonis vernalis*, *Convallaria majalis*, *Crataegus oxyacantha*, *Erysimum canescens*, *Strophanthus gratus* and *Strophanthus kombe*.

Digitoxin and the other glycosides of digitalis are obtained from the plant *Digitalis purpurea*. Its leaves, root and seeds contain the toxic glycosides, digitalin, digitoxin, digitalein, and digitonin, and other principles. From the leaves is obtained the glycoside digitalin, which, when pure, consists of fine white acicular crystals, has no odour, and possesses a bitter taste. Digitalin and digitoxin are the principal poisonous constituents. Digitalin is a cumulative poison. Its action is upon the heart, with prolongation of the systolic period in the cardiac cycle. It regulates the rhythm of the heart by depressing both excitability and conductivity. In toxic doses there is increased excitability of the heart with extrasystoles. It has been used homicidally.

Symptoms

These are nausea, vomiting, which may not, however, commence for two or three hours after taking the poison, followed by abdominal pains, and, perhaps, diarrhoea. The pulse-rate becomes remarkably slow and irregular. Consequent upon this condition of the heart, there is a feeling of faintness and praecordial oppression, the respirations become slow and sighing, the patient becomes drowsy, and the condition may gradually deepen into coma. Convulsions may precede death.

Treatment

The patient should be kept warm and at rest in bed. Atropine, 0·6 mg, should be given hypodermically, and stimulants or sedatives used as indicated by the condition of the patient. Potassium chloride may be given by mouth and, when indicated, lignocaine intravenously.

Post-mortem findings

The post-mortem findings are not characteristic.

Fatal dose and time of death

The fatal dose of digitalis (dried leaf) is probably a few grams. Digitoxin in quantities as small as 2 mg may prove fatal. If the victim survives beyond a day recovery is usually complete.

DIMETHYL SULPHATE

Dimethyl sulphate is a dense (1·33 g/ml) oily liquid which is colourless when pure but is often yellow due to impurities. It is almost insoluble in water and is hydrolysed by it to methyl alcohol and sulphuric acid. This material is used in the organic chemicals synthesis industry.

Symptoms

The symptoms of acute poisoning result from involvement of the central nervous, or cardio-vascular, system. The vapour also affects the kidneys and blood. Exposure to fumes causes lachrymation and coughing followed by convulsions, paralysis, and coma. Poisoning may also result from swallowing the fluid. A notable feature of poisoning by this substance is the delay in the onset of the symptoms following exposure and the rapidity of death after the manifestations of toxic symptoms.

Treatment

Any dimethyl sulphate in the skin should be washed off with copious amounts of soapy water for some considerable time (about 15 minutes). Any corrosion of the skin should then be treated as a burn. Treat other symptoms generally as they occur. Depressants should not be given.

Post-mortem findings

The mucous membranes may show corrosion similar to that found after sulphuric acid ingestion. Pulmonary oedema, liver and kidney damage may be present.

Analytical findings

The detection of excess sulphate may be significant, but interpretation must be carried out against the normal levels or those found after medication.

Fatal dose and time of death

The fatal dose is probably somewhat under 5 g. The safe level of the vapour in air is 1 p.p.m. Serious delayed intoxication may result from exposure to concentrations significantly above this. Death may be delayed for some days after exposure.

DINITROPHENOL

The material usually found is a mixture of isomers. The commonest, 2,4-dinitrophenol, is a yellow solid which is only very slightly soluble in water. The chief use is as a pesticide or weed killer. It can also be used as a slimming agent when taken internally, as it increases the metabolic rate. Many cases of poisoning have occurred. It aids the combustion of fat without exerting much effect on the protein constituents of the body. Some people may be sensitive to its use.

Symptoms

The symptoms of poisoning include flushing, with a feeling of warmth, sweating, and dyspnoea in acute cases. In the more chronic form of poisoning, debility, impaired vision, due to cataract, and peripheral neuritis are frequent.

In acute poisoning, pulmonary congestion and oedema, mild nephritic symptoms, and tachycardia have been reported. The hepatic and renal cells are frequently injured.

Treatment

This consists of gastric lavage with a 5 per cent solution of sodium bicarbonate, or a solution of 1 in 2,000 potassium permanganate. Dextrose and normal saline should be given intravenously. For cataract, ascorbic acid has been recommended. In certain cases, oxygen may be administered to relieve dyspnoea, and an ice pack employed to reduce febrile symptoms. The use of pentnucleotide has been suggested.

Postmortem findings

Purvine[49] reports the post-mortem findings in a suicidal case of a woman of thirty-six. These included congestion of the lungs, spleen, and kidneys. The gastric mucosa and the mucosa of the duodenum and upper part of the ileum showed small haemorrhagic areas. The tubular epithelium of the kidneys was swollen, the cells of the tubules were degenerated, and there was congestion of the glomeruli. Tainter and Wood[50] have reported that in one case the onset of rigor mortis was rapid, the body being rigid within ten minutes after death. In their experience, ecchymotic haemorrhages in the pericardium, endocardium, and pia-arachnoid membrane, may be found.

Analytical findings

Tissues or fluids may be analysed. In the case reported by Purvine a blood concentration of 120 mg dinitrophenol per 100 ml was reported.

Fatal dose

The fatal dose is about 1 g.

Note. 1. Di-nitro-*o*-cresol is a yellow solid which is very slightly soluble in water. This material which is used as a herbicide (DNOC) has properties and actions similar to di-nitro-phenol. Farago[51] reports a suicide where 30 g was ingested. The levels of dinitro-*o*-cresol found in the post-mortem materials were as follows:

Liver	31 mg/100 g
Blood	21 mg/100 ml
Urine	8 mg/100 ml

2. Picric acid (trinitrophenol) is a yellow solid which is slightly soluble in water. It is used in the manufacture of explosives and fireworks and in the dye industry. Industrial poisoning usually occurs by inhalation of fumes or dust. Clinically, it is used in the treatment of burns and certain skin conditions, but poisoning from this cause is unusual.

The symptoms are of a catarrhal nature, accompanied by epigastric pain, giddiness, and stomatitis. When swallowed, the symptoms are those of gastro-intestinal irritation. The skin will show a yellowish colour in varying degree.

Treatment consists of gastric lavage and the administration of albuminous fluids.

ERGOT

Ergot (*Secale cornutum*) is a fungus (*Claviceps purpurea*) which affects the ripe grains of certain cereals, especially rye, turns them black, and renders them poisonous. It contains at least 0·05 per cent of ergot alkaloids calculated as ergotoxine.

The action of ergot is that of a true ecbolic and emmenagogue. Among the active constituents of ergot are ergotinine, ergotoxine, ergotamine, ergotaminine, and ergometrine; in addition, histamine and tyramine are present. Ergotoxine promotes contraction of the human uterus at the end of pregnancy, but has little effect during the course of gestation. By contracting the arterioles, it eventually causes gangrene. It is the most important factor in ergot poisoning. Ergotamine has similar properties. Ergometrine is the principle chiefly responsible for the action of ergot on the uterus. Within a few minutes of its administration, it causes prolonged muscular contraction of the uterine muscle which is specially sensitive following delivery. It differs from the other alkaloids in ergot on account of the fact that it is less active in the production of gangrene.

Few fatal cases from acute poisoning have been recorded, and then only when large quantities of the drug have been taken. Von Storch[52] has reviewed a number of cases in which untoward sequelae have developed following the prolonged use of ergotamine tartrate on therapeutic grounds. In forty-two cases the sequelae were serious, and were similar to the milder form of convulsive ergotism. Overdosage appeared to be responsible in most instances.

Symptoms

The principal symptoms are pain in the stomach, nausea, vomiting, with or without haemorrhage, a weak, rapid pulse, a feeling of oppression in the chest, subnormal temperature, coldness of the body, muscular cramps, with impairment of sensation, gangrene of the toes or fingers, convulsive movements, stupor, delirium, convulsions, and coma.

Chronic symptoms include gastro-intestinal irritation, nervous exhaustion or excitement, sometimes amounting to mania, and dry gangrene of the fingers and toes.

Treatment

Free gastric lavage with diluted tannic acid, a purgative dose of magnesium sulphate or castor oil, mild stimulants, inhalations of amyl nitrite, and restoration of body heat. Intravenous dextrose has been recommended on account of hypoglycaemia often present in ergotism.

Post-mortem findings

The internal signs are extravasations of blood in the stomach, liver, kidneys, and abdominal cavity, together with evidence of gangrene of the fingers and toes.

Fatal dose and time of death

The fatal dose is probably about 1 g. However, ergotamine has produced serious conditions when only 40 mg have been used over a number of days. The safe limit is probably the order of 2 or 3 mg per day. Death may occur several days after poisoning.

Illustrative case

McKay[53] reports the case of a woman, aged thirty, who, thinking herself pregnant, obtained a 12-ounce bottle which she was told contained ergot, for the purpose of procuring abortion. She finished the contents of the bottle in a week, but without the desired effect. She got a stronger mixture, finishing it in seven days. Before it was finished her arms began to ache, her skin to itch, and her fingers to swell. Her left index finger became cold and showed cyanosis at the tip. The remaining fingers of this hand and also those of the other hand were similarly affected, and later several of them became gangrenous as far as the distal joints. She failed to abort.

ETHYL ALCOHOL (*Ethanol, alcohol*)

The term alcohol in popular use refers to ethyl alcohol, which is a colourless volatile liquid (b. pt 78°C) with a characteristic odour. It is used widely as a solvent and fuel and large quantities are ingested for its 'pleasant' effect. The available forms for this latter purpose cover almost all dilutions with water but are mainly below 50 per cent. These proliferate further under innumerable colours and flavours. The following Tables give an outline of the concentration of various types.

The ease with which alcohol can be obtained in a personally attractive form may result in the temptation to over-indulge. Fortunately alcohol is not very toxic and it does not, by itself, cause many fatalities. Somewhere in the region of a bottle of whisky taken rapidly is necessary to cause death in an average adult. However, as alcohol does appear to enhance the action of other drugs (e.g. barbiturates), fatalities of the types involving drugs and alcohol are common. Alcohol may cause

Table 7.   Common Beverages

Material	Approximate alcohol concentration (% v/v)
Shandy	under 1
Beers	2 to 6
Table wines	10
Fortified wines	16 to 20
(e.g. Sherry, Port) . . .	
Low-strength liqueurs . .	34 to 40
Standard spirits	
(e.g. whisky, gin) . . .	40
High proof spirits and liqueurs .	up to 57

Table 8.   Less Common Beverages

Material	Alcohol concentration %v/v	Comment
Home-made beer . .	5	These three drinks are rather richer sources of alcohol than is generally appreciated
Tonic wines. . .	15 to 18	
Home-made wines .	10 to 15	
'Red Biddie' . .	usually 10 to 40	A mixture of red wine and 'methylated spirits'
Various alcohol-based solvents . . .	over 75	May contain other organic solvents
Various cleaning or cosmetic materials with an alcohol base	all concentrations	May contain a wide variety of other solids, and liquids

people to be unable to save themselves from injury or death when normally they could be expected to do so.

Generally toxic effects follow ingestion, but inhalation and injection have also been responsible. When ingested it is absorbed from the stomach and upper intestine. This occurs rapidly when the stomach is empty, and the greater part of the alcohol will be absorbed within the first hour after ingestion. The rate of absorption will be affected by a variety of factors, including the condition of the stomach wall, the presence of food in the stomach, the quantity of alcohol taken, and its concentration in the drink. The presence of food in the stomach will retard absorption, milk being especially efficacious in this direction. A more rapid and complete absorption is to be expected with concentrated alcoholic drinks as compared with the dilute forms. Individuals habituated to alcohol may absorb it faster. After absorption the alcohol is rapidly distributed throughout the body, being least in the fatty tissues and bone. The concentration in blood reaches its peak within a half to one hour.

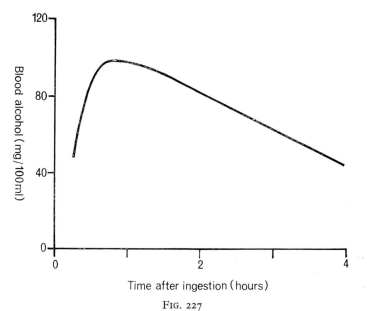

FIG. 227

The variation of blood alcohol level with time after a dose of 2·5 ml of 70° proof spirit per kg (6 fl oz/11 stone)

Alcohol is metabolised chiefly in the liver by an oxidation process. Renal or hepatic insufficiency may result in a lower handling capacity. The rate of destruction is reasonably constant for an individual and is of the order of 15 mg/100 ml of blood/hour. Unchanged alcohol is excreted in urine, sweat, saliva, and expired air and may be detected and measured in them. The amount removed by these means is small compared with the amount metabolised. Figure 227 shows a typical variation of blood alcohol levels with time. Statutary limits of 80 mg alcohol/100 ml blood and 107 mg alcohol/100 ml of urine have been fixed, over which it is an offence to drive a vehicle on a public road. Blood levels are also important because they are used as the basis for calculating the minimum dose taken. Table 9, below gives a list of concentrations and equivalent intake of 70° proof spirit in an eleven-stone man. Attempts to reduce the blood alcohol level by ingesting fructose are ill advised, as trials showed that no reduction takes place and there is an increased risk of nausea.

Table 9.   Alcohol Levels and Estimated Dose
of 70° Proof Spirit

| Level mg/100 ml | Minimum consumed vol. 70° proof spirit | |
	fluid oz	ml
50 . .	2·3	70
100 . .	4·6	140
200 . .	9·3	280
300 . .	13·9	420
400 . .	18·6	560
500 . .	23·2	700

Symptoms

Alcohol produces changes in the mental and physical processes accompanied by a degree of toxaemia. There is considerable personal variation in the reaction to alcohol and the time of onset of symptoms. Experiments on subjects drinking half a pint (284 ml) of whisky (70° proof) over a period of twenty minutes gave reactions varying from coma to no visible effect.

Small doses (under 120 ml of whisky) result in stimulation and a masking of inhibitions. Hesitancy disappears and there is a loss of circumspection and self-criticism. It should be noted, however, that these reactions are catalysed by the drinking environment. A sober person entering a party at which alcohol is freely available is instantly aware of an excess of noise and lack of inhibition though this disappears as his own blood alcohol rises.

Experiments on groups of people result in a similar state of affairs. Co-operation is less than would be expected and there is a decidedly informal atmosphere with much giggling by both males and females. Repeating the experiments on the same subjects but one at a time, results in markedly different behaviour although the blood levels are the same. There is complete co-operation but the subjects tend to be sleepy.

Large doses (280 ml) of whisky resulted in a similar situation but much more marked in all aspects. The physical disturbances consist of an inability to perform simple co-ordinated actions, the inco-ordination affecting the finer movements initially and thereafter showing itself in the simple acts of walking and balancing and the use of the upper limbs. Muscular fatigue develops more quickly and the reaction time to stimuli is lengthened. The speech becomes slurred in character until in the more advanced stages incoherence is present. The pupillary reactions are important. With well-established intoxication the pupils are usually dilated and sluggish in their reaction to light and accommodation. They may, however, be contracted and small, especially in the comatose stage. It is noted that at all times while conscious the subjects know exactly what they are doing or saying even when their actions or words are by no means normal. If the subject became nauseated all co-operation and interest is lost though tests not requiring co-operation can still be made. The subjects do not care what is done to them or what is happening. It is felt that in this state a person would not really care if he were involved in an accident or not.

In the comatose stage the chief signs are: deep unconsciousness; pallor of face, with occasionally some degree of cyanosis of lips; subnormal temperature; regular deep, but not stertorous breathing, and contracted pupils which become dilated with stimulation of the patient. This last reaction is known as Macewen's test and is absent in head injuries and other comatose states.

In the paralytic stage of acute alcoholic poisoning, there is commencing medullary paralysis, shown by such symptoms as slow, stertorous respiration, cold, clammy, cyanotic skin, dilated pupils, abolished reflexes, and almost imperceptible pulse. Death occurs from paralysis of the cardiac, or respiratory centres, or from the effects of pulmonary oedema.

Diagnosis of insobriety

If a legal limit of alcohol in blood or other material is fixed for the purpose of restricting certain activities, then diagnosis, from the point of view of the law, is a matter of analytical chemistry. Otherwise a number of tests are made on the subject to ascertain if his normal performance is impaired. Table 10 gives a selection of suitable tests which may be applied provided the examiner is satisfied that impairment is due to alcohol.

Being arrested and examined for drunkenness is a harrowing experience for an ordinary member of the public and he may not behave normally under these conditions. This must be allowed for in forming any conclusion, even if a second examination gives results at variance with the first one.

None of the tests give a conclusive result and under experimental conditions the only consistent result is an average increase in reaction time over the normal. Many subjects show positive results for a few tests but none gives a positive result for all the tests. The only test

Table 10.   Tests Used in the Diagnosis of Insobriety

Test	Details	Comments
Behaviour	General deportment and behaviour State of dress and any stains or soiling Speech and ability to say 'tongue-twisters' and difficult words Self-control	Important, as these are nearly always affected in cases of intoxication
Awareness	Memory for recent events Performance of a few simple arithmetic problems	The interpretation of this is difficult
Temperature	Read axillary temperature	May be useful in eliminating effects of disease
Skin	Note whether dry, moist, flushed or pale	Face is usually flushed and moist in earlier stages. With approaching coma pallor is present
Mouth	Record if smell of alcohol Abnormalities General state	In early stage there may be excess salivation. Later the mouth becomes dry
Eyes	General state Visual acuity Reaction to light Check convergence Nystagmus	May be injected. Reaction to light and accommodation becomes increasingly sluggish. Nystagmus is a valuable positive finding
Ears	Check for hearing defects	
Gait	Manner of walking Reaction to a command to turn Manner of turning	
Stance	Ability to stand with eyes open. Ability to stand with eyes shut	Alcohol impairs these at various levels. The effect may depend very much on the individual's 'natural' muscular control
Muscular co-ordination	Place finger on nose Place finger to finger Pick up medium-sized objects from floor Ability to button or unbutton garments Writing (which hand)	

Test	Details	Comments
Reaction times	Test if instrument available	These are always impaired; the difficulties are: the use of the instrument and knowledge of the individual's standard performance

giving a positive result for all subjects is that for nystagmus, and this is not present at any consistent time after consumption of the alcohol.

The final opinion should be based on the tests as a whole and may offer the examiner a difficult problem, especially if he is inexperienced.

Alcohol driving and the law

The ingestion of alcohol causes a drop in reaction time, efficiency, and the ability to instantly appreciate the dangers of a given situation. There is also an unjustified increase in confidence. These effects result in a dangerous lowering of the ability to control a motor vehicle. The Road Traffic Act, 1972 contains legislation which restricts driving by persons who have taken alcohol or drugs. This act includes sections dealing with impairment due to alcohol or drugs and with exceeding a statutory blood (or urine) alcohol limit.

The diagnosis of alcoholic intoxication, on clinical grounds alone, depends on the combination of a number of symptoms and signs which can be attributed only to alcohol, no single one of them being peculiar to this condition, except the odour of alcohol from the breath.

It is well known that an individual can react differently to the same amount of alcohol under different circumstances, and that the same amount of alcohol can produce different effects on different people under the same circumstances. Moreover, certain factors, such as the presence of food in the stomach, physical or mental fatigue, and the concentration of the alcohol in the drink, all can influence the absorption and action of the alcohol. Mentally unstable subjects, epileptics, and those who have suffered cerebral trauma at some earlier date may show an excessive reaction to small amounts of alcohol.

The combination of drugs of the barbiturate group and alcohol can enhance the symptoms of intoxication due to an additive action, and these drugs themselves, in overdosage and in chronic poisoning, may present a clinical picture similar to alcoholic intoxication. Further, a person who has taken no drink or drugs may well be thoroughly upset and act abnormally when taken off to the local police station.

All these points complicate the final decision and often result in a wide variation in expert opinion.

The law is as follows:

THE ROAD TRAFFIC ACT, 1972

Driving, or being in charge, when under influence of drink or drugs

5.—(1) A person who, when driving or attempting to drive a motor vehicle on a road or other public place, is unfit to drive through drink or drugs shall be guilty of an offence.

(2) Without prejudice to subsection (1) above, a person who, when in charge of a motor vehicle which is on a road or other public place, is unfit to drive through drink or drugs shall be guilty of an offence.

(3) For the purposes of subsection (2) above a person shall be deemed not to have been in charge of a motor vehicle if he proves that at the material time the circumstances were such that there was no likelihood of his driving it so long as he remained unfit to drive through drink or drugs.

(4) For the purposes of this section a person shall be taken to be unfit to drive if his ability to drive properly is for the time being impaired.

(5) A constable may arrest without warrant a person committing an offence under this section.

Driving, or being in charge, with blood-alcohol concentration above the prescribed limit

6.—(1) If a person drives or attempts to drive a motor vehicle on a road or other public place, having consumed alcohol in such a quantity that the proportion thereof in his blood, as ascertained from a laboratory test for which he subsequently provides a specimen under section 9 of this Act, exceeds the prescribed limit at the time he provides the specimen, he shall be guilty of an offence.

(2) Without prejudice to subsection (1) above, if a person is in charge of a motor vehicle on a road or other public place having consumed alcohol as aforesaid, he shall be guilty of an offence.

(3) A person shall not be convicted under this section of being in charge of a motor vehicle if he proves that at the material time the circumstances were such that there was no likelihood of his driving it so long as there was any probability of his having alcohol in his blood in a proportion exceeding the prescribed limit.

(4) In determining for the purposes of subsection (3) above the likelihood of a person's driving a motor vehicle when he is injured or the vehicle is damaged, the jury, in the case of proceedings on indictment may be directed to disregard, and the court in any other case may

disregard, the fact that he had been injured or that the vehicle had been damaged.

Evidence on charge of unfitness to drive

7.—(1) In any proceedings for an offence under section 5 of this Act, the court shall, subject to section 10 (5) thereof, have regard to any evidence which may be given of the proportion or quantity of alcohol or of any drug which was contained in the blood or present in the body of the accused, as ascertained by analysis of a specimen of blood taken from him with his consent by a medical practitioner, or of urine provided by him, at any material time; and if it is proved that the accused, when so requested by a constable at any such time, refused to consent to the taking of or to provide a specimen for analysis, his refusal may, unless reasonable cause therefor is shown, be treated as supporting any evidence given on behalf of the prosecution, or as rebutting any evidence given on behalf of the defence, with respect to his condition at that time.

(2) A person shall not be treated for the purposes of subsection (1) above as refusing to provide a specimen unless—

(a) he is first requested to provide a specimen of blood, but refuses to do so;

(b) he is then requested to provide two specimens of urine within one hour of the request, but fails to provide them within the hour or refuses at any time within the hour to provide them; and

(c) he is again requested to provide a specimen of blood, but refuses to do so.

(3) The first specimen of urine provided in pursuance of a request under subsection (2) (b) above shall be disregarded for the purposes of subsection (1) above.

Breath tests

8.—(1) A constable in uniform may require any person driving or attempting to drive a motor vehicle on a road or other public place to provide a specimen of breath for a breath test there or nearby, if the constable has reasonable cause—

(a) to suspect him of having alcohol in his body, or

(b) to suspect him of having committed a traffic offence while the vehicle was in motion;

but no requirement may be made by virtue of paragraph (b) above unless it is made as soon as reasonably practicable after the commission of the traffic offence.

(2) If an acident occurs owing to the presence of a motor vehicle on a road or other public place, a constable in uniform may require any

person who he has reasonable cause to believe was driving or attempting to drive the vehicle at the time of the accident to provide a specimen of breath for a breath test—

(a) except while that person is at a hospital as a patient, either at or near the place where the requirement is made or, if the constable thinks fit, at a police station specified by the constable;

(b) in the said excepted case, at the hospital;

but a person shall not be required to provide such a specimen while at a hospital as a patient if the medical practitioner in immediate charge of his case is not first notified of the proposal to make the requirement or objects to the provision of a specimen on the ground that its provision or the requirement to provide it would be prejudical to the proper care or treatment of the patient.

(3) A person who, without reasonable excuse, fails to provide a specimen of breath for a breath test under subsection (1) or (2) above shall be guilty of an offence.

(4) If it appears to a constable in consequence of a breath test carried out by him on any person under subsection (1) or (2) above that the device by means of which the test is carried out indicates that the proportion of alcohol in that person's blood exceeds the prescribed limit, the constable may arrest that person without warrant except while that person is at a hospital as a patient.

(5) If a person required by a constable under subsection (1) or (2) above to provide a specimen of breath for a breath test fails to do so and the constable has reasonable cause to suspect him of having alcohol in his body, the constable may arrest him without warrant except while he is at a hospital as a patient.

(6) Subsections (4) and (5) above shall not be construed as prejudicing the provisions of section 5 (5) of this Act.

(7) A person arrested under this section, or under the said section 5 (5), shall, while at a police station, be given an opportunity to provide a specimen of breath for a breath test there.

(8) In this section 'traffic offence' means an offence under any provision of this Act except Part V thereof or under any provision of Part III of the Road Traffic Act 1960 or the Road Traffic Regulation Act 1967.

Laboratory tests

9.—(1) A person who has been arrested under section 5 (5) or 8 of this Act may, while at a police station, be required by a constable to provide a specimen for a laboratory test (which may be a specimen of blood or of urine), if he has previously been given an opportunity to provide a specimen of breath for a breath test at that station under subsection (7) of the said section 8, and either—

(a) it appears to a constable in consequence of the breath test that the device by means of which the test is carried out indicates that the proportion of alcohol in his blood exceeds the prescribed limit, or

(b) when given the opportunity to provide that specimen, he fails to do so.

(2) A person while at a hospital as a patient may be required by a constable to provide at the hospital a specimen for a laboratory test—

(a) if it appears to a constable in consequence of a breath test carried out on that person under section 8 (2) of this Act that the device by means of which the test is carried out indicates that the proportion of alcohol in his blood exceeds the prescribed limit, or

(b) if that person has been required, whether at the hospital or elsewhere, to provide a specimen of breath for a breath test, but fails to do so and a constable has reasonable cause to suspect him of having alcohol in his body;

but a person shall not be required to provide a specimen for a laboratory test under this subsection if the medical practitioner in immediate charge of his case is not first notified of the proposal to make the requirement or objects to the provision of a specimen on the ground that its provision, the requirement to provide it or a warning under subsection (7) below would be prejudicial to the proper care or treatment of the patient.

(3) A person who, without reasonable excuse, fails to provide a specimen for a laboratory test in pursuance of a requirement imposed under this section shall be guilty of an offence.

(4) Nothing in the foregoing provisions of this section shall affect the provisions of section 7 (1) of this Act.

(5) A person shall not be treated for the purposes of subsection (3) above as failing to provide a specimen unless—

(a) he is first requested to provide a specimen of blood, but refuses to do so;

(b) he is then requested to provide two specimens of urine within one hour of the request, but fails to provide them within the hour or refuses at any time within the hour to provide them; and

(c) he is again requested to provide a specimen of blood, but refuses to do so.

(6) The first specimen of urine provided in pursuance of a request under subsection (5) (b) above shall be disregarded for the purposes of section 6 of this Act.

(7) A constable shall on requiring any person under this section to provide a specimen for a laboratory test warn him that failure to provide a specimen of blood or urine may make him liable to imprisonment, a

fine and disqualification, and, if the constable fails to do so, the court before which that person is charged with an offence under section 6 of this Act or this section may direct an acquittal or dismiss the charge, as the case may require.

In this subsection 'disqualification' means disqualification for holding or obtaining a licence to drive a motor vehicle granted under Part III of this Act.

Ancillary provisions as to evidence in proceedings for an offence under s. 5 or 6

10.—(1) For the purposes of any proceedings for an offence under section 5 or 6 of this Act, a certificate purporting to be signed by an authorised analyst, and certifying—

    (a) the proportion of alcohol or any drug found in a specimen identified by the certificate, and

    (b) for the purposes only of proceedings for an offence under the said section 5, in the case of a specimen of urine, the proportion of alcohol or of that drug in the blood which corresponds to the proportion found in the specimen.

shall subject to subsection (3) below, be evidence of the matters so certified and of the qualification of the analyst.

(2) For the purposes of any proceedings for an offence under the said section 5 or 6, a certificate purporting to be signed by a medical practitioner that he took a specimen of blood from a person with his consent shall, subject to subsection (3) below, be evidence of the matters so certified and of the qualification of the medical practitioner.

(3) Subsections (1) and (2) above shall not apply to a certificate tendered on behalf of the prosecution unless a copy has been served on the accused not less than seven days before the hearing or trial, nor if the accused, not less than three days before the hearing or trial, or within such further time as the court may in special circumstances allow, has served notice on the prosecutor requiring the attendance at the hearing or trial of the person by whom the certificate was signed.

A copy of a certificate required by this subsection to be served on the accused or of a notice required by this subsection to be served on the prosecutor may either be personally served on the accused or the prosecutor (as the case may be) or sent to him by registered post or the recorded delivery service.

(4) In any proceedings in Scotland for an offence under the said section 5 or 6 a certificate complying with subsection (1) or (2) above and, where the person by whom such a certificate was signed is called as a witness, the evidence of that person, shall be sufficient evidence of the facts stated in the certificate.

(5) Where, in proceedings for an offence under the said section 5 or 6 the accused, at the time a specimen of blood or urine was taken from or provided by him, asked to be supplied with such a specimen, evidence of the proportion of alcohol or any drug found in the specimen shall not be admissible on behalf of the prosecution unless—

(a) the specimen is either one of two taken or provided on the same occasion or is part of a single specimen which was divided into two parts at the time it was taken or provided, and

(b) the other specimen or part was supplied to the accused.

(6) A constable requesting any person to consent to the taking of or to provide a specimen of blood or urine for analysis shall offer to supply to him, in a suitable container, part of the specimen or, in the case of a specimen of blood which it is not practicable to divide, another specimen which he may consent to have taken.

(7) In this section 'authorised analyst' means any person possessing the qualifications prescribed by regulations made under section 89 of the Food and Drugs Act 1955, or section 27 of the Food and Drugs (Scotland) Act 1956, as qualifying persons for appointment as public analysts under those Acts, and any other person authorised by the Secretary of State to make analyses for the purposes of this section.

11. *Detention of persons while affected by alcohol*

Any person required to provide a specimen for a laboratory test under section 9 (1) of this Act may thereafter be detained at the police station until he provides a specimen of breath for a breath test and it appears to a constable that the device by means of which the test is carried out indicates that the proportion of alcohol in that person's blood does not exceed the prescribed limit.

Interpretation of ss. 6 to 11

12.—(1) In sections 6 to 11 of this Act, except so far as the context otherwise requires—

'breath test' means a test for the purpose of obtaining an indication of the proportion of alcohol in a person's blood carried out by means of a device of a type approved for the purpose of such a test by the Secretary of State, on a specimen of breath provided by that person;

'fail', in relation to providing a specimen, includes refuse and 'failure' shall be construed accordingly;

'hospital' means an institution which provides medical or surgical treatment for in-patients or out-patients;

'laboratory test' means the analysis of a specimen provided for the purpose;

'the prescribed limit' means 80 milligrammes of alcohol in 100 millilitres of blood or such other proportion as may be prescribed by regulations made by the Secretary of State.

(2) A person shall be treated for the purposes of sections 6 and 9 of this Act as providing a specimen of blood if, but only if, he consents to the specimen being taken by a medical practitioner and it is so taken and shall be treated for those purposes as providing it at the time it is so taken.

(3) References in sections 8, 9 and 11 of this Act to providing a specimen of breath for a breath test are references to providing a specimen thereof in sufficient quantity to enable the test to be carried out.

(4) For the purposes of the said section 6 and this section 107 milligrammes of alcohol in 100 millilitres of urine shall be treated as equivalent to 80 milligrammes of alcohol in 100 millilitres of blood, and the power conferred by subsection (1) above to prescribe some other proportion of alcohol in the blood shall include power to prescribe a proportion of alcohol in urine which is to be treated as equivalent to the prescribed proportion of alcohol in the blood.

13. *Person liable to be charged with offence under s. 5, 6 or 9 not liable to be charged with certain other offences.*

A person liable to be charged with an offence under section 5, 6 or 9 of this Act shall not be liable to be charged—

(a) under section 12 of the Licensing Act 1872, with the offence of being drunk while in charge, on a highway or other public place, of a carriage, or

(b) under section 70 of the Licensing (Scotland) Act 1903, with the offence of being drunk while in charge, in a street or other place, of a carriage.

Application to the Crown

188.—(1) Subject to the provisions of this section—

(a) Part 1 of this Act,

. . . .

shall apply to vehicles and persons in the public service of the Crown.

Application of ss. 6 to 11 to persons subject to service discipline

189.—(1) Sections 6 to 11 of this Act, shall in their application to persons subject to service discipline, apply outside as well as within Great Britain and have effect as if—

(a) references to proceedings for an offence under any enactment included references to proceedings for the corresponding service offence;

(b) references to the court included a reference to any naval, military or air force authority before whom the proceedings take place;

(c) references to a constable included references to a member of the provost staff;

(d) references to a police station included references to a naval, military or air force unit or establishment;

(e) references to a hospital included references to a naval, military or air force unit or establishment at which medical or surgical treatment is provided for persons subject to service discipline;

(f) in section 8 (1) the reference to a traffic offence included a reference to the corresponding service offence;

(g) in section 9 (7) the reference to disqualification were omitted and for the reference to directing an acquittal there were substituted a reference to finding the person in question not guilty without further proceeding with the case; and

(h) in section 10, subsection (4) were omitted.

(2) In relation to persons for the time being subject to service discipline the power to arrest conferred on a constable by section 5 (5) of this Act shall also be exercisable by a member of the provost staff and shall be so exercisable outside as well as within Great Britain.

(3) In this section—

'corresponding service offence', in relation to an offence under any enactment, means an offence under section 42 of the Naval Discipline Act 1957 or an offence against section 70 of the Army Act 1955 or section 70 of the Air Force Act 1955 committed by an act or omission which is punishable under the enactment or would be so punishable if committed in Great Britain;

'member of the provost staff' means a provost officer or any person legally exercising authority under or on behalf of a provost officer;

'persons subject to service discipline' means persons subject to the said Act of 1957, to military law or to air force law and other persons to whom section 42 of the said Act of 1957 or section 70 of either of the said Acts of 1955 for the time being applies;

'provost officer' means a person who is a provost officer within the meaning of the said Act of 1957 or either of the said Acts of 1955.

(The relevant penalties under the above Act are given in Appendix V.)

Notes

The following general points should be borne in mind by the medical practitioner:

1. Under the above act it is customary to have a medical examination if the charge is one of impairment.

2. The purpose of the examination is to attempt to reach an opinion as to whether the accused's apparent abnormality is due to drink, drugs, a combination of both, injury or illness.

3. It is essential that the consent of the accused should be obtained before proceeding to the examination. When possible the examination should be repeated when the accused has had time to recover from the effects of the consumption of alcohol.

4. The consent must be obtained in the presence of an impartial witness. The examination is then conducted in private and the points suggested in Table 10 can be used as a guide.

5. The doctor may be asked immediately after the examination to say whether the accused is impaired due to drink. He should not do this unless he is prepared to uphold his opinion against a blood or urine alcohol level which may not indicate agreement with his findings.

6. It is accepted that those who are habituated to alcohol can develop a degree of tolerance to it. While the physiological mechanism of this tolerance is not properly understood, the feature is frequently over-emphasised. Although the habituated individual may show much less evidence of intoxication than an abstainer, he is as likely to be unfit to control a motor vehicle properly when his blood alcohol concentration exceeds 150 mg/100 ml (0·15%).

7. If the accused refuses to be examined any opinion must be guarded.

8. It is necessary to obtain consent before taking blood or urine for analysis.

9. Blood samples must be taken by a practising doctor.

10. The specimen may be capillary blood taken by a skin puncture or venous blood taken with a syringe.

11. A suitable antiseptic which does not contain alcohol should be used.

12. If a skin puncture is used the blood should be allowed to drip into the containers.

13. Enough blood should be taken so that a sample suitable for analysis is available for the accused (at least 0·5 ml per sample for alcohol only and at least 10 ml per sample for drugs).

14. The containers should contain a suitable preservative.

15. The doctor has professional discretion about the site of sampling.

16. The lid of the sample container should be carefully secured.

The following general points should be borne in mind by the analyst:

1. The analyst must be sure that all his reagents and equipment are properly prepared for the analyses. Standards must be carefully checked.

2. The analyst should examine the sample received to see that it is properly sealed. He should also note any signs of damage whether they appear accidental or not.

3. The sample should be in reasonable condition. If kept too long blood appears as a blackish liquid. Excessive exposure to heat causes blood to set in the form of a light brown jelly-like material.

4. Both the conditions noted in 3 or a faulty seal may cause loss of alcohol or even leave the sample so that it cannot be analysed. Storage under normal conditions may result in an average fall of about 2 mg/100 ml per week. Occasionally there is no fall in the alcohol level.
5. Urine samples are much less trouble but are more easily tampered with.
6. The analyst should look out for the presence of other alcohols and solvents when carrying out the analysis.

Treatment

The stomach can be evacuated by lavage, with a weak solution of sodium bicarbonate. The intravenous administration of vitamin B6, 50 to 100 mg, may effect a rapid recovery or may restore a comatose patient to a near conscious state. In a proportion of cases coramine, 3 to 5 ml, can be given slowly, intravenously under medical supervision. Where there is dangerous respiratory depression oxygen can be administered continuously, the body warmth being maintained.

Post-mortem findings

In fatal cases there is congestion of the brain and internal organs, some of which may show cloudy swelling. On opening the cavities of the body, a distinct vinous odour is frequently noted. The gastric mucosa is congested and the contents have a vinous odour, especially after washing the stomach with warm water. The bladder is usually distended. On microscopical examination of the organs, fatty changes may be seen.

Analytical findings

Ethyl alcohol may be measured in any material available but blood and urine are those usually examined. The urine alcohol concentration found is normally accepted as being about 1·3 times the level in the blood. Blood levels are often reported after being derived using this conversion, but there has been some criticism with respect to live subjects[54] and there are often wide variations in post-mortem samples due to the progressing failure of the organism before death. As a result it is better to deal with either blood or urine as available without attempting any conversion except perhaps to enable a rough guide to the minimum dosage to be calculated.

The methods of sampling and storage are important, as poor handling techniques may be the basis of questioning a reported value. At the post-mortem examination care should be taken so that no contamination of samples can take place. Contamination may easily arise and sometimes does if concentrated solutions of alcohol from the stomach are spilled. The post-mortem diffusion of this alcohol from the stomach is also a possibility. Urine should always be taken if available as it is less likely to be contaminated and the suggested bacterial formation of ethyl alcohol does not complicate the picture. Incubation of post-mortem blood samples at 37°C for seven days can result in rises of as much as 40 mg ethyl alcohol per 100 ml of blood. The majority of samples show no change. If bacterial production has occurred by-products of the reaction may be found on analysis and a warning obtained. Alcohol concentrations may fall slightly on storage and it is accepted that an average fall of 2 mg/100 ml/week can be expected in blood stored under the conditions of the samples taken for the Road Traffic Act 1972, section 9.

Fatal dose

The fatal dose is in the region of 250 ml of ethyl alcohol, i.e. about one bottle of whisky (70° proof) taken over a short period. Table 11 gives a list of blood levels and probable effects.

Table 11. The Relation of Blood Alcohol to the Symptoms Produced

Blood alcohol (mg/100 ml)	Effects
50	Not many signs other than a flushed face. An inexperienced drinker may 'show off' while driving in company and so cause an accident
50 to 150	Talkative, fall in inhibitions and self-criticism, boisterous. Probably dangerous in control of a car
150 to 250 (280 ml (½ pint) of whisky taken)	Inco-ordination and all the above much more marked. In no condition to drive
200 to 300	Glassy eyes; reaching the stage of coma
300 to 400 (570 ml (1 pint) of whisky taken)	Coma; noisy breathing, low temperature
400 to 500	Paralytic; in danger of dying

Notes. 1. In dealing with the analyses of a very large number of defence samples of blood for driving offences it was found that only a few per cent of clients reported drinking alcohol in the quantities which the analyses indicated. This appears to be a rather convenient though unavailing effect on the memory.

2. Ethylene glycol (Glycol) is a colourless liquid which boils at

198°C. It is miscible with water in all proportions. It is freely available as a solvent and in the form of anti-freeze for water-cooled engines. Poisoning has occurred from accidental drinking of a comparatively large quantity or from its use as a substitute for ethyl alcohol in drinks. One hundred millilitres has been suggested as a fatal dose. Within the body it is oxidised to oxalic acid, and then to glycollic acid. In acute poisoning, the toxic effects are probably due to oxalic acid poisoning and depression of the central nervous system. The symptoms are vomiting, cyanosis, prostration, convulsions, coma, and respiratory failure. Severe kidney damage may occur, with extensive injury to the epithelium of the convoluted tubules, and lead to urinary obstruction and uraemia. Pons and Custer[55] have reported their experience of ten cases of fatal poisoning among soldiers who drank anti-freeze solution of the ethylene glycol type (Prestone) as an alcoholic beverage. Apart from one case, death occurred in from twenty-two to forty-four hours. In two cases there was incontinence of urine and faeces, in four, severe convulsive seizures, and in three, strabismus. In four cases the spinal fluid was blood tinged. Autopsy showed in all cases extensive oxalate crystallosis of the renal tubules, the kidneys were swollen, and the liver was enlarged. In all cases there was a moderate or marked pulmonary oedema. The authors have also seen a further eight fatal cases with similar findings. When death occurred within twelve hours, the renal damage was minimal, but if the patient lived for five days after ingestion, significant renal changes were present.

Treatment consists of gastric lavage; intravenous calcium gluconate; administration of alkalis and fluids; artificial respiration and oxygen therapy if indicated.

FLUORIDES AND HYDROFLUORIC ACID (*Hydrogen fluoride*)

Properties and uses

Pure concentrated hydrofluoric acid is a colourless liquid with an acrid vapour. The specific gravity is about 1·15. This material is necessary in many industrial processes and its use is expanding. It is not used in the home or in medicine. Sodium fluoride is the commonest salt and is usually in the form of a white powder which is reasonably soluble in water (4·2 g/100 ml at 18°C). This material and sodium silico-fluoride may be found in the home as part of insecticide powders or rodent killers.

Symptoms

Acute. The fumes from the acid are extremely irritant to the respiratory passages and lungs and cause pain in the throat, laryngitis, and bronchitis. There is also vomiting and collapse. Ulceration of the conjunctivae, nose, mouth, and gums is often produced. When the gas comes into contact with the skin, severe burns, which heal slowly, result. Sodium fluoride or sodium silico-fluoride is a protoplasmic poison which paralyses cellular respiration and deprives tissue of calcium by forming non-ionisable calcium fluoride. When it is swallowed, symptoms of gastro-intestinal irritation in acute cases may be very severe, vomiting, purging, and griping being common manifestations. There is dyspnoea, and respiration becomes rapid. The pulse becomes weak, and muscular cramps in the legs, sensory disturbances, paralysis, tremors, and convulsions may follow. Albuminuria is common. Unconsciousness precedes death from respiratory failure. When the acid is swallowed, the symptoms are similar, but there is usually a greater involvement of the respiratory passages and lungs due to the liberation of fumes.

Chronic. In cases of chronic fluorism, mottling of the dental enamel is characteristic, and sclerosis of the bones may result from fixation of calcium due to fluorine. Gastric symptoms may also occur.

Treatment

When fluorides have been swallowed, gastric lavage with lime-water, milk, or medicinal charcoal in suspension, should be employed. The use of calcium washes is recommended as this converts any fluoride ion to the insoluble calcium fluoride which is relatively non-toxic. Calcium should be given intravenously to counteract calcium losses due to combination with the fluoride ion. The administration should be continued for some time to allow for delayed reactions. Glucose should also be given intravenously to counteract hepatic glycogen depletion.

Post-mortem findings

When fluorides have been swallowed, there is usually a haemorrhagic gastritis with oedema and corrosion of the gastric mucosa and a dark crimson discoloration of the rugae. The upper part of the small intestine is frequently involved.

The acid produces such signs as ash-grey bleaching of the buccal mucosa, and denudation of the epithelium of the tongue, pharynx, and oesophagus. The gastric mucosa is in a similar condition to that already described, but there may also be marked corrosion and blackish discoloration, with submucosal haemorrhages. When the fumes have been inhaled, the respiratory passages and lungs are chiefly implicated and pulmonary congestion and oedema, together with congestion of the larynx and trachea, will be present.

Analytical findings

Fluoride concentrations may be measured in tissues and fluids and interpreted against the normal levels (Appendix III). In his extensive review Waldbott[56] mentions the depression of blood calcium levels as a result of fluoride exposure.

Fatal dose and time of death

The fatal dose is in the region of 5 to 10 g of sodium fluoride. With respect to the other fluorides, the more soluble ones approach the above level of toxicity and the less soluble ones are proportionally less toxic. Salts like calcium fluoride which are of very low solubility are virtually non-toxic. The maximum permitted level of hydrogen fluoride in the air is 3 p.p.m. Death occurs at any time from a few hours to days and depends on the severity of exposure.

Illustrative cases

Lidbeck, Hill, and Beeman[57] report a case of acute sodium fluoride poisoning in a hospital from the accidental use of 'roach' powder instead of powdered milk in mixing scrambled eggs. The mistake caused 263 cases of acute poisoning, 47 of which ended fatally. In many cases blood was present in the vomitus and stools. Death in most cases occurred two to four hours after ingestion. In some cases in which death was delayed and in some which recovered, there was paralysis of deglutition, spasm of the extremities, and carpopedal spasm. The egg mixture contained 3·2 to 13 per cent of sodium fluoride.

In 1930, smoke from a number of factories became mingled with a fog which hung over the Meuse Valley. Several thousand persons developed pulmonary symptoms and there were sixty deaths, chiefly among the elderly members of the community. Fluorine was regarded as the probable chemical cause of this, the 'Belgian Fog Disaster'.

Notes. 1. The toxicology of fluorine poisoning is the same as that for fluorides, but the maximum permissible level of this gas in air is only 0·1 p.p.m.

2. Fluoroacetamide and sodium fluoroacetate are used as rodenticides and poisoning by them resembles fluoride poisoning. There is a latent period ($\frac{1}{2}$ to 2 hours) before the onset of symptoms.

FORMALDEHYDE

Formaldehyde is a colourless gas which dissolves in water. It is this solution in water called 'Formalin' which is commonly known.

The concentrated liquid is colourless and contains about 40 per cent formaldehyde. On keeping at low temperatures a white polymer separates out from solution but may redissolve if the temperature is raised. The vapour has a characteristic, very pungent odour.

Formalin is used for disinfecting rooms, for preservative purposes and has a number of industrial applications. In the home it may be met with in the form of a woodworm killer.

Symptoms

The vapour provokes intense irritation of the mucous membranes and conjunctivae. Dyspnoea, bronchitis, and oedema of the lungs may also occur. Death from the effects of inhalation of fumes is exceptional. When strong solutions are brought into contact with the skin, dermatitis may result. Anuria is an occasional complication. When formalin is swallowed there is pain in the mouth, throat, and epigastrum. There may be vomiting and diarrhoea and the subject may be drowsy or collapse.

Treatment

Free gastric lavage with tepid water and a solution of ammonium acetate or diluted ammonia (1 ml in 150 ml of water). Some of this solution should be left in the stomach to combine with formaldehyde to form hexamine. When fumes have been inhaled, treat as for other irritant gases.

Post-mortem findings

The upper air-passages and lungs may be congested and oedematous. There may be bleaching of the tongue with eroded areas and haemorrhagic patches. The lower end of the oesophagus, the stomach and first part of the duodenum may be discoloured, excoriated, and indurated. The mucosa may show patchy desquamation and be thrown into folds. The blood vessels of the brain may be congested with punctate haemorrhages in the substance of the brain. Degenerative changes may also be found in the brain, liver, kidneys, and heart.

Analytical findings

Formaldehyde may be found in any of the fluids or tissues but is often absent due to its rapid oxidation. This oxidation proceeds by way of formic acid.

Fatal dose and time of death

The fatal dose of formalin is probably in the region of 30 to 60 ml. The maximum allowable concentration in air is 5 to 10 p.p.m., but much higher concentrations may be tolerated for short periods.

Death can occur at any time up to two days. Survival beyond this period is normally followed by recovery.

Illustrative case

A woman swallowed about 120 ml of a 40 per cent formaldehyde solution. She was collapsed and drowsy, but when roused, complained of great pain in the mouth, throat, and epigastrium. There was a strong odour of formalin from her breath. The stomach was washed out with 300 ml of water containing 4 ml of liquid ammonia. She vomited some blood-tinged fluid. She then became restless and emotional, and the pulse deteriorated. Later in the evening she became unconscious and died. Post-mortem examination showed a bleaching of the surface of the tongue, with eroded areas and haemorrhagic patches. The upper air-passages were markedly congested and definitely oedematous. The right chambers of the heart were engorged with dark blood. Both lungs and bronchi were acutely congested and oedematous. The gastric mucosa was congested and showed patchy desquamation. It was somewhat leathery to the touch.

GASEOUS AND VOLATILE POISONS

Irritant gases may be classified as follows:

Subgroup I includes those gases which act primarily upon the upper respiratory tract, for example, ammonia, hydrochloric acid fumes, sulphuric acid fumes, hydrofluoric acid gas, and formaldehyde.

Subgroup II includes those which act upon the respiratory tract, but also spread their action to the deeper structures, for example, sulphur dioxide, chlorine, bromine, iodine, and hydrogen sulphide.

Subgroup III includes those which act primarily on the lungs and only to a much less extent upon the upper respiratory tract, for example, nitrous fumes, phosgene, phosphorus trichloride, and arsenic trichloride.

Subgroup IV includes those which are not altered or destroyed by contact with the tissues of the respiratory tract, for example, the fatty hydrocarbons, their alcohols, ethers, and halogen substitution products, where important symptoms are induced by their action following absorption into the blood.

GOLD AND ITS COMPOUNDS

The metal and its salts have widespread, but specialised, uses in industry. Only the metal is commonly found in the home. The salts are used in medicine in the treatment of rheumatoid arthritis. The metal may be regarded as non-poisonous but death can occur from the use of the salts.

Symptoms

The toxic reactions comprise diarrhoea, vomiting, albuminuria, exfoliative dermatitis, aplastic anaemia, and occasionally agranulocytosis. Idiosyncrasy is quite common.

Treatment

The treatment consists in the administration of sodium thiosulphate either orally or by injection. British Anti-Lewisite (B.A.L.), dimer-captopropanol, is an effective antidote. In addition, treatment has to be directed along general and specific lines.

Post-mortem findings

In addition to the above symptoms, focal or confluent hepatic necrosis, necrosis of the renal tubular epithelium, peripheral neuro-pathy, and blood dyscrasias should be mentioned.

Analytical findings

Any of the fluids or tissues may be analysed for gold. A list of normal levels is given in Appendix III.

HYDROCHLORIC ACID *(Muriatic acid, Spirits of Salt)*

Properties and uses

The concentrated acid is a colourless fuming liquid with a pungent odour. It is more dense than water, having a specific gravity of about 1·2. The dilute acids look like water but may have the typical odour. The acid is used widely in industry but is not often found in the home, though it is contained in a number of soldering fluxes. Small quantities of hydrochloric acid are occasionally prescribed in medical practice.

Symptoms and treatment

These are described under Corrosive Poisons.

Post-mortem findings

The parts of the mucous membrane which have come in contact with the acid show, at first, a dirty-white or ash-grey colour, which later turns brown or black. Perforation of the stomach is not so frequently found as in the instance of sulphuric acid. In addition to the discoloration of the mucous membrane, patches of erosion, of varying depth and size, will also be found.

Analytical findings

These are usually restricted to an estimation of the total amount of hydrochloric acid present. Interpretation must be careful because of the natural presence of hydrochloric acid in the stomach and the abundance of chloride ion in the tissues.

Fatal dose and time of death

Death has followed ingestion of 4 ml but the fatal dose is probably 15 ml, though recovery following 90 ml has been reported. The fatal period is from four to thirty hours.

Illustrative cases

A woman, aged fifty, swallowed 90 ml of hydrochloric acid with suicidal intent. Six hours later she was taken to hospital in a collapsed condition. There were no signs of corrosion of the mouth or tongue. She died about eight hours after taking the poison. Post-mortem examination showed marked lesions of the epiglottis; the larynx was red, oedematous, and necrotic. The throat was markedly involved. The mucous membrane of the oesophagus was almost entirely destroyed. The external surface of the stomach was black in colour, there being haemorrhage into the peritoneal cavity. There was no perforation of stomach. Internally, its whole surface was almost black, this being more marked at the pyloric than the cardiac end. The duodenum at its commencement was involved.

A man, aged twenty-three, was admitted to hospital for oesophageal stricture. Four years previously he had swallowed about 120 ml of hydrochloric acid. Gastrostomy was performed, but he died ten days later. Post-mortem examination showed a stricture of the oesophagus, 6·5 cm above the cardiac end of the stomach. It was of a hard, fibrous, and annular character, and admitted a No. 15 catheter. There was also a similar stricture at the pylorus, which scarcely admitted a fine probe. The stomach was greatly hypertrophied and pouched at its cardiac end. The oesophagus showed only a slight degree of pouching.

HYDROGEN CYANIDE (*Hydrocyanic acid, Prussic acid*) AND CYANIDES

Hydrogen cyanide is a colourless liquid which is less dense than water (0·7 g/ml) and mixes with it in all proportions. The pure liquid boils at 26°C and the vapour has a strong odour variously described as peach-blossom, laurel-water, or bitter almonds. Hydrogen cyanide is a very weak acid but it does form cyanides of the form NaCN (sodium cyanide). Hydrogen cyanide is easily liberated from such compounds by the action of stronger acids. There are a number of complex cyanide compounds, e.g. $Fe(CN)_6^{3-}$ (ferricyanide), but these tend to be much less toxic, depending on the stability of the complex.

Amygdalin and emulsin exist in the kernels of various fruits, such as peaches, plums, and bitter almonds, and react upon one another in the presence of water to form hydrocyanic acid. It is also found in the leaves of cherry-laurel, a preparation of which is used medicinally, and which contains about 0·08 to 0·1 per cent. In oil of bitter almonds it is present in much larger percentage than in preparations from other fruits, the quantity of acid varying up to 10 per cent, but, for pharmacopoeial purposes, the amount of acid is adjusted to contain from 2 to 4 per cent. Eating bitter almonds has produced toxic effects on more than one occasion.

Sodium and potassium cyanide are used industrially in connection with electro-plating, coating silver, case hardening of steel and iron, and in tanning. Calcium cyanide is used as a fertiliser.

Of preparations likely to cause poisoning, oil of bitter almonds, potassium cyanide, used in photography, electro-plating, and gold-recovery, and hydrocyanic acid itself are the most common. Laurel-water has also caused poisoning.

Hydrocyanic gas, or hydrogen cyanide, in high concentration is a fulminant poison which causes very rapid death by paralysing the respiratory centre in the brain. In low concentration it may be detoxicated in the body as quickly as it is absorbed. The gas is capable of being absorbed by the skin, especially when moist with perspiration due to its ready solution in water, and that it is dangerous to remain too long in a high concentration even when wearing a respirator.

The fumigation of premises with hydrogen cyanide is a common practice. By the Hydrogen Cyanide (Fumigation) Act, 1937, which is applicable to both England and Scotland, whenever any accident occurs which occasions loss of human life or personal injury as the result of the fumigation of any premises or article, the person by whom, or by whose agent, the fumigation was carried out shall forthwith send, or cause to be sent, to the Secretary of State, notice of the accident and of the loss of human life or personal injury. The Hydrogen Cyanide (Fumigation) Regulations, 1951, make detailed provision as to the precautions to be taken in carrying out the fumigation of ships and premises.

Symptoms

These, to some extent, depend on the preparation which is swallowed, and its quantity. In large doses, the acid produces death almost immediately. There is rapid loss of consciousness and muscular power. Prolonged and deep, but jerky, respirations, cyanosis, irregular pulse, palpitation, coldness of extremities, dilated pupils non-reactive to light, convulsive seizures, and death form the usual clinical picture. A small quantity of fine froth may appear at the mouth.

In poisoning by potassium cyanide the rush of events is not quite so sudden, and minutes elapse before the symptoms commence. The principal symptoms include giddiness, dyspnoea, dilated and fixed pupils, convulsive seizures, and insensibility. The face is cyanosed, the jaws may be tightly clenched, the respirations are jerky, and the pulse is small and rapid. Death results from paralysis of the respiratory centre in the brain.

When a high concentration of hydrogen cyanide is inhaled a fatal result ensues in a few minutes. Vertigo, palpitation, and dyspnoea commence after a few breaths have been taken, and the subject falls to the ground in a state of unconsciousness. Convulsions usually occur, and death supervenes from paralysis of the respiratory centre and circulatory failure. When low concentrations are inhaled, there are usually transient symptoms of headache, vertigo, nausea, and mental confusion.

Hydrocyanic acid and the cyanides must be regarded as true protoplasmic poisons since they arrest the activity of all forms of living matter by inhibiting tissue oxidation and suspending vital functions. Asphyxia is caused by inhibition of tissue respiration, which accounts for the bright colour of the blood in the venous system, since oxygen is not abstracted from it by the tissues and it thus returns to the veins in arterial condition. Such poisons not only inhibit the enzymic activities, but also act upon the central nervous system.

Repeated exposure to non-lethal doses of cyanide may produce such clinical manifestations as headache, vomiting, diarrhoea, chronic cachexia, and mental disturbances.

Cyanide is metabolised quite rapidly to thiocyanate and in this form it is excreted.

Treatment

The principle to be aimed at in treatment is to convert haemoglobin into methaemoglobin so that the cyanide will combine with the latter compound to form non-toxic cyanmethaemoglobin.   10 ml of a 3 per cent solution of sodium nitrite should be administered slowly intravenously.   This should be followed by 25 ml of a 50 per cent solution of sodium thiosulphate intravenously and repeated if necessary.   If the above treatment is not available, inhalation of an ampoule of amyl nitrite, every three minutes, should be used.   p-Aminopropiophenone, or PAPP, has recently been recommended as an antidote since it apparently acts by forming methaemoglobin which then removes the cyanide ions from the tissues by the formation of cyanmethaemoglobin.

Following this line of treatment, when the poison has been swallowed, there should be immediate use of the stomach tube, and free lavage with warm water either alone or containing a 5 to 10 per cent solution of sodium thiosulphate, or a mixture of the sulphates (ferrous and ferric) of iron followed by a solution of potassium carbonate, to form Prussian blue, which is inert.   Emetics may be used if a tube is not available.   Ammonia inhalations, artificial respiration, and oxygen should be given to stimulate respiration.

Post-mortem findings

The face, including the lips, is of reddish colour and the body surface frequently shows pinkish, irregular patches which are not so pronounced as in carbon monoxide poisoning.   Internally, the signs are remarkably negative, except that the lungs and right side of the heart are engorged.   The odour of prussic acid will probably be perceived on opening the chest cavity, and from the contents of the stomach.   The mucous membrane of the stomach may be of a reddish colour, and the other organs, together with the blood, are usually of the same shade.   Cyanides are rapidly altered in the body after death since they unite with sulphur to form sulphocyanides.

Analytical findings

Fluids or tissues may be analysed for cyanide, bearing in mind that the method should distinguish between cyanide and sulphocyanide which is normally present in small amounts.   Bonnichsen and Maehly[58] report on some thirty-one fatal potassium cyanide ingestion cases where analyses of blood was carried out. The range found was 0·4 to 16·0 mg CN^- per 100 g of blood and the mean value was 3·5 mg/100 g. They also report on seven poisonings involving other cyanide sources and here the range is from 0·2 to 0·5 mg/100 g.   Tompsett[59] reports two non-fatal cases where the blood levels found on hospital admission were 0·36 and 0·21 mg HCN/100 ml of blood.   Reported values for tissues such as brain, kidney, and liver are in the same range as those quoted by Bonnichsen for blood.

Fatal dose and time of death

The smallest dose which has proved fatal is 40 mg of the anhydrous acid. However, recovery has followed doses of 80, 140, and 300 mg. It may be taken that the fatal dose is somewhat under 100 mg of the anhydrous acid. 8 ml of oil of bitter almonds killed a man in seventeen minutes. 300 mg of potassium cyanide have killed but recovery from larger doses is reported. Hydrogen cyanide concentrations about 120 p.p.m. are fatal within an hour and 3,000 p.p.m. are rapidly fatal. When a large dose of the acid is swallowed death may occur almost immediately. In acute poisoning, two to five minutes may elapse, but when smaller doses of the cyanides have been taken, death may not result for from twenty minutes to an hour. In a case of suicide, in which a woman swallowed a weak preparation of the acid, death did not ensue for forty minutes. In another suicidal case, life was prolonged for three and a half hours after swallowing the poison which was mixed with milk. A case of fatal poisoning[60] with a solution of potassium cyanide absorbed through the skin of the legs due to its accidental presence in rubber boots has been reported.

HYDROGEN SULPHIDE (*Sulphuretted hydrogen*)

Hydrogen sulphide, one of the most poisonous of gases and found in many industries, is a colourless gas with an odour resembling rotten eggs and may be evolved whenever organic material decomposes. It is heavier than air and tends to collect in vats and cellars. When mixed with air it is inflammable. The oil industry is a common source of accidental poisoning. Poisoning by inhalation occurs in workmen employed in chemical works, and in connection with sewers. While sewer-gas is a mixture of several gases, hydrogen sulphide is undoubtedly the most lethal. When sewers are badly ventilated, oxygen is reduced, nitrogen increased, and carbon dioxide is present in large amount, together with the sulphides of hydrogen and ammonia. The symptoms of poisoning depend on the proportion of those gases present. When concentrated mixtures are inhaled, there is profound depression of the central nervous system and death may be immediate. If diluted lividity is usually well marked, and there are fixation of pupils and insensibility, often accompanied by convulsions. Even in small percentages, hydrogen sulphide prejudices the health of those constantly exposed.

Symptoms

This is both an irritant and general poison. Its immediate lethal toxicity is not much below that of hydrocyanic acid. The symptoms of acute poisoning develop quickly and consist of dyspnoea, cyanosis, and other asphyxial signs, due to stimulation of the vagus nerve, and direct irritant action upon the alveolar mucous membrane of the lungs which causes a progressive pulmonary oedema.   Convulsions are frequent.   Hydrogen sulphide does not combine with oxyhaemoglobin, but only with methaemoglobin, and the presence of sulphaemoglobin is largely the result of post-mortem changes.   The gas also acts upon the nervous system, and in cases of subacute poisoning, psychic manifestations may develop and accompany bronchitis, and other symptoms of respiratory tract irritation.   In cases of acute poisoning, the cause of death is asphyxia, the result of paralysis of the respiratory centre.

Treatment

In acute cases the principal line of treatment is the administration of artificial respiration and the use of oxygen.   Bronchitis and bronchopneumonia require the usual lines of treatment when they arise as complications.

Post-mortem findings

These are chiefly asphyxial signs.   An odour of the gas will be perceptible, and putrefaction is rapid.   There will be evidence of respiratory irritation and the lungs will be congested and oedematous. In some cases the tissues and liver may present a greenish-grey or ashen tint due to the post-mortem combination of hydrogen sulphide and methaemoglobin.

Analytical findings

These are complicated by the possible presence of hydrogen sulphide as a decomposition product.

Fatal dose and time of death

A concentration of between 100 and 400 p.p.m. causes irritation of the eyes, nose, and throat, one of 500 p.p.m. will induce headache, giddiness, excitement, inco-ordination in walking, diarrhoea and painful micturition, after about thirty minutes, a concentration exceeding 500 p.p.m. will cause severe poisoning, while concentrations of 1,000 to 3,000 are rapidly fatal.

Note.   The intense smell of hydrogen sulphide is no guide to the concentration, as the ability to detect it falls rapidly with time of exposure.

INSECTICIDES—ORGANOCHLORINE

A large number of chlorinated hydrocarbons are available for use as pesticides. The most common for garden use are DDT (dichloro-diphenyltrichloroethane) and BHC (hexachlorocyclohexane). Many more are used in agriculture, a few of the more common being Aldrin, Chlordane, Dieldrin, and Heptachlor. Poisoning may be caused by ingestion or absorption by way of the skin. The toxicology is often complicated by the action of the organic liquid in which the material is dissolved.

Symptoms

The symptoms vary a little from compound to compound but may be generalised as emesis, excitement and tremors, and possibly convulsions.

Treatment

Treatment includes gastric lavage with water or vigorous scrubbing with soapy water to remove skin contamination. Convulsions are controlled with normal anticonvulsants.

Post-mortem findings

The most significant finding is liver damage. Fatty degeneration of the myocardium and kidney damage may also be found.

Analytical findings

The organochlorine compounds may be found but interpretation should take into account the possibility of general contamination from the environment, especially if the subject was industrially exposed. Most levels are below 10 p.p.m.[61] but healthy adults have been reported as having over 500 p.p.m. chlorocarbon in their fat.

Fatal dose and time of death

The chlorinated hydrocarbons are on the whole less toxic than the organophosphorus compounds. The toxic doses vary from about a gram in the case of Aldrin to somewhat over 30 g in the case of DDT. The fatal period varies from a few hours to two days.

INSECTICIDES—ORGANOPHOSPHORUS

Some dozens of organic phosphates are now available for use as pesticides. By far the most common in garden use is malathion.

Many others are used in agriculture, some of the more common ones being parathion, malathion, demeton-s-methyl, dimenthoate, and TEPP. Organic phosphates inhibit cholinesterase, thus permitting an accumulation of acetylcholine. Toxic reactions result from absorption by way of the stomach, lungs, open wounds, or contact with mucous membranes, the eyes, or the skin.

Symptoms

The symptoms include headache, salivation, giddiness, and blurred vision. The pupils may be pinpoint and non-reactive. The victim may believe that he is going blind. There may be nausea and abdominal cramps, vomiting, sweating, muscular twitchings, delirium, coma, and death.

Treatment

The principal line of treatment is to inhibit the action of the poison by the administration of atropine sulphate together with other therapeutic measures. The recommended dose of atropine sulphate depends on the stage of poisoning and varies from $\frac{1}{2}$ to 2 mg by intramuscular injection, or by the intravenous route in very serious cases. As an initial dose, $\frac{1}{2}$ to 1 mg should be administered subcutaneously and at two-hourly intervals if the condition of the patient remains unsatisfactory. In addition, a specific cholinesterase reactivator should be given intramuscularly or intravenously as early as possible. For this purpose P.A.M. (2-pyridine aldoxine methiodide) should be used. A dose of 1 g as a 5 per cent solution in water by intravenous injection has been recommended.

Post-mortem findings

The pupils may be contracted and there may be severe pulmonary oedema. Cases have occurred where there has been frothing at the mouth and nose resembling drowning (see p. 155).

Analytical findings

There are two analytical approaches. The first is concerned with the reduced blood cholinesterase activity. The second deals with the search for the actual organic phosphate. The first is used as a diagnostic aid and the second for the identification of the poison and its concentration. These phosphates are not natural products of the metabolism but may be present in small amounts due to food contamination so the interpretation of the analysis results should take this into account. A fall to 20 per cent of the cholinesterase levels is usually found when symptoms are present.

Fatal dose and time of death

The fatal dose of the organic phosphorus insecticide varies widely from compound to compound. The selection in Table 12 illustrates the likely values.

Table 12. Fatal Doses of Organophosphorus Insecticides

Material	Estimated fatal dose
Chlorthion	Tens of grams
Dimefox	Under a gram
Dimenthoate	Tens of grams
Ethion	Over a gram
HEPT	Tens of milligrams
Malathion	Tens of grams
Parathion	Tens of milligrams
Systox (Demeton) . . .	Tens of milligrams
TEPP	Tens of milligrams

Somewhat under 10 g of malathion have caused death but the fatal dose is probably nearer 60 g.

Van Hecke[62] and others report the death of a young man within an hour of ingesting 300 to 500 mg of parathion. Deaths have been reported following exposure of the skin during handling of parathion and the other highly toxic compounds for agricultural purposes. The time factor in these cases is of the order of a day.

Note. Tri-ortho-cresyl-phosphate is used in industry as a plasticiser for pyroxylin lacquers, and in the recovery of phenol residues from gas-plant effluents. It is a colourless, odourless, oily-looking liquid of low volatility. Cases of industrial poisoning have occurred. It is a lethal poison if swallowed in sufficient quantity, the fatal dose being about 1 g/kg of body-weight. The first symptoms are gastro-intestinal disturbances which are followed by a symptomless period. Some ten to fourteen days after ingestion, further symptoms develop, namely, general weakness, tingling, burning, and tenseness of hands and feet. Paralysis of these extremities next supervenes, termed 'Jake paralysis,' which is irreparable and can only be treated symptomatically or orthopaedically. Severe cases are bed-ridden. In order of frequency, the muscles affected are those supplied by the sciatic nerve, the intrinsic muscles of the hands, and the radial extensors.

In 1930–31, fifteen thousand persons were affected with 'ginger-paralysis' in California, due to drinking ginger liqueur containing this compound. Ten persons died. The substance has been found in cotton-seed oil.[63] Triphenyl phosphate apparently has similar toxic properties.

IODINE

Iodine is a black crystalline solid which is only slightly soluble in water but dissolves in a solution of potassium iodide. This is a deep brown liquid as is the alcoholic solution. Solutions in solvents such as carbon tetrachloride are pink. Iodine when heated does not melt but changes directly to the gas which is dense and has a violet colour. Liquid preparations of iodine, such as the liniment or tincture, have been used for suicidal purposes, and cause corrosion of the parts with which they come in contact on swallowing. Iodine vapour is very irritant to the respiratory tract. Its potassium salt, largely used in medicine, has given rise occasionally to dangerous symptoms. In these cases, the doses were not exceptionally large, and the exaggerated action would seem to be associated with personal idiosyncrasy.

Symptoms

When iodine is swallowed the symptoms are those of a corrosive and irritant poison. Inflammation of the mucous membrane of the mouth, pharynx, oesophagus, and stomach, accompanied by dark brown or yellowish staining of the parts, an intense, burning pain in the mouth, oesophagus, and stomach, vomiting, and signs of shock commonly occur.

Treatment

Treatment consists of free gastric lavage with starchy fluids, and the rest of the treatment should be conducted along general lines.

Post-mortem findings

The findings are typical of a corrosive poison.

Analytical findings

Iodine may be detected but, if not found, a quantitative evaluation of iodide gives a useful indication.

Fatal dose

4 ml of the tincture has caused death but recovery has followed ingestion of 30 ml. Maximum permissible concentration in the air is about 0·1 p.p.m.

IODOFORM

Iodoform is a yellow, crystalline solid with a characteristic odour. It is only slightly soluble in water but readily soluble in alcohol. It is used in medicine as a mild antiseptic. Systemic intoxication may result from use over a large area of skin.

Symptoms

The symptoms include headache, nausea, confusion, delirium, coma, and death. Taken by mouth there may be gastro-intestinal irritation accompanied by skin eruptions and a rise of temperature.

Post-mortem findings

The post-mortem findings include nephritis and fatty degenerative changes in the liver.

Fatal dose

The fatal dose is estimated to be in the region of 2 g.

IRON AND ITS COMPOUNDS

Iron is the most widely used and available metal. The commonest salts are ferrous sulphate and ferric chloride and both have caused a number of deaths especially among children. In the home, the source of iron poisoning is from one of the many 'iron' preparations used in medicine. Sugar-coated tablets containing either ferrous sulphate or a salt of some organic acid (e.g. ferrous succinate) are typical.

Symptoms

The clinical manifestations usually consist of vomiting, thirst, restlessness, and collapse. The vomited material may be of a brownish colour or may, after a short period, contain fresh or clotted blood.

Hurst[64] reports the case of a woman, the subject of severe simple achlorhydric anaemia following gastro-jejunostomy, who was treated by the administration of 11 g of iron ammonium citrate daily, and who suffered an acute cerebral attack, closely resembling lead encephalopathy, after she had been under treatment for three weeks.

Although a similar case has not previously been recorded, the symptoms were regarded as due to iron poisoning. The patient completely recovered and was subsequently given smaller doses of iron, when finally the anaemia disappeared.

It should be noted that fatal collapse may follow apparent recovery, so the patient must be watched for forty-eight hours. A dangerous and later complication in children is the development of pyloric stenosis. Operation has been performed successfully in a number of these cases.

Treatment

Gastric lavage with sodium bicarbonate to convert the ferrous sulphate to ferrous carbonate. An emetic should be given and the intake of bland fluids encouraged. In addition, the application of warmth and the use of cardiac stimulants form the principal line of treatment. When breathing is embarrassed, the use of oxygen is frequently beneficial. A course of penicillin treatment should be rapidly initiated when pneumonic complication threatens. The use of edathamil has been recommended.[65] Desferrioxamine is a more effective chelating agent. The recommended treatment is given in a leading article of the *British Medical Journal*.[66]

Post-mortem findings

The stomach may contain coffee-ground material, since it is very often the seat of an acute haemorrhagic gastritis. The intestinal tract shows a varying degree of vascular engorgement and oedema, while the contents reveal blackish-coloured staining. Degenerative changes, verging from cloudy swelling to complete necrosis, are found in the liver, which may have assumed a yellow tint. The kidneys are frequently in a state of cloudy swelling, while small, irregular haemorrhages may be present on the surface of the heart, lungs, thymus, and aorta. Pneumonic consolidation of one or more lobes of the lungs is not an infrequent finding.

Analytical findings

Apart from massive amounts of iron found in the stomach any levels found in the fluids or tissues must be interpreted carefully against the normal concentration. A list of the normal concentrations is given in Appendix III.

The levels found three days after ingestion of over 6 g of iron in the form of ferrous fumarate were as given in Table 13.

Table 13.   Iron in Post-mortem Materials

Material	Iron content
Whole blood	68·4 mg/100 ml
Brain (wet)	36·1 μg/g
Liver (wet)	236 μg/g
Kidney (wet)	55·3 μg/g

Fatal dose and time of death

The fatal dose is uncertain due to the resultant vomiting, but is probably in the region of 5 g iron, in the form of some soluble salt, for adults.   In the case of a fifteen-year-old girl quoted below, death occurred three days after ingestion of over 20 g of ferrous fumarate. Forbes[67] has published an interesting paper in which he describes details of two fatal cases of acute ferrous sulphate poisoning in children aged three years and one year.   In the first of these the child was thought to have swallowed fifty tablets each containing 200 mg of ferrous sulphate and in the second, thirty to thirty-five tablets of the same preparation.   Death occurred after some fifty-three and thirty hours, respectively.   In both cases some tablets were returned in the vomitus.

Illustrative case

A fifteen-year-old girl ingested over 20 g of ferrous fumarate tablets. She soon became ill and her condition worsened until she died three days later.   Post-mortem examination showed the tongue stained with altered blood.   There was a considerable quantity of this material in the larynx and trachea.   The stomach and the whole length of the alimentary canal also contained the altered blood.   The liver was pale with bright yellow areas of necrosis.   The gall-bladder was filled with tarry bile.   There were multiple haemorrhages in the parietal pericardium and the visceral pericardium.   The analytical findings are quoted in Table 13.

IRRITANT POISONS

General action

The onset of signs and symptoms, which is variable, is usually within half an hour to an hour.   They are indicative of gastro-intestinal irritation, and consist of severe pain over the epigastrium and abdomen, associated with, or followed by continuous and painful vomiting and diarrhoea. The vomited matter at first consists of normal stomach contents, but later becomes bilious in character and may be of a 'coffee-grounds' appearance due to altered blood. Over the track of the oesophagus there is a feeling of heat and constriction which provokes thirst, but drinking only induces further vomiting. The diarrhoea consisting at first of loose stools, and later of stools mixed with blood, accompanied by tenesmus, is severe and urgent. After some time the patient begins to show signs of shock, the pulse becomes thready and irregular, the skin clammy and cold, and cramps may affect the muscles of the limbs. During this period the mind of the patient remains clear, but unconsciousness, preceded or succeeded by convulsions, usually precedes death. The period before death is variable, depending upon the quantity of poison taken, and the condition of the patient at that time. Death may be due to cardiac failure through involvement of the myocardium, by the direct action of the poison, or indirectly by the effects of general prostration.

Fluid is lost from the blood which becomes concentrated, and the blood-pressure falls. The fluid loss is due to vomiting, diarrhoea, sweating, and inability to drink.

Post-mortem findings

These consist of inflammatory changes chiefly in the stomach, and frequently in the duodenal and rectal portions of the intestinal tract, especially in the latter.

LEAD AND ITS COMPOUNDS

The principal salts of lead which produce toxic effects are the acetate, the oxide converted into the oleate, in the form of diachylon, the carbonate or white lead, the tetroxide or red lead, the yellow chrome or chromate of lead, and lead arsenate. The chloride and nitrate, not being easily procured by the public, do not bulk so largely in medico-legal work. All lead salts are less irritant in action than those of arsenic, but the acetate and chromate are more irritant than the other lead salts. Chronic lead poisoning is quite common in the industries in which lead is used or handled in one form or another, for example, in lead-grinding works, potteries, paint factories, diamond-cutting, japanning, lacquer works, dye-works, in which lead chromate is used, coach-building, tinning, and enamelling works, plumbing, file making, and in electric accumulator works. Lead may gain access to the body by inhalation, ingestion, or by the skin when damaged. Lead poisoning is a notifiable disease and its occurrence must be reported to the Home Office. Inhalation of lead dust or fumes is most frequent in industry, more especially in the manufacture of white lead, the smelting of metals, and ship-breaking in which oxy-hydrogen burners are in use. It has been estimated that workers may inhale lead fumes to the extent of 215 mg of lead in eight hours' work with oxy-hydrogen flame upon paint, when employed in breaking up ships, thus severe symptoms of lead intoxication may appear quickly. Lead vapour is liberated from lead when it is heated to temperatures above 700°C.

Symptoms

Acute. Lead acetate and other lead salts in large doses produce an astringent metallic taste in the mouth, a burning, pricking sensation in the throat and oesophagus, and a similar sensation in the stomach, with pain, succeeded after an interval by nausea and vomiting, the vomited matter being latterly streaked with blood. Diarrhoea may supervene early. There is dryness of the fauces and great thirst. Colicky pains develop in the abdomen, the abdominal walls are tense and contracted, and the pains are relieved by pressure. Instead of looseness of the bowels, there may be constipation, the stools being black, and having a very offensive odour. Symptoms of collapse set in before death. Should, however, the case be protracted, arthralgia may develop, and there are likely to be numbness and paralysis of the limbs. Convulsions, delirium, or coma may precede death.

Chronic. These may be summed up as follows: Colic, which is very intense; general malaise, prostration, anaemia, debility, and loss of weight; obstinate constipation; gradual emaciation; anorexia; sallowness of face; in most cases, there is a blue line on the gums, but this is not constant. In the presence of oral sepsis, the line appears close to the gum margin. The line is not seen in the presence of healthy teeth, in edentulous subjects or at points where teeth are absent. The blue colour is due to the action of sulphuretted hydrogen generated by decomposing protein food around septic teeth in the presence of circulating lead. A blue line may also be met with in mercury and bismuth poisoning. The pulse is usually slow and hard and the blood pressure elevated, the result of constriction of the vessels caused by the action of lead on the neuro-vascular system. The nervous symptoms, almost characteristic, are 'wrist-drop', due to paralysis of the extensors and supinators of the forearms, accompanied by muscular atrophy, tremors, cramps, and shooting pains in the limbs. We have seen several cases, occurring among pottery-dippers, in which the scapular muscles and those of the arms were very atrophied. There may be paralysis of the limbs.

Early mental changes may manifest themselves and include headache, irritability, and lethargy. Lead encephalopathy sometimes occurs, especially in young subjects. This disturbance of cerebral function may give rise to recurrent convulsions, and progressive mental deterioration.

In a large number of cases of acute and chronic poisoning, punctate basophile staining of a number of the red cells will be found, and there is diminution of haemoglobin and of the red cells. Punctate basophile staining may occasionally be seen in poisoning by benzol and aniline. The polymorphonuclear leucocytes are decreased and lymphocytes increased. There may be evidence of vacuolation of the red cells and poikilocytosis.

Treatment

In the acute phase, the stomach must be emptied by emetics, or preferably by stomach tube. The ingoing water should be mixed with magnesium sulphate, to give a concentration of 0·6 per cent. This forms the insoluble sulphate. After the preliminary treatment has been completed, demulcent drinks and milk should be given, and the remainder of the treatment regulated as symptoms indicate. High colonic lavage may be usefully employed. Morphia may be given to relieve abdominal pain.

Former treatment was directed to the process of 'de-leading'. This was effected by raising and lowering the calcium intake, the excretion of lead, deposited in the bones, being controlled and its elimination regulated to obviate serious recurrent symptoms of lead poisoning during the process.

Calcium disodium ethylene diamine tetra-acetic acid (EDTA; edathamil or versene) has been used successfully in the treatment of both acute and chronic poisoning. This is a chelating agent which takes lead from the blood and forms an inactive soluble complex which is excreted in the urine. This preparation is best administered by slow intravenous drip in 5 per cent glucose saline and in a concentration of not more than 3 per cent of versene. In adults, 1 g is given twice daily for five days. After an interval of a few days, this course may be repeated.

Post-mortem findings

After acute poisoning, the appearances are chiefly those of gastro-enteritis. The gastric mucosa is congested. There may be eroded patches. In chronic poisoning, the kidneys are of small, granular, and contracted type. The left ventricle in such cases is frequently hypertrophied and the vessels show arterio-sclerotic changes.

Analytical findings

When large quantities of lead are taken into the body, excretion does not maintain an equilibrium and lead becomes stored. The poison is mainly excreted into the colon and, to a lesser extent, through the kidneys. If the rate of excretion equals that of absorption there may be no signs of poisoning. Only a part of the lead which is swallowed is absorbed into the general circulation. Non-soluble compounds are excreted in the faeces but soluble compounds are carried to the liver, where some is stored and the remainder distributed to other body tissues. Lead is stored in the bone marrow as triple phosphates, and when the acid content of the blood is increased, becomes soluble and in part may be excreted through the ordinary channels. In chronic lead poisoning there is substitution of lead for calcium, the result of the retention of lead in the bones, and an increased elimination of calcium in the urine. There appears to be a close analogy between lead and calcium with regard to distribution, storage, mobilisation, and excretion, and it has been shown that the state of calcium nutrition, the acid–base equilibrium, and the state of activity of the parathyroids are important factors in determining whether lead is stored in bone without toxic effect or is passed into general circulation with resultant tissue damage.

To establish the absorption of lead in the body by its presence in the faeces is fallacious since such a finding only establishes exposure to lead. Its absorption can only be established by its detection in the blood serum and urine in amounts which exceed those that could occur in persons not exposed to lead.

Normal values for lead in human tissue are given in Appendix III.

Fatal dose and time of death

The fatal dose is uncertain but may be in the region of 10 g in the case of a salt such as lead acetate, though recovery from greater amounts are recorded. Death may occur in any time within a few days. The minimum daily intake which results in chronic poisoning is about 1 to 2 mg.

Illustrative cases

Chronic poisoning has resulted from lodgment of bullets in the body, ingestion of lead from the paint on toys, solution of lead from the glaze of a container used for home-made wine, and contamination of food prepared in a frying pan repaired with solder. The following case of attempted murder by poisoning shows some unusual features. A man was charged with having poured white lead into a cup of milk which he placed beside his wife, so that she might drink it; having given her a chocolate filled with metallic mercury; and having on previous occasions filled a number of pills, intended for his wife, with brass filings, white lead, and copper wire, which were swallowed by her.

The bottle of milk was found to contain 5·5 g of white lead, and the chocolate, over 200 mg of metallic mercury. The interior of the pills had been drilled out, and filled either with finely powdered brass or copper and then plugged or entirely filled with white lead. The amount of lead in the pills depended upon the size of the plug or the amount of filling, and varied from 12 mg to over 60 mg in each pill.

The symptoms from which the woman suffered were abdominal pains with constipation and, later, continuous diarrhoea, loss of appetite, and cachexia.

The accused was found guilty on the charges except that of administering the chocolate.

Note. An organic compound of lead called lead tetra-ethyl is employed in fuel for motor cars, with which it is mixed to about 0·1 per cent by weight to counteract 'pinking', and on inhalation in sufficient quantity is extremely toxic. It is a colourless fluid with a sweetish odour and emits a vapour at ordinary temperature. Apart from inhalation, poisoning may be induced by absorption through the skin surface following contamination with the liquid. Poisoning in acute form chiefly affects the central nervous system and includes such symptoms as headache, nervousness, irritability, mental excitement, vertigo, tremor, insomnia, delusions, hallucinations, maniacal attacks, delirium, and convulsions. There may be slowing of the pulse rate, falling of the blood-pressure and body temperature, nausea, vomiting, and diarrhoea which is more frequent than constipation. Muscular pains and twitchings, fatigue, and general weakness are common. The symptoms in chronic poisoning are very similar to those of chronic lead poisoning.

In the treatment of severe cases, there should be a liberal intake of fluids, and normal saline or a 5 per cent solution of dextrose in normal saline will be found beneficial. Intravenous administration of from 2 to 4 g of a 2 per cent solution of magnesium sulphate has been recommended in cases of delirium.

Post-mortem findings are not specific. The brain and lungs are often congested. The liver and kidneys may show degenerative changes.

MANGANESE AND ITS COMPOUNDS

Manganese is used in the chemical, ceramic, glass, dye, and varnish industries. It is also used as a deoxidising and desulphurising agent, and in the preparation of manganese steel. Industrial poisoning may occur through handling, or by the inhalation of dust, especially during the process of grinding. Manganese is also used in the manufacture of 'dry' cells. The compound most often found in the home is potassium permanganate, which is a dark purple crystalline material which dissolves in water to give an intense pink- to purple-coloured solution. Potassium permanganate has a very limited medical use as a cleansing agent for suppurating wounds.

Symptoms

The signs and symptoms of chronic poisoning are lassitude, drowsiness, slight dyspnoea, weakness and trembling, Parkinsonism, and disturbances of gait and speech. The voice is dull and monotonous, the face mask-like, and the gestures stereotyped. Steppage gait and Rombergism may be evident. Other symptoms include excessive salivation, irritability, impairment of sexual function in the male, and emotionalism. Manganese toxaemia produces progressive bulbar paralysis, amyotrophic lateral sclerosis, and diffuse nodular hepatic cirrhosis. Differential diagnosis between post-encephalitic Parkinsonism, multiple sclerosis, and chronic manganese poisoning is sometimes necessary, and a history of exposure will help to elucidate the matter. In the Annual Report of the Chief Inspector of Factories, 1943, reference is made to a fatal case of poisoning in a man engaged in welding tram lines. He used an electrode containing 14 per cent manganese under poor conditions of ventilation.

Potassium permanganate is so widely used that its possibility as a toxic agent is often overlooked. It is a powerful oxidising and corrosive agent and fatal poisoning has occurred in a number of cases by ingestion either in the solid state or in strong solution. Dilute solutions may cause gastro-intestinal irritation. In concentrated form, this substance may affect the cardio-vascular system or the central nervous system and may produce mild corrosion. Willimott[68] reports a fatal case following urethral injection of 200 ml of a 10 per cent solution, equivalent to 20 g of the solid salt. Ascending from the bladder to the umbilicus was adhesive peritonitis, and the bladder mucosa was the seat of corrosions varying in size from a pin-head to a half-crown piece.

Ulceration of the vagina has resulted from the insertion of a tablet of potassium permanganate for the purpose of inducing abortion. A review of the attempted abortions seems to indicate that the reputed abortifacient action does not exist.

Treatment

When the substance has been swallowed gastric lavage, using charcoal, should be employed. Calcium disodium EDTA may be used as a chelating agent. Calcium gluconate (10 ml of a 10 per cent solution, daily), intravenously, has been recommended.

Post-mortem findings

Potassium permanganate shows corrosive effects in the stomach with the characteristic blackish-brown deposits of manganese dioxide formed by the destruction of the permanganate by the organic materials. There may be necrosis of any mucous membrane which has been in contact with the material.

Analytical findings

As manganese is one of the essential trace elements, interpretation of manganese levels must take into account the normal concentrations. A list of these is given in Appendix III.

Fatal dose

Acute poisoning by manganese is almost unknown. However, the estimated fatal dose of potassium permanganate is in the region of 10 g.

MERCURY AND ITS COMPOUNDS

Mercury and its compounds are used very widely in industry and agriculture. It is used extensively in dentistry and is present in most teaching and industrial laboratories. The liquid metal is a curiosity and very attractive, resulting in its introduction to many homes. This is a significant hazard, as any mercury metal left exposed to the air in ordinary room conditions is a source of considerable amounts of mercury vapour which will cause chronic poisoning in anyone exposed to it for prolonged periods.

Cases of industrial mercurial poisoning, some of them fatal, occur from time to time. Poisoning by mercury in industry is notifiable and its occurrence must be reported to the Home Office. When mercury enters the system in the metallic state it is comparatively innocuous unless in a finely divided form, when it will produce a toxic result. Inhalation of mercury dust or vapour may induce poisoning. The mode of absorption from the lungs is in doubt, but it is probable that the mercurial vapour dissolves in the fluid of the moist surfaces and thus is absorbed by the blood. It has been reported that the problem of mercurial poisoning in a Californian mine was overcome by spraying all mine floors, walls, timber, piping, wire, and ladders with lime-sulphur solution, thus converting the free mercury vapour and dust present into insoluble sulphide. Removal of mercury contamination is very difficult and cases of recurring poisoning are known when subjects re-enter environments which supposedly have been decontaminated. Mercurial salts are used clinically for both external and internal treatment. Mercuric chloride or corrosive sublimate, which is sometimes used as a disinfectant, is a frequent source of poisoning. It has an acrid and metallic taste, and one part of it is soluble in about fourteen parts of water at ordinary temperature.

Vaginal douching with corrosive sublimate may produce poisoning with fatal result.

The preparation of corrosive sublimate in the form of soloids has given rise to several cases of accidental poisoning.

The other poisonous mercurial salts are mercuric oxide or red precipitate, mercuric ammonium chloride or white precipitate, mercuric potassium iodide, mercuric nitrate, and mercuric cyanide.

A number of fatal and almost fatal reactions following the intravenous injection of mercurial diuretics has been recorded. The reaction in some of the cases was so sudden that the patient was dead before there was time to remove the needle from the vein, while in others it was characterised by convulsions, dyspnoea, cyanosis, coma, and death. The cause of death remains obscure, although a number of theories have been advanced. Some consider that the reaction is anaphylactic and connected with alteration of blood protein in nephrosis, and others that these drugs exercise a deleterious effect on the heart. It has also been thought that excessive doses may have been given, that the drugs have been continued after they have already produced toxic effects, or that the drugs have been administered to patients likely to die at any moment. It is advised that, before administering this treatment, the relatives should first be warned of the risk, and such restoratives as adrenalin and coramine should be available before the injection is given.

Poisoning may also arise from absorption of mercurial preparations applied to the skin.

It should be noted that although mercurous chloride (calomel) is generally regarded as non-toxic, its administration in teething powders is thought to have some connection with pink disease. It appears that a small percentage of the population may be sensitive to mercury exposure. As a result it is occasionally found that in a group exposed to mercury a few show severe symptoms when their colleagues show little or no reaction.

Symptoms

Acute. The symptoms frequently assert themselves soon after the poison is swallowed. A metallic, bitter taste is perceived in the mouth, with a sense of constriction or suffocation in the throat, accompanied by a feeling of heat, which extends down the oesophagus to the stomach. Pain, experienced in the region of the stomach, increased by pressure, is followed by nausea and constant vomiting. After the ordinary stomach contents have been evacuated, the vomit consists of blood-stained tenacious mucus. There is profuse diarrhoea, with severe tenesmus, the stools being composed latterly of blood-stained mucus. The pulse becomes small, feeble, and irregular, the skin cold and clammy, respiration difficult, and syncope, convulsions, and general insensibility usually precede death. Urinary secretion is either entirely suppressed or scanty in amount. The urine frequently contains albumin and blood. Elimination of the poison occurs through the mucosa of the intestinal tract and by the kidneys. These organs are therefore much affected by irritation. Elimination also occurs by the salivary glands, bile, and skin. Uraemic convulsions are rare.

Chronic. The principal signs and symptoms are: Progressive anaemia, gastric disorders, salivation, inflammation and tenderness of gums, with ready bleeding, and tremors chiefly affecting the muscles of face, hands, and arms. Some measure of paralysis may also be present. When workers are exposed to fumes of mercuric nitrate, the teeth become blackened, eroded, and loosened, due to recession of the gums. Later they may fall out. Mercury vapours may be inhaled by workers in certain processes in connection with preparation of metals.

When the poison is administered internally in repeated sublethal doses, the following signs and symptoms manifest themselves. The patient experiences a metallic taste and suffers from colicky abdominal pains, anorexia, nausea, vomiting, chronic diarrhoea, and general depression. The gums are swollen and may slough in patches, salivation is present, the teeth become loosened, and the salivary glands are swollen. An inflammatory line on the gums round the upper teeth may be seen, although this is frequently absent, and there is often much breath foetor. The patient becomes emaciated, suffers from general muscular tremor, and the effects of fully developed peripheral neuritis. Nervous manifestations frequently supervene and include morbid fears, mental depression, loss of memory, acute mania, and paralytic dementia. Renal complications are common. Before death the patient may be subject to mental disturbance accompanied by hallucinations. There may be skin eruptions.

Treatment

Treatment should be employed without delay, since the poison is rapidly absorbed and damage to the kidneys may occur quite quickly. The stomach should be emptied by gastric lavage or emesis. Rosenthal[69] reports that sodium formaldehyde sulphoxylate has saved nine out of twelve dogs from a fatal dose of corrosive mercuric chloride. When used in ten human cases of acute poisoning, recovery occurred without appreciable kidney damage. Dimercaprol (B.A.L.) is recommended as an effective treatment for mercury poisoning. An alternative chelating agent is penicillamine.

Symptomatic treatment should be given as indications arise. A lowered blood chloride level should be treated by intravenous administration of physiological saline. In certain cases, saline with 5 per cent dextrose administered intravenously may prove very beneficial.

Post-mortem findings

The tongue is white and sodden in appearance, and the mouth generally has a whitish colour. The mucous membrane of the pharynx, oesophagus, and stomach is more affected than that of the mouth. It may show a whitish or bluish-grey colour, and is inflamed or ulcerated in parts. In the stomach, especially, there is more or less general evidence of inflammation, there may be considerable extravasation of blood, and the muscular coats are often so softened that it is difficult to remove the organ without rupturing them. The mucosa of the intestines more or less shares in the inflammatory condition, and the caecum, colon, and rectum may be the seat of marked inflammatory action. Perforation of the stomach is rarely found. Histological changes, involving renal tissue, will probably be present in the endothelium of the vessels situated in the glomeruli, and the epithelial cells of the uriniferous tubules may show a varying degree of necrosis. Ogilvie[70] has recorded the results of an investigation respecting the condition of rabbits poisoned by corrosive sublimate. He found general congestion of the kidneys. The convoluted tubules and ascending limbs showed grades of injury which varied from cloudy swelling to coagulative necrosis and calcification. The liver was also congested and cloudy. Swelling and sometimes hydropic degeneration were present. Congestion of the spleen was accompanied by some destruction of the lymphoid cells. The changes in the myocardium consisted of congestion, cloudy swelling, and general patchy, fatty degeneration.

Analytical findings

When interpreting analytical results the average level of mercury in tissue (Appendix III) should be borne in mind, together with the wide

availability of mercury-containing materials and the growing environmental contamination.

Fatal dose and time of death

The time of death is very variable and usually extends to several days.
200 mg of corrosive sublimate have killed a child, and a similar dose
an adult.   This amount may be reckoned as the minimum fatal dose.
Recovery has, however, followed doses of 600 mg, 1·25 g, 2 g and after
larger doses; and of the red oxide, 2 g.   Much depends on the extent
of the prevention of absorption of the mercury by its being bound by
albumen and the amount removed by emesis or gastric lavage.

Illustrative cases

A girl, aged seventeen, swallowed 30 ml of acetic acid, and an unknown amount of added red oxide of mercury.   The amount taken
was thought to have been 2 g.   Her symptoms were stertorous breathing, vomiting of frothy fluid, without blood, pain in the throat and
stomach, and frequent blood-stained evacuations from the bowel, very
often copious, clots being passed.   The patient was conscious, but
collapsed.   There was very slight corrosion of the mouth.   There
were no convulsions.

She died within thirty hours after taking the poison.   A post-
mortem examination was made eight hours after death.   The oesophagus was inflamed and congested, and the stomach intensely so.   At
the pyloric end was a large blackened patch of erosion, the mucous
membrane being destroyed.   The duodenum showed patchy congestion, but was not ulcerated.

Millar[71] records the case of an unmarried woman who was in the
habit of using mercuric chloride tablets dissolved in water as a vaginal
douche, and inserted one tablet containing 500 mg of that salt without
water into the vagina at bedtime.   By 10 a.m. next day she complained
of pain and swelling of the vulva and by 1 p.m. was suffering from
severe abdominal pain, followed by persistent vomiting and diarrhoea.
At 7 p.m. the pain, diarrhoea, and vomiting had become worse.   Next
day a considerable amount of blood was passed in the stools and there
was suppression of urine.   She was thirsty and very drowsy.   On the
following day the gums were swollen, inflamed, spongy, and of dark
colour, the breath being foetid.   Diarrhoea, pain, and vomiting persisted.   The symptoms became progressively worse and swelling of
the salivary glands appeared, with active salivation.   She died on the
evening of the sixth day.   Post-mortem examination showed slight
jaundice, some evidence of irritation of, and a few small haemorrhages

in, the stomach, also necrosis and gangrenous ulceration of portions of the mucous layer of the intestines, with submucosal haemorrhages.

A young man swallowed, with suicidal intent, twenty-four or twenty-five soloids, each of which contained 60 mg of mercuric potassium iodide. Vomiting quickly ensued, and was encouraged. After treatment, including emetics, oils, and white of egg, he recovered.

Dérobert[72] reports a case of poisoning in a man of eighty-five by self-administered mercuric sulphate. Post-mortem examination did not disclose evidence of irritative lesions of the oesophagus, larynx, or trachea. The gastric mucosa was of brown colour, congested, and haemorrhagic.

Lewinski[73] records details of a case of suicide by swallowing a quantity of a 1 per cent solution of mercuric cyanide. Typical symptoms of mercurial poisoning followed and the woman died from uraemia after five days. Autopsy showed evidence of subacute mercurial poisoning.

Analysis of hair and nail from a dentist gave values of 171 and 558 μg/g respectively. His assistant had a hair concentration of 50·8 μg/g and a nail concentration of 286 μg/g. Further inquiry showed the presence of salivation, tremors, insomnia, and character change. It was found that over the years small pools of mercury had formed under the flooring, especially near a heater, and this resulted in a high mercury level and the symptoms of chronic poisoning.

A schoolboy took about 2co g of mercury (quite a small volume) from school to his home where he played with it. The result was a fair distribution over the living-room carpet. This primary hazard was intensified by very efficient dispersal as a result of vacuum cleaning. Soon after, all the members of the family presented at hospital where chronic mercury poisoning was diagnosed.

METHAQUALONE

This material is used as a sedative and hypnotic. It has no analgesic effect itself but it is said to potentiate the analgesic effects of other drugs such as codeine. The hypnotic effect is rather less than that of quinalbarbitone.

Symptoms

The symptoms include nausea, gastric irritation, and vomiting. Muscle twitching, hypertonia, cardiac arrhythmia, tachycardia, or myocardial infarction may be present, and respiratory depression is a possibility.

Treatment

Treat as for barbiturate overdosage.   Matthew and others[74] describe the successful treatment of Mandrax poisoning in 116 subjects by conservative management.

Post-mortem findings

These are non-specific and are those expected for barbiturate poisoning.

Analytical findings

Methaqualone may be found in tissues and fluids.   The levels found are usually in the region of a few milligrams per cent.   In a typical fatal poisoning the values found were:

Blood	1·8 mg/100 ml
Liver	3·8 mg/100 g
Urine	0·5 mg/100 ml

Fatal dose

The fatal dose is probably in the region of 5 g, though recovery from larger quantities has been reported.   In the fatal poisoning quoted above 6 g were ingested.

Note.   The majority of fatal poisonings involving methaqualone have resulted from ingestion of Mandrax, which is a mixture of methaqualone (250 mg) and diphenhydramine hydrochloride (25 mg). Possibly this combination is more toxic than methaqualone alone.

METHYL ALCOHOL (*Methanol*)

This is a colourless volatile liquid (b. pt 65°C).   It is widely used as a solvent and occurs in various concentrations and purities.   It is most commonly available to the public as 'mineralised methylated spirits'. This is ethyl alcohol containing 9·5 per cent of wood naphtha (this is a crude form of methyl alcohol derived from the destructive distillation of wood) and 0·5 per cent pyridine together with a small amount of petroleum oil.   The mixture which is coloured with methyl violet forms an opaque mixture with water.   This material and in fact any alcohol-containing mixture is ingested for its intoxicating effect.   In Glasgow a mixture of red wine and methylated spirits called 'Red Biddy' is sometimes drunk.

The Methylated Spirits (Sale by Retail) (Scotland) Act of 1937 makes it unlawful to sell by retail any methylated, or surgical spirit, unless the seller is an authorised seller, or the seller's name is on the local authority's list and an entry is made in a book kept for the purpose, and the purchaser signs the entry or delivers a signed order.

Symptoms

The symptoms of acute poisoning by methyl alcohol include drowsiness, nausea, vomiting, vertigo, headache, sometimes epigastric pain, and visual defects, frequently succeeded by blindness. There are cardiac depression, dyspnoea, cyanosis, cold sweats, subnormal temperature, confusion, delirium, convulsions, and unconsciousness, followed by coma and death.

Methyl alcohol frequently remains in the body for several days and is excreted in the breath and in the urine. It is oxidised to formic acid and formaldehyde and large quantities of lactic and other organic acids are formed. As a result the patient suffers from marked acidosis. Death has followed the ingestion of 30 ml, but cases have recovered after drinking more than ten times this quantity. It is generally held that the consumption of ethyl alcohol counters the effects of methyl alcohol and a reason advanced is that the former displaces the latter from its intracellular attachments and thus checks its oxidation to formic acid, the substance held to be primarily responsible for the acidosis.

Treatment

Gastric lavage with 4 per cent sodium bicarbonate is combined with administration of copious fluids. The eyes should be protected from strong light. Treatment should be that of acidosis due to the production of formic acid. Chew, Berger, Brines, and Capron[75] founding on their experience recommend the use of massive doses of sodium lactate. To check the downward progress of the carbon dioxide combining power of the plasma, 160 ml of a molar solution ($11 \cdot 2$ per cent) of the lactate, in a litre of an isotonic solution of the three chlorides, is given intravenously. When sodium lactate is not at hand, 50 g sodium bicarbonate in 1 litre of 5 per cent of freshly prepared glucose can be substituted. They suggest, however, that the lactate is preferable since it yields the sodium ion more slowly into the system. Sodium bicarbonate is given by the mouth in doses of 4 g every fifteen minutes for four doses or, if the patient is unconscious, by stomach tube. This routine may have to be repeated three to four times to raise the combining power from 10–20 to 40–50 volumes per cent. Where there are no facilities for checking the plasma bicarbonate, the urinary reaction may be used as a guide to the administration of the alkali.

Continued treatment with sodium bicarbonate, 2 g an hour, is recommended while the urinary pH is below 7·0, and 2 g every two hours when the pH has reached 7·0.   Of thirty-one cases so treated, after taking an average of 222 ml of methyl alcohol, only five died, of whom four were moribund when first seen.   In order to reduce the metabolism and allow excretion ethyl alcohol may be given.   The initial dose is about 1 ml/kg of a 50 per cent solution orally followed by 0·5–1 ml/kg every two hours for four days.   If the response to treatment is unsatisfactory it may be necessary to use haemodialysis.   When there is dangerous respiratory depression, oxygen and artificial respiration should be used until the natural colour has been fully restored.

Post-mortem findings

The heart, liver, and kidneys may show parenchymatous degeneration.   Histology may show oedema of the retina and optic nerve.

Analytical findings

The alcohol may be measured in any of the tissues but usually only blood levels are sought.   In many cases both ethyl and methyl alcohols are present and the analytical method must be able to distinguish them. After a dose of 435 ml of 95 per cent methanol, post-mortem blood contained 290 mg/100 ml, and the urine contained 485 mg/100 ml.[76]

Fatal dose

The fatal dose is variable.   Death has been reported after 30 ml but recovery has followed as much as ten times this volume.   The concentration of the vapour in air should not exceed 200 p.p.m.

Illustrative case

In 1942, a number of fatalities, due to drinking synthetic methyl alcohol mixed with industrial spirit obtained from leaking casks, occurred in Glasgow.   In some of the cases, many hours elapsed before the onset of acute illness accompanied by severe abdominal pain. The patients passed into coma and death resulted from paralysis of the respiratory or cardiac centres.   In one of the Glasgow hospitals eighteen cases were treated, but seven of these proved fatal.   Four eyes were examined, post-mortem, and the chief histological findings were oedema of the retina and optic nerve head, but no changes were seen in the optic nerve itself.

Methyl Bromide (*Bromomethane*)

This gas is used as one of the components in the manufacture of pigments, in the preparation of antipyrin, in certain fire extinguishers, and as a fumigant for insects.   It is practically odourless, but its thermal decomposition products are almost irrespirable.   When the vapour is inhaled toxic symptoms occur.

Symptoms

The early symptoms are headache, giddiness, vomiting, and drowsiness.   Following these, there is usually a period of intermission, which may last for quite a long time.   After this, there is full development of the manifestations of poisoning.   These include motor and sensory paralysis, inco-ordination, visual disturbances, slurring speech, mania, delirious states, convulsions, pulmonary oedema, with dyspnoea and cyanosis, and death.

Treatment

Artificial respiration may be required together with the administration of oxygen.   The use of adrenalin or glutathione has been recommended as a line of treatment.

Post-mortem findings

Since methyl bromide affects the vasomotor system, all the organs, including the brain, will be found in a state of congestion on post-mortem examination.

Analytical findings

Methyl bromide may be estimated in tissues and fluids.   In a fatal accident, a value of 34 mg/100 ml of blood was reported.   In a suicide[77] the value found for methyl bromide in lungs was 105 mg/100 g.   Methyl bromide may not be found in the body due to conversion to methyl alcohol and bromide ion.   Detection of bromide ion is used to circumvent this, but the results must be interpreted against normal or medicinal bromide levels.   In the latter case, the levels found may well obscure any produced from methyl bromide exposure.   Values of bromide ion in whole blood in the region of 10 mg/100 ml have been found in fatal poisoning.   Drawneek and others[78] report values of 0 to 15.3 mg sodium bromide/100 ml of serum in eleven symptomless men working with methyl bromide fumigation apparatus.   One subject with a value of 18.7 mg/100 ml showed symptoms of poisoning.

Fatal dose and time of death

The maximum allowable concentration is 20 p.p.m. There is a latent period before development of symptoms. This may vary up to a day depending on the severity of the exposure. Poisoning may result from absorption through the skin.

METHYL CHLORIDE

Methyl chloride is a colourless gas with a sweet aromatic odour which is only detectable in toxic concentrations. This gas is used as a refrigerant and, being more dense than air, may tend to collect in pockets.

Symptoms

The onset of symptoms is insidious and weakness and staggering are frequent. Nausea, vomiting, confusion, abdominal pain, coma, and convulsions complete the picture of serious poisoning. Toxic effects are readily shown by absorption through the skin.

Treatment

Artificial respiration may be required together with the administration of oxygen. Methoxamine hydrochloride may be used to maintain blood-pressure.

Post-mortem findings

The post-mortem signs include congestion and oedema of the lungs, petechial haemorrhages in the pericardium and pleurae, hyperaemia of the gastro-intestinal vessels, and cloudy swelling of the kidneys, together with congestion and oedema of the brain.

Analytical findings

Methyl chloride may be sought in post-mortem material but may not be found due to the rapid conversion to methyl alcohol and chloride ion.

Fatal dose and time of death

The safe concentration in air is about 100 p.p.m. Severe poisoning may occur in exposure to over 1,000 p.p.m. for any length of time. At low concentrations symptoms may be delayed for some time. Death usually supervenes within two or three days or not at all.

NAPHTHALENE

This is a colourless crystalline solid with the characteristic odour of 'moth balls'.   It is obtained from the middle fraction in the distillation of coal-tar and has properties similar to benzene.   It is used chiefly in the dye industry and for its preserving properties for woollen goods.   The vapour pressure of naphthalene is appreciable at room temperature, so over-exposure due to inhalation may occur.

Symptoms

The symptoms of poisoning are abdominal pain, frequency of micturition, cyanosis, muscular twitchings, drowsiness, and jaundice with marked brown coloration of the urine.   An ataxic gait is not uncommon in the earlier stages.   Naphthalene is a skin irritant.

Treatment

Gastric lavage, a purgative dose of magnesium sulphate, and demulcent drinks, devoid of oils and fat, form the principal lines of treatment.

Post-mortem findings

Kidney damage due to blocking with precipitated haemoglobin may be present.   Hepatic necrosis has also been reported.

Analytical findings

Naphthalene may be found in any of the tissues or fluids.

Fatal dose

The fatal dose is in the region of a few grams.   The safe concentration in air is not established but is probably in the region of 10 to 25 p.p.m.

Note. *Chlorinated naphthalene.*   When naphthalene is chlorinated a waxy substance is produced, which is used in industry as an insulating coat on electrical wires and for limiting the action in plating metals. 'Seekay' wax is used in waterproofing, flameproofing, for insect pests and fungus, also for bitumen blending, sealing and impregnation of condensers, coils, etc.   Overheating of the wax causes increased quantities of the fumes to be evolved.

Chlorinated naphthalene waxes frequently give rise to inflammation and irritation of the skin, especially acne, and breathing of their vapours or air containing fine particles of the wax may cause serious illness. Persons with liver damage are more susceptible to poisoning. Toxic jaundice is not an infrequent manifestation produced either by an acute or subacute necrosis of the liver, or by acute yellow atrophy. Continued exposure gives rise to jaundice, and slight oedema of the eyelids and ankles. When the liver is seriously involved, the area of dullness is diminished, and the urine becomes dark brown in colour and contains bile. Purpuric rashes, involving the lower abdomen and legs, may be seen.

Post-mortem findings include bile staining of the kidneys and minute areas of necrosis in the pancreatic fat. The chief lesion is found in the liver, usually greatly reduced in size, which may vary in weight from 1,200 g to 650 g or less. The capsule is usually wrinkled, and histological examination shows the acute stages of yellow atrophy.

NICKEL CARBONYL

Carbon monoxide forms compounds with metals called carbonyls. The most common of these is nickel carbonyl used in the preparation of nickel. It is a colourless liquid (sp. gr. 1·38) which boils at 43°C. The vapour has been estimated as being fifteen times more toxic than carbon monoxide. In the presence of moisture, the inhaled gas becomes dissociated and thus finely divided particles of nickel are deposited over the respiratory epithelium and are absorbed into the circulation. Poisoning occurs in the industrial process of manufacture by inhalation of fumes or by working with the fluid.

Symptoms

Acute nickel carbonyl poisoning is a two-phase process. Initially there is headache, lassitude, sickness, and constriction over the chest. There may be visual disturbances, tremors, insomnia, and a metallic taste. The second phase is characterised by dyspnoea, bronchitis, and bronchopneumonia with cough and blood-stained sputum. Elimination of the poison is by way of the intestines and kidneys.

Treatment

Remove from exposure and treat cyanosis with oxygen. Dimercaprol may be used as a chelating agent. Keep the patient at rest and treat other symptoms as they arise.

Post-mortem findings

These may be summarised as including congestion and oedema of the lungs, which show haemorrhagic areas; fatty degeneration of the heart, liver, and kidneys; and haemorrhagic areas, with degenerative changes and thrombi in some of the vessels in the brain, especially in the region of the corpus callosum, medulla, and in the upper part of the spinal cord.

Analytical findings

Nickel may be found in the tissues, especially the lungs, but interpretation against a normal level is required.   A list of normal levels is given in Appendix III.   Sunderman and Kincaid[79] report values of 0·17 to 0·41 µg nickel per ml of urine within twenty-four hours of severe exposure.   Bayer[80] reports values of 0·52 and 4·0 µg nickel per ml of post-mortem urine.

Fatal dose and time of death

The maximum permissible level in the atmosphere is 1 p.p.m. Death usually occurs between the fourth and twelfth days after exposure.

Note.   There is a cancer risk from exposure to nickel carbonyl.

NICOTINE

The plant *Nicotiana tabacum* contains the alkaloid nicotine to which its toxic effect, even by smoking, is due.   This alkaloid is a colourless liquid (b. pt 247°C) which is soluble in water.   It has a pungent acrid taste, and on exposure to air and light develops an amber tint.   Cases of acute poisoning are comparatively rare, but subacute and chronic poisoning may result from excessive use of tobacco.

Nicotine poisoning may be caused by absorption either through intact or broken skin, by inhalation or ingestion.   Poisoning by absorption through the skin has followed the use of an insecticide containing 40 per cent of free nicotine.   It has also followed the swallowing of wine containing 80 per cent of nicotine.   Cases of industrial poisoning, due to commercial preparations such as fertilisers, insecticides, and fumigants, have also occurred.

Symptoms

When nicotine is absorbed in poisonous amount, the principal symptoms are those of successive central and peripheral stimulation. Nausea, sickness, tachycardia, cardiac irregularity, praecordial oppression, severe prostration, and cardio-vascular collapse are experienced. There may also be convulsions, delirium, irregularity of respiration, dyspnoea, and coma.

Treatment

Gastric lavage and adrenalin medication. Artificial respiration and oxygen inhalations may be necessary.

Post-mortem findings

When nicotine has been swallowed, the signs are usually those of asphyxia. The mucous membrane of the oesophagus and stomach may be congested.

Analytical findings

Nicotine may be found in the tissues and body fluids of most people who smoke tobacco, and this should be borne in mind when interpreting results. Fatal levels in blood and tissues are in the region of 1 mg/100 ml.

Fatal dose and time of death

The fatal dose of nicotine is in the region of 40 mg. This quantity is contained in about two cigarettes, but most is destroyed in smoking. On ingestion of tobacco the nicotine does not appear to be absorbed very well. Death may occur any time from a few minutes to a few hours.

Illustrative case

An unusual case of absorption is recorded by Gill.[81] A convict was admitted to prison, and four hours later was found in a state of collapse and suffering from nausea, vomiting, and paralysis of both legs. The cause of his illness was regarded as due to 30 g of cut tobacco concealed in his rectum, and which he had been unable to remove. The man recovered.

NITRATES

The commonest nitrates are those of sodium, potassium, calcium, and ammonium. These are colourless, odourless crystalline solids which are soluble in water. They are used widely in industry and agriculture. They might be found in the home where they have some use as garden fertilisers. Potassium nitrate is sometimes present in gargles, often mixed with potassium chlorate. The nitrates are commonly present in fireworks.

Symptoms

The signs and symptoms consist of vomiting accompanied by severe gastric pain, and sometimes diarrhoea with blood-stained stools; symptoms of collapse, lividity of face, and insensibility are followed by death.

Treatment

Free lavage; demulcent drinks; stimulants; warmth to body; and treatment of prominent symptoms. Methylene blue is used to treat severe methaemoglobinaemia.

Post-mortem findings

The mucous lining of the stomach is bright red or brownish-red in colour. The mucous membrane is injected. The blood may be chocolate-coloured due to the presence of methaemoglobin.

Analytical findings

The stomach contents should be tested for nitrates. Detection of nitrates in blood and tissues is difficult due to decomposition and the presence of related nitrogen compounds which interfere. Nitrites and nitrates have some use as preservatives and may be present from this source.

Fatal dose and time of death

The fatal quantity is in the region of 30 g. Death may take place from a few hours to a day after ingestion.

NITRIC ACID (*Aqua fortis*)

Properties and uses

The concentrated acid is a colourless fuming liquid with a specific gravity of about 1·5. The acid is widely used in industry in a range of strengths and purity. The strong commercial acid is often coloured pale yellow to deep orange, due to the presence of nitrogen peroxide. The dilute acid looks like water.

Nitric acid produces characteristic yellow stains in contact with skin or other organic materials. Nitric acid is seldom found in the home. Its use in medicine is limited to wart removal; however, this is not common.

Symptoms and treatment

These are described under Corrosive Poisons.

Post-mortem findings

The affected mucous membranes show yellowish discoloration, and the degree of corrosion is very marked. On account of the fumes which are liberated, death is frequently caused by congestion and oedema of the lungs. Capillary bronchitis is quite a frequent complication.

Analytical findings

These are usually restricted to the measurement of the amount of acid found.

Fatal dose and time of death

Death usually occurs within twenty-four hours and may be as soon as an hour and a half after ingestion. The smallest recorded dose is 8 ml, though recovery (but with major damage) has been reported after 10 ml.

Note. The commonest irritant nitrogen oxides are nitrogen dioxide (N_2O_4) and nitric oxide (NO), which reacts with air to form the dioxide. The so-called nitrous fumes, which are mixtures of nitrogen oxides, are coloured red-brown or yellow-brown due to the presence of the dioxide, which is an intense red-brown colour. These fumes react with water to form mixtures of nitric and nitrous acids.

Many industrial processes result in the liberation of nitrous fumes. Other sources are exposed nitric acid, incompletely burned nitro-explosives, and the heat-induced reaction of nitrogen with oxygen from the air. In one case,[82] a number of men were employed in a ship in heating a heavy steel crosshead. Two large oxyacetylene burners were used, each consuming about 200 cubic feet of oxygen and acetylene per hour. The compartment was of about 5,000 cubic feet capacity and was ventilated by air injected from a blower together with two compressed-air jets. After about forty minutes, several of the men collapsed and one of them died in hospital about thirty-two hours later. The symptoms were typical of nitrous fumes. In autogenous welding, due to the generation of great heat, the oxygen and nitrogen of the atmospheric air combine to form oxides of nitrogen. The post-mortem findings consisted of massive oedema with commencing pneumonia. The blood was darker than usual. The lungs were of yellowish-brown colour.

The principal danger of inhalation of nitrogen oxide is that dangerous or fatal oedema of the lungs may follow an inhalation, not regarded as significant at the time on account of the fact that respiratory irritation has not been experienced since only the deeper parts of the respiratory tract are involved. When the fumes come into contact with moisture in the respiratory system they are converted into nitric and nitrous acids, and thus a caustic effect is produced with resultant congestion of the lungs and inflammatory oedema. In such cases nitric acid may be found in the blood.

The usual symptoms are severe cough, pain in the chest, vomiting, dyspnoea, cyanosis, and a reddish-brown sputum. In addition to massive inflammatory oedema of the lungs, there may be oedema of the brain, swelling of the liver, and necrosis of the kidneys.

NITRITES

These include sodium and potassium nitrite and the organic nitrites such as amyl nitrite. Inorganic nitrites have been used as preservatives. The organic compounds are used in medicine as vasodilators.

Symptoms

Inhalation of the volatile compounds causes headaches and fainting. Cyanosis and methaemoglobinaemia may be present and shock-like symptoms may develop.

Treatment

Treatment includes gastric lavage and oxygen or artificial respiration as necessary. Venous return should be aided by exercise and methaemoblobinaemia should be treated with methylene blue (1 to 2 mg/kg —intravenous). Blood transfusion has been used successfully.

Post-mortem findings

The most significant finding is the presence of chocolate-coloured blood due to the production of methaemoglobin.

Analytical findings

Stomach contents should be examined for nitrite, bearing in mind the possibility of nitrite as a contaminant of nitrate.

Fatal dose and time of death

The fatal dose is probably about 2 g, though recovery following approximately 10 g of amyl nitrite has been reported. The fatal period is variable, being about two hours, but death has occurred after seven days.

Note. A number of organic nitrites are described independently under the appropriate headings.

NITROBENZENE

Nitrobenzene is a yellow liquid (sp. gr. 1·2), with a pleasant odour, which is almost insoluble in water. The material is used widely in the organic chemicals industry and explosives industry.

Symptoms

The symptoms of poisoning show a wide range of variation, and since the substance is a typical example of a nitro-derivative of benzene they are given in some detail to avoid repetition when analogous substances are dealt with.

A sense of fullness and throbbing in the head with flushing of the face is experienced. There is often a burning sensation in the throat, a feeling of tightness in the chest, and there may be visual disturbances. In cases of acute poisoning, an ashen-blue cyanosis, progressive in character, develops. Many workers have reported that the cyanosis has developed without previous symptoms and without the victim being aware of any change. Nausea, vomiting, dyspnoea, giddiness, prostration, convulsions, coma, and death, describe a fatal issue. Methaemoglobin is present in the blood which is of dark colour, and a reduction in the number of blood cells, which show degenerative changes, will be found.

The stability of methaemoglobin prevents it from performing the normal function of haemoglobin, which is the transportation of oxygen in the body. On this account tissue asphyxia is caused. If methaemoglobin is in large amount, part of the haemoglobin is irremediably damaged, the red cells are broken up and their contents are diffused in the blood plasma. Profound anaemia may follow even a single intense exposure. Some of the methaemoglobin passes into the urine and produces a characteristic reddish-brown or chocolate colour. Haemoglobin loss through the kidneys is particularly serious since it causes a depletion of the body's store of iron, necessary for the formation of new haemoglobin and fresh corpuscles.

Treatment

The stomach should be washed out with water containing magnesium sulphate if the material has been ingested. The use of oxygen is recommended and blood transfusions may be necessary. A 5 to 10 per cent solution of glucose in normal saline may be given intravenously. Methylene blue is used to treat severe methaemoglobinaemia.

Post-mortem findings

These include marked congestion of the meninges and brain, a dark or chocolate colour of the blood, with engorgement of the chambers on the right side of the heart. The scented odour of nitrobenzene may be perceived in the lungs and stomach.

Analytical findings

Nitrobenzene may be sought in tissues or fluids, but exposure is usually judged by the extent of methaemoglobin formation in the blood. Values of methaemoglobin much over 50 per cent indicate severe exposure and the possibility of death.

Fatal dose and time of death

The fatal dose of nitrobenzene is about 1 g and the safe concentration in air is 1 p.p.m. Death may occur any time up to a day, thereafter recovery is likely.

Note. Dinitrobenzene, which is found widely in the manufacture of explosives, is sometimes a cause of poisoning. It is a yellowish solid which is readily absorbed through the skin. The symptoms and toxicity are similar to nitrobenzene.

NITROGLYCERINE (*Glyceryl trinitrate*)

This is a dense (1·6 g/ml), colourless to yellow oily liquid which is very slightly soluble in water and has a sweet taste. It is unstable and either heat or concussion will cause it to explode. The characteristic use is in explosives such as dynamite. In medicine, it is used as a relaxant for involuntary muscle. Typically it is administered sublingually for the treatment of angina pectoris. Absorption is by way of the skin or mucous membranes.

Symptoms

Toxic effects include headache, gastro-intestinal irritation, faintness, insomnia, dryness in the throat, dyspnoea, bronchitis, and mental excitement. Cyanosis and methaemoglobinaemia may be present.

In chronic poisoning tremors and neuralgic pain are common. Handling may produce ulceration of the finger-tips and below the nails.

Treatment

Immediate gastric lavage is recommended and exercise of the extremities to aid venous return. Skin contamination is removed by scrubbing with soap and water. Oxygen and artificial respiration may be necessary. Methaemoglobin formation may be treated with methylene blue. Blood-pressure should be maintained.

Post-mortem findings

The findings are non-specific but the chocolate-coloured blood may be used as an indicator if the general history involves exposure.

Analytical findings

It may not be possible to find nitroglycerine due to the rapid decomposition in the tissues. The stomach content is probably the best place to search.

Fatal dose and time of death

Death has followed 2 g glyceryl trinitrate. Death occurs within a few hours, thereafter recovery is usual though death may occur after some days from respiratory failure. The maximum permitted concentration in the atmosphere is about 0·5 p.p.m.

Note. Cordite is a combination of nitrocellulose and nitroglycerine, with the addition of about 5 per cent of mineral jelly. It is used as an explosive. Poisoning from cordite frequently occurs and is shown by such symptoms as tachycardia, palpitation, irregularity of the action of the heart, giddiness, dyspnoea, especially on exertion, and general debility.

The cause of death in fatal cases is asphyxia. To evade service in the Forces, malingerers have been known to suffer from toxic manifestation due to self-administration.

OPIUM

Opium consists of the inspissated juice of *Papaver somniferum,* and contains a large number of alkaloids, including morphine, narcotine, codeine, narceine, papaverine, thebaine, apomorphine, anarcotine, and others, several of which are highly poisonous, also the neutral substance called meconin, and meconic acid. The principal alkaloids used in medicine, and obtained from opium, are morphine, codeine, and apomorphine, of which the first two act as narcotics or sedatives, and the last chiefly as an emetic. Opium and morphine enter into the composition of a number of official preparations as well as of proprietary medicines, for example, Chlorodyne, Nepenthe, and others. Heroin is a derivative of morphine.

Symptoms

These appear earlier from the use of morphine than from crude opium or its preparations, and may be divided into two groups, namely, those indicative of excitation of the higher nerve-centres, and those indicative of narcosis. When a case calling for treatment comes under notice, the former symptoms will usually have passed away, and the latter are fully developed. The latter symptoms especially, therefore, call for consideration. They consist of an overpowering drowsiness which gradually becomes deeper until it ends in profound coma from which no stimulus can arouse the patient. In the earlier stages, however, the person may be partially roused. In the later stages the muscles become relaxed, the pulse is small and weak, and the breathing laboured, noisy, and perhaps irregular, and finally, shallow and slow. The temperature is subnormal. The face is pale, cold, sometimes bedewed with clammy perspiration, and the pupils are strongly contracted, almost to pin-head size. Death may follow the deepening of narcosis, or may be preceded, especially in children, by convulsive seizures.

Occasionally there may be a remission of the symptoms for a short period, but when this occurs they usually return in their original severity, and the person may die.

The symptoms of morphine poisoning may be complicated or masked by the morphine having been taken with other drugs.

Infants and young children are most susceptible to the influence of opium and morphine, and the administration of these drugs to children should be avoided. Very small doses of laudanum have proved fatal.

Self-administered injections of morphine in overdose may produce poisoning. One must therefore be alive to this form of administration, and examine for evidence of puncture marks on parts of the body available for self-administration.

Morphinism is more prevalent in persons who have a psychopathic tendency, or an unstable nervous system. After a period, there is usually evidence both of physical and moral deterioration. Addicts develop a marked tolerance to the drug and are able to take quantities which would have fatal consequences in those unaccustomed to its use. Untruthfulness, dishonesty, and mental deterioration are commonly found. When under the influence of the drug, addicts appear calm and composed; when, however, the effect wears off, they become restless, irritable, and cantankerous. Withdrawal symptoms include delirium and hallucinations.

Treatment

This must be regulated by the circumstances of each individual case. If the poison has been swallowed, there must be free gastric lavage, first with tepid water, the return being retained for analysis, and then with potassium permanganate solution (0·2 g/l). Lavage should be continued for several hours.

Even in cases in which morphine has been administered hypo-dermically, the permanganate treatment should be adopted since morphia is excreted by the stomach.   It is important to remember that permanganate must not be used in too strong solution, as it is slightly corrosive.   The use of medicinal charcoal is also beneficial.

Although potassium permanganate will oxidise the alkaloid present in the stomach, it will also be necessary to combat the toxic effects of the amount absorbed.

Atropine sulphate 0·6 mg may be injected hypodermically, but it must be used with caution to prevent depression following stimulation of the respiratory centre.

In all cases of poisoning the body warmth must be restored by ap-propriate measures, and it is unwise to subject a patient to vigorous or prolonged muscular exercise.   It is more helpful to rouse him by sustained attention.   In the immediate absence of a stomach tube, emesis should be promoted and encouraged by the readiest emetic. Artificial respiration and inhalations of oxygen may be administered as circumstances indicate.   The airway should be kept clear and the patient catheterised.   Coramine, 5 to 10 ml of 25 per cent solution, may be given intravenously.

Two drugs have been introduced as antagonists to morphine action. These are N-allyl-normorphine, and amiphenazole.   The former substance is a specific antidote to morphine and related opium alkaloids. It should be administered by the intravenous route in single doses of 10 to 40 mg.   Excessive amounts may heighten existing respiratory depression.   Amiphenazole is in use to combat the respiratory depres-sant effects of morphine.   This substance has been marketed under the trade name Daptazole, and may be used as an antidote in morphine poisoning.   It should be injected intramuscularly in doses of 10 mg at ten-minute intervals until a total of 50 mg has been given.   Anti-biotics should be administered in cases of prolonged unconsciousness.

Post-mortem findings

The post-mortem signs will be those of coma, or comatoasphyxia. If the case has been untreated, and opium or laudanum has been swallowed, the odour of the drug may be perceived in the stomach. It should not be forgotten that opium may be introduced to the body by channels other than the stomach, as, for instance, by the rectum.

Analytical findings

The fluids normally analysed are blood, urine, and bile. In a number of fatal poisonings the levels quoted for these fluids have been up to a few mg per 100 ml.

Fatal dose and time of death

One drop of laudanum has killed on more than one occasion, and compound tincture of camphor containing 3 mg of opium has produced the same result. Children have, however, occasionally recovered from large doses: from 450 mg of opium, from one and two teaspoonfuls of laudanum, and from 3·6 ml of liq. morphinae. We have seen recovery in a child of nine months, after fifteen drops of laudanum, without recourse to treatment.

250 mg of opium and 60 mg of morphia, respectively, may be regarded as probable fatal doses in those not addicted. Recovery has, however, followed treatment when 24 g of opium and 3·3 g of morphine acetate, respectively, have been taken. In a case, which we treated, recovery followed the swallowing of the contents of one and a half bottles of Collis Browne's Chlorodyne.

Death may occur within forty-five minutes. This happened in the case of a woman who had swallowed 30 ml of laudanum. The usual period is from nine to twelve hours, but it may extend to two days. In one case where 10 g of a liquid preparation of opium were injected into an adult instead of ten drops, death did not occur till two days later.

In addicts, the fatal dose may be as much as ten times higher.

Note. Etorphine (M99) and acetorphine (M183) are very powerful narcotic analgesics, and it is dangerous to taste or smell them.

Oxalic Acid *(and oxalates)*

Properties and uses

The pure acid is a reasonably soluble (9·5 g/100 ml water at 15°C), colourless crystalline solid, similar to 'Epsom salts' in appearance. It is used in a number of industries and is occasionally found in the kit of the enthusiastic home woodworker who uses it as a bleach. In the home, it is occasionally used as a cleaning agent for ink or iron stains.

Oxalic acid reacts with calcium ions in the body to form the insoluble calcium oxalate, thus causing a serious depletion of calcium. The crystals of calcium oxalate may be visible in the microscopic inspection of the victim's blood.

Symptoms

If a large dose of the acid is taken, the following signs and symptoms are commonly found, namely, a burning, acrid taste on swallowing, dysphagia, vomiting, which is severe and continuous, and a burning sensation in the oesophagus and stomach. Occasionally a feeling of suffocation, with lividity of face and hurried respiration, may be experienced. Collapse is rapid. The vomited material at first consists of normally coloured stomach contents mixed with a varying amount of mucus, but as sickness continues, the colour becomes greenish-black or almost black due to the presence of altered blood. In addition to the foregoing manifestations, there are pain and tenderness over the abdomen. If the case is of short duration, the intestinal tract is not affected, but when life is prolonged, purging and tenesmus may be present. The pulse becomes feeble and irregular, and not infrequently the patient complains of a sensation of numbness in the limbs. Convulsions often precede death. The character and severity of the symptoms depend upon the amount and the concentration of the acid swallowed. When in concentrated solution, the acid acts as a corrosive.

Treatment

Consists in first washing out the stomach and thereafter administering chalk, or lime in milk, or other demulcent drinks in small concentrated quantities. Saccharated solution of lime, in 30 ml doses, frequently repeated, is recommended and also intravenous injections of calcium chloride or gluconate. Urinary output should be checked to detect the possibility of renal damage and fluid intake controlled as found necessary. Treat shock and respiratory depression by oxygen inhalation.

Post-mortem findings

If the dose is large and the acid is in concentrated form, all the parts which have come into contact with the acid are softened, white, and corroded, or may be stained with blackish or reddish streaks. White corroded areas may be found at the corners of the mouth, on the lips, tongue, and lining of the cheeks. The oesophagus is markedly congested, and in patches, the lining membrane is frequently corroded and partly detached. The stomach contains a dark brown, glairy fluid, which has an acid reaction, and the mucous membrane is corroded and detached in varying degree; the blood-vessels in the submucous layer may be seen distinctly because of their dark-coloured contents. The stomach also shows intense congestion. Perforation is rare, but occasionally occurs. The upper part of the intestinal tract may also show evidence of a haemorrhagic necrosis. Since this poison is excreted by the kidneys, they will show marked congestion or cloudy swelling if death has been delayed sufficiently long. In such cases death is frequently due to anuria and uraemia. Concentration of oxalate in the kidneys may produce necrosis of the renal tubules.

Analytical findings

Oxalate may be looked for in any of the body fluids or materials. In the interpretation, it should be borne in mind that there is a 'normal' level. Hodgkinson and Zarembski[83] quote a value 9 to 24 mg excreted per day and say that the oxalic acid content of tissue seldom exceeds 1·0 mg/100 g.[84] Curry[85] quotes the following values found in three cases of fatal oxalate poisoning.

1. Liver 5 mg per cent, blood 7 mg per cent, brain 0·3 mg per cent
2. Blood 6·6 mg per cent
3. Blood 2 mg per cent

In a non-fatal poisoning reported by Tompsett,[86] 56 g of potassium hydrogen oxalate (salts of sorrel) were ingested. The four-hour urine sample gave a value of 10·5 mg oxalic acid/100 ml.

Fatal dose and time of death

A boy of sixteen died in eight hours after a dose of 4 g. Recovery, however, has followed the ingestion of 14, 42, and 50 g. Death in three minutes has been recorded when the subject took 40 to 50 g of oxalic acid. The fatal dose is probably above 15 g.

Illustrative cases

In one case where about 14 g was taken by mistake for Rochelle salt, the patient became ill within three minutes and suffered from severe pain in the oesophagus and stomach, vomiting, and partial unconsciousness; later, purging, and severe pains in the loins and back. He recovered. The same dose, however, proved fatal in another instance. A young woman took by mistake, for Epsom salts, a quantity of salt of sorrel.   She died before assistance could be obtained.   One patient recovered, following prompt treatment, after 28 g had been taken.

In another case, a woman of thirty-nine took, in error for a stomach powder, a quantity of salts of lemon which she dissolved in milk. Thereafter she vomited, perspired freely, and complained of burning pain in the epigastrium and oesophagus.   The woman died within an hour of taking the poison.   Post-mortem examination showed that the palate and the edges of the tongue and their under surfaces were of white appearance.   The pharynx was congested and contained clear tenacious mucus.   The oesophageal mucosa was of slate colour and there was patchy exfoliation.   The outer surface of the stomach was inflamed and the organ contained a moderate quantity of dark-coloured fluid.   A brownish-black gelatinous substance covered the gastric mucosa and was composed of mucus and altered blood.   The mucosa was inflamed and some corroded and softened patches were visible.   The lining of the duodenum showed some inflammation.   The amount of the poison consumed was not known.

Note.   Potassium tetroxalate (acid potassium oxalate, salts of sorrel, salts of lemon) is a colourless, crystalline solid, with an acid taste, which dissolves reasonably in water ($1 \cdot 8$ g/100 ml at $13\,°$C).

It has uses similar to oxalic acid and has the same biological effect. It is dealt with under oxalic acid and may be assumed to be interchangeable with it from the point of view of toxic reactions.   Weights must be adjusted, however, to allow for the higher molecular weight of the compound.

PARALDEHYDE (*para-acetaldehyde*)

Paraldehyde is a colourless liquid (b. pt $124\,°$C) with a penetrating odour.   It is soluble in water and has almost the same density ($0 \cdot 994$ at $20\,°$C).   This substance is used for inducing sleep, and is also administered rectally as a basal hypnotic for the purposes of anaesthesia. The normal dose is up to 10 ml orally or by injection or up to 30 ml rectally.   Though paraldehyde is one of the safest basal hypnotics, a number of fatalities have occurred due to overdosage as a result of mistaken concentrations or as a result of decomposition on storage.   Both these points should be checked carefully before administration. Paraldehyde not infrequently becomes a drug of addiction and tolerance builds up with use, though evidence of mental deterioration may develop.

Symptoms

There may be some symptoms of gastric irritation.   After acute overdosage the effects are prolonged unconsciousness, respiratory difficulty, cyanosis, and pulmonary oedema.

Treatment

Treatment consists of gastric lavage and the use of oxygen. The airway must be kept clear. Every effort should be made to arouse the patient, but he should not be submitted to muscular exertion. The patient should be kept warm, and antibiotics administered to obviate pulmonary complication.

If the administration of paraldehyde has been by rectum, high colonic or rectal lavage should be employed as soon as possible after the purpose of the paraldehyde has been served.

Post-mortem findings

On opening the body at autopsy there is usually a strong odour of paraldehyde. Examination may reveal congestion of the meningeal vessels, brain, and lateral ventricles, which may contain an excess of clear fluid. The lungs and abdominal organs may also show congestion.

Analytical findings

Paraldehyde may be demonstrated and measured in any of the materials submitted for analyses. The measurement is usually as acetaldehyde, as the polymer is easily broken down. Acetaldehyde levels in excess of 50 mg/100 ml of blood may be regarded as dangerous. In a report by Copeman[87] of twelve fatal paraldehyde poisonings, the average liver and kidney levels of acetaldehyde were 52 mg/100 g and 40 mg/100 g respectively.

Fatal dose and time of death

The fatal dose is very variable. Recovery has followed ingestion of 60 ml, but death has been reported with much lower doses. If the subject lives for forty-eight hours recovery is likely.

Note. Metaldehyde is a solid polymer of acetaldehyde which sublimes at 112°C and is insoluble in water. It is available commercially as a solid fuel, often in the form of white tablets which children have mistaken for sweets. Fatal poisoning has occurred from both accident and suicide. The ingestion of six tablets has caused death in adults. The symptoms of poisoning are those of acute gastro-intestinal irritation, stupor, coma, tonic then clonic muscular contractions and convulsions. Death may be delayed for several days.

Treatment consists of free gastric lavage with an alkaline solution, saline purgation, and artificial respiration and inhalations of oxygen. Attention should also be directed to the treatment of symptoms.

The post-mortem findings consist of gastro-intestinal inflammation, congestion of the brain, and cloudy swelling of the liver and kidneys.

PARAQUAT

This is a translocated herbicide but has the effect of a contact herbicide. It is available widely to the home gardener as the proprietary product 'Weedol'. There are also a number of products available for agricultural use, which contain either paraquat or a paraquat/diquat mixture.

Symptoms

Shortly after ingestion there may be vomiting of blood-stained material and possibly bloody stools. Thereafter, the subject may feel quite well for a day or two though there may be some local irritant action in the mouth or throat. The next stage of the poisoning is the development of cyanosis and possibly anuria. Some shadows in the lungs may be visible on x-ray examination. These symptoms progress till death from severe respiratory distress.

Treatment

Gastric lavage should be used immediately, but there is no way of reversing the deterioration of the lungs once it has begun.

Post-mortem findings

There may be enlargement of the liver and the kidney may be soft, pale, and swollen. The lungs, however, show the most significant changes. They are congested and oedematous, and intrapulmonary and subpleural petechial haemorrhages may be present. Microscopic examination shows proliferation of the epithelial cells of terminal bronchioles.

Analytical findings

The analytical findings may not be of much value, as death is usually delayed beyond a week during which time most of the paraquat is eliminated. Daniel and Gage[88] quote a 90 per cent elimination within twenty-four hours and Gage[89] states that 10 per cent of the ingested material is excreted in the urine. Tompsett[90] quotes values of 125, 15, and 35 μg paraquat/100 ml of urine taken ante-mortem some time in the week before death of a subject who had taken a mouthful of paraquat concentrate by accident and immediately spat it out. Values for paraquat in post-mortem tissue examined are as given in Table 14.

Table 14. Paraquat in Post-mortem Materials

Post-mortem material					Case 1[91]	Case 2[90]
Blood	.	.	.	.	. 20 μg/100 ml	—
Urine	.	.	.	.	. 1·6 μg/100 ml	—
Brain	.	.	.	.	. Not detected	—
Fat .	.	.	.	.	—	Not detected
Heart	.	.	.	.	—	Not detected
Kidney	.	.	.	.	. 580 μg/100 g	95 μg/100 g
Liver	.	.	.	.	. 60 μg/100 g	20 μg/100 g
Lung	.	.	.	.	. 160 μg/100 g	Not detected
Muscle	.	.	.	.	—	40 μg/100 g
Spleen	.	.	.	.	. 140 μg/100 g	—

Case 1   Death after 4 days   Case 2   Death after 10 days

Fatal dose and time of death

The fatal dose is uncertain. Recovery after 2·8 g is reported, but death has followed 0·2 g (injected) and in a few cases 'a mouthful', of which most was spat out. This is probably equivalent to a gram or two. The fatal period varies from about four days to two weeks.

Illustrative case[92]

A mouthful of agricultural concentrate paraquat solution was taken by mistake. The subject went immediately to hospital, where at one hour after ingestion an emetic caused blood-stained, undigested food to be vomited. After six hours the subject felt well and, apart from developing a sore throat, this condition lasted for two days. On the third day, cyanosis was present. This increased over the next two days, the subject becoming more resistant to treatment with oxygen. Thereafter, the cyanosis increased and there was a cardiac arrest on the eighth day followed by death, three hours later.

Notes. 1. Death is due to a disease process characterised by cellular proliferation of the lungs.[93]
2. The majority of deaths result from accidental ingestion due to storing the paraquat in food containers e.g. lemonade bottles.

PETROLEUM DISTILLATES (*Petrol, paraffin, etc.*)

Petroleum contains gaseous and liquid constituents. When distilled fractionally, ether, petrol, paraffin, and kerosene are obtained. The fractions which distil below 150°C include petroleum ether, petrol, naphtha, and benzine, which are poisonous when swallowed or when their vapours are inhaled. Benzine is much less toxic than benzene and should not be confused with it.

These materials are widely used as solvents and fuels and are easily available.

Symptoms

When the fumes from the more volatile of these fluids are inhaled, nausea, headache, vertigo, and sometimes vomiting occur, and unconsciousness may supervene. On regaining consciousness, or even prior to losing consciousness, there may be mental confusion or excitement with or without violence. Convulsions sometimes occur. In fatal cases cyanosis, unconsciousness, and profound coma precede death. When these fluids are swallowed, the signs are those of gastro-intestinal irritation, and in fatal cases a state of coma will merge into death.

Treatment

When the vapour has been inhaled artificial respiration and oxygen are recommended. Atropine sulphate and caffeine sodium benzoate may be used.

If the material has been swallowed, gastric lavage is recommended. Colonic irrigation may be of value. The patient should be kept warm.

Post-mortem findings

The post-mortem findings include pulmonary oedema and the appearance of acute gastro-enteritis. If the poisoning has taken place over some time, there may be kidney or liver damage.

Analytical findings

The typical hydrocarbon mixtures may be found in the fluids or tissues. It may be possible to identify the material by the distribution of the different components, but there may well be a shift in the balance due to the loss of the lighter boiling fractions.

Fatal dose and time of death

The fatal dose is uncertain. As little as 10 ml may prove fatal, but recovery has followed ingestion of more than ten times this figure. The safe concentration in air is under 500 p.p.m. Values of 1 or 2 per cent in air may be regarded as dangerous to life.   Death may occur at any time from an hour or two to a day.

Illustrative cases

Nunn and Martin[94] have recorded seven cases of petrol poisoning in children.   In two of the fatal cases, the outstanding clinical picture was increased respiration and rapid pulse-rate.   Cyanosis, stupor or coma, and crepitations throughout the lungs were present.   Death occurred within an hour and a half of swallowing the fluid, the quantity of which was not ascertained.   Post-mortem examination showed oedema of the lungs, the alveoli of which were filled with fibrin and serous exudate. Fatty degenerative changes were present in the liver and the stomach contents emitted a strong odour of petrol.   They have also reported sixty-five cases of poisoning by kerosene in children.   9·2 per cent of the cases were fatal.   The children lived from two to eighteen hours after swallowing, or aspirating the substance, and in all there were definite clinical evidences of pathological changes in the lungs, namely, crepitations, rapid and shallow respiration and cyanosis.   Convulsions occurred in two fatal and in two non-fatal cases.   The treatment administered, in the various cases, consisted of removing the kerosene by emesis or by gastric lavage, together with the administration of laxatives.

PHENACETIN

Phenacetin is a white crystalline powder which is very slightly soluble (1 in 1,700) in water.   This analgesic is easily available in many commercial forms and mixtures and is often consumed in large quantities. At one time it was considered to be a safe antipyretic but idiosyncrasy was not infrequent.

Symptoms

The symptoms of acute overdosage include sweating and gastric irritation.   There may be a fall in blood-pressure and temperature, and cyanosis of a pronounced bluish-black colour affecting the skin and mucous membranes may be present.   The urine may be chocolate-coloured due to the presence of methaemoglobin.   There may be circulatory collapse and death from respiratory failure.

Chronic poisoning results in abdominal pains, haemolytic anaemia, and methaemoglobinemia.   There may be skin rashes and low blood-pressure.   Renal damage characterised by interstitial nephritis with papillary necrosis and tubular degeneration has occurred and has caused death.   Withdrawal symptoms may develop when the drug is withheld from a patient after extended use.

Treatment

Absorption of the drug should be hindered by the use of milk. The stomach should be washed out and the patient kept warm. Cyanosis can be treated with methylene blue and ascorbic acid. Transfusions and oxygen should be given as necessary. Support against kidney damage should be considered.

Post-mortem findings

The typical finding in acute poisoning is the brownish colour due to methaemoglobin. In chronic poisoning the kidney damage described above is the most significant finding.

Analytical findings

There are a number of analytical methods available for use on biological materials. These involve the detection of phenacetin or its metabolite paracetamol or p-aminophenol, which is the product of acid hydrolyses of paracetamol. Levels quoted for paracetamol are about 9 mg/100 ml serum and for p-aminophenol in the region of 4 to 25 mg/100 ml serum.

Fatal dose and time of death

The fatal dose is variable but is probably over 5 g. Death occurs very quickly or may be delayed for some days.

Note. Paracetamol, one of the main metabolic products of phenacetin, is considered to show only mildly toxic reactions, though the estimated fatal dose is of the same order as phenacetin.

PHENOL (*Carbolic acid*) AND RELATED MATERIALS

Properties and uses

The pure material is colourless crystalline solid with a characteristic odour and a sweet burning taste. It is reasonably soluble in cold water (6·7 g/100 ml at 16°C) and completely miscible about 66°C. It mixes with alcohol in all proportions and is soluble in glycerine. Phenol is not a true acid and does not redden litmus paper. If the pure material is exposed for some time it develops a pink tinge. A crude form of phenol called carbolic acid is available. This is usually a dark brown, oily-looking liquid with the characteristic odour of phenol. It also contains cresols. Phenol is a popular disinfectant and is sold as Jeyes' disinfecting fluid, Izal, and many other proprietary compounds. Crude cresol (cresyl oil or cresylic acid) may be used as a disinfectant instead of phenol and is employed in the preparation of numerous products such as cresol soap or saponified cresol and creoline.   Lysol consists of 50 per cent v/v of solution of cresol in a saponaceous solvent, such as saponified linseed oil.   Carbolic acid acts as a mild corrosive and anaesthetic upon the skin and mucous membranes when in either the crystalline form or in strong solutions.   It gives a white, bleached, and puckered appearance to the skin at the point of application, the epidermis is destroyed, and a yellowish-brown or brown staining results.   It sometimes produces gangrene when applied as a dressing to the fingers

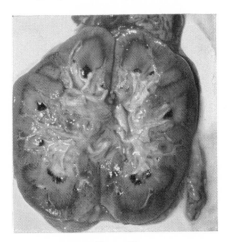

FIG. 228

Haemorrhages in kidney in lysol poisoning

and toes.   In addition to the local action, it also produces a remote action on the central nervous system.

Symptoms

These are intense burning pain in the mouth, throat, and stomach, vomiting of frothy mucus, which may be neither severe nor continuous, coldness and clamminess of the skin, contraction of the pupils, and lividity of the lips.   Stertorous, hurried, or laboured breathing, a small, thready pulse, subnormal temperature, and early onset of insensibility are also prominent manifestations.   In many cases, the odour of the acid may be detected in the breath, though not in every case.   There may be signs of corrosion on the lips and at the corners of the mouth, the marks being of a pale brown or yellowish colour.   The symptoms depend in some measure upon the concentration swallowed.   If a strong solution has been taken, death may follow quickly, with or without vomiting, and with rapidly intervening coma and stertorous breathing, but if a dilute solution has been used, the symptoms supervene only after absorption and are not usually so rapid in onset. It should be remembered that, owing to the local anaesthetic action of this acid, symptoms of irritation, such as pain and vomiting, are not so prominent as in poisoning by oxalic acid or the mineral acids.

Death usually results from respiratory or cardiac failure due to paralysis of the respiratory or cardiac centre.

Treatment

The objects of the treatment are first, to limit the absorption of the poison; secondly, to sustain the patient; and thirdly, to aid the elimination of the poison from the system. Thorough gastric lavage, using a 10 per cent solution of glycerine in water or plain water, should be carried out without delay and continued until the washings no longer emit an odour. When lavage has been completed, a quantity of medicinal liquid paraffin should be left in the stomach, and since it is not absorbed it is preferable to vegetable or animal oils. Egg albumen, since it precipitates phenol, will delay absorption. The airway should be kept unobstructed. Oxygen inhalations are frequently useful. Other treatment should be along general lines. Intravenous 5 per cent saline-glucose may be given in certain cases. When necessary, rectal feeding should be adopted for some days.

Post-mortem findings

Those parts of the skin surrounding the mouth, and the mucous membrane of the lips and mouth, with which the poison has come into contact, show a pale brown or yellowish staining. This, however, will depend upon the strength of the poison used; for example, a 1 per cent solution produces no effect whatever, a 2 per cent solution a slight staining only observable on careful examination, a 4 to 5 per cent solution a whitish discoloration, which is likely to disappear within six hours, whereas a strong solution of the acid or the pure acid causes a white slough. When impure carbolic solutions are swallowed the colour of the stain will be more or less affected. The mucous membranes of the oesophagus and stomach are also more or less similarly affected. The action of carbolic acid upon the gastric mucosa is characteristic. The mucous membrane forms projecting folds, is more or less brownish in colour, and looks leathery. On opening the abdominal cavity, the odour of phenol can usually be detected, owing to the fact that after death some of the acid passes through the walls of the stomach. For this reason, the peritoneal covering of the stomach is

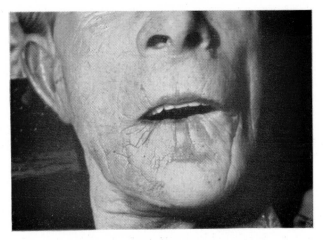

FIG. 229A

Discoloration on face caused by lysol poisoning

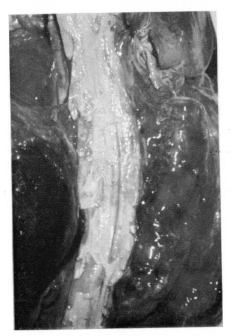

FIG. 229B

Desquamation of mucous membrane of oesophagus in lysol poisoning

injected. A varying portion of the upper part of the small intestine may show evidence of corrosion and injection of the vessels. The odour of the acid is, however, most marked on opening the stomach, and its contents may be found to consist of blood-stained mucus. When a fairly crude cresol preparation has been swallowed the odour may prove very misleading, since it is atypical and may suggest the presence of creosote due to the cresylic acid. The lungs, the abdominal viscera, and brain, are frequently congested. The urine is of greenish-black colour. Death may result from carbolic acid due to its absorption through the unbroken skin, from the effects of inhalation of its fumes, or from rectal and vaginal injections.

Analytical findings

Phenol may be separated and measured in all fluids and tissues of the body though often the analysis is not asked for. In a fatal poisoning case the level found in blood was approximately 9 mg per cent.[95] When crude cresol preparations are used cresol may be found. In one such case the stomach contained 3 g of cresol and the urine 0·1 g. In another case of lysol poisoning the results found (reported as cresol) were as follows:

Stomach contents	3·2 g
Blood	19 mg/100 ml
Liver	48 mg/100 g
Urine	30 mg/100 ml

Fatal dose and time of death

4 ml has killed in twelve hours. Recovery, however, has followed large doses; in one case, from 30 ml of 90 per cent phenol, in another, from 180 ml of crude carbolic acid, and in a third, of a child aged two, from 15 ml of crude acid containing 30 per cent carbolic acid.

Recovery, after prompt treatment, has followed the swallowing of about a pint of Jeyes' fluid. Creolin and lysol also produce toxic effects. Many cases of fatal poisoning have been recorded.

The toxicity of carbolic acid is about eight times greater than that of lysol.

Death from carbolic acid usually occurs within three hours after the poison has been taken. It has, however, followed in three minutes, and it has been retarded for sixty hours.

Illustrative cases

Miller[96] reports the case of a youth, aged eighteen, suffering from ringworm on the right shoulder, the scapular region, and over the left arm and trunk, who had a mixture of camphor and carbolic acid rubbed over the affected areas. Before this procedure was completed the youth became faint and giddy. The mixture was diluted and the application continued. The youth then became dyspnoeic, staggered to the floor, and was helped to bed, where he died within fifteen minutes after the commencement of the application. Post-mortem examination showed that both lungs were congested and in a state of acute pulmonary oedema. The mouth was filled with frothy blood.

Consden[97] reports a case where a workman fell into a vat of phenol and was contaminated as far as the thighs. He was removed and hosed down, but his clothes were not removed till he was taken to the wash room. He became drowsy shortly after his fall and was almost unconscious by the time he reached the wash room. He died there, thirty minutes after falling into the vat.

A poorly nourished, elderly woman was last seen at 14.00 hours when she was in good health. At 10.30 hours on the following day, she was found in bed apparently asleep but breathing very heavily. The woman was taken to hospital but was dead on arrival. The levels found on analysis are those quoted under analytical finding for the lysol case.

Note. *Pyrogallol (pyrogallic acid).* This substance is commonly used in photography, and in the manufacture of hair dyes and marking inks. It has very toxic properties, not only when swallowed but even when it is absorbed through the skin. Cases of poisoning from both causes are recorded. Its toxic effect is serious since, like several other poisons, it has a haemolytic action, destroying the red corpuscles and liberating the haemoglobin into the plasma. Dyspnoea, subnormal temperature, coma, and altered blood in the urine, which is brown in colour, are outstanding manifestations. On post-mortem examination the blood is generally of a brownish-red tint. Treatment consists of free lavage of the stomach; oxygen, stimulants, maintenance of body heat and transfusion.

PHENOTHIAZINES

The typical drug of this group is chlorpromazine. Among many others are acepromazine, chlorprothixene, fluphenazine, haloperidol, perphenazine, prochlorperazine, promazine, thioproperazine, thioridazine, and trifluoperazine. These materials are used as tranquillisers, i.e. to calm a subject without producing hypnosis. Apart from this, they have anti-emetic, antihistaminic, and adrenalytic actions in various degrees. For example, promethazine is commonly listed and used as an antihistamine.

Symptoms

The general side effects of these drugs may include dryness of the mouth, tachycardia, blurred vision, and oedema.   The effects of acute poisoning include drowsiness, postural hypotension, together with the side effects quoted above.   There may also be nausea, fever, and coma. Chronic poisoning may produce leukopenia or agranulocytosis.   There may be ulceration of the gums, tongue, and pharynx, fever, and disorientation.   Other symptoms include jaundice, sensitivity to sunlight, corneal and lens pigmentation.   Central nervous system effects such as convulsions are general.   Death can be caused by ventricular fibrillation.

Treatment

Discontinue drugs and use gastric lavage.   Treat symptoms as they arise but do not use convulsant stimulants.   Convulsions may be controlled with pentobarbitone.   Antibiotics may be used to combat secondary infections.

Post-mortem findings

The findings are non-specific.   There may be liver damage after chronic poisoning.

Analytical findings

Chlorpromazine levels of less than 1 mg per 100 ml may be found in the blood after death.   The liver levels may be much higher and may reach values of up to 50 mg/100 g.   The other drugs of this group cause serious poisoning at similar levels.

Fatal dose

The fatal dose is not known, but may be estimated as several grams, though severe symptoms have occurred with much less.

PHOSGENE (*Carbonyl chloride*)

Phosgene is a dense colourless gas, with a characteristic odour, which liquifies at about 8°C.   It is used in the dye and pharmaceutical industries and in metallurgy.   It has also been used in chemical warfare. Phosgene owes its toxicity to the fact that it is readily split up in the presence of water into hydrochloric acid and carbon dioxide.

Symptoms

Toxic concentrations in the air cause severe irritation of the entire respiratory tract. Very high concentrations may cause immediate death by suffocation. Lower concentrations cause progressive oedema of the lungs to such an extent that death occurs from asphyxiation or possibly heart failure. Symptoms may take some hours to develop.

Treatment

The treatment recommended is that given under chlorine.

Post-mortem findings

The essential lesions produced are pulmonary oedema, rupture of the pulmonary alveoli, and concentration of the blood.

Fatal dose and time of death

Death may be almost immediate if the concentration is high, but less severe doses result in death between a few hours and two days later. The maximum concentration allowable is 1 p.p.m. At concentrations of over 50 p.p.m. death may follow in as little as thirty minutes after exposure.

PHOSPHINE (*Hydrogen phosphide*)

This gas, heavier than air, is colourless, irritating, possesses a most unpleasant odour, reminiscent of rotten fish, and is highly toxic. Poisoning may occur industrially when the gas is liberated as a by-product. Ferrosilicon, used in the production of steel, may liberate both phosphine and arsine when brought into contact with moisture. Fatal results have been caused in this way. Poisoning may also occur in those engaged in the preparation and use of calcium phosphide.

Symptoms

The onset of symptoms is rapid after inhalation. The symptoms include oppression over the epigastrium, where a burning or piercing sensation may be felt, and breathing becomes rapid at first, but, later, slow and laboured. Nausea, vomiting, an odour of the gas in the breath, giddiness, profuse perspiration, convulsions, delirium and coma are frequently present. Death occurs from either cardiac or respiratory failure. There may be bronchitis, inflammation, or oedema of the lungs.

Post-mortem findings

The post-mortem appearances are engorgement of the lungs, liver, and covering membranes of the brain, also engorgement of the heart with dark-coloured blood.

Analytical findings

Phosphine is rapidly oxidised in the body and, as a result, may not be found on analysis.

Fatal dose and time of death

The dangerous concentration of this gas is probably in the region of a few parts per million.   Death may occur up to a week after exposure.

PHOSPHORUS

Two allotropes of phosphorus are used in industry.   One is a white or yellow waxy solid, and the other a dark red powder.   If exposed to air, white phosphorus forms a white opaque crust.   This allotrope melts at about 44° and ignites in air at about 30°C, i.e. it may well ignite if handled or kept in a pocket.   The resulting burns are very painful and heal very slowly.   People constantly exposed to the action of phosphorus fumes are liable to suffer from caries and rotting of the bones of the jaw and nose (phossy jaw).   On account of its inflammability, yellow phosphorus is kept under water in which it is almost insoluble.   A unique property of yellow phosphorus is that it glows in the dark when exposed to air.   The red isotope is relatively inert and is considered non-toxic.

Since the use of phosphorus rat poisons was introduced in vermin control a number of homicidal and accidental deaths have taken place.

Symptoms

Acute.   Phosphorus, an active protoplasmic poison, which depresses cellular oxidation and causes widespread fatty degeneration when swallowed in poisonous dose, causes pain in the stomach, which may, however, not be marked, but which is usually succeeded by vomiting. The patient may complain of a garlic taste in the mouth, and a garlic odour may be perceived in the breath.   There is an acrid, burning sensation in the throat and oesophagus, accompanied by great thirst. The vomited material is usually dark in colour, dark green, coffee-coloured, or black, has a garlicky odour, and, if exposed in the dark, becomes luminous or phosphorescent.   The faeces are also dark and luminous. Diarrhoea may or may not be present. Signs of shock develop, the pulse becomes small, irregular, feeble, and, at times, imperceptible, there is cold, clammy skin, anxious, pinched face, and subnormal temperature. Coma or convulsions usually precede death. In most cases, however, the progress is not continuous to a direct fatal termination. There is usually an intermission in the severity of the symptoms, so much so, at times, as to give the impression that recovery has taken place.

Sooner or later, it may be two or more days, fresh symptoms appear. Jaundice develops, the epigastric pain, not yet passed away from the original attack, increases in severity, and the abdomen becomes distended. On examination the liver will be found enlarged, as probably also the spleen. Vomiting returns. Haemorrhages from the nose, or from other mucous surfaces, or subcutaneous haemorrhages appear. The urine becomes scanty, strongly acid in reaction, high-coloured, and contains blood, albumin, bile and sometimes sugar. The nervous system becomes implicated, and sleeplessness, pains in the head, together with other manifestations, appear. The faeces are pale or clay-like in colour. Gradually the patient becomes more prostrate, the pulse becomes weaker, irregular, and more compressible, and some degree of pyrexia sets in. Prior to death, convulsions or coma may appear. The clinical picture may be suggestive of acute yellow atrophy of the liver.

Chronic. These usually result from inhalation rather than from ingestion. Gastro-intestinal symptoms are prominent, excreta and breath have a garlic odour, the red and white cell counts are increased, and the liver is enlarged. Anaemia, jaundice, fragility of bones, bronchitis or bronchopneumonia, necrosis of jaw, 'phossy-jaw', and general prostration may, and probably will, be evident in the more severe cases as time passes. 'Phossy-jaw' is a condition of suppurative osteomyelitis of the maxilla or of the mandible with multiple sinuses and resultant considerable disfigurement.

Treatment

Early use of the stomach tube, and free lavage with a 0·5 per cent solution of potassium permanganate, will exert an oxidising effect upon the phosphorus. A dilute solution of copper sulphate, 1 g to 4·5 l of water, may be used instead. Evacuation of the bowels is important. Any fall in serum calcium may be treated with calcium gluconate. Severe liver damage may be treated with hydrocortisone as well as dietary measures. Alkaline drinks and dextrose should be given, but oils, fats, and eggs should be withheld.

Post-mortem findings

The appearances generally are those of a highly irritant poison, consisting of inflammation or erosion of the mucous membrane of the pharynx, oesophagus, stomach, and intestines.   The stomach may contain dark-coloured fluid, consisting of mucus and altered blood, which may have a garlicky odour.   The contents may be luminous in the dark.   The liver, enlarged and usually of yellowish colour, is the seat of marked fatty degeneration and quite frequently shows a softened condition.   Its colour varies.   On microscopical examination, extensive destruction of the liver cells is found, and evidence of fatty degenerative changes is marked.   Haemorrhagic extravasations are commonly found.   Fatty degeneration of the musculature of the heart, of voluntary muscle fibres, and of the kidneys is present.

Analytical findings

Elemental phosphorus may be found in any tissues examined.   As the free element is not normally present, any amount indicates poisoning.

Fatal dose and time of death

The fatal dose is in the region of 50 to 100 mg, but Fletcher and Galambos[98] report two non-fatal poisonings where the weights ingested were 715 mg and 350 mg.   The fatal period may be as long as a week or as little as twelve hours.

Illustrative case

A 43-year-old man was admitted to hospital three days after ingesting 1·2 g of yellow phoshorus in the form of rat poison.   Within a few hours of taking the poison his skin felt hot and flushed.   He said he had much flatulence suggestive of having eaten onions.   The next day there were no symptoms.   On the third day, he became mildly jaundiced and vomited black syrup-like material which contained altered blood and mucus.   In hospital next day vomiting continued in spite of gastric lavage with permanganate.   He became oliguric and had persistent diarrhoea.   On the day after admission there was a series of convulsions followed by spastic then flaccid quadriplegia and death.

POISONOUS PLANTS AND EXTRACTS

1. BRITISH POISONOUS PLANTS

Poisoning by plants or seeds is usually accidental and involves mistakes in identification of roots and vegetation for cooking purposes, or the use of plants when they have developed poisonous properties. The typical example of the latter is the potato tuber which has become green due to exposure to light or which has begun to sprout. In this condition, poisonous materials such as solanine are produced. A number of children are poisoned due to eating berries and seeds which may have attracted them. The only answer to this problem is training, as the attractive poisonous seeds are widely available. Table 15 below gives a small selection of plants which may cause poisoning and includes the more dangerous species. Also listed are the common names, poisonous parts, and the typical poison found in the plants. This poison is usually part of a series of related substances which generally have similar actions.

Symptoms and treatment

The symptoms and treatments for the plants listed in Table 15 are given under the typical poison which the plants contain. (Table 16 or alphabetically in the general list.) The symptoms do not characterise the poisons by their actions very well, so it is necessary to investigate the history of the case closely to find the source concerned. This may be difficult because the victim must have made a reasonable mistake in the first place and may well consider the material he ingested to be safe.

Post-mortem findings

Any vegetable remains found during treatment should be retained for investigation even if they look quite common and innocuous. Generally the post-mortem appearances of the organs will not point to a specific source.

Analytical findings

All material available should be investigated but the field is very large. If any vegetable material is present this should be identified first by observing the detailed structure and then submitted to an analytical investigation. Thereafter the tissues and fluids may be processed.

Fatal dose and time of death

These are given in Table 16 where available, but they must be treated with great caution when applied to vegetable material, as the content varies widely with time and place of growth and the human metabolism reacts variably in absorption of the pure as opposed to the unextracted

Table 15.   British Poisonous Plants

Family	Plant	Common name	Poisonous parts	Typical poison
Cucurbitaceae . . .	Bryonia dioica*	White bryony	root and berries	bryonin
Leguminosae . .	Laburnum anagyroides*	Laburnum, Golden rain	all parts	cytisine
Liliaceae . .	Colchicum autumnale	Autumn crocus, Meadow saffron, Naked ladies	all parts	convallarin
Liliaceae . .	Convallaria majalis	Lily of the valley	all parts	convallarin
Oleaceae . .	Ligustrum vulgare*	Privet	leaves and berries	ligustrin
Polygonaceae .	Rheum rhaponticum	Rhubarb	leaves	oxalates
Ranunculaceae .	Ranunculus species	Buttercups and Crowfoots	all sappy parts	protoanemonin
Ranunculaceae .	Helleborus foetidus	Stinking hellebore	all parts	helleborin
Ranunculaceae .	Helleborus niger	Black hellebore, Christmas rose	all parts	helleborin
Ranunculaceae .	Aconitum napellus	Monkshood, Aconite, Wolfsbane	all parts	aconitine
Rosaceae . .	Prunus laurocerasus*	Cherry laurel, Common laurel	all parts	hydrogen cyanide
Scrophulariaceae .	Digitalis purpurea	Foxglove	all parts	digitoxin
Solanaceae . .	Datura stramonium	Thorn-apple, Devil's apple, Jimsen weed	all parts	hyocyamine, hyoscine, atropine

Family	Species	Common name	Part	Toxin
Solanaceae	*Hyocyamus niger*	Henbane	all parts	hyocyamine, hyoscine, atropine
Solanaceae	*Atropa belladonna**	Deadly nightshade, Dwale, Belladonna, Banewort	all parts	hyocyamine, hyoscine, atropine
Solanaceae	*Solanum dulcamara**	Woody nightshade, Bittersweet	all parts	solanine
Solanaceae	*Solanum nigrum**	Black nightshade, Garden nightshade	all parts	solanine
Solanaceae	*Solanum tuberosum*	Potato	stem, leaves and green sprouting tubers	solanine
Solanaceae	*Lycopersicum asculentum*	Tomato	stem and leaves	solanine
Taxaceae	*Taxus baccata**	Yew	leaves and buds	taxine
Thymeleaceae	*Daphne laureola**	Spurge laurel, Wood laurel	all parts	mezerinic acid
Umbelliferae	*Conium maculatum*	Hemlock	all parts	coniine
Umbelliferae	*Circuta virosa*	Cowbane, Water hemlock	all parts	cicutoxin
Umbelliferae	*Oenanthe crocata*	Water dropwort	all parts	oenanthetoxin

*Illustrated

Table 16. Plant Poisons

Plants typically containing	Symptoms	Treatment	Remarks
Solanine	As for atropine	As for atropine	Fatal dose is of the order of 200 mg of solanine.
Taxine	Dizziness, anaesthesia and convulsions followed by death due to depressant action on the heart or respiratory failure. If yew is ingested there may be abdominal pain due to irritant oils.	Gastric lavage and artificial respiration. Oxygen may be required. Control convulsions.	Death may be very rapid after ingestion of small amounts of yew.
Mezerinic acid	Burning sensation in mouth and stomach, vomiting, a rapid weak pulse, great prostration possibly followed by collapse and death.	Treat as for an irritant poison	
Coniine	Gastro-intestinal irritation, muscular weakness and gradually increasing paralysis due to depression of the motor nerves. Breathing becomes slow. Coma or convulsions supervene and the patient dies of asphyxia due to paralysis of the respiratory centre.	Gastric lavage with a dilute tannic acid solution. Artificial respiration and oxygen may be required. Convulsions should be controlled.	Post-mortem appearances are those of asphyxia. Gastro-intestinal irritation may be found. Very small amounts of Hemlock may cause serious poisoning. Onset of symptoms is very rapid.

Cicutoxin		As for coniine	
Oenanthotoxin		As for coniine	
Bryonin	Burning sensation of mouth and stomach, vomiting, diarrhoea, collapse, coma, and death.	Gastric lavage and treat as for an irritant poison.	Degenerative changes of liver, kidneys, and brain may be found at the post-mortem examination.
Cytisine	Nausea, vomiting, purging, giddiness, dilatation of pupils, tachycardia, subnormal temperature, coma, convulsive twitches and convulsions.	Gastric lavage, artificial respiration, and stimulants.	Gastro-intestinal irritation and asphyxia signs at the post-mortem examination. May be kidney damage. Children have died within 8 to 14 hours after eating laburnum seeds.
Colchicine	Vomiting and diarrhoea, abdominal pains, weakness, convulsions, and coma followed by death by paralysis of the respiratory centre. There may be haematuria or complete suppression of urine.	Gastric lavage with dilute solution of tannic acid. Medicinal charcoal given repeatedly. Glucose-saline intravenously, atropine (0·6 mg) hypodermically, and stimulants.	Post-mortem signs are those of irritant poisons. The kidneys may show degenerative changes.
Convallarin		As for digitoxin	
Ligustrin	Vomiting, diarrhoea, weak thready pulse, subnormal temperature, muscular twitchings or convulsions.	As for irritant poisons	May be renal damage.
Helleborin		As for digitoxin	
Protoanemonin	This is a severe irritant poison and the subject exhibits typical symptoms.	As for irritant poisons	

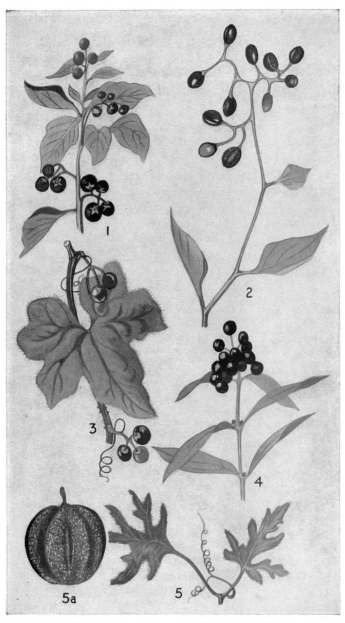

FIG. 230. **Poisonous berries and seeds**

1. *Solanum nigrum* (black nightshade). 2. *Solanum dulcamara* (bitter-sweet or woody nightshade). 3. *Bryonia dioica* (common bryony). 4. *Ligustrum vulgare* (privet). 5a. Fruit of colocynth. 5. *Citrullus colocynthis* (colocynth or bitter apple)

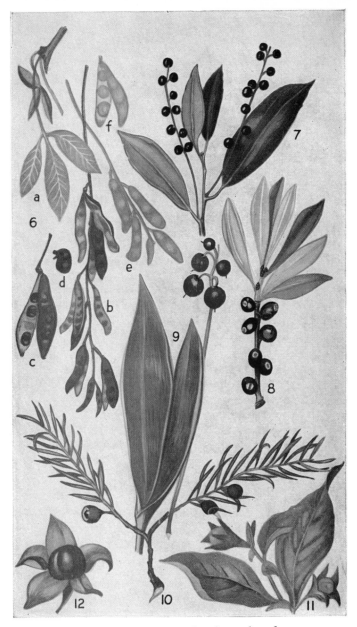

FIG. 231. **Poisonous berries and seeds**

6. *Laburnum vulgare* (laburnum)—*a*, leaves; *b*, ripe pods; *c*, ripe pod; *d*, ripe seed; *e*, unripe pods; *f*, unripe pod. 7. *Prunus lauro cerasus* (cherry-laurel). 8. *Daphne laureola* (spurge laurel). 9. *Convallaria majalis* (lily of the valley). 10. *Taxus baccata* (yew). 11. *Atropa belladonna* (belladonna). 12. Fruit of belladonna

Table 17. Poisonous Vegetable Extracts

Material (and source)	Symptoms	Treatment	Remarks
Curarine (Strychnos toxifera)	The voluntary muscles become paralysed and as the muscles of respiration become involved asphyxia develops.	Prostigmine is the antidote. 2 ml of a 1 in 2,000 solution intravenously is recommended. Artificial respiration with oxygen inhalations should be used until the drug is eliminated.	Poisoning does not occur by ingestion. Absorption is through some wound and death follows rapidly.
Gelsemine (Gelsemium sempervirens — yellow jasmine)	Symptoms include dilated pupils, impaired speech, muscular inco-ordination, convulsions, and death due to respiratory paralysis.	Empty stomach and wash with dilute tannic acid. Keep warm and use stimulants. Artificial respiration and oxygen as necessary.	
Lobeline (Lobelia inflata — Indian tobacco)	As for nicotine	As for nicotine	
Physostigmine (Physostigma venenosum — Calabar bean)	Symptoms include contracted pupils, increased peristalsis, depression of the central nervous system, and twitching of the voluntary muscles. There may be paralysis of the voluntary muscles when large doses are taken and death may be caused by paralysis of the respiratory centre.	Gastric lavage with 4 g potassium permanganate in 10 litres of water. Atropine sulphate (1·25 mg) may be injected. Artificial respiration may be required. Stimulants may be given.	The fatal dose is somewhat under 10 mg of the pure drug.

Pilocarpine (Pilocarpus jaborandi)	Symptoms include lachrymation, perspiration and excretion of mucus, giddiness, thirst, dyspnoea, laboured breathing, convulsions, and death from respiratory paralysis.	Similar to physostigmine	The fatal dose is probably in the region of 60 mg.
Quinine (Cinchona calisaya)	These include vomiting, pyrexia, oliguria, cardiac irregularities, deafness, and blindness. In large doses there is depression of the cardiac and respiratory centres. The general view of quinine as an abortifacient is that it stimulates the tone and contractions of the uterus unless the dose is toxic when it has a depressing effect. In the later stages of pregnancy, especially, quinine exerts a stimulating action on the uterine musculature.	Gastric lavage or emesis is required. Treat other symptoms as they arise.	Idiosyncrasy plays an important part in most serious poisonings. The fatal dose is probably in the region of 1 g. Quinacrine and chloroquine behave similarly.
Strophanthin (Strophanthus kombe)	As for digitoxin	As for digitoxin	More rapid in action.
Veratrine (Veratrum sabadilla)	A tingling sensation of mouth and oesophagus which becomes general and is followed by numbness. This is followed by vomiting, diarrhoea, colic, collapse, convulsions, and death by respiratory failure.	This includes gastric lavage, medicinal charcoal, and maintenance of temperature. Stimulants and artificial respiration may be necessary. Atropine may be used.	About 1 g of plant tissue may be dangerous.

Table 18.   Vegetable Irritants

Material	Source	Action	Remarks
Aloes (Aloin)	Aloe ferox	Purgative in action.	Overdose produces excessive diarrhoea and intestinal irritation.
Apiol	Carum petroselinum (Parsley)	Used in combination with other materials (e.g. ergot) for amenorrhoea and kindred ailments.	Overdose may cause polyneuritis, nephrosis, uraemia, or encephalopathy. This material has been used as an abortifacient.
Camphor	Cinnamomum camphora	Used in the form of liniments and spirit.	Symptoms include vomiting, convulsions, stertorous breathing, cyanosis of the lips, and coma.
Colocynth	Citrullus colocynthis* (Bitter apple)	Drastic purgative action.	Overdose causes excessive purgation and intestinal irritation. It has been used in an attempt to produce abortion.
Crotin oil (Crotin)	Croton tiglium	This is an irritant and vesicant.	Overdose causes vomiting, violent diarrhoea, and abdominal pain. There is some evidence that it has been tried as an abortifacient.
Eucalyptus oil (Cineole)	Eucalyptus polybractea	This is used as a popular remedy for nasal catarrh.	Overdose is characterised by gastro-intestinal irritation accompanied by cerebral excitation, convulsions, and coma. Death may occur from respiratory paralysis.
Nutmeg (Myristicin)	Myristica fragrans	Used mainly as the ground kernel in cooking. It has an irritant action.	Overdose results in a considerably increased pulse-rate and faintness. There may be contractions of the pregnant uterus. The material has been used in attempts to produce abortion.

Pennyroyal (Pulegone)	*Mentha pulegium*	This has an irritant action. The irritant action on the urinary system may cause reflex uterine contractions and, as a result, there have been attempts to use this material as an abortifacient.
Santonin	*Artemisia maritima*	This material is used as an anthelmintic and is an irritant. Symptoms of poisoning include giddiness, nausea, vomiting, diarrhoea, abdominal pain, trembling, frequency of micturition, with tenesmus, burning sensation at the urinary meatus, yellow urine when acid (red when alkaline), and perhaps haemoglobinuria. Colour vision disturbances may be present. In fatal cases coma and convulsions precede death. Chronic poisoning was sometimes seen in absinthe drinkers—the principal effect being degenerative changes of the central nervous system. This material has been used as an aphrodisiac.
Savin	*Juniperus sabinae*	The action is that of an irritant. In large doses it sometimes produces abortion, accompanied by serious toxic manifestations, principally gastro-intestinal in character. Haematuria may be present.
Turpentine (Pinene)	*Pinus sylvestris*	This is an irritant material. Symptoms include burning sensation in the mouth and stomach, vomiting, diarrhoea, cerebral excitement, coma, and death.

* Illustrated

material.   There is also the fact that most poisonous plants contain more than one active toxic agent.

Note.   There are many other poisonous plants growing wild in Britain and many cultivated as garden flowers.   Publications giving notes on microscopic identification of poisonous plants are available. Her Majesty's Stationery Office[99] publishes a detailed description booklet of plants and their actions with a few black and white illustrations.   Blandford Press[100] publishes a small book illustrating 133 poisonous plants in colour and giving brief summaries of the plants and their toxic actions.

2. POISONOUS VEGETABLE EXTRACTS

This section deals with a selection of the less important poisonous extracts from plants which do not grow naturally in Britain, but are easily available and in some cases very toxic.   The more important materials such as cocaine and opium are described in the general list. Poisoning results from ingestion of the vegetable material or the extract, except in the case of curare when poisoning is through exposure of an open wound to the drug.   The poisons and their sources are listed in Table 17.

Symptoms and treatment

The symptoms and treatment vary and each is described in Table 17 or referred to a drug in the general list.   These should be approached with caution if the subject has ingested plant material, as there may be more than one active poison present.

Post-mortem findings

The findings are of a non-specific nature and the cause of poisoning must be sought in the case history.

Analytical findings

Any vegetable materials should be examined to try to discover the identity before analysis is made.   If the source is plant material there may be more than one dangerous substance in active quantities.

Fatal dose and time of death

The values available are given in Table 17, but they must be considered variable when plant material is involved, as absorption may not be as easy as in the case of the pure substance and there may be other poisonous materials acting at the same time.

3. VEGETABLE IRRITANTS

This section deals with oils and solids extracted from vegetable sources. A selection of materials is given in Table 18 together with a typical source plant. These substances have innocent uses such as flavouring food, the preparation of purgative mixtures, and the formulation of liniments. However, they have been used for less legal purposes such as attempting to procure abortion, and these uses are noted in the Table under the heading of 'remarks'.

Symptoms

The action of these drugs is listed in Table 18 and is generally that of an irritant poison. The signs found after known overdosage are also described.

Treatment

The treatment is basically that for an irritant poison. Other symptoms should be treated as they arise.

Post-mortem findings

Deaths are rare and the findings are generally non-specific.

POTASSIUM HYDROXIDE AND SODIUM HYDROXIDE
(*Caustic potash and Caustic soda*)

Appearance and properties

These are waxy, white solids which rapidly absorb moisture from the air. The material is soapy to the touch when moist or in solution and corrodes the skin.

These alkalis are used widely in industry and may be present in the home, e.g. caustic soda is a common constituent of materials for clearing blocked drains. It has only trivial use in medicine as a wart remover or cuticle solvent.

Symptoms

Ingestion results in burning pain of the mouth, throat, and stomach. The lining becomes swollen and may slough. The surface of the mouth, tongue, and lips becomes reddened and eroded. Vomiting occurs which may contain altered blood. Usually shock develops with cold, clammy skin and a feeble and rapid pulse. Oesophageal stricture may well be an aftermath of the ingestion.

Treatment

Dilute acids such as vinegar, lemon juice, or tartaric acid, and demulcent drinks should be administered. Olive oil may be given freely or egg albumen may be employed. A stomach tube should not be used.

Post-mortem findings

Post-mortem appearances are indicative of a corrosive poisoning.

Analytical findings

These are usually limited to the determination of the amount of alkali in the stomach.

Fatal dose and time of death

The fatal dose is very uncertain but is probably somewhat under 10 g. Death has occurred after a few hours.

Illustrative cases

A man swallowed a quantity of strong caustic potash solution in mistake for ginger beer, and although he recovered from the acute symptoms, he later suffered from partial oesophageal stricture.

Willimott[95] reports the case of a person who swallowed 4 g of the solid dissolved in half a tumbler of water. Vomiting, pain in the mouth, throat, and stomach, and collapse followed. Death occurred in about twenty-nine hours. The lips and mucosa of the mouth, tongue, and pharynx were swollen. The mucosa of tongue and pharynx was of deep chocolate colour.

RADIOACTIVE SUBSTANCES

Radioactive atoms are those which have unstable nuclei but otherwise have chemical properties identical with normal atoms. These nuclei eventually disintegrate to a stable form which is usually, but not necessarily, another element. In this disintegration process a charged particle or particles and/or γ-radition is given off.   This radiation causes intense ionisation of, and therefore destruction of biological material.

There are a small number of elements which as they occur in nature contain a radioactive isotope (e.g. radium, uranium, potassium) and a large number of artificially produced radioactive isotopes (e.g. Co^{60} Sr^{90}, i.e. cobalt with an atomic mass of 60 and strontium with an atomic mass of 90).   Atoms are isotopes when they are the same chemical element (i.e. same atomic number) but have different atomic masses.

Damage may occur if someone is exposed close to an unshielded radioactive material.   In the extreme case of direct contact, damage may be great from relatively small sources.   There are extensive legislation and a number of recommended codes of practice for controlling the use of radioactive materials, and over-exposures are not common.   However, a number of incidents have occurred.   A typical example was the exposure of workers involved in the painting of watch and clock hands and dials with self luminous pigments containing radium.

Symptoms

The external symptoms resemble dermatitis.   There may also be 'burns', ulceration, and possibly skin cancer.   Alopecia, loss of fingerprint patterns, and the development of cataract are also reported. Internally there may be tissue damage and alteration with the development of malignant tumours.   When radioactive heavy elements have been ingested with subsequent deposition in the bones there may be severe damage locally.   As a result of the local concentration of the bones, tissue close by may develop malignant tumours.   A common effect is destruction of the bone marrow.

The symptoms may develop within a few days but may be delayed for years, depending on the intensity of the exposure.   Repeated exposures are cumulative.

Treatment

Remove from exposure and decontaminate the body surface if necessary.   Aid the excretion of particular element involved if possible. Treat other symptoms as they arise.

Dangerous dose

Not all radioactive isotopes have the same hazard rating.   In a single exposure by ingestion or inhalation the risk of damage is proportional to the amount of radioisotope, its rate of disintegration, and the time it is retained within the body.   The International Atomic Energy Agency publish a report[101] which gives information on the division of the various radioactive isotopes into different classes of toxicity.

SILVER NITRATE

Properties and uses

The pure substance is a colourless, crystalline solid. Organic materials which have been in contact with this material turn black due to the formation of metallic silver. The action is very much faster in the presence of light or a chemical reducing agent. Silver nitrate is used widely in industry and to some extent in medicine as an antiseptic or for its caustic properties. Its most common occurrence in the home is as a wart remover, or among the chemicals of a photographic enthusiast.

Symptoms

The solid or concentrated liquid acts as a corrosive to a limited extent.

Treatment

Sodium chloride (about 1 in 50 of water) solution causes silver nitrate to form the non-toxic silver chloride. After this treatment the stomach may be emptied by emesis or gastric lavage.

Post-mortem findings

The mouth, lips, mucous membranes, and stomach lining are stained grey-white to black and corroded.

Analytical findings

The amount of silver in the stomach can be estimated. Tissue values should be compared with normal values (Appendix III).

Fatal dose

The fatal dose is about 2 g, but recovery from much larger quantities has been reported.

STRYCHNINE

This is a colourless crystalline solid (m. pt 268°C) which is very slightly soluble in water (0·016 g/100 ml at 25°C) and has a very bitter taste perceptible at a dilution of 1 in 70,000. The salts formed with the mineral acids are easily soluble in water. Strychnine and brucine are extracted from the seeds of *Strychnos nux vomica*. It is used in tonics and as a poison for animal pests.

Symptoms

Strychnine has a selective action on the central nervous system and produces a condition of irritability of the reflex centres of the spinal cord. When a poisonous dose has been swallowed, the following symptoms appear after an interval which may vary from a few minutes to an hour. An intensely bitter taste is perceived in the mouth and soon afterwards there is a sensation of suffocation, accompanied by twitching of the muscles of the neck, body, and limbs, followed by severe tetanic convulsions which involve all the muscles of the body. During this state the muscles become stiff and rigid, so that the body is thrown into an arch, only the back of the head and heels touching the bed or ground. This condition is known as opisthotonos. In some cases, the body-curve is in the opposite direction, called emprosthotonos, or the body may be curved laterally, pleurosthotonos. Owing to the tetanic contraction of the thoracic muscles, breathing becomes difficult and imperfect, and the face in consequence becomes markedly cyanosed. As the result of the contraction of the muscles at the angles of the mouth risus sardonicus is produced, the lower jaw becomes firmly shut or fixed by the contracted condition of the masseters, the fingers are clenched in the palms of the hand, the feet arched inwards, and the eyes staring and wild looking. This tonic spasm lasts from half a minute to two minutes, and then there is a remission of symptoms. During a spasm the patient is in complete possession of his senses, and experiences acute pain. During the remission he lies in a calm but weakened condition, and may fall asleep. During the convulsive seizure the pupils become dilated, but in the period of remission they resume their normal condition, which, relative to the former state, appears to be one of contraction.

After a variable interval, depending upon the severity of the toxic effects and often as the result of some trivial cause, such as someone walking across the floor, a touch, or even a draught of cold air, another attack similar to the first comes on. In cases proceeding to a fatal issue the intervals of remission are short, in less severe cases they may be longer. Death usually supervenes either during a spasm from asphyxia induced by fixation of the chest wall, or from exhaustion due to the repetition of attacks. Death, therefore, may follow very shortly after the spasms appear, or it may be delayed for some hours.

In tetanus, or lockjaw, fixation of the lower jaw is one of the earliest and most enduring symptoms, but in strychnine poisoning it is only part of the general tetanic contraction of the body muscles, and passes off with the muscular relaxation during the period of remission. Indeed there is no other set of phenomena, from disease or poison, which is exactly comparable to that which follows the absorption of strychnine in the body.

A case of intermeningeal spinal haemorrhage has been reported where the similarity of the symptoms to strychnine poisoning were such as to warrant the withholding of a certificate of death until post-mortem examination.

Symptoms of strychnine poisoning appear even if the poison is applied externally and is absorbed.   In one case, the application of 5 mg of strychnine to the eye produced toxic effects in about three to four minutes.

Strychnine poisoning has occurred through mistakes in prescriptions by chemists.

Homicidal administration has given rise to some well-known cases, including those of William Palmer, William Dove, Silas Barlow, George Horton, Walter Horsford, Thomas Neill Cream, and Jean Pierre Vaquier.

Treatment

Anaesthesia should be induced as soon as possible in view of the fact that convulsive seizures are induced by almost any form of treatment.   As soon as the patient is under its influence, the stomach tube should be used and free gastric lavage performed, with a solution of potassium permanganate in water, 4 g in 9 l.   To follow, medicinal charcoal and water are recommended, and these may be freely given and renewed from time to time.   Light anaesthesia should be continued for long periods, if necessary, and for as long as the convulsions threaten to return.   Sedatives such as chloral hydrate may be administered. Haggard and Greenberg[102] assert that there is true antagonism between the action of sodium phenobarbitone and strychnine.   Kempf, McCallum, and Zerfas[103] report eleven cases successfully treated with sodium amytal, or pentobarbital sodium, given intravenously. They advise that only a quantity sufficient to put the patient to sleep should be given, or if convulsions are present, only enough to stop them.   They are of the further opinion that, when such drugs are administered, gastric lavage is both unnecessary and inadvisable until after the patient is asleep.   A mild convulsion should be awaited before repeating the dose of amytal.   Stalberg and Davidson[104] state that intravenously sodium amytal is a definite life-saving measure.   In conjunction with this treatment, they also use avertin anaesthesia by rectum, and this reduces the quantity of sodium amytal required.   One patient received five injections of sodium amytal, a total of 3 g, intravenously, and four rectal injections of avertin, each 250 mg.   Five capsules of sodium amytal were also given by the mouth.   The patient had taken 110 mg of strychnine. The convulsions lasted for five and a half days and did not commence until forty-nine hours after ingestion of the strychnine. Wheelock,[105] following the treatment of a suicidal case, states that the results were so dramatic that in future cases sodium amytal and sodium phenobarbitone should at least be tried. The patient had taken 60 mg of strychnine.

Artificial respiration and oxygen inhalations may also be necessary. Other symptoms should be treated as they arise.

Post-mortem findings

The most constant appearances of the internal organs consist of engorgement of the lungs, the vessels of the brain and spinal cord, but there are no typical signs.

Analytical findings

Strychnine may be found in the fluids and tissues but only in very small quantities. The urine, brain, and spinal cord are recommended tissues for analysis. The whole of the spinal cord is required. The values given below were obtained from two fatal poisonings. Case 1 (Illustrative case below) died in hospital after extensive treatment and Case 2 was found dead.

Table 19. Strychnine in Post-mortem Materials

Material	Case 1	Case 2
Blood . . .	1 μg/100 ml	60 μg/100 ml
Urine . . .	770 μg/100 ml	—
Stomach contents .	0·1 μg	108 mg
Liver . . .	0·1 μg/100 g	27 μg/100 g
Kidney . . .	7 μg/100 g	40 μg/100 g
Brain . . .	47 μg/100 g	+ve
Spinal cord . .	180 μg/100 g	190 μg/100 g

Fatal dose and time of death

Although alarming symptoms have on more than one occasion been initiated by 5 mg, 15 mg is the smallest fatal dose which has been recorded. 30 mg has also produced fatal results. Recoveries after prompt treatment have, however, followed large doses.

Death may supervene almost immediately. This happened in the case of a druggist who took 100 mg, along with nux vomica powder. Life may, however, be prolonged for several hours after the onset of symptoms.

Illustrative case

A man forcibly administered an unknown amount of strychnine to a young boy.   He then released the boy, who arrived home about thirty-five minutes later and vomited shortly after.   He was seen by a doctor at that time but no symptoms were observed.   One and a half hours later an emergency call described the boy as being stiff in bed.   He was taken to hospital where a diagnosis of strychnine poisoning or hysteria was made.   Three and a quarter hours after ingestion of the strychnine the boy was seen by a consultant anaesthetist who described him as suffering from clonic and tonic convulsions and opisthotony.

Treatment included stomach washing, intermittent positive pressure respiration, triple-strength plasma given continuously, and the administration of paraldehyde (4 ml intramuscularly), gallamine triethiodide (80 mg intravenously), thiopentone sodium (200 mg rectally), methylamphetamine hydrochloride (60 mg intravenously over a period of four hours for four incidents of cardiac arrest), atropine (0·6 mg) followed by prostigmine (2·5 mg) to reverse curarisation, and calcium gluconate (7 ml intravenously).   Eight hours after ingestion of the strychnine the boy was placed in a ward.   At this time his breathing was normal and there were no fits.   He died thirty minutes later.   The postmortem levels of strychnine are given in Case 1 above.

Note.   Brucine, which is extracted from the same plant as strychnine, differs from it in action.   It produces at first slight convulsive seizures, but these pass off quickly, the chief action being paralysis of the motor nerves and narcotism, thus resembling the action of curare or conium. It possesses only about one-eighth of the toxic effect of strychnine.

SULPHONAMIDES

The sulphonamides were used in the treatment of streptococcal infections, especially of haemolytic type, and in a wide variety of conditions due to other infective organisms.   The main use now is in the treatment of urinary tract infections and certain forms of meningitis. The compounds most commonly used are sulphamezathine, sulphadiazine, sulphaguanidine, and sulphacetamide.   Sulphaguanidine has proved of great value in cases of acute bacillary dysentery and infective diarrhoea, and sulphacetamide, or albucid, in infective eye conditions. The principal action of the sulphonamides lies in their effectiveness in inhibiting the reproduction of bacteria by impeding their metabolism.

Symptoms

The toxic effects assume a wide variety, and include gastro-intestinal irritation, giddiness, mental depression, and disturbances of vision.

Agranulocytosis is sometimes a dangerous and fatal complication in the over-prolonged use of these drugs. Hepatic miliary necrosis has occurred in a number of fatal cases. Some cases have developed methaemoglobinaemia and sulphaemoglobinaemia. These conditions cause marked cyanosis.

Sulphapyridine, sulphathiazole, and sulphadiazine are more prone to cause anuria than sulphanilamide. Anuria may result from deposition of crystals in the renal tubules or pelves of the kidneys. The following precautions should be adopted as routine with regard to sulphonamide administration. The fluid intake must be maintained at a high level, the condition of the blood should be carefully watched, and the drug should be discontinued on the approach of serious toxic symptoms.

Treatment

Use gastric lavage or emesis and give large volumes of fluid to aid excretion if kidney function normal, otherwise treat for anuria. If aplastic anaemia is present transfusions may be necessary.

Post-mortem findings

The liver, heart, and kidney may have necrotic lesions and the liver may show degenerative changes.

Analytical findings

The normal therapeutic level of these compounds in blood is somewhat under 10 mg/100 ml. The drug appears in the urine with significant but varying proportions depending on whether the drug is in the acetylated form.

Fatal dose

Severe toxic reactions have resulted from therapeutic doses, but the single fatal dose appears to be some tens of grams.

SULPHUR DIOXIDE

Sulphur dioxide is a colourless gas which has a pungent odour and an irritant effect when inhaled. Poisoning may occur during the process of manufacture, as the result of its employment in certain metallurgical and chemical works, or when the gas is used either for the purpose of disinfection or refrigeration. It is not as toxic as hydrogen sulphide.

Symptoms

Irritation of the eyes, nose, and respiratory tract, an acid taste in the mouth, bronchitis, bronchopneumonia, oedema of the larynx and lungs, a livid colour of the mucous membranes, and symptoms of gastro-intestinal irritation are usually found.

Treatment

Removal to fresh air; artificial respiration, which should be continued for a very considerable period, even in apparently hopeless cases; oxygen inhalations, restoration of bodily warmth, and stimulants.

Post-mortem findings

There will be asphyxial signs and evidence of irritation of the respiratory passages.

Analytical findings

Sulphur dioxide is rapidly changed in the body to sulphite and subsequently sulphate. It is unlikely that other than a quantitative estimation is of value and even this may not be obtainable.

Fatal dose

The maximum allowable concentration is 5 p.p.m. 500 p.p.m. is dangerous and, above this, death occurs rapidly.

SULPHURIC ACID (*Oil of vitriol*)

Properties and uses

The concentrated acid is a colourless, odourless, oily liquid with a specific gravity of about 1·8. This acid reacts violently with water with the liberation of large quantities of heat. The dilute acids are quite mobile and look like water. More concentrated acids sometimes called 'oleum' are available, but these fume strongly in air. The acid as used in industry is in a variety of strengths and purities. In the home, the commonest source is the acid (sp. gr. 1·2) for use in lead accumulators. Medical use is uncommon but small doses are sometimes prescribed.

Symptoms and treatment

These are described under Corrosive Poisons.

Post-mortem findings

The mucous membrane of the stomach will show a varying degree of blackish discoloration depending both upon the concentration and the amount of the acid swallowed. From post-mortem diffusion, the corrosive action may occasionally be observed in the peritoneal cavity. The oesophagus will also show areas of dark sloughing, and the larynx is frequently involved. When death is delayed, lesions may also be found in the duodenum.

Analytical findings

These are usually restricted to the finding and measurement of sulphuric acid in the stomach. As sulphate is a normally found ion in the body, the amount of acid found must be significantly large.

Fatal dose and time of death

2 ml has killed a child about one year old in twenty-four hours. The smallest fatal dose in an adult is probably 4 ml, but recovery has followed a dose of 15 ml. Death may occur in as little as one hour but more usually within eight to sixteen hours or later if the stomach has not been perforated. Death from shock, however, may be instantaneous, but life may be prolonged for weeks or months. Septic pneumonia is a possible complication. Only about one-third of all victims recover.

Note. Concentrated sulphuric acid has been used on a number of occasions for the disposal of human remains. The most recent case was that of Haigh (executed 1949).

THALLIUM AND ITS COMPOUNDS

The compounds of thallium, a heavy metal, may be found in zinc salts or in crude sulphur. Industrially, it is used in dyeing and glass manufacture. It is also an ingredient of certain vermin poisons. Therapeutically, it has been advocated for the treatment of ring-worm in the form of thallium acetate and it is used as a depilatory in certain preparations, occasionally causing poisoning. Thallous sulphate, which is a soluble colourless crystalline solid, is the most commonly used compound. When dissolved in water this material is not noticeable. Thallium has been used as a homicidal agent and its use in this connection would seem to be increasing.[106] The incidence is greater on the continent, Matthys and Thomas[107] having reported twenty cases during the period 1947 to 1958. Hausman and Wilson[108] report in detail over fifty cases of which four are murders.

Symptoms

This powerful poison repeated in small doses has a cumulative effect. Chronic poisoning injures the endocrine glands. Peripheral neuritis and alopecia are outstanding manifestations. General malaise, headache, drowsiness, depression, and insomnia are other symptoms.

Acute poisoning, resulting from swallowing the substance, is characterised by stimulation of the heart followed by depression which causes death from cardiac failure. There may be nausea, sickness, colic, diarrhoea, and albuminuria. Hyperaesthesia, impaired vision, ataxia, convulsions, and delirium or dementia complete the clinical picture.

Treatment

The stomach should be emptied either by stomach tube or by an emetic. A purgative dose of magnesium sulphate should be given. Intravenous injection of potassium iodide is recommended. Sodium thiosulphate, slowly administered, intravenously, 20 ml of a 3 per cent solution, daily, will cause gradual elimination of thallium in the urine.

Fluids, especially milk, should be given by mouth, and the patient should be kept warm.

Post-mortem findings

The findings at post-mortem examination are not significant.

Analytical findings

Thallium may be sought in any of the tissues, but those commonly investigated are urine, kidney, and liver. In the cases reported the urine values vary from 2 to 9 μg/ml, the kidney from 2 to 74 μg/g, and the liver from 13 to 68 μg/g. Reported normal values are under 0·4 μg/g.

Fatal dose and time of death

The fatal dose is about 1 g of a soluble salt. Death follows a fatal dose in two days to two weeks depending on the amount ingested.

Illustrative case

Hausman and Wilson[108] report the following case of a woman who was given an unknown quantity of thallous sulphate. Initially a burning sensation in the feet radiating to the knees was recorded. By the fifth day, she had severe leg pains and could not walk. Thereafter her condition deteriorated and she became lethargic and unresponsive until the eleventh day, when she died.

TIN AND ITS COMPOUNDS

The commonest use of tin is the preparation of tinplate. The use of the powdered metal or its oxide in medicine has now almost disappeared. Use in the home is restricted to tinned food containers where there is only a slight danger of interaction of the contents with the tinplate.

Symptoms

The salts of tin cause gastro-intestinal irritation such as nausea, vomiting, pain in the abdomen, diarrhoea, and prostration. A metallic taste may be experienced.

Treatment

Treatment consists of gastric lavage, demulcent drinks, and symptomatic measures.

Post-mortem findings

Gonzales and others[27] reported a case where the post-mortem examination revealed a congested and inflamed intestine and stomach with pseudomembrane formation. Sub-endocardial haemorrhages in the left ventricle were present and there was terminal bronchopneumonia.

Analytical findings

The tissues may be analysed for tin and interpreted against the normal background. This is somewhat under $1 \mu g/g$.

Fatal dose and time of death

The minimum fatal dose of soluble tin salts is not known but is estimated to be in the region of 3 to 5 g. Tin hydride is said to be more toxic than arsine. Stannic chloride, which hydrolyses to produce hydrochloric acid, has a corrosive action.

The fatal period in the case quoted by Gonzales and others[27] was two days.

TRINITROTOLUENE (*Trotyl, TNT*)

The pure material is a colourless solid (m. pt 81°C) which is almost insoluble in water. This substance is used extensively as an explosive and poisoning may occur during its manufacture by ingestion, inhalation of the dust or vapour, or absorption through the skin.   The principal source of poisoning is by inhalation.

Symptoms

A sago-grain, irritating dermatitis with exfoliation is produced by handling the powder or mixtures which contain it, particularly when the skin is perspiring, and is prone to occur in workers at the commencement of their employment.   Mixtures of trotyl with hygroscopic salts, such as amatol, a mixture of trotyl and ammonium nitrate, may be absorbed through the skin and cause poisoning.   The toxic action of trinitrotoluene is similar to that caused by the other nitro- and amino-derivatives of toluene and benzene.   It is capable of causing toxic jaundice.

Among the early symptoms are drowsiness, headache, and nausea. Some measure of cyanosis, which is of a bluish-grey colour, due to anilism, affects the lips.   Later there are likely to be abdominal pain, loss of appetite, gastritis, a feeling of oppression over the chest, and dyspnoea.   Staggering gait, palpitation, and rapid pulse-rate may be added to the picture.   The advent of toxic jaundice makes the prognosis serious since this symptom indicates liver damage or necrosis.   In very acute cases, unconsciousness may take the place of drowsiness, with perhaps convulsions, and there is likely to be marked toxic jaundice. Occasionally during the early stage of recovery from an attack of a subacute nature, amblyopia, with limitation of the field of vision and colour, has been observed.   Aplastic anaemia may occur among TNT workers.

The period of employment before the manifestation of toxic symptoms has been found to vary from several days to weeks, the time being related to circumstances of the working surroundings and individual conditions.

It has been suggested that the selective effect of TNT on the different organs should be attributed to acquired differences in tissue susceptibility.

The action of this particular poison is primarily centred on the blood and is haemolytic.   Methaemoglobin is present.   Microscopically, the red cells assume forms closely resembling those found in pernicious anaemia.   Neutrophil leucopenia and lymphocytosis are common features.   The leucoblastic function of the bone marrow is progressively involved.   Should the methaemoglobin in the blood become considerable, the liver is unable to remove it and methaemoglobinaemia is established, the blood tending to become chocolate-brown in colour, and hence the cyanosis of the patient is deepened in tint.

The dermatitis of TNT resembles vesicular eczema, accompanied by swelling and itching of the affected parts.   It commonly appears first on the skin of the hands, wrists, and forearms, but it may also be present on parts, usually covered by clothing, to which the dust has gained access.

Treatment

Remove skin contamination by working well with soap and water. Ingested material requires gastric lavage or emesis.   Intravenous calcium gluconate and a high-calcium diet are recommended.   Oxygen may be used to combat cyanosis.

Post-mortem findings

In fatal cases the liver is frequently the seat of yellow and red necrosis. In a number of instances, this organ, although enlarged in the earlier stages, is found to be very atrophied and to weigh as little as from 550 to 850 g when examined post-mortem.

Fatal dose and time of death

The fatal dose is probably in the region of 1 g.   The maximum allowable concentration in air is 1·5 mg per cubic metre.

ZINC AND ITS COMPOUNDS

The toxic effects of zinc are confined to the use of two salts of the metal, namely, the sulphate, the action of which is irritant, and the chloride, which is corrosive.   Zinc fumes also exercise a toxic action upon persons engaged in such occupations as zinc and copper smelting. The commonest form of sickness by a compound of zinc is the so-called 'brass-founders' ague' or 'metal fume fever' which results from the inhalation of freshly sublimed zinc oxide.   This condition, however, is not specific to zinc, since copper, iron, beryllium, magnesium, and other metals may cause the same condition.

Ingestion of zinc compounds is not usually fatal on account of their effective emetic action.

Zinc chloride may be found in the home in the form of a soldering flux.   Zinc stearate is used in dusting powders and is a possible source of excess zinc.   Other common zinc compounds used in medicine are the oxide and the basic carbonate (calamine).

Symptoms

The symptoms of zinc sulphate poisoning are principally those of gastro-intestinal irritation, and consist of vomiting, pain in the stomach and abdomen, diarrhoea, and, when a considerable quantity has been swallowed, collapse. Zinc sulphate has been taken in mistake for Epsom salts.

The symptoms of zinc chloride poisoning are of a somewhat different nature on account of the corrosive character of this salt. These are an immediate burning sensation in the mouth, throat, oesophagus, and stomach, with vomiting, diarrhoea, and symptoms of shock.

The symptoms of chronic poisoning are closely allied to those of lead and copper.

Treatment

Gastric lavage is the first procedure. Sodium bicarbonate in tepid water should be administered freely. Milk and egg drinks should also be given. Calcium sodium edetate is a suitable chelating agent. In addition, the case should be treated symptomatically.

Post-mortem findings

When zinc sulphate has caused poisoning, the gastro-intestinal mucosa will show patches of congestion, variable both in degree and extent. There may be a yellowish discoloration of the oesophagus and stomach. In some cases, the stomach may show patches of submucosal haemorrhage and erosion. The small intestine may be similarly affected. When zinc chloride has been swallowed, signs of corrosion may be present. The action of this salt is mainly local and corrosive, the tissues with which it passes into contact being affected. The degree of absorption is relatively slight and is in inverse proportion to its corrosive action.

Analytical findings

Zinc is an essential trace element and the levels found must be interpreted against the normal levels present in the tissues. A list of normal concentrations is given in Appendix III.

Fatal dose and time of death

The fatal dose is somewhat under 5 g for the chloride and probably double for the sulphate. In fatal cases death may occur at any time up to seven days.

References

1. POLSON, C.J. & TATTERSALL, R.N. *Clinical Toxicology*, p. 76. London: English Universities Press, 1959.
2. TOWNSEND. *Br. med. J.*, **1**, 382, 1943.
3. DEROBERT & GASCOIN. *Annls Méd. lég. Crimin. Police Scient.* **30,** No. 5, 289, 1950.
4. CAPLIN. *Lancet*, **2,** 95, 1941.
5. KEATING. *Anaesthetic Accidents.* London: Lloyd-Luke, 1956.
6. BAILEY HAMILTON. *Lancet*, **1,** 5, 1947.
7. PATTY, F.A. *Industrial Hygiene and Toxicology*, vol. 2. New York: Inter-science, 1949.
8. ISRAELS & SUSMAN. *Lancet*, **1,** 509, 1934.
9. KAYE. *Handbook of Emergency Toxicology.* Springfield, Illinois: Thomas, 1954.
10. SMITH, H. *J. forens. Sci. Soc.* **4,** 192, 1964.
11. SHULMAN, SHAW, & CASS. *Br. med. J.*, **1,** 1238, 1955.
12. LOUW & SONNE. *Lancet*, **2,** 961, 1956.
13. WORLOCK. *Br. med. J.*, **2,** 1099, 1956.
14. CLEMMESEN. *Lancet*, **2,** 966, 1956.
15. LASSEN. *Lancet*, **2,** 338, 1960.
16. BOGAN, J. & SMITH, H. *J. forens. Sci. Soc.*, **7,** 37, 1967.
17. MORTON. *Lancet*, **2,** 738, 1945.
18. SAUER. *J. Am. med. Ass.*, **102,** 1471, 1934.
19. PATTY, F.A. *Industrial Hygiene and Toxicology*, vol. 2. New York: Inter-science, 1949.
20. GERARDE, H.W. *Toxicology and Biochemistry of Aromatic Hydrocarbons.* Amsterdam: Elsevier, 1960.
21. BROWNING, E. *Toxicity of Industrial Metals*, 2nd ed. London: Butter-worth, 1969.
22. TEPPER, L.B., HARDY, H.L., & CHAMBERLIN, R.I. *Toxicity of Beryllium Compounds.* Amsterdam: Elsevier, 1961.
23. ROE. *J. Am. med. Ass.*, **101,** 352, 1933.
24. DOWDS. *Lancet*, **2,** 1039, 1936.
25. GOLDBLOOM & GOLDBLOOM. *J. Pediat.*, **43,** 631, 1953.
26. VALDES-DAPENA, M.A. & AREY, J.B., *J. Pediat.*, **61,** 531, 1962.
27. GONZALES, T.A., VANCE, M., HELPERN, M., & UMBERGER, C.J. *Legal Medicine, Pathology and Toxicology*, 2nd ed. New York: Appleton-Century-Crofts Inc., 1954.
28. PFEIFFER, C.L., HALLMAN, L.F.,& GERSH, I. *J. Am. med. Ass.*, **128,** 266, 1945.
29. SHAW, R.F. *Bull. int. Ass. forens. Toxicol.*, **3,** No. 2, 3, 1966.
30. EVANS. *Br. med. J.*, **1,** 173, 1960.
31. NICKOLLS & TEARE. *Police J.*, **28,** No. 1, 34, 1955.
32. SHILLITO, DRINKER, & SHAUGHNESSEY. *J. Am. med. Ass.*, **106,** 669, 1936.
33. MARTLAND. *J. Am. med. Ass.*, **103,** 645, 1934.
34. GETTLER & MATTICE. *J. Am. med. Ass.*, **100,** 92, 1933.
35. HANSON & HASTINGS. *J. Am. med. Ass.*, **100,** 1481, 1933.
36. HAGGARD & GREENBERG. *J. Am. med. Ass.*, **100,** 200, 1933.
37. HENDERSON & HAGGARD. *Noxious Gases.* American Chemical Society, Monograph series No. 109. New York, 1927.
38. McGUIRE. *J. Am. med. Ass.*, **99,** 988, 1932.
39. TOMPSETT, S.L. *Bull. int. Ass. forens. Toxicol.*, **4,** No. 4, 2, 1967.
40. JAIN, N.C., KAPLAN, H., & FORNEY, R.B. *Bull. int. Ass. forens. Toxicol.*, **4,** No. 4, 3, 1967.

41. BONNICHSEN, R. & MAEHLY, A.C. *J. forens. Sci.*, **11**, 414, 1966.
42. TIMPERMAN, J. & MAES, R. *J. forens. Med.*, **13**, 123, 1966.
43. HARRIS, T. *J. forens. Sci. Soc.*, **7**, 176, 1967.
44. GADDUM. *Pharmacology.* London: Oxford University Press, 1940.
45. SEMPLE, PARRY, & PHILLIPS. *Lancet*, **2**, 700, 1960.
46. BEHRENS. *Med.-leg. crim. Rev.*, **6**, No. 2, 209, 1938.
47. SIMPSON, K. *Taylor's Principle and Practice of Medical Jurisprudence*, 12th ed. London: Churchill, 1965.
48. BARBER. *Guy's Hosp. Rep.*, **84**, 267, 1934.
49. PURVINE. *J. Am. med. Ass.*, **107**, 2046, 1936.
50. TAINTER & WOOD. *J. Am. med. Ass.*, **102**, 1147, 1934.
51. FARAGO, A. *Bull. int. Ass. forens. Toxicol.*, **6**, No. 1, 2, 1969.
52. VON STORCH, *J. Am. med. Ass.*, **111**, 293, 1938.
53. McKAY. *Br. med. J.*, **2**, 365, 1906.
54. MORGAN, W.H.D. *J. forens. Sci. Soc.*, **5**, 15, 1965.
55. PONS & CUSTER. *Med.-leg. Crim. Rev.*, **14**, parts 3 and 4, 141, 1946.
56. WALDBOTT, G.L. *Acta med. scand.*, suppl. 400, 1963.
57. LIDBECK, HILL, & BEEMAN, *J. Am. med. Ass.*, **121**, 826, 1943.
58. BONNICHSEN, R. & MAEHLY, A.C. *J. forens. Sci.*, **11**, 516, 1966.
59. TOMPSETT, S.L. *Bull. int. Ass. forens. Toxicol.* **2**, No. 3, 2, 1965.
60. *Toro. S. Ist. di Med. Leg. e delle Assicur.*, Univ. Di Torino Minerva Medico-Leg. (Torino), **75**, No. 5, 158–61, 1955.
61. Editorial, *J. Am. med. Ass.*, **202**, 981, 1968.
62. VAN HECKE, W., DERVEAUX, A., & HANS-BERTEAU, M.J. *J. forens. Med.*, **5**, 68, 1958.
63. HOTSTON. *Lancet*, **1**, 207, 1946.
64. HURST. *Guy's Hosp. Rep.* **81**, 243, 1931.
65. *J. Am. med. Ass.*, **170**, 677, 1959.
66. Leading Article. *Br. med. J.*, **1**, 439, 1966.
67. FORBES. *Br. med. J.*, **1**, 367, 1947.
68. WILLIMOTT. *Br. med. J.*, **1**, 58, 1936.
69. ROSENTHAL. *J. Am. med. Ass.*, **102**, 1273, 1934.
70. OGILVIE. *J. Path. Bact.*, **35**, No. 2, 743, 1932.
71. MILLAR. *Br. med. J.* **2**, 453, 1916.
72. DÉROBERT. *Med.-leg. crim. Rev.*, **5**, No. 2, 227, 1937.
73. LEWINSKI. *Med.-leg. crim. Rev.*, **5**, No. 2, 228, 1937.
74. MATTHEW, H., PROUDFOOT, A.T., BROWN, S.S., & SMITH, A.C.A. *Br. med. J.*, **2**, 101, 1968.
75. CHEW, BERGER, BRINES, & CAPRON. *J. Am. med. Ass.*, **130**, 61, 1946.
76. OGATA, S. and others. *Jap. J. leg. Med.*, **16**, 242, 1962.
77. OLLIVIER, H. & QUICKE, J. *Annls Méd. lég. Crimin. Police scient.*, **42**, 160, 1962.
78. DRAWNEEK, W., O'BRIEN, M.J., GOLDSMITH, H.J., & BOURDILLON, R.E. *Lancet*, **2**, 855, 1964.
79. SUNDERMAN, F.W. & KINCAID, J.F. *J. Am. med. Ass.*, **155**, 889, 1954.
80. BAYER, O. *Arch. Gewerbepath. Gewerbehyg.*, **9**, 592, 1939.
81. GILL. *Br. med. J.*, **1**, 1544, 1901.
82. *Industrial Accidents.* No. 4, p. 14. London: H.M.S.O. 1934.
83. HODGKINSON, A. & ZAREMBSKI, P.M. *Analyst, Lond.*, **86**, 16, 1961.
84. HODGKINSON, A. & ZAREMBSKI, P.M. *Analyst, Lond.*, **87**, 698, 1962.
85. CURRY, A.S. *Bull. int. Ass. forensic. Toxicol.*, **4**, No. 3, 6, 1967.
86. TOMPSETT, S.L. *Bull. int. Ass. forens. Toxicol.*, **6**, No. 1, 2, 1969.
87. COPEMAN, P.R. v. D. R. *J. forens. Med.*, **3**, 80, 1956.
88. DANIEL, J.M. & GAGE, J.C. *Br. J. ind. Med.*, **23**, 126, 1966.
89. GAGE, J.C. *Bull. int. Ass. forens. Toxicol.*, **5**, No. 3, 1, 1968.

90. TOMPSETT, S.L. *Bull. int. Ass. forens. Toxicol.*, **7,** No. 2, 4, 1970.
91. HALL, R.A. & CARSON, E.D. *Bull. int. Ass. forens. Toxicol.*, **7,** No. 2, 5, 1970.
92. OREOPOULOS, D.G. and others. *Br. med. J.*, **1,** 749, 1968.
93. Leading Article. *Br. med. J.*, **3,** 690, 1967.
94. NUNN & MARTIN. *J. Am. med. Ass.*, **103,** 472, 1934.
95. WILLIMOTT. *Lancet*, **2,** 413, 1933.
96. MILLER. *Can. med. Ass. J.*, **46,** 615, 1942.
97. CONSDEN, R. *Bull. int. Ass. forens. Toxicol.*, **4,** No. 4, 4, 1967.
98. FLETCHER, G.F. & GALAMBOS, J.T. *Archs. int. med.*, **112,** 846, 1963.
99. FORSYTH, A.A. *British Poisonous Plants.* Ministry of Agriculture, Fisheries and Food, Bulletin 161. London: H.M.S.O., 1969.
100. NORTH, P. *Poisonous Plants and Fungi in Colour.* London: Blandford Press, 1967.
101. *A Basic Toxicity Classification of Radionuclides.* International Atomic Energy Agency. Tech. Rep. Ser. No. 15, Vienna, 1963.
102. HAGGARD & GREENBERG. *J. Am. med. Ass.*, **98,** 1133, 1932.
103. KEMPF, McCALLUM, & ZERFAS. *J. Am. med. Ass.*, **100,** 548, 1933.
104. STALBERG & DAVIDSON. *J. Am. med. Ass.*, **101,** 102, 1933.
105. WHEELOCK. *J. Am. med. Ass.*, **99,** 1862, 1932.
106. PRICK, SMITH, & MULLER. *Thallium Poisoning.* London: Cleaver-Hume, Press, 1955.
107. MATTHYS & THOMAS. *J. forens. Med.*, **5,** No. 3, 111, 1958.
108. HAUSMAN, R. & WILSON, W.J. *J. forens. Sci.*, **9,** 72, 1964.

Chapter 20

FOOD POISONING

FOOD poisoning in its epidemic form is properly the concern of the Medical Officer of Health, though in special circumstances medico-legal issues may be involved, particularly in the sporadic case. In its widest sense the term implies poisoning by articles of food, due either to contained toxic principles, metallic or otherwise, or to pathogenic micro-organisms. The more usual implication is that of illness due (1) to invasion of the body by members of the Salmonella group of bacteria or their toxins, (2) to the presence in the food of toxins formed by certain coagulase-positive staphylococci, or (3) toxins due to the spore-bearing and increasingly prevalent anaerobe *Clostridium welchii*, Type A. The severe and usually fatal illness due to the anaerobic Clostridium botulinum is regarded separately, though the mechanism of transmission of botulism is, for practical purposes, the same as that of the other bacterial forms.

Food poisoning is now notifiable in terms of the Clean Food Regulations which became operative on 1st August 1956.

Bearing in mind the wide sense of our title it will for the present purpose be most convenient to group the types of food poisoning as Food Idiosyncrasy, Vegetable Poisons including Fungi, Animal Poisons including Shellfish, Chemical Poisons, and Bacterial Food Poisoning including Botulism.

Food idiosyncrasy

This may be defined as supersensitivity to certain articles of diet, generally protein in nature, as a result of which their consumption is sollowed by illness, the common symptoms of which are nausea, vomiting, diarrhoea, fleeting joint pains, and the presence of an exanthem, usually urticarial in character. Victims of this condition rarely allege food poisoning.

Vegetable poisons

These are of wide occurrence in nature though happily restricted in Britain. The leaves of rhubarb may occasion a fatal illness from their oxalic acid content. Certain of the vetches, notably *Lathyrus sativus*, appear to play a part in the causation of a malady attended by paraplegia and muscular weakness and known as lathyrism, though it is now suggested that the condition is to some extent a deficiency disease. The berries and leaves of *Atropa belladonna* and the pods of *Laburnum vulgare* all of which may be eaten by children, are further examples of non-fungus vegetable poisons. In one case of interest recorded some years ago belladonna leaves became accidentally admixed with sage employed to stuff a roast and produced symptoms of atropine poisoning within ten minutes.

The toxic principle solanine is present in concentrated form in prematurely gathered and sprouting potatoes. An outbreak of solanine poisoning in Cyprus involving fifty persons proved to be due to the eating of potato shoots which, it transpired, contained five times more solanine than did the tubers.

The so-called 'mushroom poisoning' results from the ingestion of certain toxic fungi which resemble *Agaricus campestris*, the edible mushroom. The species mainly involved in this country are *Amanita phalloides*, in which case the incubation period is some ten hours, and *A. muscaria*, with a latent period of two to six hours. The general symptoms include gastro-enteritis, prostration, delirium, and finally coma. There may in addition be nephritis or even anuria. Poisoning by *A. phalloides*, of which some three hundred fatal cases are on record, may be attended by a mortality of 50 per cent. Death from *A. muscaria* is, however, rare. The alkaloid muscarine isolated from *A. muscaria* and the amanita toxin of *A. phalloides* are probably not the sole toxic factors concerned. Muscarine, which is antagonistic to atropine, appears to stimulate the post-ganglionic parasympathetic receptors, resulting in diminution in the rate and force of the heart and contraction of the pupils, together with disturbance of accommodation.

The post-mortem appearances in fungus poisoning are marked postmortem lividity, engorgement and inflammation of the gastro-intestinal mucosa, and hyperaemia of the meninges. Rigor mortis may be appreciably diminished.

Ergotism is a specialised type of vegetable poisoning due to *Claviceps purpurea*, a fungus parasitic on the rye plant. The disease may occur in epidemic form, as at Manchester some years ago, when upwards of two hundred persons were affected. In 1951, in France, some two hundred persons suffered from suspected ergot poisoning resulting from contaminated bread.[1] Symptoms, which are associated with the eating of infected rye flour, may be local, including vasomotor constriction and even gangrene of the extremities, or generalised in the nervous system with formication and paroxysmal convulsions. The suspect flour when heated with a strong solution of potassium hydroxide yields the herring-brine odour of trimethylamine.

The general treatment of fungus poisoning is for the most part symptomatic. Emetics may be given, and lavage of the stomach either with plain warm water or with dilute solutions of potassium permanganate has been found helpful. Morphine is useful for the abdominal

712 MEDICAL JURISPRUDENCE

cramp. Oxygen may be required when asthmatic crises predominate, and intravenous saline may be employed to combat collapse. Stimulants should be given in ergotism.

Poisoning by honey, which occurs from time to time, is due to toxic substances gathered by the bees from species of azalea, oleander, and rhododendron. It is of historic as well as current interest and is quoted by Xenophon.

Animal poisons

These, as here described, must not be confused with certain products of decomposition which appear in dead meat and which may produce illness; but are to be regarded rather as toxic principles present in the living animal. They are perhaps most common among the fishes. The roe of pike and the musculature of sturgeon are poisonous during the spawning season.

Poisoning by *Mytilus edulis*, the edible mussel, has been recognised for more than a century. A mild form of the illness, showing a very short incubation period, often only a few minutes, and characterised by intensely itchy urticaria, with asthma on occasion, is known as 'musselling' and is most probably an allergic response.

A neurotoxic form of the disease is also recognised. The toxin has been ascribed to plankton, but the question is so far unsettled. In a Glasgow case[2] three persons who ate mussels suffered from numbness of the mouth and fingers, nausea, vertigo, and ataxia. Symptoms in each case developed within two hours and all had recovered by the third day. The death rate from toxic mussel poisoning in Europe in recent years has been just over 18 per cent, but the mortality in American cases is only one-third of that figure.

Chemical poisons

Among trade processes of food manufacture which utilise chemicals, the hydrolysis or inversion of starch to sugar by commercial sulphuric acid has a place. The acid, made from iron pyrites, which is invariably contaminated with arsenic, contains the poison and may thus transmit it to the finished food product. Beer and confectionery which may contain invert sugar have been responsible for outbreaks of arsenical poisoning. Baking powder 'improved' with acid calcium phosphate may derive arsenic from the same source. The varnish used to laquer tinplate containers, and to polish sweets, has also yielded the poison. Arsenic may reach apples too when its solution is employed as an insecticide in orchards. Prosecutions have been made for the presence of prohibited amounts of arsenic, on apples, alleged to have been due to spraying of trees. Cider, beer, lemonade, or other plumbosolvent liquid stored in lead tanks or bottled in siphons containing lead fittings may occasion poisoning by this metal. Tea, cheese, and other tinfoil-wrapped commodities may in like manner become contaminated. Aluminium is nowadays largely taking the place of tin in the manufacture of wrapping foils. Lead-glazed vessels may yield their metal to foods cooked in them. Rathmell and Smith[3] record a unique case of acute plumbism in a child, aged twenty-two months, after drinking orange juice from toy dishes which by analysis showed a lead content. Lead solder in domestic cooking utensils may occasion lead poisoning. Poisoning by tin usually results from solution of the metal from un-lacquered tinplate containers by acid fruits or shellfish. It is worth noting in such cases that the solid part of the contents may contain more tin than the liquid. 125 mg of tin may constitute a poisonous dose. Enamels containing antimony in the form of Sb_2O_3, used as an opacifying agent, have sometimes been attacked and dissolved by lemonade and other acid drinks, with the production of illness. In one such outbreak, for example, sixty-five nurses were poisoned by lemonade which had been made from the fresh fruit in cheap white-enamelled jugs. There were no fatalities. Zinc is rarely a cause of poisoning, but consumers of dessert fruits such as apples which have been cooked in zinc receptacles have before now received emetic doses of the metal. Various metallic poisons formerly occurred in foodstuffs as dyes or preservatives, including salts of antimony, arsenic, cadmium, chromium, copper, lead, mercury, and zinc as colouring matters, and boron and salicylic acid as preservatives. Cases of poisoning by cadmium deriving from refrigerator fittings have lately been reported. The Public Health (Preservatives, etc., in Food) Regulations, 1925–40, prohibit all save scheduled colours, and limit the preservatives to benzoic and sulphurous acids and sodium or potassium nitrite, and these only in specified amounts in certain foods.

Other examples of chemical food poisoning include illness due to the use of cutlery cleaned with cyanide plate powder, and the 'ginger paralysis', which occurred in the United States and was caused by the adulteration of fluid extract of ginger with tri-o-cresyl phosphate.

Bacterial food poisoning

Infections such as typhoid fever, dysentery, scarlet fever, and diphtheria may be borne by articles of diet, and are thus, technically, examples of food poisoning. The foodstuffs mainly involved are milk, ice-cream, shellfish, green vegetables, and soft fruits.

More often, however, the illness is true bacterial food poisoning, formerly known as ptomaine poisoning. The term is a misnomer, since ptomaines, chemical substances related to amines, are harmless when administered by the mouth. Bacterial food poisoning is mainly due to various strains of the Salmonella group, of which more than 400 sero-types have been isolated.   The organisms multiply in the intestine, producing acute enteritis, and may also cause a general bacteriaemia.   It is difficult to place the causal agents in an order of frequency, but the commonest in this country are *S. typhimurium, S. enteritidis* (Gärtner's Bacillus), *S. thomson,* and *S. dublin.*   Man is rarely if ever a carrier of Salmonella infection, save in the most transient way during convalescence, but certain of the domestic animals, including cattle, sheep, and pigs, are often infected clinically or subclinically.   Rats and mice may also harbour the pathogens for considerable periods and may thus be a reservoir of infection for the human subject and for meat animals.

The general symptoms of Salmonella infection are abdominal cramp, vomiting, and diarrhoea.   The bacteria are present in the intestine during the attack.   From 50 to 100 per cent of persons partaking of the food are affected, but the case mortality is on the whole low and varies from 1·1 to 1·8 per cent.   The degree and course of the illness depend largely on whether the living bacillus, or its toxin, has been taken into the body.   The differential points concerned may be summarised as follows:

	When due to bacillus	When due to toxin
Incubation period	One to two days	A few hours
Course . .	Slow; lasting up to ten days	Rapid; generally over in a few hours
Symptoms . .	Predominantly colic, with diarrhoea	Predominantly cramp, usually with vomiting and diarrhoea
Pyrexia . .	Common	Rare
Prostration . .	Unusual	Common
Food . . .	Visible change in character occasionally but not usually present	Not visibly affected

The disease is most prevalent in the summer months, particularly when the living bacteria are concerned.   Toxin outbreaks do not exhibit a seasonal preponderance.   When living bacteria have been at fault they may usually be recovered from the food as well as from the vomit or faeces of the patient.   When, on the other hand, a toxin has been to blame, feeding experiments with animals alone can demonstrate its presence.

It has been estimated that almost one third of food poisoning outbreaks in Britain are due to coagulase-positive staphylococci, and are frequently associated with such commodities as artificial cream, pastry, confectionery, fish preparations, and gravy.

In investigating an outbreak of food poisoning it is essential to obtain samples of the peccant foodstuff and particularly of the individual portions served to the patient, since owing to the notoriously erratic distribution of the organisms in food, the patient alone may have received a charge of the bacteria. Material such as faeces or vomit should be sent to the laboratory with the least possible delay. Agglutinins to Salmonella strains are demonstrable in the blood after the seventh day of illness, and usually persist for a few months.

In seeking to trace the source of the illness it must be remembered that all commodities such as meat, made-up dishes, duck eggs, sandwiches, pies, and synthetic cream eaten during the previous twenty-four hours should be examined. It should also be remembered that food illness may be due to exceptionally heavy charges of organisms such as

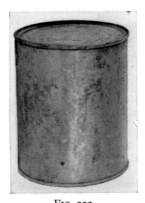

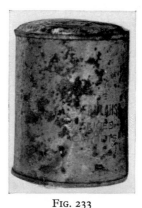

FIG. 232

Appearance of an unopened sound tin containing food. Note concave end

FIG. 233

Appearance of a 'blown' tin containing food. Note convex end

proteus and paracolon bacilli which normally are harmless. When a bacterial investigation fails to confirm the diagnosis, appropriate chemical tests should be performed.

Canned foods are from time to time the vehicles of bacterial food poisoning. When anaerobic decomposition is present the tin may be 'blown'. Canned foods contaminated by Salmonella organisms rarely present changes in appearance or taste and are not as a rule characterised by putrefactive odours.

Modern developments in the toughening of glass used in the manufacture of food containers have nowadays reduced the risk due to the inability of the older type of glass container to withstand the high temperatures of final retort-processing.

Cases of prosecution for food poisoning are reported from time to time.

It not infrequently happens that foreign bodies are by accident or carelessness included in articles of food. Nails, broken glass, pieces of string, cigarette stubs, cockroaches and the like from time to time appear. Their discovery, coupled with the fear that some of the foreign substance may already have been eaten, is sufficient in highly strung individuals to precipitate an attack of illness which may closely simulate food poisoning. Not uncommonly a medico-legal issue is raised in these cases and the practitioner has to be on his guard. In a case which came under the writer's notice the offending object was a small beetle of the genus Niptus, which is commonly present in old houses. The patient, a nervous, rather delicate female, was violently sick for a week and suffered also from diarrhoea, colic, and recurring bouts of nausea lasting over a fortnight. There was no doubt that the effect was mainly psychological. A comprehensive investigation was undertaken, including a clinical and serological examination of the patient and chemical analysis of the peccant food, in this case a soda scone. All tests for bacteria and poisonous substances were negative; and no specific agglutinins were detected in the blood.

Occasionally, crystals of ammonium-magnesium phosphate form in canned salmon and may be mistaken for glass. The addition of vinegar, in which the crystals are soluble, readily settles the question.

Botulism

(Latin: *botulus*, a sausage)

This fatal type of food poisoning is due to *Clostridium botulinum*, Types A, B, and E, a sporing anaerobe whose normal habitat is garden soil. The organism grows most readily in media of pH 5 or over, a fact which has an important bearing on the food preservation industry. The exotoxin excreted by this organism is one of the most powerful known. The disease, also known as allantiasis, is prevalent both in Middle Europe and in the United States. The outbreaks in Europe are due in most instances to meat or meat foods, whereas those in America are caused principally by vegetable, and not infrequently home-canned, products such as olives, string beans, asparagus, and similar low-acid food products. Fruits are less frequently involved. The incubation period is usually less than forty-eight hours and may be as short as four hours. The disease commonly begins with diplopia, which is rapidly followed by progressive paralysis of the eye muscles and finally those of the lids, producing complete ptosis. Involvement of the larynx soon ensues, articulation becomes faulty, and respiratory paralysis with extension to the breathing centre closes the scene. Only in a few cases is there vomiting. The unfortunate patient is usually conscious to the end. Mortality from the disease may reach 65 per cent.

Though by no means present in all instances, a rancid butter odour is often discernible in the affected foodstuff.

The outstanding British outbreak occurred in Scotland at Loch Maree in 1922, when all of eight persons who partook of sandwiches made from potted duck paste died.   The average incubation period was twenty hours.   Six of the patients were dead within forty-eight hours and the remaining two lingered for several days.   Bruce White found the duck paste rich in *Cl. botulinum*.   Antitoxic sera for Types A and B, as well as bivalent serum, are available.   The appropriate type serum should be administered immediately in all suspect cases.

References

1. *Lancet*, **2**, 436, 1951.
2. GEMMILL & MANDERSON.   *Lancet*, **2**, 307, 1960.
3. RATHMELL & SMITH, *J. Am. med. Ass.*, **114**, 242, 1940.

Chapter 21

PLANT IRRITANTS, ARROW POISONS, STINGS AND BITES

THE stinging or wounding propensity is widespread in nature both in plants and in animals. In the latter the mechanism is either defensive or is employed to stun prey.

Contact with plants

Many plants cause severe irritation when their acrid juices come into contact with the human skin. Flowers, leaves, and even barks may be concerned in the production of the lesions, which are conveniently grouped under the general title, dermatitis venenata. Clinically, the effect is commonly an acute erythema. When, as in the case of flowers, the plant has been pressed to the face so that its fragrance may be sampled, the lesion invades the features and the accompanying oedema may result in closure of the eyes. There can be little doubt that personal idiosyncrasy plays a large part in determining the occurrence of such dermatitis. Of flowers or leaves which may produce the syndrome there may be mentioned Clematis (Traveller's Joy), Chrysanthemum, Geranium, Nasturtium, Narcissus (Daffodil), and Ranunculus (Buttercup). Special mention is required for *Rhus toxicodendron*, the three-leaved poisonous ivy, sometimes termed sumach vine, which is a native of America and is known in this country as *Ampelopsis hoggii*. Rhus dermatitis is acute and is complicated by vesicles or even bullae which at times assume a pemphigoid character. Almost equally severe upon the sensitive skin are certain species of Primula, notably *P. obconica* and more especially *P. sinensis*, the Chinese primrose. As a buttonhole, at table, or in the greenhouse, primula claims its victims. That actual contact with the plant need not be necessary is illustrated by a characteristic case quoted by Sir Norman Walker.[1]

Barks and woods which may occasion papulo-vesicular dermatitis include birch, mahogany, satinwood, and teak. Sawdust of such woods employed as packing material may suffice to produce the effect.

Closely akin to the toxins of vegetable origin are the arrow poisons, of which there is a considerable range, showing both geographical and tribal variation. Besides the poisonous principles obtained from plants, venoms of insects and reptiles may be employed to smear arrow heads. In East Africa the chief plant arrow poison is that prepared by decocting and concentrating the bark of the Acocanthera shrub. Strophanthus is used in the Congo and Gold Coast. Malay tribes favour preparations of Strychnos and often use them by means of dart and blowpipe. Species of Strychnos containing the active principle curare have a vogue along the Amazon. The characteristic paralysis of the voluntary muscles and the accompanying anxiety state produced by this poison are well known.

Arrow poisons may remain long active, as is instanced by the case of a housemaid who was accidentally pierced by an Indian arrow while dusting trophies. She collapsed half an hour later and showed shallow breathing with feeble pulse. Artificial respiration was performed for two hours before consciousness was fully re-established, and some drowsiness persisted for several days.

In cases of arrow or dart poisoning, treatment, which must imperatively be immediate, consists in firm proximal ligation at the site of wounding and irrigation of the lesion with 5 per cent potassium permanganate. Stimulants are generally required and morphia is necessary as an antidote to members of the Strychnos group.

Contact with animals

The animal kingdom presents many examples of the toxic propensity, ranging from the mild irritation produced by simple aquatic forms to the lethal effect of the more poisonous snakes. Lowly examples are the stinging jelly fishes, one of which, Cyanea, or 'lion's mane', is familiar to bathers. Contact produces formication and erythema, often severe. In a case which came under the writer's notice, involving a girl aged twenty-one, contact with Cyanea occurred in the left deltoid region. Within a few minutes there was severe and spreading erythema accompanied by a burning sensation in the throat and muscular pain sufficiently severe to require morphia. Faucial spasm persisted for some hours, after which the symptoms slowly abated. The phylum Arthropoda, which ranks next above the worms, includes a variety of classes represented by the true insects, centipedes, spiders, ticks, and crustacea. The arthropods are injurious to man in various ways. The Lepidoptera include many irritant forms, mainly represented by the urticating moths whose larvae possess hairs or spines endowed with the stinging effect. The caterpillar of the tiger moth, known as the 'woolly bear', may cause severe dermatitis, and that of the puss tussock moth, swelling, nausea, and even paresis. Ingestion or inhalation of the hairs may cause serious internal disturbances.

The biting Diptera are numerous both at home and abroad. The slender mouth parts of Phlebotomus, the sand-fly, can inflict a poisonous wound. The bite of the anopheline mosquito may produce marked irritation and even sepsis, as may also the puncture of *Culex pipiens*, the common British gnat. A young medical woman was thrice bitten on the forehead by insects which from their description appear to have been culicine mosquitoes, most probably Theobaldia. Within one minute large bullae had formed in the area of the bites. Some five minutes later generalised urticaria had developed, accompanied by oedema, drowsiness, and some dyspnoea. These symptoms persisted for about eight hours and then slowly subsided. That the blood-thirsty female of Haematopota, the common cleg or horse-fly, can cause a poisoned lesion is well known, and during a summer camp the following typical case came under personal notice. A boy aged twelve, wearing the kilt and open sandals, was bitten at two places on the thigh and also below the knee and on the instep. Within three hours the affected limb was highly oedematous and showed marked vesication. The inguinal glands were slightly enlarged and there was malaise. The condition took ten days to subside and there was minor sloughing at one of the bites. In a more recent case the victim was a young woman, also bitten on the thigh, but at one place only. She complained of considerable local pain, and collapsed within a few minutes. Sloughing occurred in the wound and recovery took over a fortnight. There is good reason to believe that an allergic element is operative in most of such cases.

Perhaps the most common offenders, however, are bees and wasps, which belong to the order Hymenoptera. Bee venom is in toxic doses both neurotropic and haemolytic, though the worst effects are usually from oedema and shock. A single sting in the region of the throat may kill from suffocation: multiple stings, as from a disturbed swarm, are usually fatal. In supersensitive subjects, choking sensations, shallow breathing, cyanosis, and generalised pain may follow the sting. Cases of sudden death following wasp sting have been reported by Dyke.[2] A man aged forty-four was stung on the right temple. His face became suffused and he fell down almost immediately. When seen by a doctor twenty minutes later he was dead. At autopsy the lungs were found to be congested. The thymus was enlarged. In another similar instance the patient, a woman of sixty, was stung in the neck. She almost immediately felt ill and decided to lie down. While proceeding to her bedroom, she collapsed in the hall and died in a short time. No evidence of disease was found post-mortem. Among the Arachnida, which differ from the Insecta by having no true jaws, the Scorpions, which are capable of inflicting a sting accompanied by respiratory paralysis, cyanosis, and shock, and certain of the spiders, whose bite may be highly toxic, are outstanding. Children in North America, and in Australia, may suffer from tick fever, which resembles poliomyelitis and results from the toxic bite of Dermacentor. The bite of Latrodectus, the 'black widow' spider, is followed by abdominal rigidity which may closely simulate, and has been mistaken for, that following intestinal perforation. Opiates may be required for the severe pain.

In the treatment of severe insect bites in general, the application to the part of a solution consisting of 2 g of menthol in 30 ml of compound tincture of benzoin, followed later by zinc lotion, is recommended. Minor bites often respond to sodium bicarbonate paste, ammonia, or Eau de Javelle.   Accompanying syncope demands appropriate internal medication.

Of the poisonous fishes, Trachinus, the weever fish, and Trygon, the sting-ray, are perhaps the best known in British waters.   The weever resembles the mackerel, but is more slender.   Spines situated on the dorsal fin and gill covers are the source of the toxin, which is employed to stun prey, but which is highly irritant to the skin of man. The venom of Trygon can cause a dangerous wound, sometimes followed by paralysis and even death.   The electric organs in the head of the Torpedo ray are capable of transmitting a powerful shock.

Snakes belong to the order Reptilia, which includes the Lacertilia, or lizards, and the Ophidia, or serpents.   Of some 2,000 recorded species of Ophidia, those venomous for man are relatively few and belong to two families, the Colubridae and the Viperidae.   Snakes do not sting, as is popularly supposed.   Their poison is contained in buccal glands and is inoculated by the act of biting.   A few species, such as the spitting cobras, can eject the poison in a stream.   The venom, of which there are two kinds, is a clear, amber-tinted fluid containing modified proteins and toxic principles such as haemolysins, coagulins, and the like.   In certain of the Australian colubrines both types of venom may occur in the same reptile.   The poison of the viperine snakes acts mainly on the vascular, while that of the colubrines attacks the central nervous, system.   The mortality from all types of snake-bite is in the neighbourhood of 40 per cent, though the total annual death-rate from this cause in a country such as India may exceed 20,000.

The colubrine snakes, which preponderate amongst the poisonous varieties, include the cobra, the coral snake, the mamba, the krait, and the hamadryad or king cobra.   A bite from one of these is attended almost immediately by severe pain, rapid oedema, and inflammation of the wound, and is soon followed by apathy, paralysis, coma, and death. Should the patient survive the paralysis, recovery may be expected.

Viperines include the European viper, or adder, the Russell's viper, or daboia, the rattlesnake, and the phoorsa, all of which may produce fatal effects.   The symptoms following the bite of the daboia, for example, are local pain, oedema, and ecchymoses or other haemorrhage, together with collapse, thready pulse, and loss of consciousness.   The local lesion later becomes further aggravated and not uncommonly is the seat of suppuration, sloughing, or gangrene.   These secondary local phenomena are particularly marked in the case of the rattlesnake. The British viper produces a train of symptoms resembling those due to the daboia but of milder type.   Viper bites are, however, not infrequently fatal.

Lizards though fearsome are, save in one instance, non-poisonous. The toxic exception is the desert-dwelling genus Heloderma of which the two species *H. horridum* and *H. suspectum* are known as 'Gila Monsters'. Their bite is severe but not necessarily fatal.

Treatment of snake-bite

Local measures such as firm proximal ligation may be of some avail, particularly in cases of poisoning by a viperine. Copious lavage of the bite area with water is an important preliminary. It should be followed by incision of the wound and thorough suction either with the mouth or preferably by mechanical means. Adrenalin has been found helpful in paralytic cases, and artificial respiration is often required. Sucking of the unexcised wound is useless. Antitoxic sera, prepared from horses and known as antivenenes, are now available, but possess certain drawbacks. They must be strictly homologous. For example, viperine antivenene to, say, the daboia, is useless in cobra poisoning. The recommended intravenous dose varies from 20 to 200 ml, depending on the concentration of the serum. Concentration and dosage data accompany the package. Good results are now claimed from early intravenous injection of polyvalent antivenene serum (80 per cent colubrine with 20 per cent viperine) in cases where the species of the offending snake is not known with certainty. Dosage of antivenenes should be in inverse proportion to body weight, children receiving several times the official adult amount.

As regards general treatment it is of the greatest importance to reassure the patient, and to combat the physical shock. Black coffee, or caffeine, is beneficial. Alcohol, which can accelerate the absorption of the poison, and morphine should in all cases be avoided.

References

1. WALKER. *Introduction to Dermatology*, 10th ed., p. 119. London: Green & Son, 1939.
2. Dyke. *Lancet*, **2**, 307, 1941.

Appendix I

ANALYTICAL TOXICOLOGY

ANALYTICAL toxicology is a field in which the expert knowledge of a trained analytical chemist is required. Many basic mistakes result from inexpert use of techniques and lack of appreciation of the possibility of contamination from apparatus and other sources. Among the most common sources are detergents, water, and glassware which may have traces of materials adsorbed on the surface. Chemical reagents are seldom very pure even when recommended for analysis.

Materials for analysis are often presented in an ill-conceived assortment of containers which may not be very clean from an analytical point of view. Ideally, specially prepared, all-glass containers or disposable plastic ones should be used. Different samples should never be mixed together in one container and preserving or other solutions should be used with caution. If the analysis cannot be done immediately the materials should be placed in a refrigerator.

Analytical results

Assuming that the samples have arrived in the laboratory without contamination and are analysed expertly, there is still experimental error and the interpretation of the result to be considered.

When the analyst returns a negative result it really means that the sought-for material was not present in amounts which could be detected by the method employed. In most cases this means that there is no significant amount present but with a few drugs which are active in very small amounts (e.g. L.S.D., M-99) this is not true. To counter this, the analyst increases the amount of starting material as far as possible but even so, a small number of drugs are not found. A few materials (e.g. cannabidiol) still have no satisfactory methods of detection in body materials. If the limit of detection is below the limit of significant action a negative result may be taken at face value; otherwise evidence from the case history or clinical picture must be acted on. It is an unfortunate fact that a number of investigations are abandoned due to lack of positive analytical evidence when the circumstances suggest that no such evidence is available with present techniques. Drug concentrations which are on the borderline of detection may result in a report indicating the possible group of drugs to which the unknown belongs. Such a finding must be accepted at its face value, as detection may be possible but there may not be enough of the drug to allow further separations and positive identification procedures to be made. A more satisfactory result is one where there is enough of the drug available to allow positive identification by more than one technique. This can often be done when the amount of drug is below the level necessary for a quantitative analysis.

The most useful result is one where both the identity and concentration are given. The identity points to or confirms possible sources and the concentration allows a number of important assumptions to be made on the following points:

Fatal level. When a number of deaths have resulted from exposure to some material, an average fatal concentration in some organs or fluids is available.

Fatal dose. Collected data from a number of deaths has resulted in an average fatal dose being available. This depends on the dose form, the subject size, and the personal reaction of the victim. The relationship between tissue or fluid concentration and the amount taken is complex and the best opinion may be very inaccurate.

Time of death. It is often possible to give a rough estimate of the likely survival time after exposure to fatal amounts of various materials.

Interpretation

The interpretation of an analytical result appears to be very simple and is often made at a glance when a common material is involved. When an uncommon material concentration is encountered considerable time may elapse before an interpretation is given. This is due to the various important points which require consideration. These are as follows:

Identity. It is necessary to consider closely the analytical methods employed so that the certainty of identity can be established. A number of independent methods may well confuse the same two materials. It is the analyst's responsibility to select methods which will give the best identification. If, for any reason, complete identification is not possible he should be able to suggest other substances with which there may be confusion. A further problem arises when the found material is not identical with the ingested material due to alteration by biochemical processes. Common examples are the finding of phenobarbitone when primidone has been taken and the finding of oxazepam when diazepam has been taken. The toxicologist should be aware of such possibilities and be prepared to interpret accordingly.

Quantitative measurement. The interpretation of a quantitative measurement requires the following factors to be taken into consideration.

1. *Amount and error.* Every quantitative measurement has a degree of uncertainty and as a result, a figure quoted without the probable error can be misleading. For example, does a reported concentration of 5 mg/100 g mean somewhere between 0 and 10 or between 4 and 6 or between 4·9 and 5·1 mg/100 g? The first of these ranges is obviously unlikely but the other two could reasonably be applied to an everyday result.

Bearing this in mind it would appear that each result should be quoted as a mean value with a probable error range. The choice of method for this report requires some consideration. Strictly a mean value with its standard deviation should be quoted (when the distribution of values is 'normal'). However, it is found that a surprising number of people do not understand the significance of this type of reporting. The important point is that the recipient of the result should understand, as near as possible, what it means. A useful alternative is to quote a figure together with a reasonable range of error. The definition of reasonable is a matter for the analyst and would probably be about 2 standard deviations.

2. *Average value.* The average value is the value which is most representative of a range of values. If the range of values is small, then the average value is meaningful, but if the range is large then the average value may be quite misleading. An example is the statement that blood which contains ethyl alcohol loses an average 2 mg ethyl alcohol per 100 ml of blood per week when stored in the containers used for Road Traffic Act, 1972 samples. This tends to be interpreted in Court as meaning that all samples lose that amount and would be accurate if all samples lost slightly more or less than 2 mg/100 ml. In practice the range is much wider—some samples hardly lose any and some lose a very great deal more. Therefore, the average, though useful generally, must not be applied without serious consideration to any individual situation. This is a parallel with the preceding note on analytical results and their errors. An

average value has a variation and interpretation must take this into consideration, especially if it is being applied to a single situation which might be anywhere in the range of variation.

3. *Normal values.* If the material being analysed normally does not contain any of the sought-for substance then a positive finding indicates exposure to this substance. If the substance is a normal constituent then the analytical result requires careful comparison with the normal value. As the commonly quoted normal values are averages of many observations it follows that there is a range of values and this must be taken into consideration together with any experimental errors. For example the average arsenic content of hair is about ½ p.p.m. but the range of normal values may be up to 4 p.p.m. depending on the environment. An analytical result of 3 p.p.m. may look like over-exposure when compared with the average, but in fact when the range is considered, such a conclusion is at least doubtful.

4. *Personal variations.* The source of much of the uncertainty in the comparison of levels and judgment of the effect of fixed doses is the personal variation in response of each individual. The reaction to a therapeutic dose of substances may range from little effect to signs of overdosage. Taking this a step further the giving of a 'fatal dose' results in a significant survival rate whereas 'non-lethal' high doses sometimes result in death. These effects are due to the results of different rates of absorption, the widely different reactions of the individual organisms to the materials in question, and whether the organism is habituated to them. The commonest example of this is the obviously wide variation in effects that alcohol has on various people.

SELECTED ANALYTICAL METHODS

Four of the most common methods of analysis used by the toxicologist have been selected. These are: thin layer chromatography, colour reactions, gas chromatography, and ultra-violet spectrometry. Under these headings the techniques are described in simple terms and a suitable working example is given.

THIN LAYER CHROMATOGRAPHY

Thin layer chromatography is now one of the most widely used techniques for the separation and identification of drugs and related materials. The advantages include low costs, rapid separations, high sensitivity and the ability of the layer to withstand the action of most chemical reagents. The main disadvantage is the difficulty in obtaining reproducible results without ideal laboratory conditions. This may be overcome by the use of suitable standard materials with each experiment.

A simple outline of the technique of thin layer chromatography is given below together with a typical example of its application in drug analysis. The example chosen is the detection and identification of barbiturates.

Method

Preparation of plates. A suitable material, most commonly silica gel, is chosen for the preparation of the thin layer. A slurry is prepared by thoroughly mixing 30 g of the selected material with 60 ml of water. The chromatoplates are then prepared by spreading the slurry on to glass carrier plates of uniform thickness. Machines for spreading the layers are available commercially. They incorporate a device for varying the thickness of the layer up to 2 mm.

Usually the slurry is placed in a container which can open on to the glass plates and the layer is spread by pulling the spreader over them.   Alternatively, the layers can be prepared as follows:

Adhesive tape is fixed along the sides of a glass plate, one piece on top of the other, until the required thickness is obtained.   The slurry is then poured on to the plate and spread by pulling a glass rod along the tape surfaces, so that an even layer is left between them.   The adhesive tape is then removed.   The coated plates are air dried at room temperature for 15 minutes and then activated by heating at 110°C for thirty minutes.   After cooling in a desiccator the plates are ready for use.

In the preparation of the plates three points require careful attention:

1. The plates must be thoroughly clean.   This can be done by immersion in concentrated sodium hydroxide solution.

2. The slurry must be even and free from lumps.   This can be accomplished by sieving the powder through fine-mesh nylon gauze and then mixing thoroughly with water, using a mortar and pestle.

3. The layer should be applied evenly.   A few practice runs give confidence and improved plates.

Application of samples.   The sample for analysis is dissolved in a few drops of a suitable solvent (chloroform, ether, etc.) and the resulting solution transferred to the plates prepared as above.   The transfer is accomplished by placing the lip of a capillary tube into the solution.   Capillary action causes a small volume to be drawn into it.   The tip of the tube is then placed in contact with the layer on the plate about 2 cm from one end.   The solution is then drawn on to the plate to form a spot.   This process is repeated until all the sample is transferred to the spot, taking care that the spot diameter does not exceed 2 to 3 mm.   Four spots including standards is a reasonable number for one plate.

Development of plates.   Development of the plates is carried out in ordinary gas jars sealed with ground-glass covers.   The developing solvent is placed in the bottom of the jar to a depth of 1 cm.   The inside of the jar is lined with filter paper, soaked with the developer, to promote saturation of the atmosphere in the jar.   Before development it is best to allow the plates to reach equilibrium with the vapour in the jar.   This may be accomplished by providing small platforms at the bottom of the jars to hold the plates above the solvent mixture.   The developer is usually a mixture of solvents, which are chosen to give the greatest separation of the materials being examined.   It is also essential that the materials should be separated by the developer from any metabolites or other coextractable materials which may have followed them through the first extraction procedure.   Organic mixtures are preferred to those which contain aqueous solutions, because the development time is shorter and the layers do not break up as they tend to do when water is present.   During development the solvent is allowed to rise through the layer to a convenient distance (usually 10 to 12 cm).   The plate is removed from the tank, air dried and examined for the presence and position of the compounds under investigation.   This may be done using ultra-violet light or a chemical which reacts with the sought-for materials.

R_f values.   When the plate is being developed the solvents moving through the thin layer tend to wash the substances being analysed along with them.   The active material of the thin layer tends to hold them where they are.   The result is that the substances spread out along the plate, depending on their relative affinities for the solvent and the layer. The ratio of the distance travelled by a substance to the distance travelled by the solvent is called the 'rate of flow' or more commonly the R_f value.

R_f values are dependent on the three following factors and are not exactly reproducible:

1. The activity of the layers
2. The saturation of the chamber
3. The uniform thickness of the layer.

The order of development is always the same and so standards are run for comparison. The standard may be a mixture of substances placed on a spot beside the unknown. The position of unknown substances with relation to the known spots allows a near estimate of their identity. This may then be proved by reaction with various reagents.

Analyses for barbiturates using thin layer chromatography

Barbiturates and a few other materials may be demonstrated in biological materials using thin layer chromatography by means of the following method.

The biological samples are extracted for acid drugs (chloroform or ether extraction of acidified biological material, purification if necessary and concentration) and the resultant material taken into solution in a few drops of chloroform. This is transferred to a thin layer chromatography plate coated with silica gel 'G' (E. Merck, Germany) to a thickness of 0·25 mm. The developer used is a mixture of chloroform and acetone (9 : 1). This gives the widest distribution of barbiturates (R_f 0·3–0·8) and separates them from any metabolites or urinary constituents which may be present.

The time of development for 10 cm, using the above method, is approximately 17 minutes. This may be reduced if necessary but there is a slight loss of precision.

When the plate has been developed the barbiturates may be demonstrated as black spots by spraying the plate with a saturated solution of mercurous nitrate in water. As the plates do not develop in an exactly reproducible manner it is necessary to have standard barbiturates on the same plate so that a comparison of R_f values can be made. A list of barbiturates and R_f values is given in Table 1.

In conjunction with the R_f values the chemical reactions of the barbiturates and related compounds may be used to give the absolute identity. For this purpose the plates are sprayed with the reagents, or some of the substance may be treated with sulphuric acid after preliminary separation.

The reagents and their reactions are as follows:

Mercurous nitrate. A saturated solution (some solid should be present), is sprayed on to the plates, when black spots develop. These spots fade after a few minutes, so they should be marked immediately. This reagent reacts with all the compounds being examined, except Carbromal and Bromural, which are included because of the similarity of their action to that of the long-acting barbiturates and because they are extracted from acid solution by organic solvents.

Potassium permanganate. A 2 per cent (w/v) solution is sprayed on to the plates, when yellow-brown spots on a purple background appear. These spots indicate the presence of barbiturates with unsaturated side chains. This reagent may be applied to the plate after the mercurous nitrate.

Zwicker's reagent. 4 ml of copper sulphate solution (10 per cent w/v) are mixed with 1 ml pyridine and 5 ml water to give a clear dark blue solution. This reagent is sprayed on to the plates causing pink or green spots to appear.

Fluorescein.   10 ml of a saturated solution of fluorescein in acetic acid is mixed with 15 ml glacial acetic acid and 25 ml of 100 volume hydrogen peroxide.   This reagent must be prepared fresh as required.   The plates are sprayed initially with a sodium hydroxide solution (10 per cent w/v) (unless bromo-barbiturates are being sought) and heated to 100°C for five minutes.   They are sprayed with the fluorescein reagent and heated at 100°C for five minutes, when pink spots form.

Sulphuric acid.   A little of the substance obtained from the preliminary extraction is heated with concentrated sulphuric acid for twenty minutes at 100°C. After cooling the solution is diluted with water, re-extracted with chloroform and evaporated to about 0·1 ml.   This is placed on a chromatoplate and analysed

Table 1.   Barbiturate R_f Values

Compound	R_f	Compound	R_f
Allobarbitone . . .	0·27	Metharbital	0·55
Allylbarbituric acid . .	0·36	Methohexitone . . .	0·67
Amylobarbitone . . .	0·33	Methylphenobarbitone . .	0·59
Aprobarbital . . .	0·30	Nealbarbitone . . .	0·38
Barbitone	0·22	Pentobarbitone . . .	0·33
Bemergride	0·39	Phenobarbitone . . .	0·24
Bromural	0·26	Phenylmethyl barbituric acid .	0·12
Butallylonal	0·28	Phenytoin	0·20
Buthalitone	0·68	Probarbital	0·24
Butobarbitone . . .	0·33	Quinalbarbitone . . .	0·44
Carbromal	0·50	Thialbarbitone . . .	0·69
Cyclobarbitone . . .	0·32	Thiamylal	0·70
Doriden	0·52	Thiopentone . . .	0·68
Heptabarbitone . . .	0·31	Vinbarbitone . . .	0·28
Hexobarbitone . . .	0·50		

as an ordinary sample.   Whether the barbiturate has been destroyed or not by the acid gives a further indication of identity.

Mercurous nitrate is the most sensitive spray and reveals spots when about 1 μg of barbiturate is present.   The other reagents are less sensitive and require the following weights of material before a definite spot is seen:

Permanganate spray . . .	2 μg
Zwicker's reagent	10 μg
Fluorescein spray	10 μg

Method of identification.   The initial extract is prepared and spotted on to the chromatoplate in the following order: standard; unknown; standard; unknown; the plate is then developed and the unknown spot nearest the edge covered.   The remainder of the plate is sprayed with mercurous nitrate solution to reveal the standards and the unknown, if it is a barbiturate, Doriden, Bemegride, or Phenytoin.   If the unknown spot develops, its position is marked and the R_f calculated and compared with those listed in Table 1. The same area is then sprayed with potassium permanganate to detect un-saturated compounds.   When this is complete, the other part of the plate is sprayed with Zwicker's reagent, which reacts with two groups of barbiturates. The results obtained are compared with the reactions listed in Table 2.   If further information is required, the treatment with sulphuric acid described above may be applied. When this investigation is completed, the identity of most of the substances will be known. A few barbiturates will be impossible to distinguish, due to their similar structures and hence their similar chemistry.

When the mercurous nitrate spray fails to reveal a spot, the other part of the plate should be treated with the fluorescein spray, when Carbromal and Bromural may appear.

It is often possible to remove the spot from the plate, extract the drug from aqueous acid solution, and rechromatograph it if further tests are required and no further material is available.

COLOUR REACTIONS

Colour reactions are valuable for the identification of a drug or group to which a drug belongs. The technique involves mixing the extracted drug or pure material with a chemical reagent and noting the colour or play of colours produced. The general approach to the use of colour reagents is as follows:

1. Use a reagent of low specificity to determine presence of drug.
2. Use reagents of increasing specificity to narrow the range of possible drugs and to assign the drug to a particular group.
3. Use a reagent to differentiate these within an assigned group.
4. Confirm the identity of the drug by the use of a colour test known to be specific for it.

Identification by means of colour reactions may be combined with thin layer chromatography. In this system the drugs are relatively free from interfering biological products and extra information in the form of R_f values is available. The technique involves separation by chromatography and spraying with, or immersion in the vapour of, various chemical reagents. This gives coloured spots on a uniform background. It is often possible to overspray plates with different reagents so that further information is gained. A working example is described under the detection of barbiturates by thin layer chromatography.

Note. There is no general reaction mechanism for reagents reacting with drugs. The mode of action includes physical adsorption on to the drug, oxidation of the organic molecule, reactions resulting from the basic nature of the molecules, coloured complex formations, and reactions with individual functional groups. Often it is not understood why one reagent is a good indication of a specific group of drugs.

GAS LIQUID CHROMATOGRAPHY

Gas liquid chromatography is one of the most useful techniques available to the analytical toxicologist. It is versatile, rapid, sensitive, and can give quantitative results from small amounts of material. Apart from cost, the main disadvantage is the need for purer samples before the analyses can be made. The technique is outlined briefly below and a working example is given under the heading of 'The estimation of ethyl alcohol in blood using gas chromatography'.

General principles

As with thin layer chromatography, the separation of the drugs or other substances is achieved by allowing the materials to be washed over an active phase by a solvent. However, in this case, the active phase is usually a non-volatile liquid which is coated on to an inert solid support. The column is

Table 2. Barbiturate Reactions

Class	Compound	Mercurous nitrate	Zwicker's reagent	Potassium permanganate	Flourescein	Sulphuric acid
	Allobarbitone	+	Pink	+	—	Destroyed
	Allylbarbituric acid					
	Amylobarbitone	+	Pink	+	—	Destroyed
	Aprobarbital	+	Pink	−	—	Unchanged
	Barbitone	+	Pink	+	—	Destroyed
	Butobarbitone	+	Pink	−	—	Unchanged
	Cyclobarbitone	+	Pink	−	—	Unchanged
	Heptabarbitone	+	Pink	++	—	Destroyed
5,5-substituted barbiturates	Phenylmethyl barbituric acid					Destroyed
	Probarbital	+	Pink	−	—	Destroyed
	Nealbarbitone	+	Pink	+	—	Partially destroyed
	Pentobarbitone	+	Pink	−	—	Destroyed
	Phenobarbitone	+	Pink	−	—	Destroyed
	Quinalbarbitone	+	Pink	++	—	Destroyed
	Vinbarbitone	+	Pink		—	Destroyed

Class	Compound					
1,5,5-substituted barbiturates	Hexobarbitone	++	—	+	—	Destroyed
	Metharbital	++	Faint pink	—	—	Unchanged
	Methylphenobarbitone	++	Faint pink	—	—	Destroyed
	Methohexitone	++	Faint pink	+	—	Partially destroyed
Bromobarbiturates	Butallylonal	+	Faint pink	+	+	Destroyed
Thiobarbiturates	Thiopentone	++	Green	+++	—	Destroyed
	Buthalitone	++	Green	+++	—	Destroyed
	Thiamylal	+	Green	+	—	Destroyed
	Thialbarbituric acid	+	Green	+	—	Destroyed
Bromoureides	Bromural	—	—	++	++	
	Carbromal	—	—	++	++	
Glutarimides	Bemegride	++	—	—	—	
	Doriden	—	—	—	—	
Hydantoins	Phenytoin	+	—	—	—	

prepared by packing the resultant solid into a long thin tube usually made of stainless steel or glass. The solvent is an inert gas, usually nitrogen. The gas competes with the active stationary phase for the materials under investigation and as a result, these are separated as they move along the column. In thin layer chromatography the process is stopped after the solvents have moved a selected distance and the drugs are then shown up by chemical or other means. In gas liquid chromatography the separation takes place in a column. As a result, the drugs cannot be revealed after a set interval as in thin layer chromatography. Therefore, the process is made continuous and the drugs are detected electronically as they are washed off the end of the column. Instead of the R_f value found for substances by thin layer chromatography a new value called the retention time (R_t) is found. This is the time taken for the material to go through the column and under standard conditions is fixed.

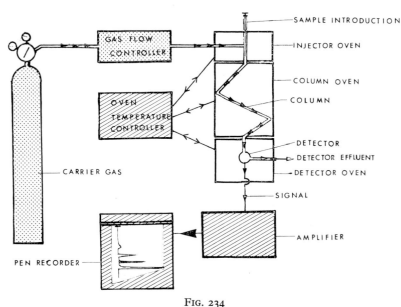

FIG. 234

Gas chromatograph layout (schematic)

Apparatus

The basic apparatus is as shown in Fig. 234 and consists of a controlled supply of inert gas (usually nitrogen). This is led to a column packed with suitable materials for separating the drugs or other substances. At the beginning of the column is an apparatus for sample introduction. This is usually a tube with a silicone rubber septum at one end through which the sample is introduced by means of a syringe and needle. After being swept through the column by the gas the sample enters a detection device. The most common device is a hydrogen/air flame with electrodes near it (flame ionisation detector). The electrodes are kept at a high voltage and the charged particles, caused by the drugs or other materials burning in the flame, carry the current across the flame. The resulting electric signal is proportional to the amount of material passing through the flame and, after amplification, may be used to form a trace on a recorder or other device so that a quantitative estimation can be made if required.

Working conditions

The following factors are important and must be taken into consideration in the operation of the technique.

1. *Carrier gas.* This is the gas which flows through the column. It must not react with the samples being analysed, the column materials or the detector materials. The most common gases are nitrogen and argon. The flow of these gases must be controlled carefully, as any variation would cause varying responses in the detector system. It is necessary to be able to set a given flow rate as required so that reproducible retention times can be obtained.

2. *Sample introduction.* The commonest technique is by injection of a solution of the sample in a volatile solvent (about 1 μl is usual). An 'injector oven' is required to vaporise liquid and solid samples in the minimum possible time before being swept on to the column as a carrier gas/vapour mixture. This oven requires a control device so that a selected temperature can be set and maintained. The temperature is usually slightly above the column working temperature. Poor injection technique or improper oven temperatures result in lower efficiency of separation.

3. *The column.* This is the place where the injected material is separated into its individual components. The separation is dependent on the amount and type of the non-volatile liquid, the solid support, the method of packing, the length of column, and the column temperature. All of these must be selected and controlled carefully otherwise a successful analysis is unlikely. The choice of conditions depends on the material being analysed and the degree of separation required and is a matter for the expert to decide.

4. *Detection.* The commonest type of detector is the flame ionisation detector described above. This requires controlled supplies of hydrogen and air for the flame and a controlled oven to keep the temperature constant and usually slightly above the temperature of the column. Any variation in these conditions results in variations in the detector's response and a loss of accuracy in the analysis.

5. The amplifier must be stable and if possible have a wide range of control so that the overall system has maximum variability. It must also have outlets suitable for driving devices such as pen recorders and integrators so that permanent records can be obtained and quantitative calculations made.

The estimation of ethyl alcohol in blood by gas chromatography

Gas chromatography is a reasonably accurate technique for finding the concentration of ethyl alcohol in small volumes (a few drops) of blood or urine. A competent analyst would expect to achieve results showing a standard deviation of less than 2 per cent in any given series of analyses of the one sample. In order to give the accused the benefit of any reasonable statistical doubt a deduction of 6 per cent (i.e. −3 standard deviations) is usually made. An outline of the method generally used is given below.

The sample. Before analysis the sample should be visually examined to determine if any tampering has taken place and to check that the blood is reasonably homogeneous. A fixed volume of the sample is then taken and mixed with a preselected volume of a solution of *n*-propyl alcohol in water (a fixed concentration solution in the region of 10 mg *n*-propyl alcohol per 100 ml of water). A standard solution of ethyl alcohol (about 80 mg ethyl alcohol/

100 ml water) is treated similarly.   The preselected volume of n-propyl alcohol solution is such that the peaks obtained on the chromatogram for the two alcohols have similar areas.   This processing of the sample is repeated at least once using different standard ethyl alcohol solutions and different proportions of sample to n-propyl alcohol solution.   The dilution of the sample with the n-propyl alcohol solution is carried out using a device called a Diluspence.

Chromatography

Two columns which give adequate separation of the two alcohols concerned, and some others if need be, are as follows.

1. A five-foot column ($\frac{1}{4}$in or $\frac{1}{8}$in) packed with 10 per cent P.E.G. 400 on Chromosorb W operating at 85 to 90°C with a nitrogen flow rate of 60 ml/min.
2. A five-foot column ($\frac{1}{4}$in or $\frac{1}{8}$in) packed with Chromosorb 101 operating at 160 to 170°C with a nitrogen flow rate of 60 ml/min.

A flame ionisation detector is used to detect the alcohols as they come off the column.

Method.   Approximately 1 μl of diluted sample or standard are injected into the column using a suitable syringe.   Separation of the two alcohols and of the alcohols from other materials takes place as they move through the column and they are detected individually as they pass through the flame ionisation detector.   The signals from the detector are amplified and drawn on a suitable recorder.   At the same time an integrator makes measurements equivalent to the amount of the alcohol present and prints the values out on paper tape.   This procedure is carried out a number of times for all the samples and standards. Thereafter the concentration of alcohol found in each sample injected is calculated by simple proportion and an average of the experimental results found. An example of the calculation is as follows:

Experimental Values

Material	Alcohol	Measurement	Ratio $\dfrac{\text{(ethyl alcohol)}}{\text{(n-propyl ,,)}}$
Standard	Ethyl n-propyl	270 300	0·900
Sample	Ethyl n-propyl	335 310	1·08

Standard: The standard ethyl alcohol solution contained 81 mg ethyl alcohol/ 100 ml water.

Calculation: The result is reached by the following simple proportion calculation.

$$\text{Concentration of sample} = \frac{\text{Ratio of sample}}{\text{Ratio of standard}} \times \text{concentration of standard}$$

In this example

$$\text{Concentration of sample} = \frac{1\cdot08}{0\cdot900} \times 81 \text{ mg ethyl alcohol per 100 ml sample}$$

$$= 97 \text{ mg ethyl alcohol per 100 ml sample}$$

ULTRA-VIOLET SPECTROMETRY

This technique is used in analytical toxicology for the identification and estimation of drugs and other materials. The method involves placing a sample of the material in a beam of ultra-violet radiation and varying the wavelength from 200 mμ to 450 mμ. Many materials absorb ultra-violet light over limited ranges in the ultra-violet spectrum. The result of plotting absorption (or transmittance) against wavelength is a graph which may have a characteristic shape with peaks and valleys. The height of a peak may be used as a quantitative measurement when compared with standard spectra.

The substances being investigated are usually in solution in dilute acid or alkali, alcohol, or other suitable solvent. The solution is held in a silica cell (usually 1 cm wide) with optically finished sides so that the radiation passes through without loss. As there may be some small interfering absorption by the containers or solvents, it is usual in practice to pass an identical beam of radiation through a matched cell containing the same solvent. The spectrum of this blank is then automatically subtracted from the spectrum of the cell containing the drug, resulting in a drug spectrum which is free from interference.

The following example shows the use of ultra-violet spectrometry as a quantitative technique.

Determination of barbiturate in blood by ultra-violet spectrometry

Barbiturates may be extracted from 5 ml of whole blood directly into 50 ml of chloroform. The chloroform is filtered and extracted with 5 ml of 0·45N sodium hydroxide. The aqueous layer is centrifuged and 1·5 ml of it added to 1·5 ml of 0·45N sodium hydroxide. The resulting solution is placed in a 1 cm cell and the absorption spectrum plotted against a 0·45N sodium hydroxide reference solution. A further 1·5 ml of the extract is added to 1·5 ml borate buffer (37·2 g H_3BO_3 + 45 g KCl per litre) and the spectrum is drawn against a reference solution prepared by mixing 1·5 ml of borate buffer solution with 1·5 ml 0·45N sodium hydroxide.

The concentration of barbiturate in the original solution is calculated from the difference in absorption at 260 mμ of the two solutions using the equation:

$$C = \frac{D \times F}{V}$$

where C is the concentration of barbiturate in mg/100 ml blood
     D is the difference in absorption at 260 mμ
     F is a calibration factor
     V is the original volume of blood.

The calibration factors for a selection of barbiturates are as follows:

Amylobarbitone	.	.	. 41·7
Butobarbitone .	.	.	. 38·8
Cyclobarbitone .	.	.	. 44·7
Pentobarbitone .	.	.	. 48·1
Phenobarbitone .	.	.	. 43·7
Quinalbarbitone	.	.	. 47·5

Note. The following conditions are necessary before the presence of barbiturates can be assumed.

1. Maximum absorbance in borate buffer solution at 238 to 240 mμ
2. Maximum absorbance in sodium hydroxide solution at 252 to 255 mμ and a minimum at 234 to 237 mμ
3. Isobestic points (where spectra cross) at 227 to 230 mμ and 247 to 250 mμ.

SELECTED DATA FOR DRUG ANALYSES

Tables of experimental results found under standard working conditions are useful for comparison purposes. A selection of such material based on the techniques described earlier has been made and is given under the following headings.

1. Thin layer chromatography—R_f values.
2. Colour reactions on thin layers.
3. Gas liquid chromatography—R_t values.
4. Ultra-violet spectrometry—Absorption maxima and minima.

THIN LAYER CHROMATOGRAPHY—R_f VALUES

The following table of R_f values is from a selection of basic drugs chromatographed on 0·25 mm layers of silica gel. The coated plates are air dried at room temperature for 15 minutes and activated by heating to 110°C for 30 minutes. The solvent used for development is a mixture (3 : 1) of chloroform and methanol. A list of R_f values for barbiturates is given in the description of the analysis of barbiturates by thin layer chromatography (Table 1).

Table 3. R Values of Drugs

Drug	R_f	Drug	R_f
Acepromazine	0·57	Benzthiazide	—
Acetophenazine	0·65	Berbamine	0·59
Acetyldigitoxin	0·93	Berberine	0·52
Adrenaline	0·00	Betaine	0·23
Alkavervir	0·45		streaked
	0·59	Bromodiphenhydramine	0·85
	0·70	Brucine	0·29
	0·82	Buphenine	0·60
	0·93	Butacaine	0·55
Amethocaine	0·72	Butyl Aminobenzoate	0·87
Aminoacetic Acid	—	iso-Butylamine	0·83
Amiphenazole	0·74		streaked
Amisometradine	0·70	Cadaverine	0·11
Amitriptyline	0·74	Caffeine	0·68
Amodiaquine	0·74	Cantharidin	1·00
Amphetamine	0·21	Caramiphen	0·18
iso-Amylamine	0·07	Carbetapentane	0·54
Amylocaine	0·87	Carphenazine	0·62
Anabasine	0·38	Cephaeline	0·51
	0·15	Cephaloridin	0·00
	0·77	Chlorcyclizine	0·90
	0·85	Chlordiazepoxide	0·87
	0·90	Chlormezanone	0·87
Antazoline	0·29	Chloroquine	0·25
Apomorphine	0·80		streaked
Atropine	0·15	Chlorpheniramine	0·32
Bemegride	0·97	Chlorpromazine	0·61
Benactyzine	0·88	Chlorprothixene	0·78
Benzocaine	0·66	Cinchocaine	0·53
Benzoquinonium Chloride	0·04	Clioquinol	0·81
	streaked	Cocaine	0·68

Drug	R_f	Drug	R_f
Codeine	0·40	Levorphanol	0·20
Coniine	0·09	Lignocaine	0·70
Cyclizine	0·84	Lobeline	0·62
Cysteine	0·00	Menthol	0·89
Demecolcine	0·80	Mepacrine	0·15
Desipramine	0·41	Mephenesin	1·00
Dextromethorphan	0·29	Mephentermine	0·13
Diamorphine	0·70	Meprobamate	0·77
Dicyclomine	0·87	Mepyramine	0·41
Diethazine	0·71	Mescaline	0·12
Digitalin	0·90	Methadone	0·56
Digitoxin	0·83	Methanthelinium Bromide	0·28
Digoxin	0·83		streaked
Dihydrochlorothiazide	0·00	Methapyrilene	0·40
Dimenhydrinate	0·47	Methaqualone	0·93
Dimethisoquin	0·83	Methotrimeprazine	0·77
Diphenhydramine	0·53	Methylamphetamine	0·38
Diphenoxylate	1·00	Methylpentynol	—
Dipipanone	0·79	Methyl Phenidate	0·63
Diprophylline	—	Metoclopramide	0·25
Doxylamine	0·28	Morphine	0·28
Droperidol	0·87	Nalorphine	0·76
Emetine	0·90	Narceine	0·28
Ephedrine	0·11	Neostigmine	0·23
Ergometrine	0·62	Nicotinamide	0·49
Ergotamine	0·97	Nicotine	0·35
Ergotoxine	1·00		0·67
Ethanolamine	0·89	Nikethamide	0·84
Ethoheptazine	0·37	Noradrenaline	0·00
Ethopropazine	0·71	Norharman	0·72
Fluphenazine	0·68	Nortriptyline	0·47
Gallamine	0·00	Noscapine	0·98
Halopyramine	0·52	Ouabain	0·97
Harman	0·61	Oxanamide	0·93
Hexamethonium Bromide	0·00	Oxybuprocaine	0·58
Histamine	0·05	Oxyphenonium Bromide	0·26
Homatropine	0·00	Papaveretum	0·26
Hydrallazine	0·31		0·42
	0·92		0·94
Hydromorphone	0·24		0·98
Hydroxychloroquine	0·11	Papaverine	0·94
Hydroxyzine	0·88	Pecazine	0·71
Hyoscine	0·74	Penthienate	0·27
Hyoscine-N-Butyl Bromide	0·19		streaked
	streaked	Pericyazine	0·53
Hyoscyamine	0·04	Perphenazine	0·72
Hypoxanthine	0·00	Pethidine	0·72
Imipramine	0·52	Phenadoxone	0·96
Isoprenaline	0·00	Phenindamine	0·87
Lanatoside C	—	Pheniramine	0·26
Laudexium	0·44	Phenmetrazine	0·58
	streaked	Phenylephrine	—

Table 3 (*contd*)

Drug	R_f	Drug	R_f
β-Phenylethylamine	0·21	Succinyl Sulphathiazole . .	0·04
Phenylpropanolamine . . .	0·13	Sulphacetamide	—
Pholcodine	0·36	Sulphadiazine	0·73
Picrotoxin	—		streaked
Pipamazine	0·56	Sulphadimidine	0·74
Pipenzolate	0·24	Sulphaguanidine	0·00
	tailed	Sulphapyridine	0·83
Piperocaine	0·71	Sulphathiazole	—
Prilocaine	0·66	Suxamethonium Bromide . .	0·00
Primaquine	0·08	Suxethonium Bromide . . .	0·00
Procainamide	0·22	Terpin Hydrate	—
Procaine	0·40	Tetraethylammonium Bromide	0·26
Prochlorperazine	0·77		streaked
Procyclidine	0·45	Thenyldiamine	0·40
Proguanil	0·00	Theobromine	0·73
Promazine	0·48		streaked
Promethazine	0·79		
n-Propanolamine	0·07	Theophylline	0·81
	streaked	Thiopropazate	0·92
Propantheline	0·35	Thioproperazine Mesylate . .	0·75
Protriptyline	0·38	Thonzylamine	0·61
Pseudoephedrine	0·12	Tricyclamol	0·15
Putrescine	0·06	Trimeprazine	0·54
Pyrathiazine	0·76	Trimetaphan Camsylate . .	0·19
Pyrimethamine	0·72		tailed
Pyrrolidine	0·91	Trimethylamine	Diffuses
Quinidine	0·52	Trimipramine	0·68
	(0·23)	Tripelennamine	0·63
Quinine	0·52	Triprolidine	0·55
Rauwiloid	0·51	Tryptamine	0·16
	0·71	Tubocurarine	0·33
	0·96	Veratrine	0·89
Reserpine	0·94	Xanthine	0·00
Strophanthin K	—	Yohimbine	0·84
Strychnine	0·33	Zoxazolamine	0·83

Note. The locating agents are iodoplatinate, acidified iodoplatinate, and iodine vapour and should be tried in that order till a reaction is obtained. The reagents are prepared as follows.

Iodoplatinate reagent. 1 g of chloroplatinic acid is dissolved in 10 ml of water and a solution of 10 g of potassium iodide in 350 ml of water is added to it. The final volume is adjusted to 500 ml with water.

Acidified iodoplatinate reagent. This is prepared as for the iodoplatinate reagent but the final volume is adjusted with diluted hydrochloric acid. For this purpose 144 ml of hydrochloric acid of specific gravity 1·18 is mixed with 96 ml of water.

Iodine vapour reagent. Solid iodine is heated to produce the characteristic purple vapour which may be blown on to the plates from a polyethylene bottle or used for immersion purposes.

Colour Reactions on Thin Layers

A number of chemical reagents react with drugs to give coloured products. Three of the most used have been chosen and the results of reaction with the selection of basic drugs are described in the following Tables. Colour reactions of barbiturates are described in the example on barbiturates given under thin layer chromatography. The colour developing reagents may be mixed directly with the drug, but the method chosen here involves spotting the drug on to a silica-gel-coated chromatography plate and spraying with the selected reagent. The drugs show up as coloured spots against a uniform background.

Table 4. Colour Reactions with Acidified Iodoplatinate

BROWN

Acetyl Digitoxin
Alkavervir (M)
Amisometradine
Amodiaquine
Anabasine
Antazoline
Apomorphine
Atropine
Bemegride
Benzoquinonium
  Chloride
Benthiazide
Berbamine
Berberine
Bromodiphenhydramine
Brucine
Buphenine
Butyl Aminobenzoate
Caramiphen
Cephaeline
Cephaloridine
Chlorcyclizine
Chloroquine
Chlorpheniramine
Cinchocaine
Clioquinol
Cocaine
Codeine
Coniine
Cyclizine
Demecolcine

Dextromethorphan
Diamorphine
Dicyclomine
Diethazine
Digitalin
Digitoxin
Digoxin
Dimenhydrinate
Dimethisoquin
Diphenhydramine
Diphenoxylate
Dipipanone
Doxylamine
Emetine
Ephedrine
Ergometrine
Ergotamine
Ergotoxine Esylate
Fluopromazine
Gallamine
  Triethiodide
Hexamethonium
  Bromide
Histamine
Hydromorphone
Lanatoside C
Laudexium
  Methylsulphate
Levorphanol
Lignocaine
Lobeline

Menthol
Mepacrine
Mephenesin
  Carbamate
Nicotine
Ouabain
Oxybuprocaine
Oxyphenonium
  Bromide
Papaveretum (M)
Pavatrine
Pecazine
Penthienate
Phenylpropanolamine
Picrotoxin
Piperocaine
Prilocaine
Procyclidine
Propantheline
Rauwolfia (M)
Rauwolfia alkaloids (M)
Succinyl Sulphathiazole
Sulphathiazole
Suxamethonium
  Bromide
Suxethonium Bromide
Tricyclamol
Trimethidinium
  Methosulphide

PURPLE BROWN

Amiphenazole
Amitriptyline
Carbetapentane
Ethopropazine
Halopyramine
Harman

Hyoscine
Hyoscine-N-Butyl
  Bromide
Imipramine
Methotrimeprazine
Narceine

Neostigmine Bromide
Norharman
Nortriptyline
Papaverine
Pethidine
Phenadoxone

3

5

Table 4   *(contd)*

PURPLE BROWN (contd)

Phenindamine	Procaine	Thiethylperazine
Pheniramine	Pyrathiazine	Thonzylamine
Phenmetrazine	Pyrimethamine	Trifluopromazine
Pholcodine	Quinidine	Triprolidine
Pipenzolate	Quinine	Yohimbine
Primaquine	Reserpine	

PURPLE

Amethocaine	Nalorphine	Thioproperazine
iso-Amylamine	Noscapine	Mesylate
Amylocaine	β-Phenylethylamine	Trimeprazine
Butacaine	Prochlorperazine	Trimetaphan
iso-Butylamine	Promazine	Camsylate
Mescaline	Pseudo strychnine	Trimethylamine
Methadone	Strychnine	Tryptamine
Methanthelinium	Sulphadiazine	Tubocurarine
Bromide	Theobromine	Tyramine
Methaqualone	Theophylline	Veratrine
Methyl Phenidate		

BLUE BLACK

Acepromazine	Isoprenaline	Sulphaguanidine
Chlordiazepoxide	Mepyramine	Sulphapyridine
Chlorpromazine	Methapyrilene	Tetraethylammonium
Fluphenazine	Morphine	Bromide
Homatropine	Perphenazine	Thenyldiamine
Hydroxychloroquine	Proguanil	Tripelennamine
Hydroxyzine	Pseudo ephedrine	
Hyoscyamine	Sulphadimidine	

BLUE

Amphetamine	Methylamphetamine	Pyrrolidine
Cadaverine	Nicotinamide	Zoxazolamine
Hydrallazine	Nikethamide	
Mephentermine	Putresine	

BLUE GREY

Caffeine

GREY

Benzocaine

(M)—Mixture of alkaloids.

Table 5. **No Reaction with Acidified Iodoplatinate Reagent**

Adrenaline	Glycine	n-Propanolamine
Betaine	Hypoxanthine	Strophanthin K
Cantharidin	Methylpentynol	Sulphacetamide
Diprophylline	Noradrenaline	Terpin Hydrate
Ethanolamine	Phenylephrine	Xanthine

Note. The preparation of this reagent is described under 'Thin layer chromatography—R_f values'.

Table 6. **Colour Reactions with Mandelin's Reagent**

RED

Acepromazine	Mephenesin Carbamate	Promazine
Antazoline	Methyl Phenidate	Promethazine
Berberine	Pecazine	Pyrathiazine
Chlorpromazine	Perphenazine	Thioproperazine
Cinchocaine	Prilocaine	Trimeprazine
Fluopromazine	Primaquin	
Gallamine Triethiodide	Prochlorperazine	

PINK

Mepyramine

SALMON PINK

Noscapine   Terpin Hydrate

ORANGE

Benzoquinonium Chloride	Pipenzolate	Trifluoperazine
Mepacrine	Propantheline	Tryptamine
Methanthelinium Bromide	Pseudo strychnine	
	Strychnine	
	Thenyldiamine	

YELLOW

Brucine	Diphenhydramine	Rauwolfia alkaloids (M)
Demecolcine	Mescaline	Yohimbine

LIME GREEN

Clioquinol

BLUE

Cephaloridin	Phenindamine	Thiethylperazine
Imipramine	Reserpine	

Table 6. *(contd)*

VIOLET

Amethocaine	Diamorphine	Noradrenaline
Amitriptyline	Dimethisoquin	Nortriptyline
Amphetamine	Hydramorphone	Oxybuprocaine
Amylocaine	Levorphanol	Papaverine
Benzocaine	Lignocaine	Pavatrine (M)
Buphenine	Methadone	Pethidine
Butacaine	Methyl Amphetamine	Phenmetrazine
Butyl Aminobenzoate	Morphine	Phenylpropanolamine
Codeine	Nalorphine	Procainamide
Dextromethorphan	Neostigmine	

VIOLET PURPLE

Thonzylamine

PURPLE

Harman	Norharman	Tyramine
Methotrimeprazine	Penthienate	

BROWN

Alkavervir (M)	Digoxin	Rauwolfia
Apomorphine	Laudexium	Trimethidinium
Berbamine	Methylsulphate	Methosulphide
Digitalin	Methapyrilene	

RED BROWN

Diethazine	Ethopropazine	Fluphenazine

VIOLET BROWN

Ephedrine	Theophylline	Tubocurarine
Picrotoxin		

BEIGE

Procaine	Tetraethylammonium Bromide

GREY BROWN

Acetyl Digitoxin

GREY GREEN

Digitoxin

WHITE

Dicyclomine	Papaveretum (M)

BRICK RED → BROWN

Ergometrine	Ergotamine	Ergotoxine Esylate

(M)—Mixture of alkaloids.

Table 7.   No Reaction with Mandelin's Reagent

Adrenaline	Emetine	Pheniramine
Amiphenazole	Glycine	Phenylephrine
Amisometradine	Halopyramine	Pholcodine
Amodiaquin	Hexamethonium	Piperocaine
Anabazine	Bromide	Procyclidine
Atropine	Histamine	Proguanil
Bemegride	Homatropine	Pseudo ephedrine
Benzthiazide	Hydrallazine	Putrescine
Betaine	Hydroxychloroquin	Pyrimethamine
Bromodiphenhydramine	Hydroxyzine	Quinidine
Cadaverine	Hyoscine	Quinine
Caffeine	Hyoscine Butyl	Strophanthin K
Cantharidin	Bromide	Succinyl
Caramiphen	Hyoscyamine	Sulphathiazole
Carbetapentane	Isoprenaline	Sulphacetamide
Cephaeline	Lanatoside C	Sulphadiazine
Chlorcyclizine	Lobeline	Sulphadimidine
Chlordiazepoxide	Menthol	Sulphaguanidine
Chloroquine	Mephentermine	Sulphapyridine
Chlorpheniramine	Meprobamate	Sulphathiazole
Cocaine	Methaqualone	Suxamethonium
Coniine	Methylpentynol	Bromide
Cyclizine	Narceine	Suxethonium Bromide
Cysteine	Nicotinamide	Theobromine
Dihydrochlorothiazide	Nicotine	Tricyclamol
Dimehydrinate	Nikethamide	Trimetaphan Camsylate
Diphenoxylate	Ouabain	Tripelennamine
Dipipanone	Oxyphenonium	Triprolidine
Diprophylline	Bromide	Veratrine
Doxylamine	Phenadoxone	Zoxazolamine

Note.   The reagent is prepared by dissolving 1 g of ammonium vanadate in 100 g of sulphuric acid (sp. gr. 1·98).   Stir before use.

Table 8.   Colour Reactions with Marquis' Reagent

RED

Chlorpromazine	Prochlorperazine	Pyrathiazine
Diethazine	Promazine	Thenyldiamine
Perphenazine	Promethazine	

CRIMSON

Pipenzolate	Propantheline

PINK

Mephenesin Carbamate	Pecazine	Thioproperazine
Mepyramine	Penthienate	Mesylate
		Trimeprazine

Table 8 (*contd*)

SALMON PINK

Acepromazine	Fluopromazine	Trifluoperazine
Ethopropazine	Terpin Hydrate	

ORANGE

Cephaloridine	Methanthelinium	Tetraethylammonium
Fluphenazine	Bromide	Bromide
Hydromorphone	Noscapine	
Levorphanol	Papaverine	

YELLOW

Amodiaquine	Gallamine Triethiodide	Reserpine
Berberine	Mepacrine	Yohimbine
Bromodiphenhydramine	Methyl Phenidate	
Demecolcine	Neostigmine Bromide	

GREEN

Digitoxin	Phenindamine

LIME GREEN

Clioquinol

TURQUOISE

Thiethylperazine

BLUE

Imipramine

VIOLET

Codeine	Dihydrocodeine	Morphine
Diamorphine	Ephedrine	Theophylline

PURPLE

Benzoquinonium	Methadone	Nalorphine
Chloride	Methotrimeprazine	

BROWN

Alkavervir (M)	Methapyrilene	Rauwolfia alkaloids
Apomorphine	Nicotine	Trimethidinium
Diphenhydramine	Pavatrine (M)	Methosulphide

FAWN

Acetyl Digitoxin	Berbamine	Rauwolfia (M)

MAUVE

Ergometrine	Ergotamine	Ergotoxine Esylate

GREY

Digitoxin	Lanatoside C

(M)—Mixture of alkaloids.

Table 9.   No Reaction with Marquis' Reagent

Adrenaline
Amethocaine
Amiphenazole
Amisometradine
Amitriptyline
Amphetamine
Amylocaine
Anabasine
Antazoline
Atropine
Bemegride
Benzocaine
Benzthiazide
Betaine
Brucine
Buphenine
Butacaine
Butyl Aminobenzoate
Cadaverine
Caffeine
Cantharidin
Caramiphen
Carbetapentane
Cephaeline
Chlorcyclizine
Chlordiazepoxide
Chloroquine
Chlorpheniramine
Cinchocaine
Cocaine
Coniine
Cyclizine
Cysteine
Dextromethorphan
Dicyclomine
Digitalin
Dihydrochlorothiazine
Dimenhydrinate
Dimethisoquin
Diphenoxylate
Dipipanone

Diprophylline
Doxylamine
Emetine
Glycine
Halopyramine
Harman
Hexamethonium
   Bromide
Histamine
Homatropine
Hydrallazine
Hydroxychloroquine
Hydroxyzine
Hyoscine
Hyoscine-N-Butyl
   Bromide
Hyoscyamine
Isoprenaline
Laudexium
   Methylsulphate
Lignocaine
Lobeline
Menthol
Mephentermine
Meprobamate
Mescaline
Methaqualone
Methylamphetamine
Methylpentynol
Narceine
Nicotinamide
Nikethamide
Noradrenaline
Nortriptyline
Ouabain
Oxybuprocaine
Oxyphenonium
   Bromide
Pethidine
Phenadoxone
Pheniramine

Phenmetrazine
Phenylephrine
Phenylpropanolamine
Pholcodine
Picrotoxin
Piperocaine
Prilocaine
Primaquin
Procainamide
Procaine
Procyclidine
Proguanil
Pseudo ephedrine
Pseudo strychnine
Putrescine
Pyrimethamine
Quinidine
Quinine
Strophanthin K
Strychnine
Succinyl Sulphathiazole
Sulphacetamide
Sulphadiazine
Sulphadimidine
Sulphaguanidine
Sulphapyridine
Sulphathiazole
Suxamethonium
   Bromide
Suxethonium Bromide
Theobromine
Thonzylamine
Tricyclamol
Trimetaphan
   Camsylate
Tripelennamine
Triprolidine
Tubocurarine
Veratrine
Zoxazolamine

Note.   The reagent is prepared by dissolving one drop of formaldehyde in 1 ml of concentrated sulphuric acid immediately before use.

GAS LIQUID CHROMATOGRAPHY—R_t VALUES

The selected basic drugs are investigated using G.L.C. and lists of retention times relative to selected standard drugs are prepared.   As the range of retention times is large it is necessary to use three standard materials at varying column temperatures so that there is no undue delay in the drugs reaching the detector. A five-foot column of 5 per cent SE 30 (a silicone gum rubber) on acid-washed Chromosorb W (60–80 mesh) treated with dimethyl-dichloro-silane is used throughout. The nitrogen flow rate is 60 ml per minute. A selection of barbiturates is also given using a six-foot column of 5 per cent SE 30 on Aeropak 30 (100–200 mesh) and a nitrogen flow rate of 60 ml per minute.

Table 10. Retention Times Relative to Codeine

(*Column temperature—200°C, R_t codeine 9·75 minutes*)

Drug	R_t relative	Drug	R_t relative
Acepromazine	2·62	Dextromethorphan	0·51
Acetyldigitoxin	0·30	Diamorphine	1·95
Adrenaline	0·03	Dicyclomine	0·45
Amethocaine	0·61	Diethazine	1·12
Amiphenazole	0·15	Digitalin★	0·05
Amisometradine	0·31	Digitoxin★	0·19
Amitriptyline	0·57	Dihydrocodeine	1·00
Amodiaquin	0·20	Dimethisoquin	0·33
Amylocaine	0·07	Diphenhydramine	0·19
Anabasine	0·61	Diphenoxylate	0·20
Atropine	0·54	Dipipanone	1·45
Bemegride	0·04	Diprophylline	1·05
Benzocaine	0·06	Doxylamine	0·26
Benzoquinonium Chloride★	0·53	Emetine	0·19
	1·30	Ergotamine	0·87
Berbamine	1·42	Ergotoxine	0·17
Berberine	0·37	Ethopropazine	1·01
Bromodiphenhydramine	0·55	Fluopromazine	0·62
Buphenine	0·85	Fluphenazine	0·28
Butacaine	1·21	Gallamine	2·26
Butyl Aminobenzoate	0·15	Halopyramine	0·74
Caffeine	0·17	Harman	0·33
Cantharidin	0·07	Hexamethonium Bromide★	0·02
Caramiphen	0·32		1·30
Carbetapentane	0·77	Histamine	0·19
Cephaeline★	1·20	Homatropine	0·37
Cephaloridin★	0·05	Hydrallazine	0·08
	0·57	Hydroxychloroquin★	0·25
	1·25	Hydroxyzine	4·92
Chlorcyclizine	0·69	Hyoscine	0·82
Chlordiazepoxide	1·49	Hyoscine-N-Butyl Bromide	0·82
Chlorpheniramine	0·34	Hyoscyamine	0·59
Chlorpromazine	1·30	Imipramine	0·70
Cinchocaine	2·80	Lanatoside C.	0·19
Clioquinol	0·26	Laudexium Methylsulphate	6·00
Cocaine	0·57	Levorphanol	0·60
Codeine	1·00	Lignocaine	0·21
Colchamine★	1·13	Lobeline	0·02
Cyclizine	0·34	Menthol	0·02
Cysteine★	0·09	Mepacrine	0·78
Desipramine	0·73	Mephenesin	0·08

Drug	R_t relative	Drug	R_t relative
Meprobamate	0·15	Piperocaine	0·29
Mepyramine	0·63	Prilocaine	0·17
Mescaline	0·10	Primaquine	0·85
Methadone	0·49	Procainamide	0·64
Methanthelinium Bromide	0·90	Procaine	0·32
Methapyrilene	0·28	Prochlorperazine	5·28
Methaqualone	0·49	Procyclidine	0·50
Methotrimeprazine	1·52	Proguanil	0·21
Methyl Phenidate	0·13	Promazine	0·87
Morphine	1·19	Promethazine	0·72
Nalorphine	1·80	Propantheline Bromide	0·99
Narceine*	0·13	Protriptyline	0·68
Neostigmine	0·13	Pyrathiazine	1·56
Nicotinamide*	0·02	Pyrrolidine	0·02
L-Noradrenaline*	0·02	Suxamethonium Bromide	0·14
Norharman	0·32	Suxethonium Bromide	0·22
	0·38	Terpin Hydrate*	0·03
Nortriptyline	0·60	Thenyldiamine	0·32
Ouabain*	0·17	Theobromine	0·12
Oxybuprocaine	0·62	Theophylline	0·27
Oxyphenonium Bromide	0·59	Thiethylperazine	1·45
Pecazine	1·79	Thonzylamine	0·62
Penthienate Methobromide	0·44	Tricyclamol Chloride	0·59
	0·54	Trimeprazine	0·80
Perphenazine	1·44	Trimipramine	0·66
Pethidine	0·13	Tripelennamine	0·31
Phenadoxone	1·62	Triprolidine	0·80
Phenelzine	0·32	Tryptamine	0·21
Phenindamine	0·51	Tyramine	0·08
Pheniramine	0·18	Veratrine	0·27
Phenmetrazine	0·05	Yohimbine	0·17
Pholcodine	0·02		1·20
Picrotoxin	0·91	Zoxazolamine	0·01
Pipenzolate Bromide	0·90		

* Solid injection.

Table 11. Retention Times Relative to Ephedrine

(*Column temperature—125°C, R_t ephedrine 4·5 minutes*)

Drug	R_t relative	Drug	R_t relative
Amphetamine	0·33	Pentamethylenediamine	0·17
D-Coniine	0·17	β-Phenylethylamine	0·33
Ephedrine	1·00	Phenylpropanolamine	0·86
Ethanolamine	0·00	Pseudo ephedrine	1·00
Isoamylamine	0·00	Pyrrolidine	0·00
Isobutylamine	0·00		0·22
Mephentermine	0·64		2·33
Methyl Amphetamine	0·50	Tetramethylenediamine	0·12
Nicotine	0·89	Trimethylamine	0·00

Table 12. Retention Times Relative to Papaverine

(Column temperature—250°C, R_t papaverine 4·75 minutes)

Drug	R_t relative	Drug	R_t relative
Chloroquine	0·71	Pseudo strychnine	2·02
Codeine	0·32	Pyrimethamine	0·02
Colchamine	1·45	Quinidine	1·06
Ergometrine	0·52	Quinine	1·00
Metoclopramide	0·61	Strychnine	2·02
Noscapine	2·23	Sulphacetamide	0·24
Papaverine	1·00	Sulphadiazine	0·58
Pavatrine	0·27	Sulphadimidine	0·79
Pecazine	0·52	Sulphapyridine	0·55
Perphenazine	0·03	Trifluoperazine	0·60

Table 13. Drugs Giving no Response with the Column and Conditions in the above Tables

Antazoline	Isoprenaline	Tetraethylammonium
Benzthiazide	Methyl Pentynol	Bromide
Betaine	Phenylephrine	Thioproperazine
Brucine	Strophanthin K	Trimetaphan
Digoxin	Succinyl	Camsylate
Dihydrochlorothiazide	Sulphathiazole	Trimethidinium
Glycine	Sulphaguanidine	Bromide
Hexamethonium	Sulphathiazole	Tubocurarine
Bromide		

Table 14. Retention Times Relative to Pentobarbitone

Column temperature—150°C, R_t pentobarbitone 2·9 minutes)

Drug	R_t relative	Drug	R_t relative
Allobarbitone . . .	0·48	Methohexitone . .	0·90
Allylbarbituric Acid . .	0·72	Methylphenobarbitone .	1·76
Amylobarbitone . .	0·90	Nealbarbitone . . .	0·52
Aprobarbital . . .	0·61	Pentobarbitone . . .	1·00
Barbitone . . .	0·38	Phenobarbitone . .	2·80
Butallylonal . . .	2·80	Phenylmethylbarbituric Acid	1·45
Buthalitone . . .	0·98	Probarbital . . .	0·43
Butobarbitone . . .	0·76	Quinalbarbitone . .	1·18
Cyclobarbitone . .	2·33	Thialbarbitone . .	1·38
Heptabarbitone . .	2·30	Thiamylal . . .	2·00
Hexobarbitone . .	1·56	Thiopentone . . .	1·35
Metharbital . . .	0·21	Vinbarbitone . . .	1·18

Table 15 (*contd*)

Drug	Absorption maxima millimicrons	Absorption minima millimicrons
Strophosid	—	—
Strychnine	*254*, 278 (inflexion), 287	227
Succinyl Sulphathiazole .	*257*, 280	224, 267
Sulphacetamide . . .	*271*, 266	238, 268
Sulphadiazine . . .	*242*, 307	228, 286
Sulphadimidine . . .	*243*, 301	226, 276
Sulphaguanidine . .	*218*, 264, 271	252, 269
Sulphapyridine . . .	239, *309*	226, 276
Sulphathiazole . . .	214, *280*	237
Sulthiame.	244	222
Suxamethonium Bromide	—	—
Suxethonium Bromide .	—	—
Tetracycline	*269*, 353	233, 299
Tetraethylammonium Bromide	—	—
Tetraethylammonium Chloride	—	—
Thenyldiamine . . .	*239*, 315	264
Theophylline	*270*, 225 (shoulder)	220, 242
Thiamine	246	—
Thiethylperazine . . .	*260*, 300	238, 287
Thiopropazate . . .	*253*, 304	225, 276
Thioproperazine Methanesulphate . .	234, *263*, 314	216, 240, 295
Thioridazine	*263*, 313	289
Thonzylamine . . .	*235*, 274, 280, 314	261, 277, 287
Tranylcypromine . .	*264*, 258, 271	236, 260, 269
Trichloroethylphosphate	—	—
Tricyclamol Chloride .	*256*, 250, 263	233, 253, 261
Trifluoperazine . . .	*255*, 305	222, 278
Trimeprazine. . . .	*251*, 301	220, 278
Trimetaphan Camsylate .	*257*, 251, 263	249, 254, 262
Tripelennamine . . .	*239*, 314	219, 263
Triprolidine	289	260
Tubocurarine. . . .	280	254
Veratrine	*260*, 292	247, 281
Yohimbine	*271*, 277, 287	241, 274, 285
Zoxazolamine. . . .	*278*, 284	247, 281

Note. When there is more than one peak present the main one is in italics.

Appendix II

USEFUL WEIGHTS AND MEASURES

Table 16. **Weights and Measures (Metric and Imperial) Conversions**

Weight

1 mg . . 0·0154 gr	1 gr . . . 64·8 mg	
1 g . . . 15·4 gr	1 dr . . . 1·77 g	
0·564 dr	1 oz . . . 28·3 g	
0·0353 oz	1 lb . . . 0·454 kg	
1 kg. . . 35·3 oz		
2·20 lb		

Volume

1 ml. . . 16·9 min	1 min. . . 0·0592 ml
0·282 fl dr	1 fl dr . . 3·55 ml
1 l . . . 35·2 fl oz	1 fl oz . . 28·4 ml
1·76 pt	1 pt . . . 0·568 l
	1 gal . . . 4·55 l
1 cm³ . . 0·0610 in³	1 in³ . . . 16·4 cm³
1 m³ . . 35·3 ft³	1 ft³ . . . 28,300 cm³
1·31 yd³	1 yd³ . . . 0·765 *m*³

Note. cm³ and ml may be regarded as interchangeable.

Length

1 cm . . 0·394 in	1 in . . . 2·54 cm
1 m . . . 39·4 in	1 ft . . . 30·5 cm
3·28 ft	1 yd . . . 91·4 cm
1 km . . 0·62 mi	1 mi . . . 1·61 km

Area

1 cm² . . 0·155 in²	1 in² . . . 6·45 cm²
1 m² . . 10·8 ft²	1 ft² . . . 929 cm²
1·20 yd²	1 yd² . . . 0·836 m²

Temperature

To convert degrees Centigrade to degrees Fahrenheit, multiply by 9, divide by 5 and add 32.

To convert degrees Fahrenheit to degrees Centigrade subtract 32, multiply by 5 and divide by 9.

Table 17. Weights and other Data of Organs

Adult organs[1]

(Average weight)

Adrenals	. . . . .	5 to	6 g
Brain— Female	. . . .	1250 ,,	1275 ,,
Male	. . .	1365 ,,	1450 ,,
Heart— Female	. . . .	250 ,,	280 ,,
Male	. . .	270 ,,	360 ,,
Kidneys— Right	. . .		140 ,,
Left	. . .		150 ,,
Lungs— Right	. . .	480 ,,	680 ,,
Left	. . .	420 ,,	600 ,,
Liver	. . . . .	1440 ,,	1680 ,,
Ovaries	. . . . .	4 ,,	8 ,,
Pancreas	. . . . .	60 ,,	135 ,,
Spleen	. . . . .	155 ,,	195 ,,
Thymus— At birth	. . . .		. 14 ,,
End of second year	. . .		. 26 ,,

Then decreases until gland disappears
A rapid diminution occurs at puberty

Uterus— Nulliparous	. . .	. 40 to 50 g
Multiparous	. .	. Increased by 20 ,,

Note. These weights should be interpreted in relation to size of subject.

Other data

Diameter of aorta . . . . . 1·7 to 3·0 cm

Uterus

Nulliparous measurements		Multiparous measurements
Length . .	7·0 cm	
Breadth . .	4·0 ,,	Increased 1 cm or more
Thickness .	2·5 ,,	
Length (cavity) .	5·0 ,,	5·7 cm

Organs of new-born child[1]

(Average weight)

Brain	380·0 g
Thymus	14·0 ,,
Heart	20·6 ,,
Lungs (together)	58·0 ,,
Spleen	11·1 ,,
Kidneys (together)	23·6 ,,
Testicles	0·8 ,,
Liver	118·0 ,,

Reference

1. Ross. *Post-mortem Appearances.* London: Oxford University Press, 1931.

Appendix III

NORMAL LEVELS OF TRACE ELEMENTS

Table 18. Normal Levels of Trace Elements in Human Tissue
(μg/g dry tissue) **and Fluids** (μg/ml)

	Blood	Brain	Hair	Heart	Kidney	Liver	Urine
Antimony . .	0·016	0·11	0·69	0·09	0·17	0·19	—
Arsenic . .	0·03	0·016	0·65	0·027	0·050	0·057	0·084
Barium . .	0·07	0·01	—	0·08	0·06	0·007	—
Beryllium . .	0·0001	0·002	—	0·002	0·002	0·0009	0·0002
Bismuth . .	0·01	0·1	—	0·08	0·09	0·07	—
Boron . . .	0·13	0·6	—	0·2	0·5	0·48	—
Cadmium . .	—	2·55	—	3·34	66·4	6·38	—
Copper . .	1·2	23·9	23·1	16·5	14·9	25·5	0·04
Fluorine . .	0·32	2	—	2	3·2	4	—
Gold . . .	0·00004	0·5	0·05	0·00013	0·5	0·0001	—
Iron . . .	475	200	130	190	290	520	0·07
Lead . . .	0·29	0·20	35	—	0·27	1·7	0·023
Manganese .	0·15	1·00	2·51	0·88	3·34	4·65	—
Mercury . .	0·02	2·94	5·52	1·76	9·03	3·66	0·023
Nickel . .	0·03	0·3	6	0·2	0·2	0·2	—
Silver . . .	0·03	0·03	0·9	0·01	0·005	0·04	—
Thallium . .	0·02	0·5	—	0·4	0·4	0·4	—
Tin . . .	0·12	2	—	0·2	0·2	0·6	0·01
Zinc . . .	7·0	39·1	173	87·9	188	169	0·5

Appendix IV

PHARMACEUTICAL AND TRADE NAMES

THE tables below contain a selection of pharmaceutical names with some of the trade equivalents for a number of the drugs mentioned in the toxicology section.

Table 19. Pharmaceutical and Trade Names of a Selection of Drugs listed alphabetically with respect to the pharmaceutical name

Pharmaceutical name	Selection of trade names
Acepromazine . .	Notensil
Amitriptyline . .	Laroxyl, Saroten, Tryptizol
Amphetamine . .	Benzedrine
D-Amphetamine .	Dexedrine, Dexamed
Antazoline . . .	Antistin, Histostab
Benzhexol . . .	Artane, Pipanol
Caramiphen . . .	Parpanit, Taoryl
Chlordiazepoxide .	Librium
Chlorpheniramine .	Chlor-Trimeton, Haynon, Piriton
Chlorpromazine . .	Largactil
Chlorprothixene .	Taractan
Cyclizine . . .	Marzine, Valoid
Diazepam . . .	Valium
Dicyclomine . . .	Merbentyl, Wyovin
Diethylpropion . .	Tenuate
Diphenhydramine .	Benadryl
Fluphenazine . .	Modecate, Moditen, Prolixin
Haloperidol . . .	Serenace
Hyoscine . . .	Pamine, Scopolamine
Imipramine . . .	Dimepressin, Praminil, Tofranil
Meclozine . . .	Ancolan
Methaqualone . .	Melsedin, Paxidorm
Methylamphetamine	Methedrine
Methylphenidate .	Ritalin
Nitrazepam . .	Mogadon
Nortriptyline . .	Allegron, Aventyl
Perphenazine . .	Fentazin, Trilafon
Phenalzine . . .	Nardil
Phenindamine . .	Thephorin
Pheniramine. . .	Daneral, Trimeton
Phenmetrazine . .	Preludin
Phentermine . .	Duromine
Prochlorperazine .	Compazine, Stemetil
Promazine . . .	Sparine
Promethazine . .	Phenergan
Propantheline . .	Probanthine
Thioproperazine .	Majeptil
Thioridazine . .	Melleril
Thonzylamine . .	Neohetramine
Trifluoperazine . .	Stelazine
Tripelennamine. .	Pyribenzamine

Table 20. Pharmaceutical and Trade Names of a Selection of Drugs listed alphabetically with respect to the trade name

Trade name	Pharmaceutical name	Trade name	Pharmaceutical name
Allegron	Nortriptyline	Neohetramine	Thonzylamine
Ancolan	Meclozine	Notensil	Acepromazine
Antistin	Antazoline	Pamine	Hyoscine
Artane	Benzhexol	Parpanit	Caramiphen
Aventyl	Nortriptyline	Paxidorm	Methaqualone
Benadryl	Diphenhydramine	Phenergan	Promethazine
Benzedrine	Amphetamine	Pipanol	Benzhexol
Chlor-Trimeton	Chlorpheniramine	Piriton	Chlorpheniramine
Compazine	Prochlorperazine	Praminil	Imipramine
Daneral	Pheniramine	Preludin	Phenmetrazine
Dexamed	D-Amphetamine	Probanthine	Propantheline
Dexedrine	D-Amphetamine	Prolixin	Fluphenazine
Dimepressin	Imipramine	Pyribenzamine	Tripelennamine
Duromine	Phentermine	Ritalin	Methylphenidate
Fentazin	Perphenazine	Saroten	Amitriptyline
Haynon	Chlorpheniramine	Scopolamine	Hyoscine
Histostab	Antazoline	Serenace	Haloperidol
Largactil	Chlorpromazine	Sparine	Promazine
Laroxyl	Amitriptyline	Stelazine	Trifluoperazine
Librium	Chlordiazepoxide	Stemetil	Prochlorperazine
Majeptil	Thioproperazine	Taoryl	Caramiphen
Marzine	Cyclizine	Taractan	Chlorprothixene
Melleril	Thioridazine	Tenuate	Diethylpropion
Melsedin	Methaqualone	Thephorin	Phenindamine
Merbentyl	Dicyclomine	Tofranil	Imipramine
Methedrine	Methylamphetamine	Trilafon	Perphenazine
Modecate	Fluphenazine	Trimeton	Pheniramine
Moditen	Fluphenazine	Tryptizol	Amitriptyline
Mogadon	Nitrazepam	Valium	Diazepam
Nardil	Phenelzine	Valoid	Cyclizine
		Wyovin	Dicyclomine

Table 21. Pharmaceutical and Trade Names of a Selection of Barbiturates

Pharmaceutical name	Trade name(s)
5,5-substituted Barbiturates	
Allobarbitone	Dial
Allylbarbituric acid	Sandoptal
Amylobarbitone	Amytal
Aprobarbital	Alurate
Barbitone	Medinal
	Veronal
Butobarbitone	Sonalgin
	Soneryl
Cyclobarbitone	Phanodorm
	Rapidal
Heptabarbitone	Medomin
Nealbarbitone	Censedal
	Nevental
Pentobarbitone	Nembutal
Phenobarbitone	Barbenyl
	Gardenal
	Luminal
Phenylmethylbarbituric acid	Rutonal
Probarbital	Ipral
Quinalbarbitone	Seconal
Vinbarbitone	Delvinal
N-methyl Barbiturates	
Hexobarbitone	Cyclonal
Metharbital	Gemonil
Methohexitone	Brietal
Methylphenobarbitone	Phemitone
	Prominal
Bromobarbiturates	
Butallylonal	Pernoston
Thiobarbiturates	
Buthalitone	Transithal
Thialbarbitone	Kemithal
Thiamylal	Surital
Thiopentone	Pentothal
	Intraval

Note. The most common mixture of barbiturates is Tuinal (Quinalbarbitone and Amylobarbitone).

Appendix V

PROSECUTION AND PUNISHMENT OF OFFENCES INVOLVING ALCOHOL UNDER THE ROAD TRAFFIC ACT, 1972

ROAD TRAFFIC ACT, 1972

SCHEDULE 4

Prosecution and Punishment of Offences

Part 1

Offences under this Act

(extract)

See Table on pages 761 and 762

1 Provision creating offence	2 General nature of offence	3 Mode of prosecution	4 Punishment	5 Disqualification	6 Endorsement	7 Additional* provisions
5 (1)	Driving or attempting to drive when unfit to drive through drink or drugs.	(a) Summarily.	4 months or £100 or both; or in the case of a second or subsequent conviction or of a conviction subsequent to a conviction of an offence under section 6 (1) or 9 (3) (where it was shown as mentioned in paragraph (i) of the entry in this column relating to that offence), 6 months or £100 or both.	Obligatory.	Obligatory.	Sections 181 and 183 and paragraph 3 of Part IV of this Schedule apply.
		(b) On indictment.	2 years or a fine or both.			
5 (2)	Being in charge of a motor vehicle when unfit to drive through drink or drugs.	(a) Summarily.	4 months or £100 or both.	Discretionary.	Obligatory.	Sections 181 and 183 and paragraph 3 of Part IV of this Schedule apply.
		(b) On indictment.	12 months or a fine or both.			
6 (1)	Driving or attempting to drive with blood-alcohol concentration above the prescribed limit.	(a) Summarily.	4 months or £100 or both; or in the case of a second or subsequent conviction or of a conviction subsequent to a conviction of an offence under section 5 (1) or 9 (3) (where it was shown as mentioned in paragraph (i) of the entry in this column relating to that offence), 6 months or £100 or both.	Obligatory.	Obligatory.	Sections 181 and 183 and paragraph 3 of Part IV of this Schedule apply.
		(b) On indictment.	2 years or a fine or both.			
6 (2)	Being in charge of a motor vehicle with blood-alcohol concentration above the prescribed limit.	(a) Summarily.	4 months or £100 or both.	Discretionary.	Obligatory.	Sections 181 and 183 and paragraph 3 of this Schedule apply.
		(b) On indictment.	12 months or a fine or both.			

1 Provision creating offence	2 General nature of offence	3 Mode of prosecution	4 Punishment	5 Disqualification	6 Endorsement	7 Additional* provisions
8 (3)	Failing to provide a specimen of breath for a breath test.	Summarily.	£50.	—	—	Sections 181 and 183 apply.
9 (3)	Failing to provide a specimen of blood or urine for a laboratory test.	(a) Summarily.	(i) Where it is shown that at the relevant time (as defined in Part V of this Schedule) the offender was driving or attempting to drive a motor vehicle on a road or other public place, 4 months or £100 or both; or in the case of a conviction subsequent to a conviction under section 5, (1) or 6 (1) or to a conviction under section 9 (3) where it was so shown, 6 months or £100 or both. (ii) Where in any other case it is shown that at that time the offender was in charge of a motor vehicle on a road or other public place, 4 months or £100 or both.	(a) Obligatory if it is shown as mentioned in paragraph (i) of column 4. (b) Discretionary if it is not so shown.	Obligatory.	Sections 181 and 183 and paragraph 3 of Part IV of this Schedule apply.
		(b) On indictment.	(iii) 2 years or a fine or both in the case of a conviction where it is shown as mentioned in paragraph (i) above. (iv) 12 months or a fine or both in the case of a conviction where it is shown as mentioned in paragraph (ii) above.			

* The additional provisions are given below.

ROAD TRAFFIC ACT, 1972
PART VII

Evidence by certificate

181—(1) In any proceedings in England or Wales for an offence under this Act to which this section is applied by column 7 of Part 1 of Schedule 4 to this Act or which is punishable by virtue of section 178 thereof or for an offence against any other enactment relating to the use of vehicles on roads a certificate in the prescribed form, purporting to be signed by a constable and certifying that a person specified in the certificate stated to the constable—

(a) that a particular motor vehicle was being driven or used by, or belonged to, that person on a particular occasion, or

(b) that a particular motor vehicle on a particular occasion was used by, or belonged to, a firm in which that person also stated that he was at the time of the statement a partner, or

(c) that a particular motor vehicle on a particular occasion was used by, or belonged to, a corporation of which that person also stated that he was at the time of the statement a director, officer or employee,

shall be admissible as evidence for the purpose of determining by whom the vehicle was being driven or used, or to whom it belonged, as the case may be, on that occasion.

(2) Nothing in subsection (1) above shall be deemed to make a certificate admissible as evidence in proceedings for an offence except in a case where and to the like extent to which oral evidence to the like effect would have been admissible in those proceedings.

(3) Nothing in subsection (1) above shall be deemed to make a certificate admissible as evidence in proceedings for an offence—

(a) unless a copy therof has, not less than seven days before the hearing or trial, been served in the prescribed manner on the person charged with the offence, or

(b) if that person, not later than three days before the hearing or trial or within such further time as the court may in special circumstances allow, serves a notice in the prescribed form and manner on the prosecutor requiring attendance at the trial of the person who signed the certificate.

(4) In this section 'prescribed' means prescribed by rules made by the Secretary of State by statutory instrument.

Proof in summary proceedings, of identity of driver of vehicle

183. Where on the summary trial in England or Wales of an information for an offence under this Act to which this section is applied by column 7 of Part 1 of Schedule 4 to this Act or which is punishable by virtue of section 178 thereof or for an offence against any other enactment relating to the use of vehicles on roads—

(a) it is proved to the satisfaction of the court, on oath or in manner prescribed by rules made under section 15 of the Justices of the Peace Act 1949, that a requirement under section 168 (2) of this Act to give information as to the identity of the driver of a particular vehicle on the particular occasion to which the information relates has been served on the accused by post; and

(b) a statement in writing is produced to the court purporting to be signed by the accused that the accused was the driver of that vehicle on that occasion,

the court may accept that statement as evidence that the accused was the driver of that vehicle on that occasion.

ROAD TRAFFIC ACT, 1972
SCHEDULE 4
PART IV

Supplementary provisions as to prosecution, trial and punishment of offences

3. A contravention occurring in Scotland of any of the provisions of this Act or of any regulations made thereunder, which is directed to be prosecuted summarily and which, if it had been triable on indictment, could competently have been libelled as an additional or alternative charge in an indictment charging a person with culpable homicide in respect of the driving or attempted driving or use of a motor vehicle, or with a contravention of section 1, 2, 5, 6 or 9 may, notwithstanding the direction aforesaid, be so libelled and may be tried accordingly.

In this paragraph any reference to a contravention of regulations includes a reference to a failure to comply with regulations.

Index

Human remains, dismemberment of, 89
  identification of, 31, 73–90
  mutilation of, 89
Human Tissue Act 1961, 43
Hydrochloric acid, 616
Hydrocyanic acid, 618
Hydrofluoric acid, 161
Hydrogen cyanide, 618
Hydrogen fluoride, 611
Hydrogen phosphide, 675
Hydrogen sulphide, 621
Hydrostatic test, 404
Hymen, forms of, 432–434
Hyoid bone, 178, 183, 188
Hyoscine, 681
Hypostasis, 114
Hypothermia, 228

I

Identification,
  age and, 75
  anthropometry, 59
  Bertillon's system of, 59
  body deformities and peculiarities, 88
  bones, 76, 79, 82, 87
  of criminals, 59
  of the dead, 31, 73–90
  by dust and debris, 70
  by finger-prints, 59
  by foot-prints, 61
  by injuries, 68
  of living persons, 73–90
  of mutilated remains, 89
  post-mortem examination and, 31
  scars in, 88
  sex in, 81
  stature and, 87
  by teeth, 73
  by teeth marks, 65
  by wounds, 68
Idiosyncrasy, and food, 710
  and poisons, 511
Ileum, rupture of, 333
Ill-treatment of children, 222
  law regarding, 210
Imbecile, carnal knowledge of, 425
Imipramine, 521
Immersion blast, 338
Impaction of foreign bodies, 164, 415
Impanelling of jury, 26
Impotence and sterility, in female, 359
  in male, 358
Incest, 451

Incised wounds, 234–238
Indecency with Children Act, 1960, 427
Indecent assault, 425, 427
Indecent exposure, 458
Indian hemp, 560
Indictment, form of, 25
Industrial guns, 288
Inebriety, 479
Infamous conduct, 5
Infant Life Preservation Act 1929, 400
Infanticide, by cold and exposure, 416
  by commission, 399
  concealment of birth and, 400
  concealment of pregnancy and, 401
  definition of, 399
  by drowning, 411
  examination of body in, 32, 403
  fracture of skull, 410, 415
  hydrostatic test, 404
  by injury, 413
  law regarding, 400
  lung conditions in, 403
  by omission, 399
  precipitate labour in, 415
  signs of live birth in, 409
  stomach-bowel test in, 408
  by strangulation, 411, 415
  by suffocation, 411
  by violence, 413
Infanticide Act 1938, 399
Inflation of lungs of new-born, artificial, 406
  natural, 404
Infra-red photography, 71, 291
Infra-red spectrometry, 71
Injury, abdominal, 268, 326, 336, 338
  benefit, 27
  bladder, 336
  bone, 324
  chest, 267
  crush, 170
  degloving, 328
  genital, 331
  head, 209, 298–314
  heart, 267, 339
  and malignancy, 339
  following medical procedure, 338
  movements following, 266, 268
  neck, 173, 175, 262–267
  perineum, 331
  rectal, 336
  spinal, 322
  urethral, 331